1984

YEAR BOOK OF

OBSTETRICS AND GYNECOLOGY®

THE 1984 YEAR BOOKS

The YEAR BOOK series provides in condensed form the essence of the best of the recent international medical literature. The material is selected by distinguished editors who critically review more than 500,000 journal articles each year.

Anesthesia: *Drs. Kirby, Miller, Ostheimer, Saidman, and Stoelting.*

Cancer: *Drs. Clark, Cumley, and Hickey.*

Cardiology: *Drs. Harvey, Kirkendall, Kirklin, Nadas, Resnekov, and Sonnenblick.*

Critical Care Medicine: *Drs. Rogers, Booth, Dean, Gioia, McPherson, Michael, and Traystman.*

Dentistry: *Drs. Cohen, Hendler, Johnson, Jordan, Moyers, Robinson, and Silverman.*

Dermatology: *Drs. Sober and Fitzpatrick.*

Diagnostic Radiology: *Drs. Bragg, Keats, Kieffer, Kirkpatrick, Koehler, Sorenson, and White.*

Digestive Diseases: *Drs. Greenberger and Moody.*

Drug Therapy: *Drs. Hollister and Lasagna.*

Emergency Medicine: *Dr. Wagner.*

Endocrinology: *Drs. Schwartz and Ryan.*

Family Practice: *Dr. Rakel.*

Medicine: *Drs. Rogers, Des Prez, Cline, Braunwald, Greenberger, Bondy, Epstein, and Malawista.*

Neurology and Neurosurgery: *Drs. De Jong, Sugar, and Currier.*

Nuclear Medicine: *Drs. Hoffer, Gottschalk, and Zaret.*

Obstetrics and Gynecology: *Drs. Pitkin and Zlatnik.*

Ophthalmology: *Dr. Ernest.*

Orthopedics: *Dr. Coventry.*

Otolaryngology: *Drs. Paparella and Bailey.*

Pathology and Clinical Pathology: *Dr. Brinkhous.*

Pediatrics: *Drs. Oski and Stockman.*

Plastic and Reconstructive Surgery: *Drs. McCoy, Brauer, Haynes, Hoehn, Miller, and Whitaker.*

Psychiatry and Applied Mental Health: *Drs. Freedman, Lourie, Meltzer, Nemiah, Talbott, and Weiner.*

Sports Medicine: *Drs. Krakauer, Shephard and Torg, Col. Anderson, and Mr. George.*

Surgery: *Drs. Schwartz, Najarian, Peacock, Shires, Silen, and Spencer.*

Urology: *Drs. Gillenwater and Howards.*

The YEAR BOOK of

Obstetrics and Gynecology®

1984

Editors

ROY M. PITKIN, M.D.

Professor and Head, Department of Obstetrics and Gynecology,
University of Iowa College of Medicine

FRANK J. ZLATNIK, M.D.

Associate Professor and Vice-Chairman,
Department of Obstetrics and Gynecology,
University of Iowa College of Medicine

YEAR BOOK MEDICAL PUBLISHERS, INC.
CHICAGO

Printed in U.S.A.

International Standard Book Number: 0-8151-6693-1

International Standard Serial Number: 0084-3911

The editor for this book was Roberta A. Mendelson and the production manager was H. E. Nielson.

Table of Contents

The material covered in this volume represents literature reviewed up to August 1983.

Introduction

Readers occasionally ask about how the YEAR BOOK OF OBSTETRICS AND GYNECOLOGY reaches its final printed form. A brief outline of the process might therefore be of interest.

The publisher subscribes to nearly all biomedical journals published in English as well as to a number in German, French, Spanish, and Italian. Each article in each journal is screened by YEAR BOOK employees and marked to indicate the YEAR BOOK for which it is appropriate. Often, an article may be marked for consideration by editors of four or more of the 25 different YEAR BOOKS. In the case of our YEAR BOOK, all articles relating to obstetrics and gynecology in the broadest possible sense are included.

Each month, a rather large box containing intact issues of specialty journals or individual articles torn from general journals arrives on our doorstep. Our task is to review these and select those we wish to include. One of us reads each paper selected and summarizes it for the other; the primary reviewer also prepares a rough draft of the editorial comment. Our major focus in selecting articles is that of relevance to clinical practice. We try to pick those that report new information or resolve controversial or contradictory data. Most of our selections represent what we believe to be the best papers published, although in some cases a study that we regard as flawed is included in order to point out its inadequacies. Although many articles are selected from United States specialty journals, each year we include many papers from general and foreign journals that ordinarily are not seen by the practitioner. Our goal is to provide the obstetrician-gynecologist with an extensive body of current information.

Articles selected are sent to the publisher for abstracting by professional abstractors. The original article and the abstract are then returned to us for verification, and at this time we put our editorial comments in final form. Toward the end of the year (October in the case of the YEAR BOOK OF OBSTETRICS AND GYNECOLOGY), we organize the articles in proper category and sequence and make one final check of the manuscript. It might seem that this would be a propitious time for a celebration but by the time the manuscript has gone to the publisher, we've already been working on the next year's book for two months!

The special articles in this year's edition concern two important topics in contemporary obstetrics and gynecology. Jennifer R. Niebyl, of Johns Hopkins University, has prepared an excellent summary of drug effects in pregnancy, with particular emphasis on clinical teratology. This general subject probably accounts for more patient questions, to say nothing of its medicolegal implications, than any other, and Doctor Niebyl is one of the nation's authorities in the area. The second article, an update on the pathogenesis, diagnosis, and treatment of endometriosis, is authored by Robert W. Kistner, Robert L. Barbieri, and Stephen Evans, of Harvard University. Doctor Kistner's name has certainly been the one most associated with this particular disease for more than a quarter century, and he has played a major role in most of the advances occurring over that period of time.

ROY M. PITKIN, M.D.
FRANK J. ZLATNIK, M.D.

Journals Represented

Acta Endocrinologica
Acta Obstetricia et Gynecologica Scandinavica
American Journal of Cardiology
American Journal of Clinical Nutrition
American Journal of Diseases of Children
American Journal of Epidemiology
American Journal of Medicine
American Journal of Obstetrics and Gynecology
American Journal of Surgery
American Surgeon
Anaesthesia and Intensive Care
Anesthesia and Analgesia
Annales Chirurgiae et Gynaecologiae
Annals of Internal Medicine
Annals of Surgery
Archives of Diseases of Childhood
Archives of Internal Medicine
Australian and New Zealand Journal of Obstetrics and Gynaecology
British Journal of Clinical Pharmacology
British Journal of Obstetrics and Gynaecology
British Journal of Surgery
British Journal of Urology
British Medical Journal
Canadian Medical Association Journal
Cancer
Clinical Endocrinology
Clinical Pediatrics
Contraception
Developmental Medicine and Child Neurology
Diabetologia
Fertility and Sterility
Gynecologic and Obstetric Investigation
Gynecologic Oncology
International Journal of Fertility
International Journal of Gynaecology and Obstetrics
Journal of Adolescent Health Care
Journal of the American Medical Association
Journal of the Canadian Association of Radiologists
Journal of Clinical Endocrinology and Metabolism
Journal of Family Practice
Journal of Nervous and Mental Disease
Journal of Occupational Medicine
Journal of Pediatric Surgery
Journal of Pediatrics
Journal of Urology
Lancet
Life Sciences

Neurology
Neuropediatrics
New England Journal of Medicine
Obstetrics and Gynecology
Pediatric Research
Pediatrics
Prostaglandins
Psychological Medicine
Psychophysiology
Quarterly Journal of Medicine
Scandinavian Journal of Clinical and Laboratory Investigation
Science
South African Medical Journal
Southern Medical Journal
Surgery
Therapeutic Drug Monitoring
Urologia Internationalis

PART ONE

OBSTETRICS

1. Maternal and Fetal Physiology

1-1 **Growth of the Birth Canal in Adolescent Girls.** Obstetric complications associated with young teenage mothers include increased risk of prolonged labor, uterine dysfunction, contracted pelvis, and cesarean section. These risks may be related to immaturity of the pelvis and the smaller size of the birth canal. Marquisa LaVelle Moerman (Univ. of Michigan, Dearborn) analyzed the growth and development of the birth canal in a longitudinal sample of 90 healthy middle-class girls aged 8 to 18 years. Examinations included physical measurement of four pelvic dimensions, detailed gynecologic history, and prior to 1950, annual radiographic study of the pelvis.

Compared with stature, the pelvic basin was found to grow more slowly and continuously through late adolescence. At menarcheal age (MA) 0 to 2, mean pelvic size was considerably smaller than mean adult pelvic size at age 18 years. Pelvic dimensions for the inlet of the pelvic basin (measure A), the interspinous diameter (measure B), and the maximum breadth of the sacral alae (measure C) for Ma 0 to 2 were significantly smaller than adult size, but the inferior breadth of the ischial tuberosities (measure D) was not significantly smaller at MA 2, compared with mean adult size. At MA 3, pelvic size for any of the four measures did not differ significantly from the adult size. Despite the likely onset of fecundity at an early MA, pelvic growth continued beyond the asymptote of stature (1% or less of growth remaining), with greater pelvic growth remaining at all ages (table).

PERCENTAGE OF GROWTH REMAINING IN YEARS AFTER MENARCHE*

	MA 0 (%)	1 (%)	2 (%)	3 (%)
Body dimensions:				
Stature	4.3	2.1	0.9	0.5
Weight	20.4	11.9	6.7	3.5
Bicristal hip diameter	9.6	5.7	3.3	1.4
Pelvic diameters:				
A. Inlet	13.0	7.0	3.9	1.7
B. Bispinous	18.2	12.6	8.9	6.0
C. Sacrum	12.4	7.4	3.2	2.4
D. Inferior ischium	14.0	5.0	3.0	0.8

*Calculated retrospectively from longitudinal series of 45 girls on basis of subject size at age 18.

(Courtesy of Moerman, M. L.: Am. J. Obstet. Gynecol. 143:528–532, July 1, 1982.)

(1–1) Am. J. Obstet. Gynecol. 143:528–532, July 1, 1982.

The growth in bicristal hip diameter closely approximated pelvic growth. Although only minor differences were observed in the size of the birth canal and in bicristal hip diameter at age 18, girls with an early menarche were appreciably shorter and heavier than their late-maturing counterparts at this age.

Immaturity of the birth canal may be of significance for obstetric risk among young primiparous teenage girls.

▶ [Several studies of adolescent pregnancy have indicated that there is an increased rate of cephalopelvic disproportion. This longitudinal study of pelvic dimensions demonstrates that the pelvis continues to grow in late adolescence after the asymptote for stature has been reached. Pelvic dimensions are related to both chronological and gynecologic (i.e., postmenarchal) ages. At menarche, younger girls have smaller pelves than older girls.] ◀

1–2 **Birth Weight and Paternal Height.** Colin W. Pritchard, Hamish W. Sutherland, and Roy A. Carr-Hill (Univ. of Aberdeen) examined the hypothesis of a relationship between paternal height and standardized birth weight by comparing the distribution of birth weights of infants born to women of given heights married to short or tall men. Data were obtained on 7,305 infants born alive between 1967 and 1971, and analyses were based on 5,834 legitimate singleton births. Birth weights were standardized for gestation, parity, and infant sex. Standardized birth weights were consistently greater for infants born to women with tall husbands.

It would appear that tall parental stature is related to favorable environmental and genetic components among those that influence birth weight. Class-related factors such as nutrition and life-style may have a role in observed differences in distributions of standardized birth weight.

▶ [Most previous studies have concluded that paternal height doesn't significantly affect birth weight, after correction has been made for maternal height. This complicated analysis of the extensive Aberdeen data suggests there is an independent effect of the father's height on birth weight. It may be environmental rather than genetic, however. In the men studied, height and socioeconomic class were positively correlated.] ◀

1–3 **Relative Contribution of Prematurity and Fetal Growth Retardation to Low Birth Weight in Developing and Developed Societies.** Low birth weight (LBW) infants accounted for 21 million or 17% of births worldwide in 1979. Those born in developing countries accounted for more than 90% of the total. Using published data on births occurring from 1965 onward, José Villar and José M. Belizán analyzed the relative contributions of prematurity (birth weight ≤2,500 gm and <37 weeks' gestation) and intrauterine growth retardation-LBW (IUGR-LBW) (birth weight ≤2,500 gm and ≥37 weeks' gestation) to the total number of infants with LBW in 11 regions in the developed world and in 25 developing areas.

The incidence of LBW was 4 times higher in developing areas than in developed countries and cases of IUGR-LBW were 6.6 times more prevalent in developing areas, but the incidence of prematurity was only twice as high (table). In the developing areas, a linear correla-

(1–2) Br. J. Obstet. Gynaecol. 90:156–161, February 1983.
(1–3) Am. J. Obstet. Gynecol. 143:793–798, Aug. 1, 1982.

INCIDENCE OF LOW BIRTH WEIGHT (≤ 2,500 GM) IN DEVELOPING AND DEVELOPED AREAS

	Population from developing countries	*Population from developed countries*	*Rate ratio*
No. of populations studied	25	11	
Total LBW (%) (average)	23.63	5.90	4.0
IUGR-LBW (%) (average)	16.97	2.57	6.6
Preterm LBW (%) (average)	6.66	3.32	2.0

(Courtesy of Villar, J., and Belizán, J. M.: Am. J. Obstet. Gynecol. 143:793–798, Aug. 1, 1982.)

tion was observed between total incidence of LBW and IUGR-LBW (Fig 1–1). However, when the total incidence of LBW was correlated with incidence of prematurity, the coefficients were not significant. In the developed countries, where the total incidence of LBW never exceeded 11% (mean, 5.9%), the results were exactly the opposite of those for developing areas. The correlation between the total incidence of LBW and IUGR-LBW was not significant, but the association

Fig 1–1.—Developing countries. Correlation between overall incidence of LBW and IUGR. Significant correlation (r = 0.95; $P < .001$; n = 25) with regression coefficient of 0.98 was found. (Courtesy of Villar, J., and Belizán, J. M.: Am. J. Obstet. Gynecol. 143:793–798, Aug. 1, 1982.)

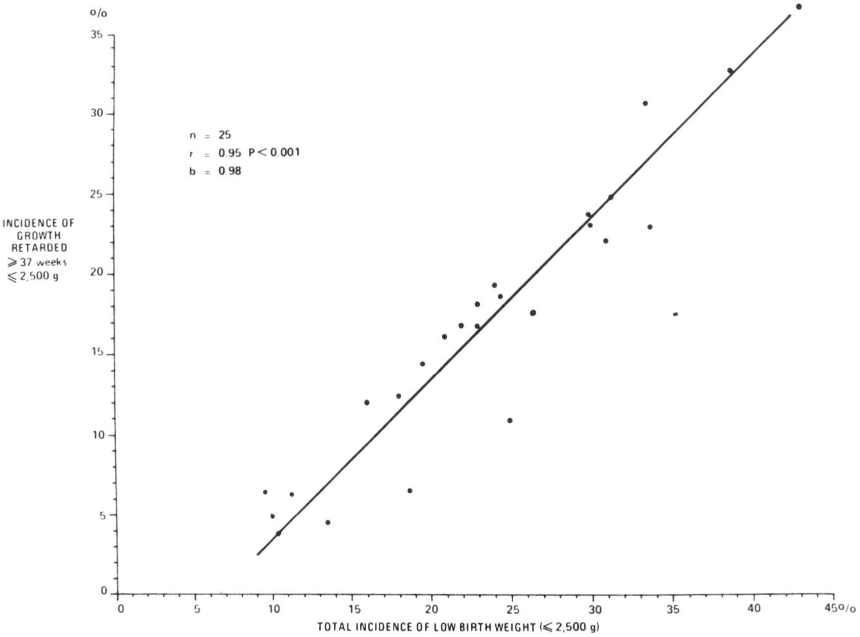

between overall incidence of LBW and rate of preterm LBW was statistically significant. Study of nonwhite births in the United States from 1963 to 1979 revealed patterns of association that were the same as those found for populations in the developing countries, despite a small decrease in the incidence of LBW.

It appears that when the incidence of LBW is greater than 10%, as it is in most developing countries, it is due almost linearly to the increase in IUGR-LBW. The proportion of premature infants remains essentially unchanged. Thus, no more than 5% to 7% of all LBW births can be expected to be premature and any higher percentage is attributable to IUGR-LBW. The observed differences between populations may be the result of environmental factors susceptible to changing socioeconomic conditions.

▶ [The differences between developed and developing areas concerning the relative contributions of prematurity and intrauterine growth retardation to the rate of delivery of low birth weight infants are illustrated in this study. In large part, differences in maternal nutritional status must explain these findngs.] ◀

1–4 **Effect of Maternal Weight Gain on Fetal, Infant, and Childhood Death and on Cognitive Development.** Dale R. Tavris and John A. Read analyzed the effect of maternal weight gain during pregnancy on fetal, infant, and childhood death and on cognitive development by assessing the pregnancy outcomes of 2,590 women who participated in the Child Health and Development Studies at the University of California, Berkeley. Long-term outcome was evaluated by comparing test scores on the Raven Colored Progressive Matrices test of 1,638 children of study subjects. Weight change during pregnancy was defined as the difference in weight between the first and the last prenatal visits.

The percentage of fetal and neonatal deaths in the low weight gain categories was much greater than that in the high weight gain categories. However, when analysis of fetal and neonatal deaths was confined to pregnancies in which delivery occurred after 244 days' gestation, there were no significant differences for various weight gain categories. The markedly greater number of deaths for low weight gain categories was fully accounted for by premature deliveries. The weight gain categories were collapsed into three groups: −24 to 4, 5 to 29, and 30 or more lb. Children whose mothers gained 5–29 lb during pregnancy scored higher on the Raven test at age 5 than those whose mothers gained less than 5 or more than 29 lb. Within the 5- to 29-lb group, there were no significant differences in test scores among the categories of maternal weight gain.

In this study, the population was not strictly comparable to that of the United States in general. A cause-and-effect relationship is not necessarily implied for the less optimal pregnancy outcome of those women who gained less than 5 or more than 30 lb. That there were relatively good outcomes for those who gained 5–9 lb does not mean that this is adequate for all women. Maternal nutrition during pregnancy is very complex and varied. Thus, the need for individualized

---

(1–4) Obstet. Gynecol. 60:689–694, December 1982.

recommendations should be kept in mind, and dangerous generalizations should be avoided.

▶ [The "bottom line" of this study seems to be that, across a very wide range of maternal weight gains, the amount of gain per se has little to do with infant outcome in terms of life-death or cognitive development. Although survival was better with more weight gain, this was due entirely to the confounding variable of gestational age at delivery (i.e., women who deliver prematurely gain less because they are pregnant for less time), and any gains of 5 lb or more were associated with equivalent scores on intellectual assessment. However, several caveats must be expressed. The most important is that weight gain is defined as the difference between weight at first (within 120 days of the last menstrual period) and last prenatal visits, and this difference may well not correlate very closely with true gestational gain in weight. Preconceptional weight is not mentioned at all (except to say that it made no difference in the Raven test scores), and this is probably every bit as strong as weight gain in determining birth weight. Finally, the data base is 15–20 years old, and only slightly more than half of the children in the study took the Raven test at age 5.] ◀

1–5 **Dietary Protein in Pregnancy: Effect on Anthropometric Indices of the Newborn Infant.** Although significant effects of diet on pregnancy outcome have been described in animals, reports relating obstetric outcome to diet during pregnancy in women in developed countries vary greatly in their results and conclusions. Frank J. Zlatnik and Leon F. Burmeister (Univ. of Iowa) assessed protein intake, as reflected by the urinary nitrogen-creatinine nitrogen (UN/CN) ratio, throughout pregnancy in 870 women with singleton pregnancies, seen initially in the first half of gestation. They were encouraged to eat well-balanced meals to appetite; weight restriction and use of diuretics were avoided. Vitamin-mineral supplements were prescribed. Intensive dietary interviews were conducted in 47 women to correlate protein intake with total caloric intake.

The mean UN/CN ratio was 16.5, and protein intake averaged 1.05 gm/kg for the study population. The mean respective daily protein intakes for groups L, M, and H (i.e., those with the lowest, intermediate, and highest UN/CN ratios, respectively) were 0.7, 1.1, and 1.5 gm/kg. Demographic features are related to the UN/CN ratio in Table

TABLE 1.—MATERNAL DEMOGRAPHIC CHARACTERISTICS BY MEAN URINARY NITROGEN-CREATININE NITROGEN RATIO GROUPS

	Group			*Statistical significance of observed differences (p values, NS = p ≥ 0.05)*		
	L (N = 87)	*M (N = 696)*	*H (N = 87)*	*L versus M*	*L versus H*	*M versus H*
Marital status (% single)	36	19	13	<0.005	<0.005	NS
Race (% black)	14	2	1	<0.005	<0.005	NS
Pay status (% nonprivate)	87	70	46	<0.005	<0.005	<0.005
Age (yr)						
Mean	21.1	23.2	25.9	<0.01	<0.01	<0.01
SD	3.7	4.8	5.0			
Maternal education (yr)						
Mean	11.4	12.8	14.8	<0.01	<0.01	<0.01
SD	2.0	3.0	3.2			
Paternal education (yr)						
Mean	12.1	13.7	16.2	<0.01	<0.01	<0.01
SD	3.0	3.9	4.1			

L = lowest urinary nitrogen-creatinine nitrogen (UN/CN) group; M = intermediate UN/CN group; H = highest UN/CN group.

(Courtesy of Zlatnik, F. J., and Burmeister, L. F.: Am. J. Obstet. Gynecol. 146:199–203, May 15, 1983.)

(1–5) Am. J. Obstet. Gynecol. 146:199–203, May 15, 1983.

TABLE 2.—MATERNAL ANTHROPOMETRIC CHARACTERISTICS BY MEAN URINARY NITROGEN-CREATININE NITROGEN RATIO GROUPS

	Group			*Statistical significance of observed differences (p values, NS = $p \geq 0.05$)*		
Anthropometric characteristics	*L* (*N* = 87)	*M* (*N* = 696)	*H* (*N* = 87)	*L versus M*	*L versus H*	*M versus H*
Height (cm)						
Mean	164	164	163	NS	NS	NS
SD	7	7	6			
Nonpregnant weight (kg)						
Mean	64.5	59.9	55.0	<0.01	<0.01	<0.01
SD	16.1	12.8	8.0			
Ponderal index						
Mean	0.24	0.22	0.21	<0.01	<0.01	<0.01
SD	0.06	0.05	0.03			
Total gain (kg)						
Mean	12.3	14.7	14.6	<0.01	<0.01	NS
SD	5.9	5.0	4.3			

L = lowest urinary nitrogen-creatinine nitrogen (UN/CN) group; M = intermediate UN/CN group; H = highest UN/CN group.

(Courtesy of Zlatnik, F. J., and Burmeister, L. F.: Am. J. Obstet. Gynecol. 146:199–201, May 15, 1983.)

1 and to anthropometric characteristics in Table 2. Women in the L group were of lower socioeconomic classes than those in the H group, weighed more before pregnancy, and gained less weight during pregnancy. Birth weights, however, were not related to dietary protein intake during pregnancy. Protein consumption also was unrelated to the length of gestation, Apgar scores, or the occurrence of anomalies, stillbirths, or neonatal deaths. Daily total calorie and protein intakes correlated significantly in the women interviewed.

This study of women in a rural Midwestern state indicates that most consumed less protein than the recommended dietary allowance of 1.3 gm/kg daily during pregnancy. Protein intake was associated with socioeconomic status, but not with physical characteristics of the newborn infants. Subtle benefits from high levels of protein intake may not have been apparent in this study. It probably is wise to continue to recommend a generous amount of dietary protein to pregnant American women. In poor populations, however, prescription of dietary protein supplements may not be the best use of available funds.

▶ [The effect of the level of dietary protein during pregnancy on reproductive performance in generally well-nourished populations remains uncertain. This study, conducted on our service, demonstrated a relationship between protein intake and both socioeconomic status (no surprise) and maternal anthropometric characteristics, but not with length of gestation or birth weight and other anthropometric indices of the newborn.] ◀

1-6 **Prenatal Dietary Supplementation of African Women and Birth Weight.** Dietary supplementation of pregnant women may be an efficient, cost-effective means of improving child growth and survival in chronically undernourished populations. Andrew M. Prentice, Roger G. Whitehead, Michael Watkinson, William H. Lamb, and Tim J. Cole examined the effects on birth weight of a groundnut-based biscuit supplement given to pregnant Gambian women. These women exhibit marked seasonal fluctuations in energy balance, with marked negative balance occurring in the wet season because of food

(1–6) Lancet 1:489–491, Mar. 5, 1983.

shortages and a high agricultural work load. The supplement of biscuits and a vitamin-fortified tea drink was offered 6 days a week under supervised conditions and resulted in a net energy increase of 431 kcal daily.

Analysis of 181 births before supplementation and 93 after supplementation was possible. In the wet season, supplementation improved birth weights by a mean of 224 gm and reduced the incidence of low birth weight infants from 28% to 5%. In the dry season, when the women were previously in positive energy balance despite an energy intake of only 60% of that recommended, supplementation had no beneficial effect on birth outcome.

High levels of nutritional supplementation can be maintained over several years in chronically undernourished populations. Very substantial benefits can be obtained from supplementation under certain conditions, but the threshold effect observed in the present study indicates the need to identify groups truly at risk for prenatal supplementation programs in developing countries. In the present population, supplementation led to a sixfold reduction in the proportion of low birth weight infants at the time of year that energy balance was negative.

▶ [This is another study indicating that any effect of nutritional supplements in birth weight is largely limited to populations with marked dietary deficiency of energy intake. In those with more nearly normal energy balance, such as are found in developed countries, the effect of supplements is negligible.] ◀

1-7 **Plasma Vitamin K_1 in Mothers and Their Newborn Babies.** Normal newborn infants have mean concentrations of vitamin K-dependent clotting factors about 30%–60% of normal adult values. Both early spontaneous bleeding and hemorrhage occurring some 4–8 weeks after birth respond promptly to vitamin K_1, with a rise in values of the affected clotting factors toward normal. M. J. Shearer, S. Rahim, P. Barkhan, and L. Stimmler (Guy's Hosp., London) assayed plasma vitamin K_1 concentrations by a method based on high-performance liquid chromatography in 30 healthy adults of both sexes aged 20–50 years; 15 healthy term mothers, 6 of whom received 1 mg of vitamin K_1 intravenously shortly before delivery; and the newborn infants.

The mean vitamin K_1 concentration in healthy fasting subjects was 0.26 ng/ml. Eight of 9 healthy term mothers had a mean vitamin K_1 value of 0.2 ng/ml, but no vitamin K_1 was detected in the cord plasma of their infants. Injection of 1 mg of vitamin K_1 just before delivery raised the maternal plasma vitamin K_1 concentrations to 45–93 ng/ml, and vitamin K_1 was detected in the cord plasma of 4 of the 6 infants, at concentrations not exceeding 0.14 ng/ml.

The large concentration gradient between maternal and neonatal plasma for vitamin K_1 suggests that it does not cross the placenta readily, or that uptake by fetal plasma is low, possibly because of low concentrations of a binding lipoprotein. The low concentrations of vitamin K present in cord plasma in normal neonates can explain

(1–7) Lancet 2:460–463, Aug. 28, 1982.

"physiologic" hypoprothrombinemia and suggest a need to review current practice with respect to vitamin K prophylaxis in the early neonatal period. Intraventricular hemorrhage, especially in premature infants, may in some cases be due to vitamin K deficiency. Administraton of vitamin K_1 for 2 weeks before delivery has prevented hypoprothrombinemia and hemorrhage in infants of epileptic women treated with anticonvulsant drugs.

▶ [This study, utilizing the modern analytic technique of high-performance liquid chromatography, demonstrates that vitamin K levels in cord blood are low. This finding probably reflects very limited placental permeability, although low fetal levels of binding lipoproteins also could be responsible. These data provide strong support for routine vitamin K administration to the newborn, a widespread practice in the United States but not (according to a statement in this article) in the United Kingdom.] ◀

1-8 **Preliminary Evidence of Effect of Calcium Supplementation on Blood Pressure in Normal Pregnant Women.** An association between calcium intake and pregnancy-induced hypertension (PIH) or preeclampsia has been proposed, because women with low calcium intakes have an increase in pressure predisposing to PIH in the later part of gestation. Jose M. Belizán, José Villar, Amely Zalazar, Laura Rojas, Daniel Chan, and Graeme F. Bryce examined the hypothesis that calcium supplementation in pregnancy can modify blood pressure in normal women. Thirty-six women aged 20–35 with normal single pregnancies were studied from 15 weeks' gestation. They received either elemental calcium in a dose of 1 or 2 gm daily or placebo in a blind study. The groups initially were demograhically and clinically comparable and had similar calcium intakes and blood pressures.

Both calcium-supplemented groups tended to have reductions in systolic blood pressure in the second trimester, whereas pressures oscillated throughout gestation in the control group. In the third trimester the systolic pressure increased in controls and in patients given 1 gm of calcium, but those given 2 gm of calcium experienced no rise in systolic pressure in the third trimester. Diastolic blood pressure showed similar trends, remaining significantly lower in the latter part of pregnancy in the group given 2 gm of calcium. No significant group differences in calcium and phosphorus levels were noted, nor were changes in parathyroid hormone concentration significant.

These findings support the hypothesis that calcium supplementation reduces blood pressure in pregnant women. Regardless of the mechanisms involved, it is clear that low calcium levels are associated with elevated blood pressure. Calcium supplementation also reduces blood pressure in nonpregnant women and in animals.

▶ [Calcium supplementation was associated with lower blood pressures in these normal pregnant women. Although a placebo was used, the authors do not state that the study was double-blind. We hope that those taking the blood pressures did not know to which groups the subjects belonged. The mechanism of the blood pressure-lowering effect of calcium is unknown; the authors think it may relate to parathyroid hormone.] ◀

(1–8) Am. J. Obstet. Gynecol. 146:175–180, May 15, 1983.

1-9 **Effect of Iron Supplementation on Serum Ferritin Levels During and After Pregnancy.** Iron is required during pregnancy for the developing fetus, the placenta, and for the increasing maternal erythrocyte mass, besides the usual daily requirements of a nonpregnant woman. David J. Taylor, Carol Mallen, Neil McDougall, and Tom Lind (Newcastle upon Tyne) measured serum ferritin and total plasma ferritin concentrations and hematologic indices during and for 6 months after normal pregnancy in 45 healthy women, 21 of whom took a preparation of 325 mg of ferrous sulfate and 350 μg of folic acid daily from 12 weeks' gestation.

Untreated women had a fall in serum ferritin concentration until 28 weeks' gestation. Most had a lower value 6 months post partum than at initial study at 12 weeks' gestation. The mean cell volume increased significantly up to 28 weeks and then declined. The hemoglobin concentration fell up to 32 weeks' gestation, but values 6 weeks post partum were similar to initial values. The effect of supplementation on serum ferritin concentration is shown in Figure 1–2. Cell volume 6 months post partum in supplemented subjects was at the baseline level. The hemoglobin concentration declined up to 28 weeks' gestation and then increased until term. Nonpregnant values were reached 6 weeks to 6 months post partum.

Routine oral iron supplementation is advisable during pregnancy, particularly after 28 weeks' gestation. Supplementation from 12 weeks' gestation will maintain normocytic erythropoiesis during pregnancy and iron stores after pregnancy. In women not receiving supplementation, microcytic erythropoiesis may develop during pregnancy and a reduction in iron stores may develop afterward. Delay of supplementation to 28 weeks' gestation might prevent the microcytic

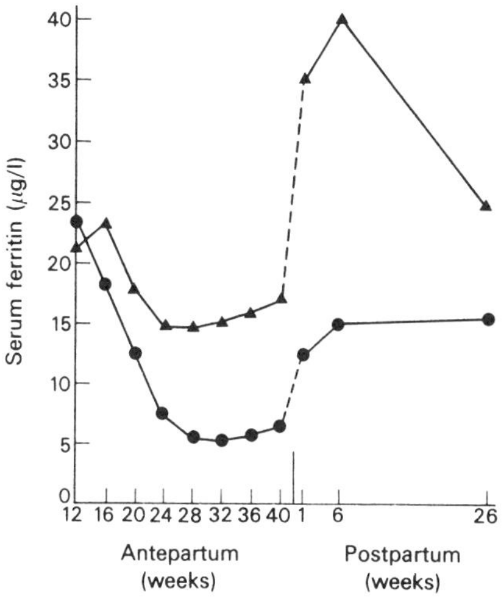

Fig 1–2.—Effect of hematinic therapy during pregnancy on serum ferritin concentrations. Triangles denote therapy group, and circles denote nontherapy group. (Courtesy of Taylor, D. J., et al.: Br. J. Obstet. Gynaecol. 89:1011–1017, December 1982.)

(1–9) Br. J. Obstet. Gynaecol. 89:1011–1017, December 1982.

erythropoiesis without causing side effects such as constipation, diarrhea, or indigestion.

▶ [In the absence of iron supplementation, serum ferritin levels fell to low levels in late pregnancy and were lower 6 months post partum than they were at 12 weeks' gestation. The authors recommend iron supplementation during the last trimester in order to prevent microcytic erythropoiesis during pregnancy and a reduction in iron stores after pregnancy.

Perhaps the Anglo-American disagreement concerning the advisabilty of supplemental iron during pregnancy is fading. It's a bloody shame!] ◀

1–10 **Use of Ferritin to Assess Need for Iron Supplements in Pregnancy.** Iron supplementation in pregnancy is routine, regardless of the individual needs of the patient, because of the difficulty in assessing iron stores accurately, easily, inexpensively, and in a noninvasive manner. J. Foulkes and D. J. Goldie (Southmead Hosp., Bristol, England) sought to determine whether measurement of serum ferritin concentration by using a direct radioimmunoassay technique can be of value in evaluating the need for iron supplements in pregnancy.

Serum ferritin levels were measured in 568 women attending a prenatal clinic at 12 to 16 weeks' gestation (Fig 1–3). Of the 501 women who participated in the study, 251 were selected randomly to receive

Fig 1–3.—Distribution of serum ferritin levels in 568 women between 12 and 16 weeks' gestation. (Courtesy of Foulkes, J., and Goldie, D. J.: J. Obstet. Gynaecol. 3:11–16, July 1982.)

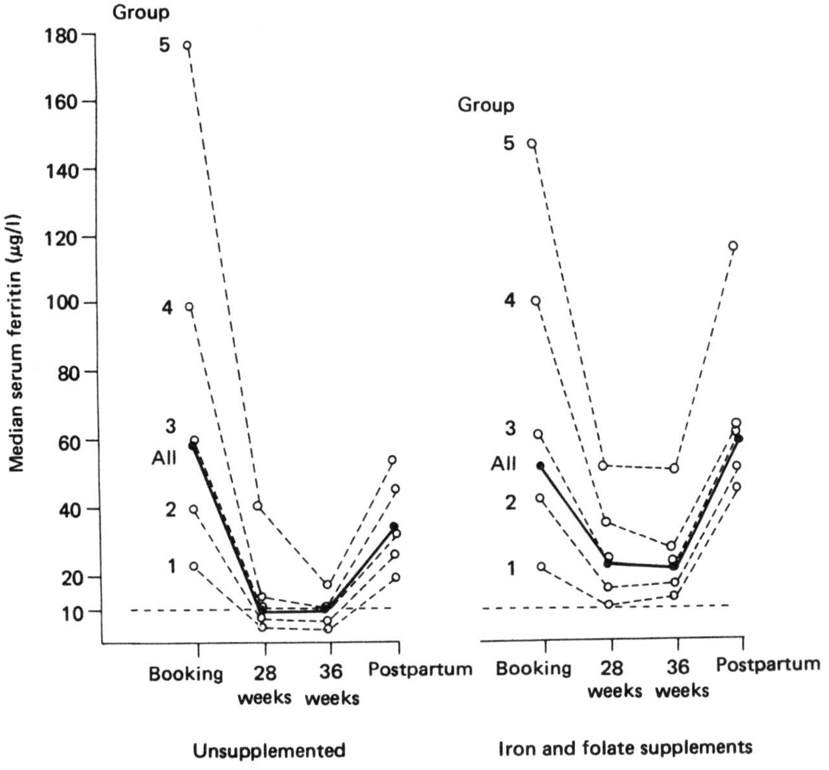

(1–10) J. Obstet. Gynaecol. 3:11–16, July 1982.

MEAN HEMOGLOBIN LEVELS IN EACH GROUP OF PATIENTS

	Group 1		Group 2		Group 3		Group 4		Group 5		*All*	
Ferritin level at booking (μg/l)	12–29		30–49		50–79		80–119		≥120			
Iron supplementation	Yes	No	Yes	No	Yes	No	Yes	No	Yes	No	Yes	No
Mean haemoglobin (g/dl)												
At booking	12·6	12·5	12·8	12·7	12·8	12·8	12·9	12·7	12·9	12·7	12·8	12·7
	n.s.		n.s.		n.s.		n.s.		n.s.		n.s.	
At 28 weeks	11·8	11·1	11·8	11·3	12·0	11·6	11·9	11·8	11·8	11·7	11·0	11·0
	$P<0·05$		$P<0·05$		$P<0·05$		n.s.		n.s.		$P<0·001$	
At 36 weeks	12·0	11·0	12·6	11·2	12·5	11·7	12·4	11·8	12·3	11·9	12·3	11·5
	$P<0·001$		$P<0·001$		$P<0·001$		$P<0·05$		n.s.		$P<0·001$	
Postpartum	12·1	11·7	12·3	11·6	12·4	11·7	12·4	11·8	11·8	12·1		
	$P<0·05$		$P<0·05$		$P<0·05$		$P<0·05$		n.s.			

Standard deviations ranged between ±0.7 and ±0.9; n.s. = not significant.
(Courtesy of Foulkes, F., and Goldie, D. J.: J. Obstet. Gynaecol. 3:11–16, July 1982.)

100 mg of elemental iron and 350 μg of folic acid daily, and 250 received no supplement.

Low initial ferritin levels were associated with higher parity, lower social class, and increased incidence of anemia in pregnancy. There was a marked fall in ferritin levels in both groups by 28 weeks' gestation, particularly in those not taking iron. The levels continued to fall in this group to 36 weeks' gestation, but those who received iron therapy maintained ferritin levels above 10 μg/L.

Although the distribution of ferritin levels were similar initially in the two groups, at 28 and 36 weeks' gestation and post partum the ferritin levels were higher in all subgroups (grouped according to initial ferritin levels) of women given iron. Mean levels of ferritin in cord blood were similar whether the women supplemented (203 μg/L) or not (186 μg/L).

As pregnancy advanced, meaningful differences in hemoglobin levels tended to emerge between supplemented and unsupplemented women with lower initial ferritin levels (table). Hemoglobin levels of less than 10.5 gm/dl developed before delivery in 59 women (12%), of whom 12 received iron and 47 did not. Of the 47 not taking iron, 41 (87%) had ferritin levels of less than 50 μg/L (median, 28 μg/L) at the initial visit.

It has been suggested that a ferritin level in early pregnancy of 130 μg/L is required for pregnancy if iron supplements are not given. The present data suggest that this is an overestimate, and that 50 to 80 μg/L is adequate. When ferritin measurements are taken at the initial visit, it is possible to identify most women who will become anemic during pregnancy. Women with ferritin levels of less than 50 μg/L should receive iron supplements during pregnancy.

▶ [Iron is easy to prescribe, but, at least for many patients, not so easy to take. The authors of this report suggest using serum ferritin levels in early pregnancy to decide who really needs iron supplementation. The incidence of anemia during pregnancy did not differ between supplemented and unsupplemented patients in the half with an initial ferritin level >50 μg/L, although, as the table indicates, there were modest differences in hemoglobin levels except in those patients with ferritin levels ≥120 μg/L. The approach recommended here is appealing. It won't save money, however. In our hospital, a ferritin assay costs $22. A 300-mg ferrous sulfate tablet costs a penny.] ◀

1–11 **Measurements of Iron Absorption From Prenatal Multivitamin-Mineral Supplements.** Iron supplementation often is provided by daily ingestion of a single multivitamin-mineral supplement containing 60–65 mg of elemental iron. Paul A. Seligman, Jennifer H. Caskey, Janet L. Frazier, Richard M. Zucker, Elaine R. Podell, and Robert H. Allen (Univ. of Colorado, Denver) encountered a number of pregnant women with iron deficiency despite the daily use of prenatal multivitamin-mineral supplements. Iron absorption from several different prenatal preparations was assessed in crossover studies of normal nonpregnant women of childbearing age by determining the rise in the serum iron level after oral iron ingestion. All had normal hematologic values. Trials were carried out in groups of 15–24 women with Stuartnatal 1 + 1, Materna 1.60, Natalins Rx, and Natafort.

Mean iron absorption from each brand of prenatal supplement was less than the required 3.5 mg, ranging from 1.8 to 3.0 mg. Absorption was significantly less than the 8.1 mg absorbed from 65 mg of iron alone. Decreased iron absorption from the supplements appeared to result from inhibition by calcium carbonate and magnesium oxide (table) and, in some instances, from poor iron release. Reformulation of 1 supplement to contain less calcium carbonate and magnesium oxide increased mean iron absorption to 4.5 mg.

The amount of iron absorbed from many prenatal multivitamin-mineral supplements appears to be significantly less than that absorbed from standard forms of iron in nonpregnant women. Bioavailability studies in pregnant women are needed to determine whether available prenatal supplements provide adequate amounts of iron during pregnancy. Dietary supplementation with an increasing number of vitamins and minerals is now recommended and used today in numerous settings, and it will be necessary to evaluate multinutrient supplements and fortified foods in terms of the bioavailability and biocompatibility of their individual components.

▶ [This study indicates that iron absorption from prenatal supplements is less than that from ferrous salts alone and, moreover, varies from one supplement to another. Part of the problem with absorption seems to be the calcium and magnesium salts present, which presumably limit iron absorption through their antacid action. When one of the products was reformulated so as to decrease the amount of calcium carbonate and magnesium oxide, iron absorption nearly doubled.

1–12 **Fluoride Tablet Supplementation During Pregnancy for Caries Immunity: Study of Offspring Produced.** Frances B. Glenn, William D. Glenn III, and Robert C. Duncan (Univ. of Miami) compared eight parameters in 375 children whose mothers drank fluoridated water during pregnancy and in 117 children whose mothers, in addition, received a daily supplement of 2.2-mg sodium fluoride in tablet form, containing 1 mg of fluoride. The 492 children were di-

(1–11) Obstet. Gynecol. 61:356–362, March 1983.
(1–12) Am. J. Obstet. Gynecol. 143:560–564, July 1, 1982.

SUMMARY OF IRON FORMULATIONS AND IRON ABSORPTION IN VARIOUS EXPERIMENTS

Iron preparation	Amount of iron ingested (mg)*	Form and amount of calcium and magnesium present (or added) at ingestion: Calcium sulfate (mg)*	Calcium carbonate (mg)*	Magnesium oxide (mg)*	Magnesium hydroxide (mg)*	Calculated mean values for iron absorption in various studies (mg): 1	2	3	4	Average
Ferrous fumarate	65					8.0	9.0		7.3	8.1
Stuartnatal	65	200		100		2.0†		1.3§	2.2†	1.8
Materna—original	60		350	100		2.8†				
Ferrous fumarate	65	(200)					9.5			
Ferrous fumarate	65		(350)				6.8†			
Ferrous fumarate	65			(100)			6.6†			
Ferrous fumarate	65	(200)		(100)			6.2†			
Ferrous fumarate	65		(350)	(100)			4.3†,‡			
Materna—reformulation A	60		350	25				3.0§		
Materna—reformulation B	60		250	25				5.0§	4.1$^{\dagger,\|}$	4.6
Natalins	60		200		100				2.4†	
Natafort	65		350	100					3.0†	

*Refers to weight of elemental iron, calcium, or magnesium, and not to weight of the entire salt. Iron is present in the form of ferrous fumarate in all prenatal multivitamin-mineral supplements.

†$P < .05$ when compared to iron alone.

‡$P < .05$ when compared to iron plus calcium carbonate and iron plus magnesium oxide.

§$P < .05$ when any one is compared to either of the other two.

‖$P < 0.5$ when compared to Stuartnatal or Natalins.

(Courtesy of Seligman, P. A., et al.: Obstet. Gynecol. 61:356–362, March 1983. Reprinted with permission from The American College of Obstetricians and Gynecologists.)

vided among four groups: a control sibling group of 210 children in multichildren families whose mothers did not receive fluoride tablets, a fluoride sibling group of 193 whose mothers received fluoride tablets during one pregnancy but not during another, an only-child group of 57 whose mothers either did or did not receive fluoride tablets, and a twin group of 32 (16 sets) with or without prenatal fluoride supplements.

Prenatal fluoride supplementation was associated with absence of decayed, filled tooth surfaces and a 99% reduction in decay; with caries-free children; with heavier birth weights for boys; with heavier birth weights, sex-adjusted; with twins and siblings being longer at birth; with fewer birth defects; and with a higher percentage of term pregnancies in twins and in siblings.

The lack of any medical or dental defects in the 117 children whose mothers received prenatal fluoride tablets corroborates the position of the Food and Drug Administration, American Medical Association, and American Dental Association that fluoride supplementation during pregnancy in this dosage range is completely safe. The virtual elimination of caries is probably due to the fact that teeth that develop in an environment with sufficient fluoride form enamel as calcium fluorapatite rather than calcium hydroxyapatite. The former is 6 to 10 times more resistant to acid dissolution and has a tight crystal structure with a smooth surface, free from pits and fissures that allow decay.

By means of nutritional counseling and supplementation, the mother-to-be may be aided in producing a child whose teeth are immune to decay. From the third through ninth months of pregnancy, a separate 1-mg fluoride tablet (2.2 mg of sodium fluoride) should be taken on an empty stomach and not followed by milk, antacids, or calcium-containing supplements.

▶ [These results seem to indicate that maternal ingestion of a fluoride supplement (for an unstated period during gestation) by women already consuming fluoridated water (at an unstated concentration) virtually eliminated dental caries in the offspring. In fact, among 117 children whose mothers took prenatal fluoride, only 1 had a decayed or filled tooth when examined at a mean age (depending on the group) of 4.7 to 7.6 years and none had any congenital defects. Moreover, infants born to women taking fluoride supplements were heavier, longer, and much less likely to be premature. One interpretation of these findings is that prenatal fluoride supplementation affords many benefits to the fetus. Another is that the supplemented and control groups may have differed in other ways than fluoride supplementation. With respect to this point, the paper states that the groups were not different in such factors as "race, . . . age, . . . poverty, . . . uneducated, no prenatal care. . ." but no supporting data are given and this information may have been difficult to verify from contact with the parents and physicians and examination of the records, particularly in a retrospective study a number of years after birth.

The issue of prenatal fluoride administration is controversial. The article abstracted above elicited a letter to the editor (*Am. J. Obstet. Gynecol.* 147:225, 1983) from Robert J. Musselman, President of the American Academy of Pedodontics, critical of the study and its conclusions.] ◀

1–13 **Zinc Nutritional Status During Pregnancy: Longitudinal Study.** Adequate maternal zinc nutrition during pregnancy is necessary for normal embryonic and fetal development in experimental an-

(1–13) Am. J. Clin. Nutr. 37:429–442, March 1983.

imals, but little is known of the effects of zinc deficiency in human pregnancy. K. M. Hambidge, N. F. Krebs, M. A. Jacobs, A. Favier, L. Guyette, and D. N. Ikle (Univ. of Colorado, Denver) assessed zinc status longitudinally in 46 pregnant middle-income women. Ten received daily zinc supplements of 15 mg as zinc sulfate. All of the women were healthy and had unremarkable medical and obstetric histories. The zinc-supplemented women had a mean age of 31 years, and the others had a mean age of 27 years.

The mean dietary zinc intake of nonsupplemented women was 11.3 mg daily and that of the supplemented women, 21.7 mg daily, representing 56% and 109% of the recommended dietary allowance, respectively. Plasma zinc levels were 17% lower in the nonsupplemented group at 2 months' gestation and continued to fall significantly thereafter. The levels did not differ significantly in the two groups at any stage of gestation. Supplemented patients had higher serum alkaline phosphatase activity. The level of prenatal iron supplementation in the control group correlated negatively with the alkaline phosphatase activity and the plasma zinc level in the second and third trimesters, respectively.

Standards for the lower limit of the plasma zinc concentration during gestation are given in the table. The plasma zinc level may be a relatively insensitive index of nutritional zinc status during pregnancy. It appears that a higher intake of zinc may be desirable and that routine prenatal zinc supplementation may prove helpful. Prenatal supplemental iron may affect the maternal zinc status adversely. Further work is needed to determine the optimal means of supplementing the diets of pregnant women.

▶ [Evidence from animal experiments and fragmentary suggestions from reported human experience imply that zinc may be an especially important trace element dur-

TENTATIVE STANDARDS FOR LOWER LIMIT OF PLASMA ZINC CONCENTRATION (90% CONFIDENCE LIMIT) AT SUCCESSIVE STAGES OF GESTATION

Mo of gestation	Plasma zinc	Z scores
	μg/dl	
2	54	−3.25
3	52	−3.45
4	50	−3.65
5	48	−3.86
6	46	−4.07
7	44	−4.27
8	42	−4.48
9	40	−4.70

Regression equation: $y = \beta_0 + \beta_1 X - t_{n-2,1-\alpha}\left[\sqrt{1 + \frac{1}{n} + \frac{(x - \bar{x})^2}{SSQ_x}}\right] S_{y \cdot x}$ where $\beta_0 = 73.61$; $\beta_1 = -2.04$; x = month of gestation; $t = 1.282$ (for 90th percentile of t distribution, with $n - 2$ degrees of freedom); $n = 175$; $\bar{x} = 5.96$; $SSQ_x = 785.5$; $S_{y \cdot x} = 11.96$.

(Courtesy of Hambidge, K. M., et al.: Am. J. Clin. Nutr. 37:429–442, March 1983.)

ing pregnancy. The situation is hampered by the lack of a test of zinc nutritional status. In this study, which indicates that customary intakes are only about half of the recommended daily allowance, plasma levels declined during gestation and did not correlate with zinc status, whereas hair levels seemed to be a more reliable index. Plasma zinc levels correlated negatively with iron intake, a finding that potentially has implications that need additional study with respect to levels of iron supplementation.

In a related investigation, Hunt and colleagues (*Am. J. Clin. Nutr.* 37:572, 1983) measured serum and hair zinc levels with and without supplementation in a Mexican-American population of pregnant women. Supplementation did not affect mean levels in serum or hair but did lower significantly the percentage of low serum values (<53.3 $\mu g/dl$) at term, suggesting that severely depressed serum levels indicate inadequate zinc nutriture.] ◀

1–14 **Serum Protein Pattern in Normal Pregnancy With Special Reference to Acute-Phase Reactants.** The classic indicators of inflammation vary widely during pregnancy, limiting their diagnostic usefulness. Kjell Haram, Kåre Augensen, and Said Elsayed (Bergen, Norway) measured concentrations of acute-phase protein reactants, total protein, and albumin and globulin fractions through pregnancy in 27 women with normal findings who delivered normal singleton infants at 37–42 weeks' gestation. The mean maternal age was 28 years. Labor was induced in 2 women. The mean gestational age was 40 weeks, and the mean birth weight, 3,419 gm. All but 2 infants had Apgar scores of 9.

The levels of α_1-antitrypsin and ceruloplasmin rose gradually during pregnancy to a peak in the third trimester. Levels of orosomucoid and haptoglobin were highest in the first and third trimesters, falling at about 24 weeks' gestation. Levels of C-reactive protein were similar to those in healthy nonpregnant individuals. The levels of α_1-globulin, α_2-globulin, and β-globulin rose from the first trimester to term, but there was little change in γ-globulin levels during pregnancy. The results are shown in Figure 1–4. Ceruloplasmin exhibited the best congruity among the acute-phase reactants; all but one of the individual patterns was similar to the mean. α_1-Antitrypsin also showed fair congruity in most cases. All but 2 women had a decrease in the total protein and albumin levels during pregnancy. About a third had a small rise in the last weeks of gestation.

Reference ranges for serum protein levels in normal pregnancy now are available. Serum levels of acute-phase reactant proteins may prove useful in diagnosing acute pathology during gestation. Determination of the ceruloplasmin level in particular should prove reliable. Currently, changes in levels of acute-phase proteins during various abnormal gestational states are under study.

▶ [This longitudinal study of serum protein concentrations during the course of normal pregnancy confirms the previously recognized fall in albumin, rise in α- and β-globulins, and lack of consistent change in γ-globulin levels. Figure 1–4 tells the story of the acute-phase reactants. Usually, C-reactive protein was undetectable. The authors apparently plan to look for changes in acute-phase protein patterns in various complications of pregnancy.] ◀

(1–14) Br. J. Obstet. Gynaecol. 90:139–145, February 1983.

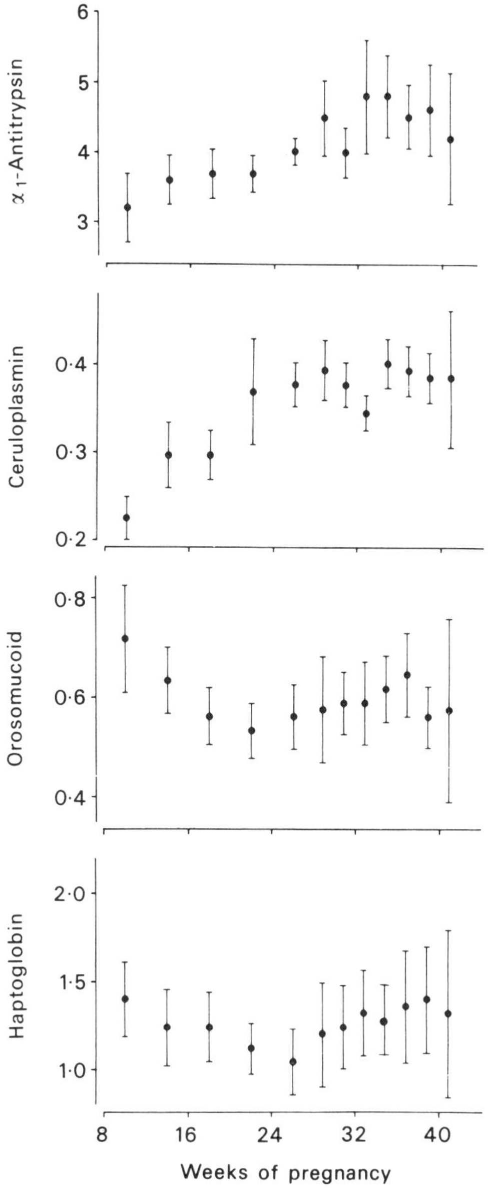

Fig 1–4.—Serum concentrations of acute-phase proteins during normal pregnancy vs. gestational ages. Values are given in gm/L as mean and 95% confidence intervals. (Courtesy of Haram, K., et al.: Br. J. Obstet. Gynaecol. 90:139–145, February 1983.)

1–15 **Pregnancy Maintenance After Early Luteectomy by 17-Hydroxyprogesterone-Caproate.** M. O. Pulkkinen (Univ. of Turku, Turku, Finland) reports data on 11 patients who had luteectomy on

(1–15) Acta Obstet. Gynecol. Scand. 61:347–349, 1982.

amenorrhea day 28 or earlier, and who underwent replacement therapy with 17-hydroxyprogesterone-caproate (17 OH-P-caproate). In human beings, luteectomy performed before luteoplacental shift provokes abortion if progesterone is not replaced. The 11 patients were hospitalized for tubal ligation and termination of pregnancy. If no abortion occurred, suction curettage was performed on the seventh postoperative day.

Two patients, both 39 years old and para 2, gravida 1, were luteectomized, 1 on amenorrhea day 17, the other on amenorrhea day 27. A dose of 250 mg of 17 OH-P on days 0 (luteectomy) and 2, or 1,000 mg on days 0 and 4 did not prevent abortion, which occurred on the fourth postoperative day. Nine other patients received 500 mg of 17 OH-P every 12 hours. One patient had an infection on the fourth postoperative day and aborted on the seventh postoperative day. This treatment prevented abortion in 6 patients but failed in 2. The failures had normal placental microscopic structure; no significant increase either in uterine activity or oxytocin or prostaglandin sensitivity occurred in those 6 cases of maintained pregnancy. In the aborted cases, the evolution of uterine activity and the increased oxytocin sensitivity after luteectomy were coincident with continuous decrease of plasma progesterone and estradiol levels.

Although pregnancy can be maintained in some patients by means of treatment with high doses of 17 OH-P caproate, this study does not provide any answer as to whether pregnancy was maintained by means of 17 OH-P, progesterone, decreased prostaglandins, or some other mechanism. Clinically, 17 OH-P-caproate cannot be considered as effective as progesterone after luteectomy, although it apparently has pregnancy-maintaining properties.

▶ [If luteectomy is performed prior to 6 weeks from conception, spontaneous abortion often results because placental progesterone production is not yet sufficient to maintain pregnancy. Although this clinical misadventure is uncommon, it does occur (e.g., bleeding corpus luteum cyst). If recognized, timely progesterone therapy at generous dosages (100 mg intramuscularly twice a day) may permit the pregnancy to continue. This article indicates that 17-hydroxyprogesterone-caproate in large doses is also effective, although there is no apparent reason to choose it over progesterone.] ◀

1–16 **Biologically Active Chorionic Gonadotropin: Synthesis by the Human Fetus.** The human placenta is a source of endorphin, adrenocorticotropin hormone, and hypothalamic releasing hormones; also, large amounts of immunoreactive human chorionic gonadotropin (hCG) occur in a variety of human fetal tissues. W. G. McGregor, R. W. Kuhn, and R. B. Jaffe (Univ. of California, San Francisco) found that fetal tissues can synthesize the α subunit, as well as the β subunit, of glycoprotein hormones and that the synthesized hormone is bioactive. Kidney tissue and, to a slight degree, liver tissue of human fetuses synthesized and secreted the α subunit, but fetal lung and muscle tissues did not. Fetal kidney and liver tissues were found previously to synthesize β hCG. Newly synthesized hormone bound to mouse Leydig cells and elicited testosterone synthesis.

(1–16) Science 220:306–308, Apr. 15, 1983.

These findings suggest that the human fetus may participate in metabolic homeostasis during its development. Although the physiologic role of hCG after the first trimester remains unclear, the finding that the fetus synthesizes bioactive hormone in the second trimester suggests a possible regulatory function. Chorionic gonadotropin stimulates dehydroepiandrosterone sulfate production by the fetal adrenal cortex, binds to microsomes from the fetal thyroid, and can bind to the human fetal testis, resulting in testosterone synthesis. Fetal hCG may, through helping regulate fetal steroidogenesis, influence the development or maintenance of tissue differentiation. Further study of the autoregulatory role of hCG during human fetal development is needed.

▶ [These interesting observations suggest that the early second-trimester fetus itself, mainly its kidney, produces hCG or at least a hormone with immunologic and biologic effects identical with hCG.] ◀

1–17 **Thyroid-Associated Components in Serum During Normal Pregnancy.** Lottie Skjöldebrand, Jan Brundin, Anders Carlstöm, and Tom Pettersson measured the levels of thyroid-associated components in serum samples, taken every 2 weeks, from 290 apparently healthy women with normal pregnancies seen at Danderyd Hospital, Danderyd, Sweden. Data regarding 3 women with extremely low levels of thyroxine-binding globulin (TBG) due to suspected inherited reasons and 2 women considered to be either hypothyreotic or hyperthyreotic were excluded.

The mean concentration of TBG increased from normal nonpregnant levels until the 24th week and remained unchanged thereafter until term. The concentration of thyroxine (T_4) increased until the 16th week and thereafter remained constant for the rest of the pregnancy. The concentration of free T_4 declined until the 20th week to values that were almost subnormal for the nonpregnant state. The concentration of triiodothyronine showed a slight but significant increase in the beginning of pregnancy and then leveled off to a constant value after the 14th week. The level of thyroid-stimulating hormone increased toward the end of pregnancy, reaching its maximum level during the last 4 weeks. The level of thyroxine-binding prealbumin (TBPA) showed constant values throughout pregnancy.

The finding that the increase in the level of the carrier protein TBG during early pregnancy was not paralleled by any increase in TBPA suggests that TBPA is not primarily a transporting protein for T_4, but possesses other functions in the metabolism of thyroid hormones. Thyroid-binding prealbumin should probably be considered a product of importance that possesses complex physiologic properties in pregnancy.

▶ [This large cross-sectional study confirms the elevation of T_4 in pregnancy associated with the estrogen-induced increase in TBG. Free T_4 levels generally remained in the normal nonpregnant range; however, the means are at the lower end of that range and many individual values were below the range. Although thyroid-stimulating hormone levels increased in late pregnancy, they remained within the normal nonpregnant limits.] ◀

(1–17) Acta Endocrinol. (Copenh.) 100:504–511, August 1982.

1–18 **Serum Free Thyroxine Concentration and Free Thyroid Hormone Indices in Normal Pregnancy.** Measurements of serum free thyroid hormone levels in pregnancy have given conflicting results, possibly as a result of the problems of indirect equilibrium dialysis. M. R. Hopton, K. Ashwell, I. V. Scott, and J. S. Harrop (Derby, England) measured serum free thyroxine (fT_4) levels by the new Amerlex and Immophase methods in 26 women at 36 to 38 weeks of normal pregnancy (mean age, 24 years), 10 women taking oral contraceptives (mean age, 25 years), and 16 healthy female controls (mean age, 32 years). These new methods for measuring fT_4 are easy to use, and the results correlate well with measurements made by equilibrium dialysis in euthyroid, hypothyroid, and hyperthyroid subjects.

Serum fT_4 levels as determined by the Immophase method were normal in late gestation. All methods gave normal results in subjects using oral contraception. Indices of fT_4 and free triiodothyronine (fT_3), derived from the Amerlex T_3 uptake, were above normal in late gestation. Both the T_4-binding globulin and T_3-binding globulin ratios were reduced.

Serum concentration of fT_4 may decline in late pregnancy, and circulating fT_4 may not be the sole determinant of thyroid status at this time. Current direct and indirect methods of assessing levels of serum fT_4 produce different patterns of change in pregnancy.

▶ [Depending on the laboratory technique used, the free T_4 levels in late pregnancy were either reduced or normal. The former finding agrees with the calculated free T_4 and, generally, with the observations of Skjöldebrand et al. presented in the preceding article.] ◀

1–19 **Plasma Renin Substrate and Estrogens in Normal Pregnancy.** The increased concentration of plasma renin substrate (PRS) concentration during pregnancy generally has been believed to be caused by estrogen. However, as bilateral oophorectomy in premenopausal women does not affect PRS concentration and there have been reports of possible variations in PRS during the menstrual cycle, the role of endogenous estrogens in the regulation of PRS concentration is not clear. To evaluate the relationship between PRS and endogenous estrogens, Ilkka Immonen, Anja Siimes, Ulf-Håkan Stenman, Jorma Kärkkäinen, and Frej Fyhrquist (Helsinki) measured serum concentrations of estradiol-17β (E_2), estriol (E_3), and renin substrate, as well as plasma renin activity, in 6 women throughout pregnancy.

As measured by exhaustive incubation of plasma with an excess of human kidney renin and radioimmunoassay of angiotensin I (AI) production, PRS concentration was within the reference range in 3 subjects and elevated in 1 at week 8 of pregnancy. At week 12, PRS concentration was elevated in all subjects and continued to increase up to about week 24, after which PRS remained relatively constant between 5,500 and 6,900 μg AI/L. After delivery, PRS concentration returned to nonpregnant levels within 6 weeks. Plasma renin activity already was elevated to 8.2 ± 4.1 μg AI/L/hour at week 8 of pregnancy and then began to decrease at week 16, reaching its lowest

(1–18) Clin. Endocrinol. (Oxf.) 18:431–437, April 1983.
(1–19) Scand. J. Clin. Lab. Invest. 43:61–65, February 1983.

value at term (3.3 ± 1.4 μg AI/L/hour). Serum E_2 and E_3 concentrations increased steadily until term. Positive correlations were observed between concentrations of PRS and E_2 ($r = .60$; $P < .001$) and between PRS and E_3 ($r = .68$; $P < .001$) for the whole group. For each subject, the correlation coefficients between PRS and estrogen concentrations ranged from 0.74 to 0.86 for E_2 and from 0.71 to 0.91 for E_3. No significant correlation was observed between plasma renin activity and estrogen concentrations or between PRS concentrations and plasma renin activity.

The results support the hypothesis that estrogens cause the increase in plasma renin substrate concentration during pregnancy and emphasize the variation in individual responses of renin substrate concentration to serum levels of estrogens. The absence of an effect of endogenous estrogens on PRS is probably the result of lower estrogen concentrations in the nonpregnant state.

▶ [This study notes a statistical correlation between plasma renin substrate and estrogen level ($r = .60$ and .68 with E_2 and E_1, respectively), findings consistent with the hypothesis that estrogen leads to the characteristic increase in plasma renin substrate with gestation. Statistical association does not necessarily mean causation, however, for the findings simply could reflect the duration of pregnancy.] ◀

1-20 **Adrenergic Stimulation of Placental Progesterone Production.** Terbutaline, a β_2-adrenergic receptor agonist, and isoproterenol, an adrenergic agonist with β_1 and β_2 effects, enhance progesterone production by placental cells in culture. Steve N. Caritis, Robert P. Hirsch, and Anthony J. Zeleznik (Univ. of Pittsburg) attempted to characterize the mechanism of this effect in 24-hour monitoring of progesterone production by cells of term human placentas obtained from women having repeat cesarean section. Both dobutamine, a β_1-adrenergic receptor agonist, and terbutaline increased progesterone production. The effects of both drugs were completely blocked by propranolol. The effect of the cyclic adenosine monophosphate (cAMP) analogue 8-bromo-cAMP in increasing progesterone production was not blocked significantly by propranolol. Methoxamine, an α-adrenergic receptor agonist, did not significantly influence placental progesterone production. The stimulatory effect of terbutaline was not significantly affected by α-adrenergic receptor blockade with phentolamine.

Placental progesterone production is significantly influenced by stimulation of β-adrenergic, but not α-adrenergic, receptors. The response may be mediated by increased amounts of intracellular cAMP. The findings may hold significance for the management of preterm labor. Stimulation of β-adrenergic receptors is likely to occur under pathologic conditions (e.g., preterm labor) when β-adrenergic agonists are administered in high doses. The efficacy of β-adrenergic receptor agonists may be attributable to increased placental progesterone production, as well as to their direct effect on myometrial contractility. Progesterone may reduce the excitation threshold in uterine smooth muscle and inhibit the propagation of electrical stimuli by affecting

---

(1–20) J. Clin. Endocrinol. Metab. 56:969–972, May 1983.

gap junction formation. It inhibits the formation of gap junctions, thereby restricting electrical impulses to their site of origin.

▶ [The results of this in vitro study indicate that β-agonists stimulate placental progesterone production. It would be interesting to know if there is a detectable effect of β-agonist therapy on plasma or placental progesterone levels. Could this be part of the mechanism of tocolytic action of β-adrenergic agents?] ◀

1-21 **Dopamine Influence on Human Uterine Activity at Term Pregnancy.** Near term, dopamine occurs in fetal plasma and amniotic fluid in high concentration, but its significance and possible effects on the pregnant uterus are unclear. J. Urban, J. Radwan, T. Laudański (Bialystok, Poland) and M. Åkerlund (Lund, Sweden) studied the effect of dopamine on uterine activity in 4 women who were postterm before spontaneous labor, 8 women at term in spontaneous labor, and 9 women who were postterm and had oxytocin-induced labor. All 21 received dopamine by intravenous infusion in a solution of 50μg in 500 ml of 5% glucose at a rate of 0.4 μg/minute/kg. Uterine activity was monitored by external tocography and fetal heart rate by external ultrasonography.

In all 4 women who were not in labor, dopamine infusion initiated uterine contractions that were regular, clearly demarcated, and had a mean frequency of 3.2 per 10 minutes. In these women, higher doses of infusion (0.6 and 0.8 μg/minute/kg) increased the response slightly but not proportionally. In the 8 women in spontaneous labor, dopamine increased the frequency of contractions after 5 to 15 minutes of infusion and usually caused a transient increase in basal tone. In the 9 women in oxytocin-induced labor, no further stimulation of uterine activity was seen when dopamine infusion was added. None of the 21 women showed any side effects or any effects of dopamine on fetal heart rate, maternal pulse rate, or maternal arterial blood pressure.

The possibility of inducing and stimulating labor with small doses of dopamine may offer some clinical advantage because it apparently has no adverse effects on uterine blood flow.

▶ [This represents a study of dopamine effects on the human uterus in vivo, and the results indicate some degree of ecbolic action. Dopamine concentrations are relatively high in amniotic fluid and may increase further near term, so perhaps this catecholamine plays some role in the physiology of parturition.] ◀

1-22 **β-Endorphin and β-Lipotropin Concentrations in Umbilical Cord Blood.** Mamdouh M. Shaaban, Tran T. Hung, David I. Hoffman, Rogerio A. Lobo, and Uwe Goebelsmann (Los Angeles) developed antiserums for human β-endorphin and β-lipotropin and also established radioimmunoassays to measure these peptides in umbilical cord plasma. Silicic acid extraction and gel chromatography were used to separate the β-endorphin from the β-lipotropin fraction, both of which were determined in umbilical venous plasma in 64 newborn infants. These peptides then were measured to assess effects of the presence or absence of labor, route or mode of delivery, and absence or presence of clinically evident fetal distress (hypoxia) on the concentration of the peptides.

(1-21) Br. J. Obstet. Gynaecol. 89:451-455, June 1982.
(1-22) Am. J. Obstet. Gynecol 144:560-568, Nov. 1, 1982.

Concentration of β-endorphin and β-lipotropin in the umbilical vein averaged 38.5 and 50.4 fmoles/ml, respectively, in 54 newborn infants without fetal distress. Concentrations measured 115 and 110 fmoles/ml, respectively, in the 10 newborn infants with apparent fetal distress. Neither presence nor absence of labor nor the route or mode of delivery was found to affect the concentration of β-endorphin or β-lipotropin in the umbilical vein. However, levels of both peptides in cord plasma were significantly elevated in fetal distress, as evidenced by prolonged bradycardia, late and prolonged variable fetal heart rate decelerations, or fetal acidosis. In 18 of 22 pairs of simultaneously measured concentrations of umbilical venous and arterial β-endorphin and β-lipotropin in newborn infants without apparent intrapartum distress, the venous β-endorphin levels (average, 40.4 fmoles/ml) were significantly higher than the arterial β-endorphin levels (mean, 28.5 fmoles/ml). No significant difference in umbilical arteriovenous concentration was found for β-lipotropin. The ratio of umbilical arterial to venous β-endorphin levels rose as absolute cord plasma β-endorphin levels increased. Both the molar umbilical venous and arterial β-lipotropin to β-endorphin ratios decreased significantly in association with intrapartum fetal distress.

These data indicate that the stress-related increase in the level of umbilical plasma β-endorphin exceeds that of β-lipotropin and may be, at least in part, of fetal origin. These data are consistent with the hypothesis that fetal hypoxia causes release of neurotransmitters such as β-endorphin, which may modulate the regulation of fetal heart patterns. These data also indicate that narcotics administered to the mother during labor and delivery do not affect levels of umbilical venous β-endorphin or β-lipotropin.

▶ [β-Endorphin is a neurotransmitter that, according to these studies, seems to be released by the "stressed" fetus or, perhaps more accurately, the placenta and that could be the mechanism of the fetal heart rate changes characteristic of hypoxia.

In a related study, Divers and colleagues (*Am. J. Obstet. Gynecol.* 144:539, 1982) found β-endorphin (but not α-melanocyte) levels in amniotic fluid to be increased with fetal growth retardation and premature labor.] ◀

1–23 **Amniotic Fluid Phospholipids After Maternal Administration of Dexamethasone.** The effect of steroids, if any, on phospholipid indices of fetal lung maturation in women treated for premature labor are unclear. Philip M. Farrell, Michael J. Engle, Richard D. Zachman, Luis B. Curet, John C. Morrison, A. Vijaya Rao, W. Kenneth Poole, and the Collaborative Group on Antenatal Steroid Therapy reviewed the amniotic-fluid phospholipid findings obtained in a multicenter trial of prenatal corticoid therapy for the prevention of respiratory distress syndrome. A significant reduction in incidence of the syndrome was found, especially in female infants, after administration of 5 mg of dexamethasone as many as 4 times at 12-hour intervals before delivery. Amniotic fluid was sampled before and about a week after intramuscular dexamethasone or placebo injections were given. Forty-five patients had amniocenteses before and after treat-

---

(1–23) Am. J. Obstet. Gynecol. 145:484–490, Feb. 15, 1982.

ment within 3–9 days of one another. Gastric aspirate samples of amniotic fluid were available from another 121 patients.

The lecithin to sphingomyelin (L/S) ratio was nearly identical initially, and no significant difference in mean levels after treatment was found in a comparison of steroid-treated and control pregnancies. Significant increases occurred in both groups during the interval between amniocenteses. No phosphatidylglycerol was detected when phospholipid levels were measured before and after administration of steroids. Absolute concentrations of both phosphatidylcholine and disaturated phosphatidylcholine increased relatively modestly in degree, which could be attributed to advanced gestational age as well as to steroid therapy.

Current measurements of fetal lung maturity do not provide a reliable means of detecting pulmonary maturational responses to steroids prenatally. Repeated amniocentesis after steroid administration is not clinically valuable in monitoring steroid therapy.

▶ [There seems to be little question that glucocorticoids in at least some instances accelerate fetal lung maturity, but whether or not the amniotic fluid indices reflect this effect is controversial, with a number of studies on either side of the issue. This report, using material derived from the National Institutes of Health collaborative study (see 1983 YEAR BOOK, p. 216), should be the final word—no effect on the L/S ratio, phosphatidylglycerol, or the ratio of phosphatidylglycerol to sphingomyelin.] ◀

1–24 **Amniotic Fluid Phospholipids and Glucocorticoids in Multiple Pregnancy.** Little is known of the amniotic fluid findings in multiple pregnancies, in which the high rates of preterm labor and elective delivery require accurate assessment of pulmonary maturity in both twins. R. J. Norman, S. M. Joubert, and M. Marivate (Univ. of Natal, South Africa) determined the phospholipid and glucocorticoid composition of amniotic fluid in 30 twin pregnancies at a mean gestational age of 37.7 weeks. Amniotic fluid was obtained at the time of cesarean section, done on standard obstetric indications. The mean maternal age was 28 years and the mean parity was 2. Nine mothers had mild hypertension. Six were in spontaneous labor with intact membranes at the time of section. Only 1 pregnancy was at less than 35 completed weeks; the patient had hypertension and fetal growth retardation detected at 32 weeks.

All 60 infants had Apgar scores of 7 or above. The mean weight of the first twin was 2,570 gm and that of the second twin, 2,531 gm. Eighteen infants were growth-retarded. None experienced respiratory distress. There were no significant differences in amniotic fluid phospholipid concentrations between the two twins before onset of labor. With onset of contractions, significant increases occurred in the lecithin-sphingomyelin (L/S) ratio and the phosphatidylglycerol-sphingomyelin ratio in the first twin compared with findings in the second. Growth-retarded infants and nonretarded siblings had comparable findings before onset of labor. Levels of amniotic fluid unconjugated glucocorticoids were similar in both twins before labor; however, during labor, concentrations in the sac of the first twin were markedly higher than those in the second. Levels of conjugated glucocorticoids

---

(1–24) Br. J. Obstet. Gynaecol. 90:51–55, January 1983.

were higher in the first twin in patients who labored, and higher in both twins than in patients not in labor. No difference in glucocorticoid concentrations was found between growth-retarded and well-grown fetuses.

The L/S and phosphatidylethanolamine-sphingomyelin ratios increase in the leading twin once labor begins. The findings support the view that the fetus itself has a major role in determining organ maturity and in initiating labor.

▶ [Twin pregnancy is a useful model for studies in reproductive biology. Prior to labor, the amniotic fluid phospholipid ratios do not differ between the sacs. This means that "maturity testing" requires fluid from only one twin. What about the situation where one twin develops respiratory distress syndrome and the other does not? In labor, the first twins had significantly higher lecithin-sphingomyelin and phosphatidylglycerol-sphingomyelin ratios than did the second twins. Glucocorticoids were also higher in the amniotic fluids of the first twins in patients in labor. This association between phospholipids and corticosteroids is consistent with the view that fetal cortisol is important in lung maturation. The differential response of twins in labor adds support to the fetal, rather than maternal, origin of the elevated corticosteroid levels in cord blood samples. If the elevated amniotic fluid corticosteroid concentrations were simply secondary to elevated maternal steroid levels due to the stress of labor, one would have expected similar values in both sacs. This was not the case.] ◀

1-25 **Antipyrine Disposition in Relation to Lowered Anticonvulsant Plasma Level During Pregnancy.** Kan Chiba, Takashi Ishizaki, Tohru Tabuchi, Takashi Wagatsuma, and Yoichi Nakazawa studied antipyrine disposition before and after delivery in 4 epileptic women in whom the ratio of the level of anticonvulsants in plasma to dosage was lowered during pregnancy and compared the results to those found in 6 nonpregnant women undergoing antiepileptic treatment and in 6 healthy women. All patients, except 1 who was treated with only phenytoin and phenobarbital, received phenytoin, phenobarbital, and valproic acid. Duration of antiepileptic treatment ranged from 10 to 21 years.

The plasma level per dosage ratio of phenytoin tended to fall during pregnancy and to rise again during the puerperium in all 4 subjects, with a trough from 4 to 6 weeks before delivery. The ratio for phenobarbital also decreased to a minimum in all patients 2–4 weeks before delivery. The ratio for valproic acid also decreased as pregnancy advanced in all patients, with a trough about 3 weeks before or 2 weeks after delivery. The antipyrine clearance at term was lower than it was early in the puerperium and about 3 months after delivery. The antipyrine clearance in nonpregnant epileptics was comparable to that found 3 months after delivery, whereas it was significantly higher than that found in healthy women.

These observations suggest that the fall during pregnancy of concentrations of anticonvulsants in plasma relative to dosage is not attributable to the enhanced oxidative process of drug metabolism. Other possible mechanisms, such as alterations in rate and extent of drug absorption, in renal drug elimination, and in drug protein bind-

---

(1–25) Obstet. Gynecol. 60:620–626, November 1982.

ing, should be explored to explain the decrease during pregnancy in the ratios of the level of anticonvulsant in plasma to dosage.

▶ [Antipyrine clearance is used as an indicator of hepatic microsomal activity. Oral contraceptive use is associated with decreased antipyrine clearance (1980 YEAR BOOK, pp. 421–422). In the present study, pregnant epileptics had decreased antipyrine clearances compared with nonpregnant epileptics. The authors suggest that this means that increased metabolism of phenytoin during pregnancy is *not* the reason for the lower plasma levels observed. Many assumptions are made here that may or may not be true, but the hint is that perhaps decreased intestinal absorption of phenytoin during pregnancy helps account for the low blood levels (1979 YEAR BOOK, pp. 76–77 and 166–168).] ◀

1-26 **Differential Inhibition of Fetal Vascular Prostacyclin and Platelet Thromboxane Synthesis by Nonsteroidal Anti-inflammatory Drugs in Humans.** Fetal vessels generate much prostacyclin (PGI_2), presumably for control of the fetal circulation, and thromboxane A_2 (TxA_2) synthesis by fetal animal lungs is lower than in adults. U.-M. Mäkilä, E. Kokkonen, L. Viinikka (Univ. of Oulu), and O. Ylikorkala (Univ. of Helsinki) examined TxA_2 generation by human fetal platelets and compared the effects of commonly used prostaglandin synthesis inhibitors on TxA_2 production and prostacyclin synthesis by human umbilical arteries. Production of TxA_2 was examined using umbilical venous blood from 13 infants of healthy mothers. Fetal PGI_2 production was assessed in a superfusion system using umbilical arteries from 27 healthy term infants.

Basal production of thromboxane B_2 (TxB_2), the stable metabolite of TxA_2, by fetal platelets was comparable to that seen in adults. Basal production of TxB_2 and 6-keto-prostaglandin $F_{1\alpha}$ ($PGF_{1\alpha}$) was comparable in all inhibition studies. Indomethacin and diclofenac inhibited both vessel wall and platelet cyclo-oxygenase more completely than did naproxen and acetylsalicylic acid. Platelet cyclo-oxygenase was 4–44 times more sensitive to these prostaglandin synthesis inhibitors than was vessel wall cyclo-oxygenase.

Neonatal platelet disturbances cannot be attributed to abnormalities in TxA_2. Thromboxane A_2 produced by fetal platelets may contribute to the regulation of fetal blood flow that is in part controlled by vasodilatory prostacyclin produced by the fetal vessels. The balance between TxA_2 and PGI_2 may be the critical factor regulating local blood flow in the fetus. The balance may be shifted toward prostacyclin dominance by the maternal use of prostaglandin synthesis inhibitors. Theoretically, these inhibitors could prevent microthrombus formation and increase fetal blood flow.

▶ [These results indicate that prostaglandin-inhibiting drugs depress thromboxane A_2 synthesis by fetal platelets and prostacyclin production by umbilical arteries. Thromboxane A_2 causes vasoconstriction and prostacyclin causes vasodilation, and the interplay between the two may be important in regulating blood flow. This is yet another reason to be cautious about nonsteroidal anti-inflammatory agents in pregnancy.] ◀

1-27 **Fetal Response to Voluntary Maternal Hyperventilation: Preliminary Report.** Maternal hyperventilation can cause transient reduction in fetal oxygen tension. Danny Navot, Yoel Donchin, and

(1–26) Prostaglandins 25:39–46, January 1983.
(1–27) Acta Obstet. Gynecol. Scand. 61:205–208, 1982.

NEONATAL OUTCOME OF 33 PATIENTS WITH REACTIVE AND 14 WITH NONREACTIVE FETAL HEART RATE

Outcome	33 cases with reactive FHR	14 cases with non-reactive FHR
Neonatal death	–	1/14 (7%)
Fetal distress in labor	3/33 (9%)	8/14 (57%)
Intrauterine growth retardation	–	4/14 (28%)
5 minute Apgar score of 7 or less	–	4/14 (28%)
Poor overall outcome	3/33 (9%)	11/14 (79%)
Good overall outcome	30/33 (91%)	3/14 (21%)

(Courtesy of Navot, D., et al.: Acta Obstet. Gynecol. Scand. 61:205–208, 1982.)

Eliahu Sadovsky (Hadassah Univ. Hosp., Jerusalem) studied the fetal heart rate (FHR) response to transient voluntary maternal hyperventilation and evaluated the results according to neonatal outcome in 50 women, of whom 10 had normal and 40 had high-risk pregnancies (postdatism, decreased fetal movement, preeclampsia, previous infertility, and other complications).

The women were tested in the semi-Fowler position at 32–42 weeks' gestation. Fetal heart rate was monitored continuously. After a baseline period, the women hyperventilated by overbreathing until extreme dizziness or faint feelings occurred (30 seconds to 5 minutes; mean, 110 seconds).

Hyperventilation caused no change in FHR patterns in 14 women. In 33 women there was acceleration of FHR or transient gradual tachycardia, or both. The other 3 patients were excluded from the study for technical reasons. As shown in the table, the neonatal outcome was good in 30 (91%) of the 33 patients with reactive FHR patterns but in only 3 (21%) of the 14 with nonreactive FHR patterns.

The FHR response to maternal hyperventilation late in pregnancy may correlate with fetal outcome. This simple, noninvasive technique for recording the FHR response to voluntary maternal overbreathing needs further study to assess its predictive clinical value.

▶ [This test of fetal well-being is similar to that proposed several years ago in which maternal exercise was used to stress the fetus, presumably by decreasing uterine blood flow. The "reactive" fetus, according to this study, responds to maternal hyperventilation with transient tachycardia. The results are interesting, but the "extreme dizziness or faint feeling" engendered by the hyperventilation makes widespread adoption of this maneuver unlikely.] ◀

2. Medical Complications of Pregnancy

2-1 **Effect of Dietary Fiber on the Oral Glucose Tolerance Test in Pregnancy.** Soluble fiber is known to blunt the increase in postprandial serum glucose in nonpregnant subjects. To assess the influence of dietary fiber on glucose tolerance in pregnancy, S. G. Gabbe, A. W. Cohen, G. O. Herman, and S. Schwartz (Univ. of Pennsylvania) carried out paired oral glucose tolerance tests (OGTTs) in the third trimester of pregnancy in 14 normal women and 4 women with diabetes mellitus. After a standard 100-gm OGTT, serum glucose and insulin levels were determined in the fasting state and at 60, 120, and 180 minutes after ingestion of the glucose load. A second OGTT was performed 3–5 days later, in which the glucose load was supplemented with 15 gm of flavored guar gum, a purified soluble dietary fiber.

All but 1 patient showed a significant improvement in glucose tolerance. After ingesting guar gum, mean serum glucose levels were significantly reduced at 1 hour, 2 hours, and 3 hours, and each of the

Fig 2–1.—Results of OGTT with and without guar gum. *Open circles,* normal OGTT on initial testing; *solid circles,* abnormal OGTT on initial testing; *solid lines,* without fiber; *dashed lines,* with fiber. (Courtesy of Gabbe, S. G., et al.: Am. J. Obstet. Gynecol.: 143:514–517, July 1, 1982.)

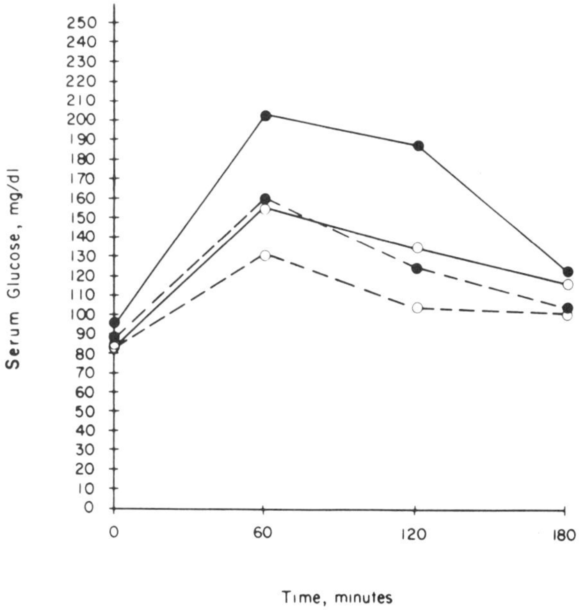

(2–1) Am. J. Obstet. Gynecol. 143:514–517, July 1, 1982.

diabetic subjects exhibited a normal glucose tolerance curve (Fig 2–1). Plasma insulin levels did not differ significantly between the standard OGTTs and those with guar gum. One patient experienced severe nausea without vomiting after receiving the guar gum and glucose mixture.

Ingestion of guar gum, a dietary fiber, may limit the postchallenge increase in serum glucose levels in pregnant subjects. The improvement noted in glucose tolerance in pregnant diabetic subjects was of sufficient magnitude to suggest a potential clinical value for dietary fiber in the treatment of gestational diabetes.

▶ [Several reports over the past several years have documented that a diet high in fiber has a salutory effect on diabetes. This study of the acute effects on the oral glucose tolerance test represents the first report of such an approach in pregnant women. The results indicate improvement in both normal women and gestational diabetics. A randomized clinical trial would now seem to be in order.] ◀

2–2 **Comparison of Glycohemoglobin Determination and the 1-Hour Oral Glucose Screen in the Identification of Gestational Diabetes.** B. D. Shan, A. W. Cohen, C. May, and S. G. Gabbe (Univ. of Pennsylvania) conducted a prospective study to evaluate the use of glycohemoglobin (HbA_1) as a screening tool for the detection of gestational diabetes in 90 subjects. At 28–30 weeks' gestation, these patients had a blood HbA_1 determination prior to diabetes screening with a 1-hour serum glucose screening test after administration of 50 gm of oral glucose. Those women with an abnormal result were then given a standard 3-hour oral glucose tolerance test.

On the 1-hour glucose screening test, 47 patients had abnormal values and 43 had normal values. Of the 43 patients with normal results, 41 had normal HbA_1 values. Eight of these patients had a strong clinical history for diabetes mellitus and underwent glucose tolerance testing; 3 had an abnormal 3-hour oral glucose tolerance test value. The 47 patients with abnormal screening values were divided into two groups: group 1 comprised 38 patients with normal HbA_1 levels, and group 2 comprised 9 with abnormal HbA_1 levels. Eleven patients (29%) in group 1 and 4 (46%) in group 2 had abnormal oral glucose tolerance test results. The sensitivity and specificity of blood HbA_1 determinations alone were 27% and 86.5%, respectively, whereas sensitivity and specificity of the combination of the 1-hour glucose screen and the HbA_1 test were 22.4% and 87.7%, respectively. There was no statistical difference between the groups.

These results suggest that although HbA_1 is an indicator of overall control, it has a very wide range with respect to the fine control of diabetes mellitus and cannot be used as a screening tool for an obstetric population. Because HbA_{1c} constitutes the greatest part of total HbA_1, the same conclusion may be inferred for HbA_{1c}.

▶ [Glycosylated hemoglobin levels reflect blood glucose levels over the prior several weeks, suggesting that their measurement might be a useful screening test for gestational diabetes. Unfortunately, this does not seem to be the case, at least according to these findings. The correlation between an elevated HbA_1 concentration and an oral glucose tolerance test was—in a word—poor.] ◀

(2–2) Am. J. Obstet. Gynecol. 144:774–777, Dec. 1, 1982.

2-3 **Maternal Diabetes and Neonatal Macrosomia: I. Postpartum Maternal Hemoglobin A_{1C} Levels and Neonatal Hypoglycemia.** Yves W. Brans, Robert W. Huff, Donna L. Shannon, and Mary Ann Hunter (Univ. of Texas, San Antonio) undertook to determine whether macrosomic neonates with and those without diabetic mothers could be distinguished by postpartum maternal hemoglobin A_{1C} concentrations. Relations among maternal diabetes, neonatal size, hypoglycemia, and postpartum hemoglobin A_{1C} concentrations were examined in 88 nondiabetic women and 73 diabetic women in White classes A to D. There were 41 nondiabetic mothers of neonates with normal growth and 47 nondiabetic mothers of macrosomic neonates, defined as weighing over the 90th percentile at birth.

The mean hemoglobin A_{1C} value in the control group was 5.7%, and the upper limit of normal was set at 7.1%, or 2 SD above the mean. Mean hemoglobin A_{1C} values were similar in mothers of macrosomic infants and mothers of normal-growing infants in both nondiabetics and the various diabetic groups. No correlation with relative birth weight was found. Class A diabetic mothers had mean hemoglobin A_{1C} values similar to those of nondiabetic mothers, but class AB diabetic mothers and class BCD patients had significantly higher mean values. In all groups, mean hemoglobin A_{1C} values were similar for mothers of infants with and without hypoglycemia. Neonatal hypoglycemia was related to both diabetes class and birth weight.

Although hemoglobin A_{1C} values in diabetics adequately reflect diabetic control over a period of 60 to 90 days, values may not be reliable as an indicator of fine tuning of diabetic control in the last trimester of pregnancy. Hemoglobin A_{1C} values may be less sensitive to changes in maternal plasma glucose concentration than the fetal glucose-insulin homeostatic axis.

▶ [The results reported here are consistent with those in two articles in the 1981 YEAR BOOK (pp. 52–53). There was much overlap in $HgbA_{1c}$ levels at delivery between diabetic and nondiabetic pregnant women and levels did not correlate with birth weight, either absolute or relative. In the present study, maternal $HgbA_{1c}$ levels did not predict the development of neonatal hypoglycemia either. The clinical utility of this determination in diabetic women in late pregnancy has not been established.] ◀

2-4 **Five Years' Experience of A "Prepregnancy" Clinic For Insulin-Dependent Diabetics.** Judith M. Steel, F. D. Johnstone, A. F. Smith, and L. J. P. Duncan (Edinburgh) report the first 5 years' experience of the first prepregnancy clinic for diabetics in Edinburgh. Patients were invited to attend the new clinic. Letters were sent to all patients aged 14–40 years who had registered with a department for diabetes. Patients who intend to become pregnant attend the clinic with their partners and are seen at the first visit in a joint consultation with an obstetrician and a physician. In subsequent visits the patients and their partners are seen by the physician only.

Ninety couples have attended the prepregnancy clinic. Eight were advised against pregnancy, 18 have been investigated for infertility, and 46 pregnancies have continued past 20 weeks. Three couples

---

(2–3) Pediatrics 70:576–581, October 1982.
(2–4) Br. Med. J. 285:353–356, July 31, 1982.

TABLE 1.—HEMOGLOBIN A_1 LEVELS IN 46 INSULIN-DEPENDENT DIABETIC PREGNANCIES*

Time	Prepregnancy clinic (n = 31)			Others (n = 15)			p
	Mean	SE	% Below 8%	Mean	SE	% Below 8%	
First attended prepregnancy clinic (n = 16)	11·77	0·47	0				
Booking	9·42	0·28	20	11·21	0·48	0	<0·005
1st Trimester	9·01	0·21	30	10·60	0·34	0	<0·001
2nd Trimester	8·05	0·12	58	9·09	0·37	33	<0·001
3rd Trimester	7·64	0·11	82	7·91	0·26	63	NS

*Normal nonpregnant range, 5 × 9% to 8 × 0%.
(Courtesy of Steel, J. M., et al.: Br. Med. J. 285:353–356, July 31, 1982.)

moved away. Those patients advised against pregnancy included those with severe nephropathy in whom the outcome of pregnancy and their own life expectancy would be poor. Those attending the prepregnancy clinic had a "heightened awareness" of the need for intensive care before and during pregnancy compared with other patients attending the clinic. The prepregnancy clinic patients had an earlier mean gestational age at which they first sought care for pregnancy than the others. Table 1 shows hemoglobin A_1 levels throughout the course of the last 46 pregnancies. Control, particularly in early pregnancy, was better in patients attending the clinic. In 43 pregnancies among women attending the prepregnancy clinic, 2 perinatal deaths occurred in viable pregnancies. One woman delivered twins at 26 weeks, with one twin dying in the neonatal period and the other dying during the first year of life. Two deaths were due to congenital abnormality (Table 2) and 3 were due to premature labor. Among pregnant diabetic patients treated by the authors during the past 6 years, 42 had not attended the prepregnancy clinic. Twenty-one of these patients delivered or were pregnant during the year the clinic was started. This group was difficult to manage during the pregnancies.

This experience of a prepregnancy clinic for diabetic patients shows that such a clinic contributed to improved management of pregnancy in this patient group by permitting better control of diabetes, particularly at the time of conception and throughout the first trimester. Objective evidence of benefit was difficult to obtain, but those women who had attended the prepregnancy clinic attended earlier and had lower hemoglobin A_1 concentrations in the first trimester than those diabetic women who had not attended the clinic.

▶ [The reported association between elevated maternal hemoglobin A_{1c} levels in early pregnancy and congenital malformations in infants of diabetic mothers suggests that rigid periconceptional blood glucose control might be helpful (1982 YEAR BOOK, pp. 37–39). This article describes the experience of a "prepregnancy" clinic for insulin-dependent diabetics. Clinic attendance was associated with lower hemoglobin A_{1c} levels in early pregnancy; the data regarding malformations are too few to permit conclusions. This is an important issue. We are sure to read more reports concerning this subject in the next few years.] ◀

TABLE 2.—MAJOR CONGENITAL ABNORMALITIES IN WOMEN INSULIN-DEPENDENT BEFORE ONSET OF PREGNANCY*

Case No	Pre-pregnancy clinic	White's classification	Clinical details	Gestation at delivery (weeks)	HbA_1 1st Trimester	Defect	Outcome
1	No	C	Social and psychological problems. Presented late in pregnancy. Poor control often omitted evening insulin	24	Presented too late	Anencephaly	Induced abortion
2	No	C	Social and psychological problems. Often omitted insulin in early pregnancy	34	13·4%	Sirenomelia (with renal agenesis)	Neonatal death (3 h)
3	No	R/F	Proliferative retinopathy treated with photocoagulation. Nephropathy. Concealed pregnancy. Very poor control. Often omitted insulin	34	Presented too late	Sacral agenesis	Urinary incontinence. Lesion only diagnosed at age 3 years
4	No	R	Proliferative retinopathy treated	35	Before assay available	Large encephalocele and microcephaly	Encephalocele surgically repaired. Good outcome on current follow-up
5	Yes	C	Well motivated. Previous fetal loss with multiple haemangiomas	38	9·5%	Transposition of great vessels, ventricular septal defect	Died at 2 months while undergoing cardiac surgery

*Class C, insulin-dependent diabetic women; age of onset 10–20 years or duration 10–19 years; no microangiopathy. Class F, insulin-dependent diabetic women; diabetic nephropathy. Class R, insulin-dependent diabetic women; proliferative retinopathy.

(Courtesy of Steel, J. M., et al.: Br. Med. J. 285:353–356, July 31, 1982.)

2-5 **Uteroplacental Blood Flow in Diabetic Pregnancy: Measurements With Indium-113m and a Computer-Linked Gamma Camera.** L. Nylund, N.-O. Lunell, R. Lewander, B. Persson, and B. Sarby, with the technical assistance of S. Thornström, measured the uteroplacental blood flow index during the last trimester of pregnancy in 41 healthy women, 14 women with insulin-dependent diabetes mellitus, and 12 women with gestational diabetes mellitus.

The women were studied in either the 30-degree left lateral recumbent or the supine position. After an intravenous bolus injection of 1 mCi of ^{113m}In-chloride, the radiation emanating from the placenta was recorded with a computer-linked gamma camera. Serial scintigrams were obtained at 10-second intervals for 240 seconds.

The uteroplacental blood flow index was about 30% lower in the supine than in the left lateral recumbent position (table). Diabetic patients in the left lateral recumbent position showed a rise time that was prolonged and a blood flow index that was 45% lower than that of the control group. Diabetic patients in the supine position also showed lower maximum activity than the control group, and the blood flow index was reduced 35%.

Diabetic patients with infants who were large for gestational age had median uteroplacental blood flow indices that were somewhat lower, but not significantly so, than diabetic patients with normal-sized infants. Women with gestational diabetes and those with insulin-dependent diabetes showed similar reductions in blood flow index. Impaired control of blood glucose was associated with a diminished uteroplacental blood flow index. In both the diabetic and control groups, a positive correlation was found between gestational age at scintigraphy and blood flow index in the supine but not the left lateral recumbent position.

There appears to be no direct relationship between uteroplacental blood flow and fetal birth weight in diabetes. The present findings support the concept that increased density of the diabetic placenta caused by enlargement of the villi may affect uteroplacental blood flow because the intervillous space would then be reduced.

▶ [As we commented previously (1981 YEAR BOOK, p. 95), the methodology, assumptions, and mathematics of this technique are complex. The table indicates the wide range of values obtained. We are not surprised that the blood flow index was greater

UTEROPLACENTAL BLOOD FLOW INDICES IN NORMAL AND DIABETIC PREGNANCIES*

	Normal pregnancy		*Diabetic pregnancy*	
Maternal position	*Left lateral (Group 1)*	*Supine (Group 2)*	*Left lateral (Group 3)*	*Supine (Group 4)*
n	24	17	12	14
Rise time (sec)	50 (20-84)	67 (35-100)	65 (30-95)	65 (50-110)
Maximum activity (counts/10 sec)	900 (420-1,540)	880 (460-1,504)	800 (369-1,620)	742 (264-875)
Blood flow index (proportional to ml/sec)	20.6 (7.4-51.3)	13.9 (6.1-30.1)	11.6 (4.3-40.0)	9.2 (4.1-16.7)

*Values given as median and range.
(Courtesy of Nylund, L., et al.: Am. J. Obstet. Gynecol. 144:298–302, Oct. 1, 1982.)

(2–5) Am. J. Obstet Gynecol. 144:298–302, Oct. 1, 1982.

in the left lateral than in the supine position, but are surprised that it did not differ between White's classes.] ◀

2–6 **Regulation of Glucose Production in Newborn Infants of Diabetic Mothers.** The physiologic basis of the changes in glucose metabolism seen in infants of diabetic mothers remains unclear. Katherine C. King, Kou-Yi Tserng, and Satish C. Kalhan (Case Western Reserve Univ., Cleveland) investigated the hepatic regulation of glucose production in infants of both normal and diabetic mothers by examining the effects of glucose infusion on systemic glucose production and utilization. Five infants of insulin-dependent diabetic mothers, 1 of a gestationally diabetic mother, and 5 normal newborn infants were examined at age 2–4 hours. Rigid metabolic control of insulin-dependent diabetes had been achieved in the third trimester of pregnancy. All patients but 1 had plasma glucose levels of 36–104 mg/dl, and 3 had normal postprandial glucose levels. Deuterium-labeled glucose was used as a tracer. After infusion of glucose at a rate of 4 mg/kg/minute for 2 hours, fractional glucose uptake was determined by giving a glucose pulse of 0.5 gm/kg.

Basal plasma glucose levels were lower in the infants of diabetic mothers than in the normal infants, but glucose production and utilitzation rates did not differ significantly. Metabolic clearance rates were 7.7 ml/kg/minute in the infants of diabetic mothers and 5.2 ml in the normal group. Infusion of glucose led to greater suppression of the endogenous glucose production rate in the normal infants. An acceleration of fractional glucose uptake was observed in the normal infants. The mean volume of distribution of glucose was 429 ml/kg.

Rigid regulation of maternal diabetes appears to normalize the rate of glucose production in infants of diabetic mothers, although intermittent maternal hyperglycemia may result in altered regulation of hepatic glucose production. The infants of diabetic mothers in this study had lower basal glucose concentrations than normal newborn infants. Two infants of diabetic mothers were large-for-gestational age despite rigorous antepartum management.

▶ [This study compares glucose production indices in normal infants and infants of diabetic mothers. The production rates were similar in the two groups, so the lower plasma glucose concentration in infants of diabetic mothers must reflect increased metabolic clearance. Endogenous glucose production was suppressed by glucose infusion, more so with normal infants than with infants of diabetic mothers. The fact that these differences existed despite tight metabolic control during the preceding pregnancies indicates that it is probably not possible to normalize fetal metabolism entirely.] ◀

2–7 **Pregnancy and Its Outcome in Women With and Without Surgical Treatment of Congenital Heart Disease.** Ruth Whittemore, John C. Hobbins, and Mary Allen Engle followed 233 women with congenital heart defects prospectively through 482 pregnancies. A total of 372 infants were followed over the first 3 years of life. One hundred eighteen women had been operated on. The proportion of pregnancies resulting in live births was not significantly influenced

(2–6) Pediatr. Res. 16:608–612, August 1982.
(2–7) Am. J. Cardiol. 50:641–651, September 1982.

by cardiac surgery, but more and larger live-born infants were born to mothers who became acyanotic as a result of reparative surgery than in those who remained cyanotic, whether or not palliative operation was performed. Placental size was abnormally large in cyanotic women in relation to birth weight, which was abnormally low.

There was no maternal mortality, and no case of infective endocarditis, stroke, or brain abscess occurred. The chance of an infant being born alive was associated with the mother's cardiac function. Mothers in fair to poor cardiac condition had more interrupted pregnancies and more cardiovascular complications during pregnancy. Nearly one third of these mothers had cardiovascular complications. Congestive heart failure occurred in 17 pregnancies. Arrhythmia was a problem in 20 pregnancies in 18 mothers. The overall incidence rate of infants with congenital heart disease was 16.1%.

Women with congenital heart disease in this series who were in excellent cardiac condition at the time of pregnancy had fewer unsuccessful pregnancies, obstetric complications, and cardiac complications than those whose cardiac status was poorer. Persistently cyanotic women should have the hemoglobin concentration and hematocrit monitored to avoid extremes of polycythemia or relative anemia. Antibiotic prophylaxis is used at the time of labor. Spontaneous labor is preferable to induction. Cyanotic women are often given oxygen throughout labor and delivery. Women should remain in the hospital for 3 or 4 days after delivery. The safest and most effective mechanical contraceptive method is the diaphragm with contraceptive gel; oral contraception is contraindicated. Depo-Provera may be useful in this setting. Tubal ligation should be done with great caution and not until several months after delivery in a patient with pulmonary hypertension.

▶ [With a declining incidence of rheumatic heart disease and increasingly effective forms of surgical treatment, the most frequent type of heart disease complicating pregnancy nowadays is the congenital variety. The analysis of this large series provides an excellent summary of the current state of the art. It is encouraging that no maternal deaths or other serious complication occurred in 233 patients through 482 pregnancies. The incidence of congenital heart disease in the offspring, 16%, is higher than that reported previously, which may reflect the careful follow-up of the infants.] ◀

2–8 **Pregnancy After Surgical Correction of Tetralogy of Fallot.** H. Singh, P. J. Bolton, and C. M. Oakley (Royal Postgrad. Med. School, London) note that uncorrected cyanotic heart disease carries a high risk in pregnancy for both woman and fetus. In a previous review of 57 pregnancies in women with uncorrected tetralogy of Fallot, there was a fetal mortality of 22% and a maternal mortality of 7%. In this study, a questionnaire asking for details of infertility, pregnancies, and miscarriages was sent to 52 patients with surgically corrected tetralogy of Fallot.

Twenty-five patients had had no pregnancies, but only 1 complained of infertility. A total of 6 miscarriages had occurred in 2 patients, both of whom had achieved at least 1 successful pregnancy.

(2–8) Br. Med. J. 285:168–170, July 17, 1982.

Two patients had had termination of pregnancy for reasons other than their cardiac disease. There were 40 successful pregnancies in 27 patients. No serious cardiac complications occurred in 31 pregnancies about which detailed information was available. Overt cardiac failure did not develop; and no patient required a prolonged hospital stay. Nine patients had mild ankle edema, but no specific treatment was necessary. The only obstetric antenatal complications were transient mild hypertension in 6 patients and mild edema in 9. Gestational age ranged from 35 to 42 weeks. Labor was induced in 5 patients; cardiac disease was given as the indication in only 1 case. Of the 31 deliveries about which detailed information was available, 15 were spontaneous vaginal deliveries. Of the 31 infants (18 boys, 13 girls), 30 were essentially normal and 1 had pulmonary atresia.

Surgical repair of tetralogy of Fallot has a low perioperative mortality, and survivors are usually much improved symptomatically. In this study, the incidence of miscarriage was no higher in patients who had undergone surgical repair than in the general population. The obstetric details suggest that pregnancy in patients with corrected tetralogy of Fallot is comparable with that in the normal population. A patient who has had a surgical correction of tetralogy of Fallot should be examined early in pregnancy. The pregnancy should be managed in the normal manner with no special precautions, provided there are no major residual defects.

▶ [Complete or near-complete surgical correction of the tetralogy of Fallot is possible, and patients with this malformation, formerly destined for early death, now can lead a relatively normal life. This questionnaire study of women who had had surgical correction found that nearly half had not conceived but almost none complained of infertility. In those who became pregnant, the outcome was astonishingly good. No maternal complications of any note were uncovered and, except for one infant with pulmonic atresia "under cardiologic surveillance," all children did well, too.] ◀

2–9 **Pregnancy in Patients With Porcine Valve Bioprosthesis.** Orally administered anticoagulants given to pregnant women with mechanical cardiac valve prostheses may be harmful to the fetus, whereas suspension of such treatment exposes the mother to an undue risk of embolic complications. Thus, the use of porcine bioprostheses is recommended in women wishing to bear children. Uberto Bortolotti, Aldo Milano, Alessandro Mazzucco, Carlo Valfre, Rosario Russo, Marialuisa Valente, Luciano Schivazappa, Gaetano Thiene, and Vincenzo Gallucci (Univ. of Padova, Padova, Italy) report the results in 7 women who became pregnant 8 times after receiving Hancock bioprostheses.

Of the 7 women, aged 14 to 31 years (mean, 24 years) at the time of valve replacement, 6 received an isolated mitral valve and 1 received a mitral valve and an aortic valve. Digoxin was used postoperatively in all patients. Sodium warfarin was administered orally for 3 months to all patients and then discontinued.

The women became pregnant at ages 18 to 35 years (mean, 28 years). The interval between valve replacement and delivery was 21 to 88 months (mean, 51.3 months). At conception, all women were in

---

(2–9) Am. J. Cardiol. 50:1051–1054, November 1982.

sinus rhythm; 6 were in New York Heart Association functional class I and 1 was in class II. Medications administered during pregnancy included digoxin in all cases, diuretics in 2, and dipyramidole in 1. Only 1 patient was given an anticoagulant during pregnancy, low-dose calcium heparin subcutaneously starting at the thirty-second week of her second pregnancy because of cardiac failure and atrial fibrillation. In 2 patients the possibility of spontaneous abortion arose around the eleventh week; both were managed successfully. Of the 8 pregnancies, 4 ended in the vaginal delivery of a healthy term baby, 1 ended in the vaginal delivery of a preterm infant who died of respiratory distress, and 3 ended in cesarean deliveries performed for obstetric indications. No maternal or fetal hemorrhagic or embolic complications occurred. One patient died 3 months after delivery in severe heart failure caused by diffuse calcification of both mitral and aortic xenografts. Another underwent successful reoperation soon after her second pregnancy because of calcific stenosis of the mitral porcine valve.

Bioprosthetic valves can be considered the most suitable devices for use in women of childbearing age because use of anticoagulants can be avoided. However, reoperation for bioprosthetic failure might be needed earlier than expected because pregnancy may favor calcification of porcine heterografts, leading to bioprosthetic failure. Therefore, close clinical and echocardiographic follow-up of these patients is recommended after pregnancy.

▶ [Porcine heart valves offer a great theoretical advantage over synthetic prostheses in that the need for anticoagulation is avoided. This review of 7 patients who conceived after bioprotheses were placed indicates that pregnancy was generally well tolerated. However, it is of some concern that calcification of the valve developed during pregnancy or the puerperium in 2 cases. Pregnancy doesn't seem to predispose to tissue calcification generally and the occurrence may be purely coincidental, but it bears watching.

A more optimistic view comes from a report by Denbow and associates (*Chest* 8:541, 1982), who described generally satisfactory outcomes of 13 pregnancies in 10 patients with homograft cardiac valves.] ◀

2–10 **Peripartum Cardiomyopathy Due to Myocarditis.** Kenneth R. Melvin, Peter J. Richardson, Eckhardt G. J. Olsen, Kieran Daly, and Graham Jackson (King's College Hosp., London) present data on 3 women, aged 21 to 28 years, with primary myocardial disease that developed during pregnancy or in the first 5 months post partum. Each had signs and symptoms of congestive heart failure without any known previous medical illness. Two had a history of an influenza-like illness and the third had an elevated titer of antibody to Coxsackie B_2 virus.

Detailed invasive and noninvasive investigations resulted in a clinical diagnosis of dilated cardiomyopathy until an endomyocardial biopsy specimen taken during cardiac catheterization showed acute inflammatory myocarditis. Immunosuppressive treatment with prednisone and azathioprine resulted in dramatic clinical improvement and disappearance of the inflammatory infiltrate in all 3 women.

(2–10) N. Engl. J. Med. 307:731–734, Sept. 16, 1982.

Myocarditis may cause peripartum cardiomyopathy because the cardiovascular system may be rendered potentially vulnerable by the increased workload of pregnancy, during which reactivation of a dormant virus or infection with a new cardiotropic agent, viral or otherwise, may result in the clinical presentation of primary myocardial failure. Viruses may cause myocarditis or act as a trigger, promoting an autoimmune reaction in the myocardium. Development of primary myocardial disease as a result of an alteration in immune function that permits viral invasion or establishment of an autoimmune mechanism for myocardial damage may be due to factors related to the effects of pregnancy on maternal immunologic tolerance.

Acute myocarditis should be suspected in patients with peripartum cardiomyopathy; this diagnosis should be either excluded or proved by endomyocardial biopsy at the time of presentation.

▶ [Peripartum cardiomyopathy is an uncommon problem. In the cases reported here, histologic myocarditis, diagnosed on endomyocardial biopsy, was present. The authors suggest a viral or autoimmune basis. Immunosuppressive therapy was apparently effective in these 3 patients.] ◀

2–11 **Pregnancy in Patients With Systemic Lupus Erythematosus.** Systemic lupus erythematosus has a predilection for women of childbearing age. Michael W. Varner, Richard T. Meehan, Craig H. Syrop, M. Paul Strottmann, and Clifford P. Goplerud (Univ. of Iowa) reviewed the outcome of 38 pregnancies in 31 patients aged 16–37 with systemic lupus. Eleven patients had had 24 pregnancies before lupus was diagnosed. Eight spontaneous abortions occurred, and there were 2 elective abortions; all 14 live-born infants survived.

The rate of spontaneous or missed abortion was 7.9%, and that of elective abortion was 10.5%. The perinatal mortality was 12.9%. One maternal death occurred 5 weeks post partum. All perinatal deaths occurred in mothers having onset of systemic lupus during pregnancy as well as nephritis or significant thrombocytopenia. Three of the 29 live-born infants were small and 1 was large for gestational age. Most of the patients whose disease was exacerbated during or after pregnancy, or was unchanged with treatment, received anti-inflammatory therapy, usually steroids. Untreated patients whose disease was unchanged during pregnancy had few manifestations involving the central nervous system, kidneys, or serosae. The cutaneous, serologic, and musculoskeletal manifestations of lupus had no prognostic value. Complement component levels did not correlate closely with the course of disease. Twelve of the 30 surviving patients underwent surgical sterilization.

The management of systemic lupus erythematosus during pregnancy does not differ substantially from that in nonpregnant patients. Immunosuppressive therapy should not be reduced or discontinued during pregnancy. Clinical parameters, renal function data, and hematologic findings are more useful than immunologic data are in assessing the course of disease during pregnancy and guiding changes in treatment. Antepartum fetal surveillance is recommended. The timing and route of delivery should be individualized.

(2–11) Am. J. Obstet. Gynecol. 145:1025–1040, Apr. 15, 1983.

Systemic lupus erythematosus itself is not an indication for section delivery. Intrauterine contraceptive devices should not be used in immunosuppressed patients, and oral contraceptives probably are contraindicated in patients with active systemic lupus erythematosus. Patients with lupus nephritis should defer pregnancy until all renal manifestations are absent.

▶ [This is a large and well-analyzed 10-year experience with systemic lupus erythematosus complicating pregnancy at one institution. It points out the gravity of disease onset *during* gestation and, in fact, all perinatal deaths occurred in patients initially diagnosed in pregnancy. The experience reported with serum complement and anti-DNA levels as indicators of disease status (i.e., about 40% accurate) is not nearly as optimistic as earlier reports would suggest (see 1981 YEAR BOOK, p. 41).] ◀

2–12 **Pregnancy Complications in Type IV Ehlers-Danlos Syndrome** were investigated by Noreen L. Rudd, Carl Nimrod, Karen A. Holbrook, and Peter H. Byers. Ehlers-Danlos syndrome type IV (EDS IV) is a distinct type of EDS with unique complications in pregnant women. Disordered production of type III collagen results in thin skin, slight joint hyperextensibility often limited to the hands, and few difficulties with scar formation. Patients may die of arterial and bowel rupture. Complications of pregnancy are severe enough to warrant consideration of early termination. At the least, all these pregnancies must be considered to be at high risk of complications.

Thirty-four persons in 14 families with EDS IV were seen in a 5-year period. Ten of the 20 women have had 20 pregnancies. Two pregnancies were interrupted, 1 because of concern about inheritance of the disease and possible complications and 1 because of colonic rupture at 8 weeks' gestation. Twelve of the 16 live-born infants had EDS IV. Two infants died during complications of delivery; 1 was normal, and the status of the other is unknown. Five women died of pregnancy-related complications, all in the peripartum period. Complications included bowel rupture, rupture of the aorta and vena cava, uterine rupture, vaginal laceration, and postpartum uterine hemorrhage. The overall risk of death in each pregnancy in this series was 25%.

The rate of maternal complications is high in pregnant women with EDS IV. Half the women in this series who were pregnant died in the peripartum period. Major complications also can occur ante partum, but the times of greatest risk are labor-delivery and the postpartum period. The possible complications should be discussed with women who are not yet pregnant. If desired, prenatal diagnosis may be feasible. Discussion of elective termination is appropriate with patients in early pregnancy. Patients first seen late in gestation should be cared for as high-risk patients and monitored closely during labor and for several days thereafter.

▶ [The Ehlers-Danlos syndrome (EDS) refers to a group of inherited connective tissue disorders of at least nine distinct types. Type IV EDS is characterized by thin, translucent skin and abnormal type II collagen production. The pregnancy performance of these patients, who were not selected because of problems in pregnancy, was abysmal. The vascular ruptures are reminiscent of those in Marfan's syndrome. If type IV EDS is suspected clinically, every effort should be made to confirm or ex-

(2–12) Lancet 1:50–53, Jan. 1/8, 1983.

clude the diagnosis biochemically in order to counsel the patient appropriately. The authors emphasize that their findings in type IV EDS are not to be expected in patients with other forms of EDS.] ◀

2–13 **Prenatal Prediction of Thrombocytopenia in Infants of Mothers With Clinically Diagnosed Immune Thrombocytopenia.** Management of pregnant women with immune thrombocytopenia is complicated by the unavailability of the fetal platelet count. Transplacental passage of antiplatelet antibodies mediates infant thrombocytopenia, and it has been suggested that measurement of maternal platelet-associated IgG might help to predict infant outcome. John G. Kelton, Martin J. Inwood, Robert M. Barr, Sidney B. Effer, David Hunter, William E. Wilson, David A. Ginsburg, and Peter J. Powers (Hamilton, Ont.) related the maternal platelet count and platelet-associated IgG level to the infant platelet count in 41 prospectively studied pregnancies (involving 44 fetuses) in 38 women, aged 18–43 years, with immune thrombocytopenia diagnosed clinically during pregnancy.

Five infants (11%) died in utero at 18–28 weeks' gestation. Of the 39 live-born infants, 15 were thrombocytopenic at delivery or immediately afterward. The level of maternal platelet-associated IgG was highly predictive of infant thrombocytopenia but maternal platelet count was not (table). Infants who were thrombocytopenic were born to 11 of 12 mothers with elevated platelet-associated IgG but to only

ASSOCIATION BETWEEN VARIOUS MATERNAL HEMATOLOGIC PARAMETERS EVALUATED AT DELIVERY AND THROMBOCYTOPENIA OF LIVE-BORN INFANTS

Maternal parameter	*No. of pregnancies*	*Thrombocytopenic infants* *No.*	*%*
Normal platelet count	6	2/7*	28
Thrombocytopenia (all)	30	13/32*	41
Thrombocytopenia (platelet count <75,000/μl)	15	7/15	47
Thrombocytopenia (all) plus elevated platelet-associated IgG	12	11/12	92
Thrombocytopenia (all) plus normal platelet-associated IgG	18	1/18	6
Elevated platelet-associated IgG, any platelet count	12	11/12	92
Normal platelet-associated IgG, any platelet count	24	4/27*	15

*Includes twins.

(Courtesy of Kelton, J. G., et al.: Am. J. Obstet. Gynecol. 144:449–454, Oct. 15, 1982.)

(2–13) Am. J. Obstet. Gynecol. 144:449–454, Oct. 15, 1982.

1 of 18 mothers with normal levels of this antibody. However, maternal platelet-associated IgG was not predictive of the severity of infant thrombocytopenia.

There was no neonatal mortality or significant infant morbidity after delivery. Of the 15 infants who had thrombocytopenia, most had quite severe deficits. In many, the platelet nadir did not occur until 2–6 days after delivery. In all but 3 infants the platelet count was above 100,000/μl within 1–2 weeks after delivery.

Measurement of platelet-associated IgG in pregnant women with immune thrombocytopenia can be used to predict infant thrombocytopenia. In this study, in contrast to some reports, maternal and infant morbidity in patients with clinically diagnosed immune thrombocytopenia was low. The reason for the high rate of fetal loss during pregnancy is uncertain. The percentages of infants in whom thrombocytopenia developed and of thrombocytopenic mothers in whom platelet-associated IgG was elevated were lower than expected from published reports. Conclusions about the relationship of maternal use of corticosteroids to infant outcome could not be made because treatment was not allocated randomly. However, such treatment did not appear to increase the platelet count in infants in this study.

2–14 **Antiplatelet Antibodies and Platelet Counts in Pregnancies Complicated by Autoimmune Thrombocytopenic Purpura.** The management of pregnancies in women with autoimmune thrombocytopenic purpura remains unclear because not all neonates are affected. James R. Scott, Neal S. Rote, and Dwight P. Cruikshank reviewed data from 44 patients during 48 pregnancies in an attempt to assess the reliability of possible means of predicting the fetal platelet count before onset of labor. Nineteen patients had previous splenectomy, and the operation was done during pregnancy in 1 patient. Twenty-four patients received 10–80 mg of prednisone daily at the time of delivery. An enzyme-linked immunosorbent assay for antiplatelet antibody was used. Fetal platelet counts were determined in scalp blood samples in a prospective series of 25 pregnancies. Labor was induced in 11 of these women.

There were no neonatal deaths; 1 fetal death occurred due to subarachnoid hemorrhage. Ten mothers with platelet counts of more than 100,000/cu mm delivered markedly thrombocytopenic infants, whereas 9 with lower counts delivered infants having normal counts. Infant platelet counts did not correlate closely with maternal treatment methods. Neither maternal nor infant antiplatelet antibody levels were consistently predictive of fetal platelet counts. The relationship between maternal and infant platelet counts in the prospective series is shown in Figure 2–2. All 5 thrombocytopenic infants had neonatal bleeding problems, but none had intracranial hemorrhage. In all cases the fetal scalp blood platelet count was predictive of neonatal thrombocytopenia.

Fetal scalp blood platelet counts can reliably determine the proper means of delivering singleton infants in patients with autoimmune

(2–14) Am. J. Obstet. Gynecol. 145:932–939, Apr. 15, 1983.

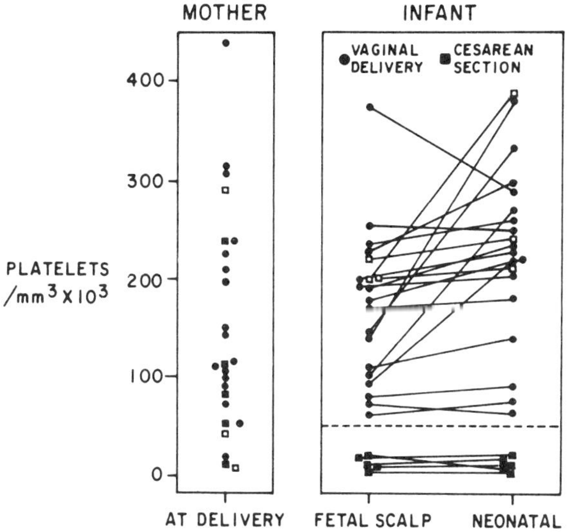

Fig 2–2.—Maternal and infant platelet counts in 25 pregnancies complicated by autoimmune thrombocytopenic purpura. Open squares represent patients who underwent delivery by cesarean section for obstetric reasons unrelated to the underlying disease. (Courtesy of Scott, J. R., et al.: Am. J. Obstet. Gynecol. 145:932–939, Apr. 15, 1983.)

thrombocytopenic purpura. This is a considerably more accurate approach than others, and abnormal bleeding did not occur from scalp puncture sites in thrombocytopenic fetuses. The technique permits safe vaginal delivery in most instances, while sparing thrombocytopenic fetuses the possible hazards of vaginal birth.

▶ [This article and the preceding one both involved measurement of antiplatelet antibodies in gravidas with immune thrombocytopenia, and the conclusions regarding clinical utility seem exactly opposite. The study of Kelton and associates seems to indicate that maternal platelet-associated IgG levels predict the risk of neonatal thrombocytopenia with a high degree of accuracy. Eleven of 12 instances in which levels were elevated resulted in thrombocytopenic infants, and 23 of 27 cases with normal levels were associated with normal babies. Yet, there are some curious aspects to this article. One wonders why the data are reported in qualitative rather than quantitative terms—i.e., platelet-associated IgG levels normal or elevated and platelet count above or below 150,000. The article states that the platelet-associated IgG level predicts the existence, but not the severity, of neonatal thrombocytopenia; because thrombocytopenia is defined as a platelet count of less than 150,000, this implies that the test does not distinguish between platelet counts of 145,000 and 5,000, conditions with greatly differing risks.

By contrast, Scott and his colleagues, using an enzyme-linked immunosorbent assay system to measure antiplatelet antibodies, found that neither maternal nor infant values consistently predicted the platelet count in the infant. They concluded that direct fetal platelet counts are still the best guide to management.

Antibody studies seem sound theoretically but until the methodologic problems are resolved, we'll follow the advice of Scott et al. and rely on the fetal platelet count.] ◀

2–15 **Newborn Infants to Myasthenic Mothers: Clinical Study and Investigation of Acetylcholine Receptor Antibodies in 17 Children.** Myasthenia gravis affects about 12% of infants born to myasthenic mothers. Its occurrence in neonates provided early evidence of

---

(2–15) Neurology (NY) 33:133–138, February 1983.

a circulating factor now thought to be maternal IgG receptor antibody. Ann Kari Lefvert and Per Olof Osterman reviewed the clinical and serologic findings in 17 infants of 15 myasthenic mothers. Two infants had typical symptoms of neonatal myasthenia gravis. Acetylcholine receptor (AcChR) antibody was detected by incubating serum or IgG with a complex of ^{125}I-α-neurotoxin from the cobra *Naja naja siamensis* and human skeletal muscle receptor.

The AcChR antibody was found in the sera of 14 of 15 mothers and in 16 of 17 infants at birth. The mother who lacked antibody had an infant without antibody in cord blood. The concentration of receptor antibody in cord blood usually was higher than that in the mother. The antibody titer fell rapidly in unaffected children, but in the 2 children with neonatal myasthenia the decline was much slower. No significant effect of α-fetoprotein was noted on the binding of AcChR antibody to receptor-toxin complex. Studies with an anti-idiotypic antibody found marked differences between idiotypes in the mother and in affected children.

These findings indicate that transient synthesis of receptor antibodies in the infant is a factor in the pathogenesis of neonatal myasthenia gravis. Treatment with cholinesterase inhibitors does not seem important in the development of neonatal myasthenia, because it can occur in infants of untreated mothers. Maternal treatment with these drugs may delay the appearance of symptoms.

▶ [A percentage of infants born to women with myasthenia gravis demonstrate transient myasthenia themselves, and it was this observation that represented the initial evidence that the disease is immunologic in nature. Presumably, maternal antibodies against acetylcholine receptors cross the placenta in affected cases. However, according to this study, the situation may not be one of simple passive immunization. First, the lack of any correlation between antibody titer and presence or severity of neonatal myasthenia is puzzling. Second, there was a difference in antibody half-life between affected and unaffected infants. Finally, differences between idiotypes in antibodies in mother and infant were observed. Taken together, these findings suggest that transient receptor antibody synthesis by the fetus or neonate, instead of or in addition to placental transfer, may be involved in neonatal myasthenia.] ◀

2–16 **Thyrotoxicosis in Pregnancy: Results of Treatment by Antithyroid Drugs Combined With T_4.** Cretinism has occurred in some cases of thyrotoxicosis in pregnancy managed by antithyroid drugs alone, but the use of supplemental thyroxine (T_4) is controversial. Ian Ramsay, S. Kaur, and G. Krassas (London) reviewed experience with such treatment in 19 thyrotoxic women, aged 21 to 39 years, studied during 20 pregnancies. Fourteen pregnancies occurred while the mothers were euthyroid during treatment with an antithyroid drug and L-thyroxine. Twelve of these women were using carbimazole. The dosage of carbimazole was adjusted to 5 mg four times daily when pregnancy was diagnosed, and L-thyroxine was increased in 11 cases to 0.3 mg daily. Patients who became pregnant and thyrotoxic concurrently received 15 mg of carbimazole three times daily until they became euthyroid and then 5 mg four times daily with 0.3 mg of L-thyroxine daily.

A total of 21 infants were delivered, with no fetal losses and with

---

(2–16) Clin. Endocrinol. (Oxf.) 18: 73–85, January 1983.

gestational ages and weights in the normal range. Apgar scores were better than in control cases. One infant had a small goiter that disappeared spontaneously in a few days. One infant each had a persistent vitelline duct and an inguinal hernia. One infant developed thyrotoxicosis on the second day and was successfully treated. Cord blood thyrotropin concentrations were higher than in control cases, but most other hormone values were similar to those in controls. Three women had variably elevated thyroid hormone concentrations at delivery, and their infants had abnormal thyrotropin values.

No fetal losses occurred in this prospective series of thyrotoxic pregnancies managed with both antithyroid drugs and T_4. The clinical and biochemical outcome of the infants has been reasonably good. A prospective, randomized comparison of antithyroid drugs alone with combined antithyroid drug and T_4 therapy in thyrotoxic pregnant patients is under way.

▶ [The results reported here are excellent, but we think they reflect the patient population (most women were euthyroid and receiving antithyroid medication prior to pregnancy) and the quality of care given during pregnancy, rather than the supplemental T_4. Because current opinion is that thyroid hormones do not cross the placenta to any appreciable extent, we do not use thyroid hormones for supplementation in our thyrotoxic patients, but use propylthiouracil alone in the lowest effective dose.] ◀

2–17 **Hyperparathyroidism and Pregnancy.** Primary hyperparathyroidism is unusual in pregnancy. When it occurs, the risks of the untreated disease must be weighed against those of surgery during pregnancy. Only 49 previous cases have been reported. Daniel K. Lowe, Eric S. Orwoll, Michael R. McClung, Mary L. Cawthon, and Clare G. Peterson (Portland, Ore.) report data on 6 pregnancies in 4 mothers who had hyperparathyroidism. Four pregnancies were completed without treatment. Two patients underwent parathyroidectomy and delivered healthy infants. Only 14 previous cases of parathyroidectomy during pregnancy have been reported. There appears to be some risk to both the mother and fetus with either a surgical or a nonoperative approach. Three of the 4 patients in this study who had primary hyperparathyroidism during pregnancy were seen in the past 4 years, probably reflecting an increased awareness of this disorder.

Nephrolithiasis is a prominent feature of maternal hyperparathyroidism, but its presence does not in itself appear to adversely affect the outcome of pregnancy. The incidence of hyperparathyroidism in pregnancy remains unknown, but it probably occurs more often than is thought. The manifestations of maternal hyperparathyroidism and its effects on the outcome of pregnancy are varied. Hypercalcemia sometimes poses a distinct threat to the mother and the pregnancy, and parathyroidectomy is clearly indicated in such cases. It is most safely done in the second trimester. In other instances hyperparathyroidism seems to be quite well tolerated by both the mother and infant. Patients with mild disease may do well when managed nonoperatively. Infants born to mothers with hyperparathyroidism, including

---

(2–17) Am. J. Surg. 145:611–614, May 1983.

those delivered after parathyroidectomy, should be observed carefully for evidence of tetany.

▶ [Recent studies have suggested that pregnant women with primary hyperparathyroidism should be treated by parathyroidectomy. The conclusion from the cases reported here was that operation is indicated only with asymptomatic hypercalcemia, and asymptomatic patients with mild hypercalcemia can be followed without operation durihg pregnancy.] ◀

2–18 **Severe von Willebrand's Disease During Labor and Delivery.** Richard A. Lipton, Jahangir Ayromlooi (Long Island Jewish-Hillside Med. Center, New Hyde Park, N.Y.), and Barry S. Coller (SUNY at Stony Brook) report their experience in the successful management of pregnancy and delivery in two patients with clinically severe von Willebrand's disease.

CASE 1.—Woman, 25, had moderately severe von Willebrand's disease since childhood. Dental extractions had been performed with plasma transfusion support without difficulty. Her first pregnancy, which resulted in vaginal delivery of a healthy infant, was managed elsewhere. It was complicated by excessive bleeding from the episiotomy site. During the last trimester of the second pregnancy there was a rise in factor VIII coagulant activity (VII:C) to 53%. Onset of labor was spontaneous. Cryoprecipitate transfusions were begun just before delivery. A healthy infant was delivered vaginally. Thirty donor units was transfused, with 20 units transfused every 12 hours for 4 days thereafter. With cryoprecipitate transfusions, levels of factor VIII:C, factor VIII ristocetin cofactor (VIII R:Cof), and factor VIII-related antigen rose. Bleeding recurred on the eighth day and the patient received 30 units of cryoprecipitate. Dilatation and curettage were performed. She then received 20 units every 12 hours for 2 days.

CASE 2.—Woman, 28, with von Willebrand's disease had a history of hemorrhage after tonsillectomy and dental extractions, as well as chronic menorrhagia. Her first pregnancy resulted in a normal vaginal delivery, but vaginal hemorrhage began several days later and was managed by dilatation and curettage. A second pregnancy required a cesarean section because of nonprogression of labor. A postpartum hemorrhage occurred. Two months later, the diagnosis of von Willebrand's disease was made, based on factor values. During a third pregnancy there was an increase in all three factor VIII activities. Before elective cesarean section, during which a healthy infant was delivered, 30 units of cryoprecipitate was transfused and then 20 units was given daily for 2 more days. No shortening of bleeding time was seen 8 hours after the first transfusion. The patient was discharged on the eighth postoperative day without having had any major postpartum bleeding.

In management of labor and delivery of those women with von Willebrand's disease, the necessity for transfusion support can be predicted by the degree to which bleeding time and factor VIII R:Cof have normalized before birth. In clinically mild von Willebrand's disease in which these indices approach normal, prophylactic transfusion is not necessary. In severe disease in which factor VIII R:Cof fails to rise to 50% of normal, prophylactic transfusion support probably should be given. For cesarean section, transfusions should be given until abdominal sutures are removed. General management should include avoidance of antiplatelet drugs and intramuscular injections and attention to blood type specificity.

(2–18) JAMA 248:1355–1357, Sept. 17, 1982.

▶ [The discussion in this article serves as a nice review of this unusual, but by no means rare, disorder. The low factor VIII levels and platelet dysfunction apparently are related to a lack of the carrier protein (von Willebrand factor) for factor VIII, best measured by the factor VIII ristocetin cofactor assay. The treatment of choice, when patients with von Willebrand's disease have abnormal bleeding or are at risk for bleeding (labor, operation), is cryoprecipitate. Factor VIII concentrates are not as effective, presumably because they contain less carrier protein. We recently operated on a patient with von Willebrand's disease. Our hematologists suggested twice-daily cryoprecipitate infusions for 7 days.] ◀

2–19 **Prenatal Screening of Pregnant Women for Infections Caused by Cytomegalovirus, Epstein-Barr Virus, Herpesvirus, Rubella, and *Toxoplasma gondii.*** Katherine Hunter, Sergio Stagno, Elizabeth Capps, and Richard J. Smith (Univ. of Alabama, Birmingham) report the findings in a service-oriented screening program designed to detect viral and parasitic infections that occur during gestation. A total of 8,140 pregnant women were screened for evidence of rubella, *Toxoplasma,* and cytomegalovirus (CMV) infection. Most subjects were urban women from the middle-upper socioeconomic sector, but urban women of low socioeconomic status and rural women also were included. Rubella immunity was assessed by hemagglutination inhibition testing. Cytomegalovirus was assessed by indirect fluorescent antibody testing or anticomplement immunofluorescence. *Toxoplasma* was studied by indirect fluorescent antibody testing, Epstein-Barr virus (EBV) by methods for viral capsid antigens, and herpesvirus by microneutralization testing.

No differences in seroimmunity to rubella were found, but susceptibility to both CMV and *T. gondii* was greater for the urban middle-class group than for the rural group. Women from the lower-class urban group had the lowest seronegativity rate for CMV and the highest rate for *T. gondii*. Susceptibilities to herpesvirus and EBV, assessed only in the middle-class urban group, were 32% and 6%, respectively. Two seroconversions to *T. gondii* occurred during pregnancy; neither infant was infected. Seroconversion to CMV occurred in up to 2% of subjects each year. Only 3 of 37 patients with primary CMV infection had clinical evidence of acute infection. All were from the urban middle-class group and had a mononucleosis-like illness during pregnancy. One pregnancy was interrupted because of first-trimester infection. One of the 2 infants had viruria, but neither had symptoms. Nearly half the infants of women with primary CMV infection were infected in utero, but only 2 infants had clinical features of congenital CMV infection.

Screening to detect immunity to both CMV infection and rubella appears to be feasible. The feasibility of screening for herpesvirus and EBV warrants further study. Because of the low rate of toxoplasmosis, patient education rather than screening may be appropriate.

▶ [The data presented here don't make a very good case for routinely screening pregnant women for these infections. Although rubella antibody testing is probably indicated as a means of identifying those women who should be immunized post partum, the figures concerning *Toxoplasma* and cytomegalovirus aren't very impressive. Two of 5,142 women studied seroconverted to *T. gondii* during pregnancy; neither infant was infected. There were 37 seroconversions to cytomegalovirus (about

---

(2–19) Am. J. Obstet. Gynecol. 145:269–273, Feb. 1, 1983.

0.5% of women tested, something over 1% of susceptible women). Seventeen infants delivered of these 37 women were infected, but only 2 showed signs of illness in the neonatal period. To be sure, some of these infected infants may manifest problems later, but the yield still seems awfully low.] ◀

2-20 **Characteristics and Management of Pregnancy in Women With Genital Herpes Simplex Virus Infection.** Recent studies indicate that cesarean section might be avoided in many women with previous genital herpes simplex virus (HSV) infection without increasing the neonatal risk. James H. Harger, George J. Pazin, John A. Armstrong, Mary C. Breinig, and Monto Ho (Univ. of Pittsburgh) examined the natural course of genital HSV infection during 83 pregnancies in 78 women. In all, 163 recurrent episodes were studied by HSV cultures of the cervix and of vulvar lesions, taken at intervals of 1–3 days. Cervical HSV cultures were obtained weekly from asymptomatic women from 32 weeks' gestation.

Recurrent genital HSV infection was documented by at least 1 positive genital HSV culture in 74% of women. Eleven contracted their initial genital HSV infection during pregnancy. The mean duration of HSV shedding in recurrent episodes was 4½ days. The results in 11.8% of cervical cultures were positive. No recurrent episodes were noted in 20 pregnancies. The mean number of recurrent lesions in all term pregnancies was 1.8. The mean interval between recurrences was about 2 months, but many intervals were less than 3 weeks. The rate of development of positive HSV cultures is shown in Figure 2–3.

Fig 2–3.—Rate of development of herpes simplex virus (HSV) cultures with positive findings. Bars indicate proportion of HSV cultures on RK_2 cells yielding positive results on each day after inoculation; the line graph displays the cumulative total of positive HSV culture results on each day. (Courtesy of Harger, J. H., et al.: Am. J. Obstet. Gynecol. 145:784–791, Apr. 1, 1983.)

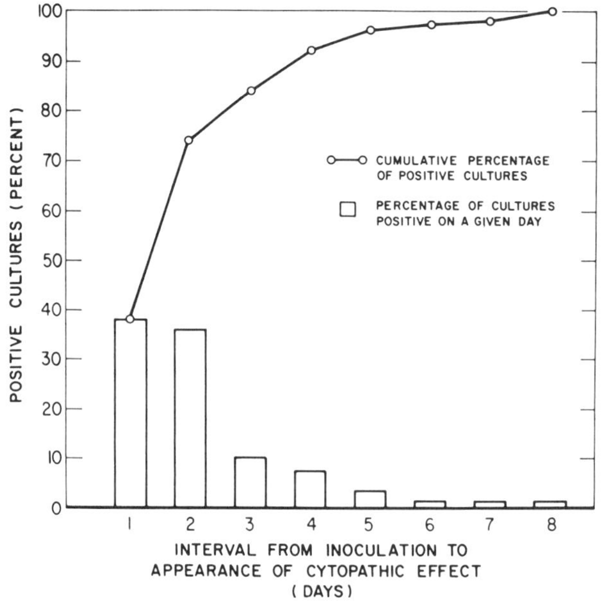

(2–20) Am. J. Obstet. Gynecol. 145:784–791, Apr. 1, 1983.

The overall cesarean section rate was 30.9%, and the rate of cesarean section to prevent neonatal HSV infection was 17.3%. No infant had evidence of congenital anomaly.

More than two thirds of these women were delivered of their infants vaginally, and no neonatal morbidity was caused by HSV. Data from frequently repeated genital HSV cultures can be used to manage pregnancies; this information will also reduce the need for cesarean section while avoiding neonatal HSV morbidity. Cultures must be obtained often because of the unpredictable and sometimes brief intervals between recurrences and the wide variation in HSV shedding at that time.

▶ [Our practice is similar to that described in this article. Patients with a history of genital herpetic infection have frequent cervical cultures performed in late pregnancy. If a patient's last culture was positive, she is delivered by cesarean section in early labor or within 4 hours of membrane rupture. Neonatal herpetic infection is devastating and, therefore, we currently support this approach, but have the feeling that we may be doing more cesarean sections than are necessary. What's needed is a better handle on the magnitude of risk to the individual neonate of vaginal delivery from an asymptomatic woman without lesions whose cervix is culture positive. Such a handle might be provided by the following article. Read on . . . .] ◀

2–21 **Incidence and Outcome of Asymptomatic Herpes Simplex Genitalis in an Obstetric Population.** The incidence of herpes simplex virus (HSV) genital infections during pregnancy has increased; however, the incidence and infectivity of subclinical cases are not yet clear. At least 33% of herpes-afflicted infants are born to asymptomatic mothers. Jonathan Scher, Edward Bottone, Edward Desmond, and Wendi Simons conducted a prospective study of an obstetric population to define factors leading to neonatal risk. Patients in the study were attending the obstetric clinic of Mount Sinai School of Medicine, New York. Patients with positive viral cultures from the genital tract at the time of delivery underwent cesarean section.

Results show that 28 of 488 (4%) routine asymptomatic patients had positive cultures for herpes simplex in the genital tract. The first 12 asymptomatic patients ranged in age from 19 to 40 years, with a mean of 27 years. Average time for viral shedding when cultures were obtained weekly from the date of first positive culture to the date of reversion of culture to negative status was 14 days. Two of 4 patients who had reversion to negative cultures had cesarean sections for obstetric reasons; 1 patient with a positive culture at the time of delivery had cesarean section for an unrelated cause. Among the other 7 patients with positive cultures, 2 patients had cesarean section; the remaining 5 had vaginal delivery. No infant in this study had neonatal herpes.

The 4% incidence of asymptomatic shedders of HSV reported in this series is higher than that reported (0.65%) by others. The differences may represent differences in populations studied. The incidence of neonatal herpes seems lower than the positive cultures would suggest. Some cases may go unreported because the usual incubation period is 4–21 days and patients are discharged from the hospital on the third day after delivery. The fact that 5 patients in this series

---

(2–21) Am. J. Obstet. Gynecol. 144:906–909, Dec. 15, 1982.

had virus in the genital tract and delivered vaginally without placental or fetal effect perhaps shows that the infectivity in asymptomatic cases is not high and management of these cases by cesarean section may have to be changed.

▶ [The incidence of herpes simplex virus isolation from asymptomatic prenatal patients found here, 4%, is (at least to our knowledge) by far the highest reported. It generally has been believed that one third of infants born through a culture-positive birth canal will acquire neonatal herpes, but that hardly seems possible if the carriage rate is as high as 4%. Therefore, it must be that the infectivity is lower than formerly believed, at least in asymptomatic cases.] ◀

2-22 **Antenatal Infections With *Candida* Species.** R. K. Whyte, Z. Hussain, and D. deSA (McMaster Univ., Hamilton, Ont.) report on the clinical, pathologic, and microbiologic features of 18 pregnancies complicated by intrauterine infection with *Candida* species. A review of previously reported cases and of the clinical aspects of the infants in this study reveals a syndrome differing from that seen in infections with a hematogenous dissemination of *Candida* species.

Discrete rounded yellow plaques, the pathognomonic changes of *Candida* species funisitis, were observed in the umbilical cord and membranes. These lesions varied in size from 0.5 to 2.0 mm and appeared in clusters (Fig 2–4). Histologic examination showed subamniotic distribution of the lesions on the cord (Fig 2–5). Numbers of organisms present varied considerably from case to case and from one lesion to another in the same case. In some plaques, organisms replicated freely on the surface; in others, they were ensheathed in fibrin and were fewer in number. None of the placentas showed evidence of inflammatory changes affecting the chorionic villi or decidual plate. All except 1 pregnancy were of short duration, 12 of them less than 28 weeks. Eight mothers had intrauterine contraceptive devices (copper in 7) present throughout pregnancy. Five mothers with previous repeated fetal losses had cervical sutures in place. When compared with controls, the cases had a predominance of foreign bodies in the cervix (72% of cases to 1% of controls). Three infants died before or within 1 hour of birth, 1 died at 6 days, and 1 died of bronchopulmonary dysplasia at 14 weeks. Of those who survived the immediate perinatal period, 4 developed a skin rash and 5 had radiologic signs of pneumonic consolidation. Three infants weighing greater than 2

Fig 2–4.—Umbilical cord showing clusters of small yellow focal lesions on amniotic surface. (Courtesy of Whyte, R. K., et al.: Arch. Dis. Child. 57:528–535, July 1982.)

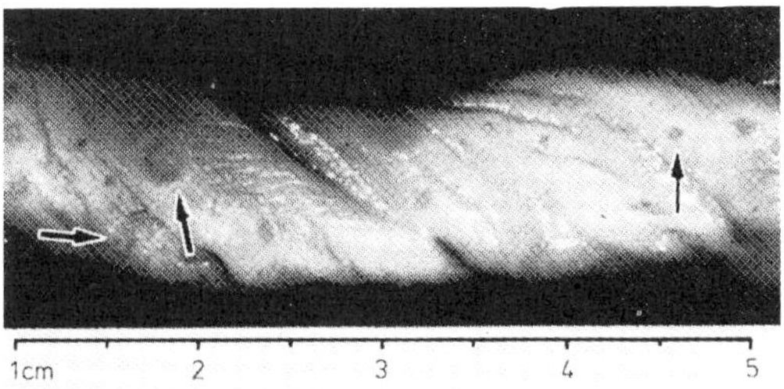

(2–22) Arch. Dis. Child. 57:528–535, July 1982.

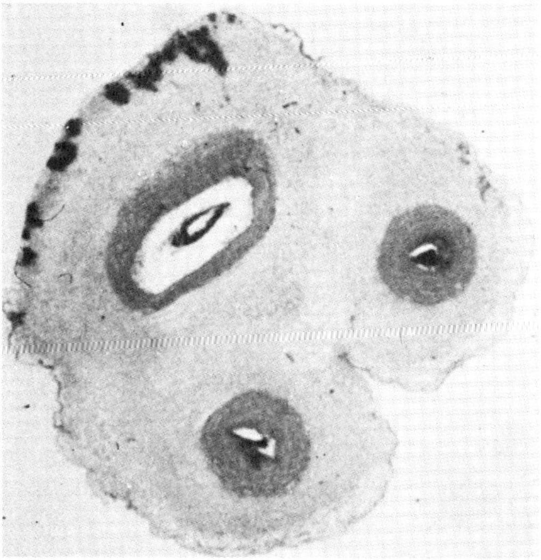

Fig 2–5.—Low-power view of transverse section of cord showing subamniotic lesions *(upper left)* strung out along the surface. Papanicolaou stain; ×16. (Courtesy of Whyte, R. K., et al.: Arch. Dis. Child. 57:528–535, July 1982.)

kg at birth were asymptomatic. All infants were treated with a combination of orally and topically administered nystatin. Eight infants in whom clinical and hematologic features suggested disseminated infection were also given systemic amphotericin B. The table shows the highest white blood cell counts and their differentials in babies who survived the immediate perinatal period. The white blood cell counts were highest in the first few days of life; in 10 cases the highest counts were recorded within the first 3 days of life.

The authors conclude that congenital infections with *Candida* species can be anticipated by their association with foreign bodies in the genital tract in pregnancy and diagnosed by careful examination of the cord and membranes at delivery. An infant of very low birth weight who develops a very high neutrophil count with immature forms may well be infected with *Candida* species.

▶ [Although vaginal candidiasis in pregnancy is common, intrauterine infection is rare. This article represents a nice summary of the problem. The association with a foreign body (intrauterine contraceptive device or cervical suture) is newly recog-

HIGHEST RECORDED WBC COUNTS FROM 15 CASES OF *Candida* CHORIOAMNIONITIS COMPARED WITH 14 CONTROLS

	Candidiasis *Count × 10⁹/l*		*Controls* *Count × 10⁹/l*		
	Median	*10–90 centile*	*Median*	*10–90 centile*	*P*
Total white cell count	62·2	23·6–91·0	20·8	15·6–35·7	<0·005
Segmented neutrophils	41·5	8·4–71·6	11·7	4·4–25·0	<0·001
Band neutrophils	2·4	0·2–19·0	0·6	0·0–5·3	<0·005
Immature neutrophils	1·7	0·0–12·8	0·0	0·0– 1·1	<0·001
Lymphocytes	8·1	5·3–13·0	5·4	2·9–12·2	<0·02

(Courtesy of Whyte, R. K., et al.: Arch. Dis. Child. 57:528–535, July 1982.)

nized. The characteristic appearance of the cord, illustrated in Figures 2–4 and 2–5, should alert the obstetrician, who, in turn, should alert the pediatrician. Neonates with *Candidia* infections typically have an unusually high white blood cell count.] ◀

2-23 **Influence of Pregnancies on Prolactinomas.** Hanns-Kristian Rjosk, Rudolf Fahlbusch, and Klaus von Werder (Univ. of Munich) used bromocriptine to treat hyperprolactinemic patients who desired pregnancy and had normal sella turcica or radiologic evidence of a microprolactinoma without suprasellar extension. Women who desired pregnancy and had large adenomas or suprasellar extension were treated by transsphenoidal surgery and in most instances with bromocriptine postoperatively. Sixty-one patients with hyperprolactinemia of intrasellar origin were included in the study and 81 pregnancies were observed in this group. Sixty-five of these pregnancies were completed with delivery at term. Twenty-two pregnancies have been observed in 13 patients undergoing surgery; 4 of these patients became pregnant without receiving bromocriptine postoperatively. The dose of bromocriptine necessary to normalize human prolactin (hPrl) levels and ovarian function was positively correlated to height of postoperative hPrl levels. In all patients bromocriptine was withdrawn as soon as pregnancy was diagnosed. During pregnancy, hPrl levels were measured every 2 weeks. During pregnancy, an increase above the hPrl increase range in normal pregnancies was only observed in 7 of 22 hyperprolactinemic women with a normal sella turcica. In patients with radiologically proved prolactinoma who did not have surgical treatment and who became pregnant after receiving bromocriptime, a rapid increase of hPrl levels was seen after withdrawal of bromocriptine. In patients with prolactinomas after operative treatment, pregnancies leading to delivery at term were observed in only 3 patients, with no rise of hPrl levels throughout pregnancy. In 6 patients who had surgery for prolactinoma, elevated hPrl levels persisted postoperatively but returned to normal levels after administration of bromocriptine, and pregnancy followed. The hPrl levels during pregnancy in bromocriptine-treated hyperprolactinemic women varied considerably, with no difference in these levels found in those patients with or without prior surgery.

A rapid fall of hPrl levels in 60 patients after termination of pregnancy indicated that estrogen stimulation does not cause persistent growth of the adenoma. In contrast, in 10% of pregnancies of hyperprolactinemic patients, a reduction of hPrl levels has been observed leading to spontaneous ovulatory cycles in 5 patients. In addition, whatever the reason for the different behavior of the hPrl levels during pregnancy may be, the findings show that adenomas within the sella turcica without suprasellar extension will never lead to complications during pregnancy, even if a tremendous increase of hPrl signals enhanced estrogen sensitivity of the prolactinoma.

▶ [Various forms of management were used in the 61 hyperprolactinemic patients described. There were 65 deliveries at term with no complications related to the pituitary. Transsphenoidal operation was undertaken in patients with macroadenomas, suprasellar extension, or prolactin levels above 5,000 μU/ml. Patients with microad-

(2–23) Acta Endocrinol. (Copnh.) 100:337–346, July 1982.

enomas and those with normal sellas were treated with bromocriptine until pregnancy was diagnosed. Prolactin levels rebounded in early pregnancy, but often were in the normal pregnant range by the third trimester. In most patients, prolactin levels decreased markedly post partum. These results support a conservative, i.e., nonoperative, approach to most hyperprolactinemic patients with microadenomas who desire pregnancy.] ◀

2–24 **Carpal Tunnel Syndrome in Pregnancy.** Fluid retention in pregnancy is often sufficient to lead to nerve compression in the wrist. To assess the incidence and severity of carpal tunnel syndrome in pregnancy, Andrus J. Voitk, John C. Mueller, Dianne E. Farlinger, and Richard U. Johnston (Orillia Soldiers' Meml. Hosp., Orillia, Ont.) interviewed by questionnaire 1,000 consecutive postpartum patients. A particularly severe case in which emergency operative decompression of the carpal tunnel was performed is also presented.

Of the 1,000 women, 335 (33.5%) reported having had symptoms in their hands during pregnancy. The symptoms were limited to the distribution of the median nerve (carpal tunnel syndrome) in 249 (74%) of those with symptoms, to the distribution of the ulnar nerve in 19 (6%), and 67 (20%) had poorly defined symptoms that did not clearly correspond to a known nerve distribution. There was little difference in maternal and fetal age, parity, and weight change between symptomatic and asymptomatic groups. Symptomatic women had twice the rate of ring removal because of swelling (73%) than asymptomatic women (36%). The rates of preeclampsia, hypertension, and edema, but not proteinuria, were somewhat higher in symptomatic women. The proportions of patients who had had wrist fracture were essentially the same in all groups and subgroups, but the prevalence of "arthritis" was twice as great among women with hand symptoms. More than 75% of the women had bilateral symptoms and 51% of the multigravidas had had similar symptoms in previous pregnancies. The symptoms were considered annoying by 51% of the symptomatic women. Hand function was impaired in 42%, 29% claimed that symptoms interfered with sleep, and 4% reported the symptoms to be intolerable. Less than 1% of the women did not consider the symptoms bothersome. Although 46% of the symptomatic patients reported their symptoms, only 16% (35% of those who complained) received advice or treatment and only 8% (17% of those who complained and 49% of those treated) obtained relief with treatment.

Because carpal tunnel syndrome in pregnant women is related to the pregnancy, it disappears with delivery. Consequently, operative decompression, which is achieved by dividing the flexor retinaculum, rarely is chosen. However, few women in this series were offered alternative therapy, and the forms of treatment used were effective in less than 50% of those treated. Surgery is definitive, can be performed with the use of local anesthesia, and has no significant associated morbidity. Because symptoms tend to recur with successive pregnancies, surgical decompression appears to have advantages over therapy with analgesics, sedatives, and diuretics, which carry risks, and over

---

(2–24) Can. Med. Assoc. J. 128:277–281, February 1983.

splints, which are inconvenient, especially to the primigravida with early, severe, bilateral involvement.

▶ [According to this survey, one third of women in late pregnancy experience some type of symptoms in their hands. In three fourths of these, numbness occurs in the distribution of the median nerve, meeting the criteria for the diagnosis of carpal tunnel syndrome. Associations with ring removal and preeclampsia suggest that interstitial fluid retention is responsible. Usually no treatment is indicated, although operative decompression rarely may become necessary.] ◀

2-25 **Pregnancy Following Gastric Bypass For Treatment of Morbid Obesity.** Kenneth J. Printen and David Scott (Univ. of Iowa, Iowa City) report that 45 patients who had undergone gastric bypass for treatment of morbid obesity became pregnant on 54 occasions; 46 infants were delivered. Two spontaneous abortions (4.0%) and 6 early terminations of an undesired pregnancy occurred; 7 infants were delivered prematurely. One child was born microcephalic and is retarded in growth and development.

In contrast to reports of infants born to mothers with jejunoileal bypass, 12 babies (more than 50% of those who could be compared with older siblings) born to mothers after gastric bypass were heavier at birth than older siblings. Another 10 infants were the first born to women who had lost more 100 lb after gastric bypass.

All but 1 of the women became pregnant more than 6 months after surgery; most patients became pregnant in the first 24 months after gastric bypass. This corresponded to the period of maximal weight loss and reversal of menstrual abnormalities associated with massive obesity. Four of the 7 patients with premature births delivered within 16 months of surgery.

Pregnancies were well tolerated by the mothers, with no excessive increase in weight loss or development of metabolic deficiencies. Five mothers continued to lose weight at an average of 15 lb during the pregnancy. In 1 case, a loss of 28 lb was associated with a premature birth. Since the gastric bypass is modeled on the Billroth II gastrectomy, additional iron supplementation was recommended during pregnancy.

Early conception after gastric bariatric surgery seems to be a risk factor for premature delivery. Although pregnancy cannot be recommended during the period of rapid weight loss in the initial postoperative period, the data indicate that neither the mother nor the fetus is unduly endangered by a pregnancy after the period of rapid postoperative weight loss.

▶ [Several articles have described pregnancy after intestinal bypass operations but this is the first, at least to our knowledge, detailing the outcome of patients who conceive after undergoing gastric bypass. The results appear quite good, probably because nearly all conceptions occurred more than 6 months postoperatively. The number of premature infants (7 of 58) seems high, but it is hard to know what this means because the manuscript states only, "Seven babies were delivered prematurely either by gestational age or low birth weight." An obstetric journal would certainly have insisted on more information concerning this point!] ◀

(2-25) Am. Surg. 48:363–365, August 1982.

3. Obstetric Complications

3–1 **Thyroid Function in Patients With Hyperemesis Gravidarum.** R. Bouillon, M. Naesens, F. A. Van Assche, L. De Keyser, P. De Moor, M. Renaer, P. De Vos, and M. De Roo (Katholieke Univ., Louvain, Belgium) report on their experience in a systematic exploration of concentrations of thyroid hormones in patients with hyperemesis gravidarum severe enough to warrant hospitalization. Thirty patients (33 pregnancies), aged 15–42 years, were studied. Mean duration of vomiting prior to hospitalization was 4 weeks and mean loss of weight was 5 kg.

Results show serum concentration of total thyroxine (T_4) to have been significantly higher in patients with hyperemesis gravidarum than in controls. Triiodothyronine (T_3) resin uptake was significantly increased in the experimental group also. Free T_4 index was much higher in patients with the disorder. In 24 of 33 (73%) pregnancies with hyperemesis gravidarum, the free T_4 index was more than 2 standard deviations above the mean of the controls (Fig 3–1). Free triiodothyronine (T_3) index was increased in only 4 of 11 hyperthyroxinemic patients. In 5 hyperthyroxinemic patients tested, no increase in serum thyrotropin was observed after injection of thyrotropin-releasing hormone. Goiter, exophthalmos, or previous history of hyperthyroidism was absent in all patients. The thyroxinemia returned to normal in 1 week to several weeks, whether or not it was treated with antithyroid drugs. Thyroid function during the period of hyperemesis had no influence on the subsequent rate of abortion or duration of pregnancy. A lower birth weight was observed in children born to hyperthyroxinemic mothers.

Hyperemesis gravidarum should be included in the differential diagnosis of elevations in free T_4 index during pregnancy and in the differential diagnosis of hyperthyroidism. The mechanism of an increased concentration of thyroid hormones in patients with the condition is still speculative, however. The need for the use of antithyroid drugs is questionable in these patients. Also, abnormal concentrations of thyroid hormones in patients with hyperemesis gravidarum should not be considered classic hyperthyroidism, but probably represent a special transient form of hyperthyroidism.

▶ [The fact that there was no increase in thyrotropin induced by thyrotropin-releasing hormone in some of these patients suggests that they were indeed hyperthyroid and that the laboratory abnormalities were not artifacts related to recent vomiting and weight loss. The timing of nausea and vomiting in pregnancy and the relationship between hyperemesis and certain "hyperplacentosis" conditions (twins, mole) hint at a relationship between human chorionic gonadotropin and hyperemesis, but previous studies haven't been able to make this connection. The findings reported here may

(3–1) Am. J. Obstet. Gynecol. 143:922–926, Aug. 15, 1982.

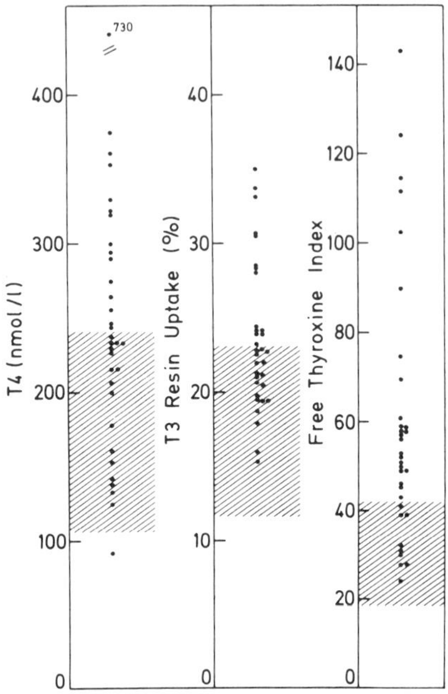

Fig 3–1.—Thyroid hormone concentrations in patients with severe hyperemesis gravidarum. Hatched areas represent the normal range (mean ± SD) obtained in 52 normal pregnant women. To convert T_4 to µg/100 ml, multiply by 0.0777. (Courtesy of Bouillon, R., et al.: Am. J. Obstet. Gynecol. 143:922–926, Aug. 15, 1982.)

rekindle an interest in chorionic gonadotropin because it is thought to have some thyrotropin-like activity. Free thyroxine should be measured in future studies of thyroid function in patients with hyperemesis gravidarum. Is there a relationship between thyroid hormone levels and the psychological factors that most of us think are important in this situation?] ◀

3–2 **Observation of an Organism Found in Patients With Gestational Trophoblastic Disease and in Patients With Toxemia of Pregnancy.** Judith Lueck, John I. Brewer, Silvio Aladjem, and Marilyn Novotny report the finding of multiple forms of a wormlike organism in patients with gestational trophoblastic disease and toxemia of pregnancy. A 3.5-µ structure was first seen during study of trophoblastic cells from a patient with choriocarcinoma, and it subsequently was found in fresh tissue specimens of choriocarcinoma and hydatidiform mole. A modified toluidine blue-O staining procedure was used to characterize the organism. Studies were done in 41 patients with mole or choriocarcinoma, 35 with preeclampsia, and 1 with eclampsia. All patients with trophoblastic disease had elevated hCG titers and evidence of active disease. Fifteen normal subjects also were studied.

The wormlike forms most often observed had an average length of 1 to 1.5 mm. Larva-like forms with an average length of 150 µ and primordial eggs and egglike forms in developmental stages, 7 to 43 µ in diameter, also were observed. The spermlike forms were 3.5 µ or smaller in size. These forms were present in contact smears prepared from peripheral blood of both groups of patients, trophoblastic tumor

(3–2) Am. J. Obstet. Gynecol. 145:15–26, Jan. 1, 1983.

tissue, placentas of patients with preeclampsia-eclampsia, and umbilical cord blood of infants of mothers with preeclampsia-eclampsia.

The forms of this organism share morphological features with several orders of helminths. Their taxonomy is unsettled; at present, the term "*Hydatoxi lualba*" is suggested. There is experimental evidence that the organism has biologic activity in mice and in beagles. It does not appear to represent an artifact.

3–3 **Experimental Induction of a Toxemia-Like Syndrome in the Pregnant Beagle.** Toxemia of pregnancy is seen in the first trimester in patients with hydatidiform mole, and the agent *Hydatoxi lualba* has been associated with the trophoblast of mole and placentas from toxemic patients. Silvio Aladjem, Judith Lueck, and John I. Brewer (Chicago) report the induction of a toxemia-like syndrome in pregnant beagles by intraperitoneal inoculation of concentrates of placentas from patients with preeclampsia-eclampsia and hydatidiform mole that contained *H. lualba.*

Pregnant dogs inoculated with either of the concentrates containing the agent developed progressive hypertension (Fig 3–2), eyeground changes of hypertensive retinopathy, proteinuria, disseminated intravascular coagulation, and hepatic dysfunction. Intrauterine growth retardation and fetal death also occurred. Hepatic periportal hemorrhage and glomeruloendotheliosis were seen in inoculated dogs. Sensitivity to angiotensin II infusion was significantly increased. *Hydatoxi lualba* was demonstrated in cardiac blood of pups of mothers inoculated with the effective concentrates. No toxemia-

Fig 3–2.—Mean diastolic pressures of pregnant dogs inoculated with concentrate II or concentrate III. Note progressive increase that reached maximum levels toward end of gestation. Concentrate I was prepared from placentas of normal pregnancies free from *H. lualba;* concentrate II was prepared from placentas of preeclamptic-eclamptic patients containing *H. lualba;* and concentrate III was prepared from evacuated hydatidiform mole containing *H. lualba.* (Courtesy of Aladjem, S., et al.: Am. J. Obstet. Gynecol. 145:27–38, Jan. 1, 1983.)

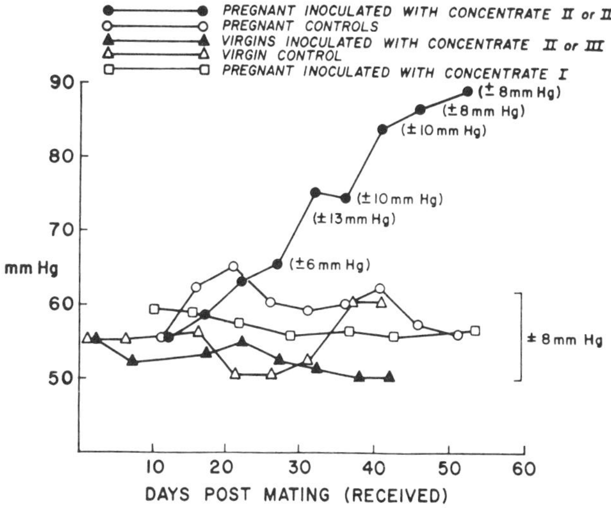

(3–3) Am. J. Obstet. Gynecol. 145:27–38, Jan. 1, 1983.

like syndrome developed in pregnant dogs given concentrate prepared from placentas of normal term pregnancies that lacked the agent or in nonpregnant dogs inoculated with concentrates containing the agent.

It appears that inoculation of concentrates containing *H. lualba* is necessary for production of a toxemia-like syndrome in the pregnant beagle. A metabolic product of the agent may be responsible, or it may stimulate the endogenous production of pressor substances. Intrauterine transmission of the agent may explain the higher rate of toxemia found in daughters of mothers who have had toxemia. The exact mechanisms involved remain to be clarified.

▶ [Wow! These are two of the most provocative articles to appear in the obstetric literature in years. A wormlike "organism" has been identified in the blood of patients with preeclampsia and trophoblastic disease. Placental concentrates containing the organism induced a toxemia-like syndrome in the pregnant beagle. The condition in the dog certainly resembles preeclampsia. The delay from inoculation to development of the pathologic process suggests that it isn't simply the infusion of a pressor substance that is involved. The preceding article doesn't list how often the various forms of the organism were recovered. No mention is made of its prevalence in control patients, but it was identified in 14 of 15 project personnel.

The bombshell represented by these articles has continued to reverberate at intervals during the months after their publication. David Heyneman, President of the American Society of Parasitologists, wrote a letter to the editor (*Am. J. Obstet. Gynecol.* 147:227, 1983) in which he expressed "astonishment" at the authors' "naiveté" in thinking that their description actually could be that of a single organism and concluded that the articles "are simply not credible."

According to a letter signed by the authors of the original article (ibid. 146:742, 1983), the dean of the medical school from which the work emanated convened a panel of three parasitologists to examine the authors' material. The panel concluded, "The objects in question are not parasites . . . . It seems likely that all are contaminants of the preparation . . . . The source of the objects is not known but it is suspected that the crystalline substances are tall and come from surgical gloves."

It appears that the famous blank plaque at the Chicago Lying-In Hospital will remain blank for the time being.] ◀

3–4 **Effective Prevention of Gestational Hypertension in Nulliparous Women at High Risk as Identified by Rollover Test.** It would appear that there is a high-risk group of pregnant women who are identified by the supine pressor test as possibly susceptible to development of gestational hypertension. This test, also known as the rollover test, is performed between 28 and 32 weeks of gestation. Ronald X. Spinapolice, Steven Feld, and John T. Harrigan performed the rollover test on 32 nulliparous women. All 32 had abnormal test results. Of these, 16 were instructed to remain in the left lateral recumbent position for at least 4 hours a day, in addition to normal bed rest on the left side. If the mean arterial pressure increased by 9 degrees or more, they were told to remain on the left side for at least 6 hours a day. The other 16 women served as controls.

The findings are shown in the table. Twelve of the 16 control patients experienced preeclampsia or hypertension between 32 and 40 weeks' gestation; 1 of the "treated" patients had an increase in pressure requiring more daytime rest. Another in the treated group experienced gestational hypertension at 38 weeks' gestation. Induction

(3–4) Am. J. Obstet. Gynecol. 146:166–168, May 15, 1983.

NUMBER OF PATIENTS WITH HYPERTENSION IN TREATED AND UNTREATED GROUPS HAVING ABNORMAL RESULTS OF ROLLOVER TEST

	No. of patients with abnormal test results	*No. of patients with hypertension*
Control	16	13
Treated	16	1

(Courtesy of Spinapolice, R. X., et al.: Am. J. Obstet. Gynecol. 146:166–168, May 15, 1983.)

of labor and premature delivery were necessary because of elevated blood pressure in 2 women.

Patients prone to the development of hypertensive disease of pregnancy can be identified early in the course, and simple intervention with increased rest in the left lateral position can effectively control the process. This approach requires minimal change in the patient's life and permits her to continue most activities. It also is a cost-effective approach; large numbers of such patients can be managed in an outpatient setting.

▶ [We're surprised! Do the results reported here mean that 4 hours per day of rest in the left lateral recumbent position from 28 weeks' gestation would virtually eliminate the subsequent development of preeclampsia? If others, utilizing random assignment of patients to rest and control groups and characterizing the patients as to the development of preeclampsia without knowledge of their assigned group, confirm these findings, then (1) a relatively simple and inexpensive intervention will do much good and (2) the rollover test will have a more important place in antepartum care than we currently think it does.] ◀

3–5 **The Incidence of Pregnancy-Induced Hypertension Is Increased Among Colorado Residents at High Altitude.** Lorna Grindlay Moore, Douglas W. Hershey, Dennis Jahnigen, and Watson Bowes, Jr. noted that both pregnancy-induced hypertension and high-altitude residence are associated with fetal growth retardation. They hypothesized that pregnancy-induced hypertension would be more common at high than at low altitude. They retrospectively collected data on the incidence of this condition in samples of about 150 women at each of three altitudes (1,600 m, 2,410 m, and 3,100 m) in Colorado.

Pregnancy-induced hypertension was more common at 3,100 m (12%) than at 2,410 m (4%) or 1,600 m (3%)($P < .01$). Proteinuria and edema in the upper extremities were also more frequent at 3,100 m than at 1,600 m (proteinuria, 28% vs. 9% [$P < .01$]; edema, 22% vs. 13% [$P < .01$]). Blood pressure during pregnancy increased with altitude among all women and among those without pregnancy-induced hypertension ($P < .05$). In a prospective study at 3,100 m, women with pregnancy-induced hypertension had no significant change in blood pressure during pregnancy prior to the onset of hypertension, whereas blood pressure decreased in the normal women

(3–5) Am. J. Obstet. Gynecol. 144:423–429, Oct. 15, 1982.

($P < .01$). Arterial oxygen saturation during the third trimester was inversely related to the degree of hypertension in women with pregnancy-induced hypertension at 3,100 m ($r = .8$, $P < .05$).

The results suggest that residence at high altitude increases the incidence of pregnancy-induced hypertension and transient hypertension. There was a shift to higher values in the distribution of blood pressures during pregnancy at the higher altitudes. A comparison of factors known to predispose women to hypertension during pregnancy failed to reveal any obvious explanation for this increased incidence. The mechanism responsible for increase in blood pressure during pregnancy at high altitudes is not clear, but appears to operate in an inverse fashion with arterial oxygen saturation in those women in whom pregnancy-induced hypertension develops. Maternal hypoxia may play a previously unsuspected role in pregnancy-induced hypertension.

▶ [This finding that pregnancy hypertension seems to vary directly with altitude is interesting and provocative. Of course, the women (and the people taking care of them) varied between the three Colorado cities, and it is entirely possible that some characteristic(s) other than altitude might be responsible. If other variables could be eliminated, indicating that altitude is the determinant, what might the mechanism be? As one possibility, it has been shown previously that chronic maternal hypoxemia leads to larger placentas, and conditions with "hyperplacentosis" (e.g., multiple pregnancy, molar gestation) seem to predispose to preeclampsia.] ◀

3–6 **Plasma Noradrenaline and Adrenaline Levels in Normal Pregnancy and in Pregnancy-Induced Hypertension.** Women who develop pregnancy-induced hypertension are more sensitive than normotensive pregnant women to various pressor agents, even before hypertension is diagnosed by conventional means, and an increase in sympathetic nervous activity has been proposed, leading to increased vascular reactivity in these women. P. G. Natrajan, H. H. G. McGarrigle, Daphne M. Lawrence, and Gillian C. L. Lachelin (London) monitored plasma catecholamine concentrations during pregnancy in 51 women who remained normotensive and in 9 who developed pregnancy-induced hypertension but were otherwise normal. The latter developed a diastolic pressure of 90 mm Hg or greater after 20 weeks of gestation, whereas the pressure had been less than 90 mm Hg before.

Results were comparable in primigavidas and multigravidas. Norepinephrine and epinephrine concentrations fell significantly during pregnancy in the normal subjects. Mean catecholamine concentrations were lower in the patients with pregnancy-induced hypertension throughout pregnancy. Postnatal values were not significantly different from those found during pregnancy. Uric acid concentrations were higher in the study group in the third trimester. Prolactin concentrations rose significantly in both groups during pregnancy. Catecholamine concentrations did not correlate significantly with blood pressure in either group. Results of the rollover test did not differ significantly in the two groups.

It appears that circulating catecholamine concentrations are not el-

(3–6) Br. J. Obstet. Gynaecol. 89:1041–1045, December 1982.

evated in patients with pregnancy-induced hypertension. The explanation for the increased sensitivity to pressor amines proposed in previous studies must lie elsewhere. The reason for the decline in circulating catecholamine values seen during pregnancy in normal subjects is unclear.

▶ [This longitudinal study suggests that overactivity of the sympathetic nervous system is not involved in the pathogenesis of preeclampsia.] ◀

3–7 **Hemoconcentration in Severe Preeclampsia.** Norvald Sagen, Oddmund Koller, and Kjell Haram (Univ. of Bergen, Bergen, Norway) examined the usefulness of hemoglobin (Hb) determinations in monitoring preeclamptic patients, because high Hb levels per se may indicate fetal growth retardation and impending intrauterine death. The last maternal Hb value before delivery was related to perinatal outcome in 87 nonanemic women, mean age 25, with severe preeclampsia; blood pressure was 160/110 mm Hg or above, and proteinuria of 5 gm/24 hours or more, with or without edema, was present. Most were primigravidas. Management included provision of a protein-rich diet, bed rest, and administration of hydralazine derivatives. Fifty-nine women had cesarean section.

Perinatal distress was diagnosed in 47 instances, and there were 6 perinatal deaths. The mean birth weight was 2,435 gm and the mean gestational age, 36.5 weeks. The weight centile and the maternal Hb value had a significant inverse correlation. Significantly increased Hb values were present in pregnancies with perinatal distress and fetal growth retardation; especially high levels were present in those whose infants died (table). In only 1 of 28 pregnancies with no signs of perinatal pathology was the maternal Hb value more than 2 SD above the mean, whereas 41 of 59 pregnancies complicated by perinatal distress or fetal growth retardation were associated with elevated Hb values. There was only 1 falsely elevated Hb value, but the sensitivity of the determination was less impressive.

LAST MATERNAL HEMOGLOBIN VALUES BEFORE DELIVERY: RELATION TO STATE OF THE NEWBORN

		Haemoglobin (g/dl)		
Perinatal state	*n*	Mean	SD	*P**
Uneventful course	40	12·60	1·11	<0·001
Perinatal distress (perinatal death inc.)	47	13·96	1·19	
Living infant	81	13·21	1·28	<0·001
Perinatal death	6	15·10	0·76	
Weight ⩾10th centile	44	12·60	1·14	<0·001
Weight <10th centile	43	14·09	1·11	

*Student's *t* test (two-tail).

(Courtesy of Sagen, N., et al.: Br. J. Obstet. Gynaecol. 89:802–805, October 1982.)

(3–7) Br. J. Obstet. Gynaecol. 89:802–805, October 1982.

Elevated maternal Hb values were associated with perinatal distress and intrauterine growth retardation in this series of severely preeclamptic women. Whether there is a causal, rather than a merely statistical, relationship between increased maternal Hb values and placental dysfunction remains unclear. Increased blood viscosity from hemoconcentration could lead to increased resistance to blood flow and placental infarct formation that would impair placental capacity and worsen the preeclamptic state. Hemoglobin determination is useful in severe preeclampsia if anemia is absent.

▶ [This observation is certainly not new, but is important. Hemoconcentration in a patient with preeclampsia portends perinatal problems.] ◀

3–8 **Pregnancy Outcome in 211 Patients With Mild Chronic Hypertension.** The appropriate management of pregnancies complicated by chronic hypertension is uncertain. Baha M. Sibai, Thomas N. Abdella, and Garland D. Anderson (Univ. of Tennessee) evaluated a conservative approach to antihypertensive drug therapy in cases of mild chronic hypertension. Drugs were discontinued at the first prenatal visit and reinstituted only if the blood pressure was persistently elevated over 160/110 mm Hg. A total of 211 pregnancies were managed in this way between 1980 and 1982. All patients were seen early in pregnancy and delivered after 20 weeks' gestation. All had blood pressure elevations to at least 140/90 mm Hg before week 20. Most patients had received antihypertensive drugs before pregnancy, and 36 were still taking them when first seen.

The mean gestational age at the first prenatal visit was 14 weeks. The mean creatinine clearance was slightly lower than is reported in normal pregnancies. About half the women had a fall in mean arterial pressure in the second part of pregnancy. Twenty-eight patients (13%) required antihypertensive medication for hypertension in the third trimester. Only 5 of the 36 patients in whom drugs were stopped at the initial visit required treatment in the third trimester. Preeclampsia developed in 10% of the group. Twenty of the 45 cesarean sections were repeat procedures. Antepartum fetal heart rate testing was useful but failed to predict some adverse perinatal outcomes. There were 2 stillbirths and 4 neonatal deaths, for an uncorrected perinatal mortality of 28/1,000 births. All perinatal deaths were of fetuses less than 1,000 gm or less than 29 weeks gestational age. Perinatal mortality in the cases of preeclampsia was 24%. Of the liveborn infants, 11.7% had an Apgar score of 5 or below at 1 minute and 6.1% had a score of 7 or below at 5 minutes.

The routine use of antihypertensive drugs appears to be unnecessary in the management of pregnant women with mild chronic hypertension. In the absence of superimposed preeclampsia, the perinatal mortality approaches that of the general obstetric population.

▶ [The outcome of pregnancy complicated by mild degrees of chronic hypertension is generally quite good unless superimposed preeclampsia develops. This complication developed in 10% of the patients in the series presented here, and this subset had incidences of perinatal death of 24% and intrauterine growth retardation of 21%. Drug therapy of the gravida with "uncomplicated" mild chronic hypertension is controversial, with some studies demonstrating benefit and others not. The present re-

---

(3–8) Obstet. Gynecol. 61:571–576, May 1983.

port describes a generally nihilistic attitude in which any antihypertensive agent is stopped at the enrollment of the patient in antenatal care and not reinstituted unless blood pressure rose to levels above 160/110. There is no control group of chronic hypertensive patients managed another way, but the outcome (uncorrected perinatal mortality rate of 28.1) is quite good and probably could not be improved on by drug therapy. We are also quite conservative about antihypertensive drugs in this condition, although not perhaps as nihilistic as the authors in that we are more likely to leave the patient on a current regimen. Our techniques of maternal and fetal evaluation and surveillance are essentially the same as those described in this article.

For a specific consideration of drug therapy by the same authors, see the following article.] ◀

3–9 **Plasma Volume Findings in Pregnant Women With Mild Hypertension: Therapeutic Considerations.** Plasma volume determination is of potential use in the management of pregnancies complicated by hypertensive disease. Baha M. Sibai, Thomas N. Abdella, Garland D. Anderson, and Preston V. Dilts, Jr. (Univ. of Tennessee) estimated plasma volume changes in 51 pregnant women with mild to moderate chronic hypertension, 11 of whom were being treated with diuretics, at 15–22 weeks' gestation. Diastolic pressures were 90–110 mm Hg. Plasma volumes were determined serially during gestation by the Evans blue dye dilution method. The validity of the single-sample method was reconfirmed in 20 patients with chronic hypertension.

Initial plasma volumes were reduced markedly in the patients taking diuretics. After discontinuance of the diuretic, plasma volume expanded to the level found in the other patients. The mean plasma volume in women not taking diuretics was the same as that in normotensive controls. Two required methyldopa for adequate control of hypertension in the third trimester of pregnancy. Two of the 11 patients previously taking diuretics required methyldopa for control later in pregnancy. Six patients (12%) became preeclamptic in the third trimester. One spontaneous abortion occurred. Four infants were small for gestational age; there was evidence of intrauterine growth retardation in 2 of these pregnancies, and 3 of the mothers had plasma volumes 2 SD below the normal mean for gestation.

Pregnancies complicated by mild to moderate hypertension have outcomes similar to those of normotensive pregnancies. Diuretics cause a marked reduction in plasma volume in these patients, which is reversed on discontinuance of treatment. After discontinuance of diuretics, few patients require other antihypertensive medications during the remainder of the pregnancy. Diuretics should not be given to pregnant patients with mild to moderate chronic hypertension.

▶ [Diuretics aren't helpful in either prevention or therapy of preeclampsia. This report suggests that pregnant women with chronic hypertension shouldn't take them either. The diuretic group had significantly lower plasma volumes when first seen than did those hypertensive pregnant women not taking diuretics. The plasma volumes increased to normal after the diuretics were discontinued.] ◀

3–10 **Serum Uric Acid Levels as an Index of Fetal Prognosis in Pregnancies Complicated by Preexisting Hypertension and Preeclampsia of Pregnancy.** Although hyperuricemia is a charac-

(3–9) Am. J. Obstet. Gynecol. 145:539–544, Mar. 1, 1983.
(3–10) Int. J. Gynaecol. Obstet. 20:401–408, October 1982.

teristic finding in preeclampsia, little is known of the value of serum uric acid determinations in identifying fetuses at risk in pregnancies complicated by hypertension, preeclampsia, or both. Thankam R. Varma (St. George's Hosp. Med. School, London) examined the relation of plasma urate concentration and blood pressure to perinatal mortality in 200 cases of preexisting hypertension and 200 of preeclampsia. A rise in plasma urate concentration was defined as an increase of 60 μmole/L or more from baseline on two or more consecutive occasions and a maximum of at least 330 μmole/L. Normal values were obtained in 50 pregnant patients.

Perinatal mortality was markedly higher when the maternal plasma urate concentration was elevated, generally in association with severe preeclampsia of early onset or superimposed on preexisting hypertension. Maternal hypertension without hyperuricemia, even if severe, was not associated with a poor prognosis for the fetus. Where hyperuricemia was present, the fetal prognosis was poor regardless of the blood pressure. Perinatal mortality was higher in cases of preeclampsia than in those of preexisting hypertension. One fifth of the patients with preexisting hypertension had moderately severe hypertension. Superimposed preeclampsia was present in 45% of this group.

The serum urate concentration appears to be a reliable index of fetal welfare when pregnancy is complicated by preexisting hypertension, preeclampsia, or both. An increased urate concentration helps distinguish preeclampsia from essential and other chronic forms of preexisting hypertension complicating pregnancy. In cases of moderately severe preexisting hypertension and preeclampsia, the urate concentration is significantly increased, and the rates of intrauterine growth retardation, fetal distress in labor, and perinatal death are increased. Patients with mild preeclampsia have a better fetal outcome than those with moderately severe involvement, but the fetal outcome is unsatisfactory when preeclampsia is associated with high or increasing urate concentrations.

▶ [It long has been appreciated that preeclampsia is accompanied by a tendency to hyperuricemia, and attention has been redirected in recent years to this sign as an index of fetal status in pregnancies complicated by hypertension (see 1977 YEAR BOOK, p. 28). The authors of this report, noting a correlation between high serum uric acid levels and adverse fetal outcome (morbidity, mortality, and impaired growth), conclude that uric acid is a useful prognostic test. We don't disagree, but we regard it simply as a "marker" of preeclampsia, and thus a correlation with fetal outcome simply reflects the fact that the fetus does less well with preeclampsia than with chronic hypertension and with severe as opposed to mild preeclampsia.] ◀

3–11 **Use of Glucocorticoids in Pregnancies Complicated by Severe Hypertension and Proteinuria.** In 1972, Liggins and Howie advised against the use of prophylactic glucocorticoid therapy for the prevention of idiopathic respiratory distress syndrome in pregnancies complicated by hypertension and proteinuria. R. F. Lamont, P. D. M. Dunlop, M. I. Levene, and M. G. Elder (Hammersmith Hosp., London) reviewed the outcome of a change in policy in the administration of

---

(3–11) Br. J. Obstet. Gynaecol. 90:199–202, March 1983.

antepartum glucocorticoids in 53 pregnancies complicated by severe hypertension and proteinuria during a 2-year period. In the first part of the study, 32 infants of less than 34 weeks gestational age were delivered to mothers who did not receive antepartum glucocorticoids. In the second part, 24 infants of less than 34 weeks gestational age were delivered to mothers who did receive antepartum glucocorticoids.

There were no marked differences in the severity of maternal disease, gestational age at delivery, birth weight, and obstetric management between groups. Overall, the incidence of idiopathic respiratory distress syndrome (IRDS) was similar in treated and untreated groups. However, the incidence of IRDS was considerably less in the treated group delivered at 30–33 weeks. The incidence of intraventricular hemorrhage was also lower in the treated group, especially in those delivered at 26–29 weeks. In the group receiving glucocorticoids, 88% of the infants were alive at the time of discharge from the neonatal unit, compared with 72% of the infants in the group not treated ante partum. There was no evidence that glucocorticoid therapy had any adverse effects on the mothers' condition or on fetal outcome.

It is concluded that the antepartum administration of glucocorticoids to the mother does not pose an increased risk to the fetus and may reduce the risk of IRDS and subsequent intraventricular hemorrhage in pregnancies complicated by severe hypertension and proteinuria requiring delivery before completion of 34 weeks of pregnancy.

▶ [In their important article that started it all (*Pediatrics* 50:515–525, 1972), Liggins and Howie cautioned against the use of antepartum steroids for fetal lung maturation in patients with preeclampsia, because they observed an excess of fetal deaths in steroid-treated patients with this complication. Not so, according to this retrospective study. We view severe preeclampsia as an indication to effect delivery. The inherent delay associated with antepartum steroid therapy may not be in the best interests of the fetus.

Use of corticosteroids for lung maturation remains controversial in the United States. "Users" apparently need no longer regard hypertension as an absolute contraindication.] ◀

3–12 **Effects of Maternally Administered Magnesium Sulfate on the Neonate.** Parenteral magnesium sulfate is used widely in the United States to treat pregnancy-induced hypertension. It effectively prevents seizures and has a wide margin of safety for the mother and fetus. Karen W. Green, Thomas C. Key, Ronald Coen, and Robert Resnik (Univ. of California at San Diego) examined the effects of intravenous magnesium sulfate on maternal and neonatal calcium and magnesium homeostasis because of reports of neonatal depression in infants of treated mothers. The series included 24 women with pregnancies at 37–43 weeks. Sixteen had pregnancy-induced hypertension requiring magnesium therapy. A dose of 4 gm of magnesium sulfate was given intravenously over 20 minutes, followed by 1 gm/hour by infusion. Control patients received saline or Ringer's lactate intravenously during labor.

(3–12) Am. J. Obstet. Gynecol. 146:29–33, May 1, 1983.

Magnesium levels rose from 1.6 mg/dl to 3.6 mg/dl in treated patients. Maternal calcium levels were lower at delivery in both groups, but the reduction was greater in the magnesium-treated group (14.5% vs. 3.1%). There were no group differences in birth weights, Apgar scores, or respiratory rates. Umbilical cord blood magnesium levels were increased in study infants, but calcium levels were similar in the two groups. Neurologic status also was comparable in the two groups of infants, although the tone of the neck extensors was reduced in study infants on the first day of life.

No adverse effects of magnesium of newborn infants were found in this study when infusions of 1 gm/hour followed a 4-gm loading dose in the treatment of pregnancy-induced hypertension. Infant depression in this setting may be a result of asphyxia or prematurity. The effects of larger amounts of magnesium, currently recommended to produce therapeutic magnesium levels in the mother, require further study.

▶ [This careful study confirms the vast clinical experience that magnesium sulfate therapy is very well tolerated by the newborn. The findings are similar to those of a study presented in the 1982 YEAR BOOK (p. 90).] ◀

3–13 **Magnesium Deficiency-Induced Spasms of Umbilical Vessels: Relation to Preeclampsia, Hypertension, and Growth Retardation.** The pathophysiology of preeclampsia remains unclear, but hypomagnesemia has been observed, and decreased magnesium and increased calcium ion have been described in placentas from women with preeclampsia or eclampsia. Burton M. Altura, Bella T. Altura, and Anthony Carella (SUNY, Downstate Med. Center) attempted to determine whether spasm of the umbilical vessels can be produced by magnesium deficiency. The effects of sudden withdrawal of Mg^{2+} and hypermagnesemia (2.4–9.6 mM) on vascular tone and vasoactive drug-induced responses in umbilical arteries and veins taken from cords of 34 pregnant women at term spontaneous delivery were studied.

Sudden withdrawal of extracellular Mg^{2+} resulted in a rapid increase in tension in the umbilical arteries and veins in 30 of 34 cases. Sudden increases in Mg^{2+} led to a concentration-dependent relaxation in all vessels tested. Withdrawal of Mg^{2+} potentiated the constrictor effects of bradykinin, serotonin, angiotensin II, and prostaglandin F_2. Increased Mg^{2+} suppressed the constrictor actions of bradykinin, PGF_2, and angiotensin II and decreased that of serotonin.

Effects of extracellular Mg^{2+} concentration on vascular tone appear to reflect its influence on membrane permeability of Ca^{2+}, binding, and translocation and membrane stability. Progressive hypomagnesemia in pregnancy can lead to progressive vasoconstriction and spasms of umbilical and placental vessels and other peripheral vessels in the pregnant mother and fetus. An adequate magnesium ion intake can prevent these events. The findings help explain the high infant mortality in regions with soft drinking water and soil lacking Mg^{2+} as well as the favorable effects of magnesium sulfate in pre-

---

(3–13) Science 221:376–378, July 22, 1983.

eclampsia. The familial tendency to develop preeclampsia and eclampsia is consistent with the present findings, because the level of Mg^{2+} in some tissues is under genetic control.

▶ [In this in vitro study, there was an inverse correlation between the magnesium level and the reactivity of the umbilical vessels. Theoretically, this might explain why magnesium sulfate is of clinical value in preeclampsia. However, clinicians know that magnesium sulfate treatment generally has little effect on the blood pressure level itself.] ◀

3–14 **Results of a Management Protocol for Premature Rupture of the Membranes.** Richard L. Berkowitz, E. Laurence Hoder, Richard M. Freedman, David T. Scott, and Mark C. Maltzer (Yale Univ.) report the results of a management protocol for women with premature rupture of the membranes (PROM) between 27 and 36 weeks' gestation. Prior to 33 weeks' gestation, patients were hospitalized and observed for signs of infection; labor was induced if amnionitis was diagnosed. After 33 weeks' gestation, patients with vertex presentations underwent elective induction of labor after 16 hours of PROM. Amniocentesis was not performed, corticosteroids were not administered, and tocolysis was not used.

A total of 58 patients delivered neonates between 33 and 36 weeks' gestation. Fourteen (24%) of these were delivered with PROM of less than 16 hours (group 1). In this subset there were 5 cesarean sections, 3 inductions, and 6 cases of rapid premature labor. Three women (21.5%) had amnionitis. All 14 neonates in group 1 survived; 3 had moderate respiratory distress syndrome (RDS).

Forty-four patients delivered between 33 and 36 weeks' gestation with PROM of longer than 16 hours. In this subset there were 10 cesarean sections and 34 vaginal deliveries (group 2). The only neonatal death in group 2 occurred 48 hours after vaginal delivery at 34 weeks; severe intracranial hemorrhage and moderate RDS were present in the infant. The 1 case of amnionitis (2.3%) in group 2 was not associated with fetal sepsis.

A total of 50 patients delivered neonates between 27 and 33 weeks' gestation. Nine delivered with PROM of less than 16 hours, including 2 cesarean sections, 2 inductions, and 5 cases of premature labor (group 3).

Forty-one neonates were delivered between 27 and 33 weeks' gestation after PROM of more than 16 hours (group 4), including 13 cesarean sections, 5 inductions, and 23 cases of vaginal delivery after premature labor. One neonate in group 4 died; severe RDS and intracranial hemorrhage were present. There were 9 cases of amnionitis in this group (21.9%).

The overall perinatal mortality was only 2.8% for this study population, and 2 of the 3 deaths occurred in infants delivered at 27 and 28 weeks' gestation, respectively. These data suggest that elective induction after 16 hours of PROM beyond 33 weeks' gestation is extremely unlikely to result in delivery of a neonate with severe RDS. If conducted properly, a policy of elective induction will not necessarily increase the incidence of operative deliveries. Documented fetal

(3–14) Obstet. Gynecol. 60:271–276, September 1982.

sepsis was infrequent and was not usually a source of fetal morbidity and mortality.

▶ [The approach used here in managing premature rupture of the membranes was a fairly aggressive one—induction at 33 weeks' gestation or beyond. The authors conlude, "The results in the present series are remarkably good . . ." but we're not so sure. There were 58 patients in the group with gestations at 33–36 weeks, some of whom surely would have been delivered with any management protocol because of spontaneous labor, cord prolapse, amnionitis, and similar indications. Thus, the occurrence of *only 1* neonatal death due to prematurity and its complications in something less than 50 patients induced more-or-less electively is not to be dismissed lightly. Moreover, the article gives no indication of neonatal morbidity, as opposed to mortality, and prematurity-associated conditions such as hyperbilirubinemia, hypoglycemia, hypocalcemia, and feeding difficulties must have occurred as a result of preterm birth. Finally, the cesarean section rate of nearly 25% merits comment. The article states that only a small proportion of cesarean sections "might possibly have been avoided if induction had not been part of the protocol." However, we find it hard to agree with this judgment when the reasons for cesarean delivery included breech, repeat cesarean section, and fetal distress during induction.] ◀

3–15 **Maternal and Fetal Serum Prolactin Levels in Cases of Premature Rupture of Membranes.** Premature rupture of the fetal membranes (PROM) is a major cause of prematurity and therefore of fetal morbidity and mortality. The cause of PROM is unknown in most cases. High prolactin concentrations have been demonstrated in amniotic fluid and in chorion-decidua. M. Ron, U. Beller, J. Ori, M. Ben-David, and Z. Palti (Jerusalem) determined fetal and maternal serum prolactin concentrations in 20 first pregnancies with PROM admitted at 36 to 40 weeks. Premature rupture was defined as rupture of the fetal membranes at least 2 hours before the onset of contractions. All pregnancies and births were normal. Twenty first normal births without PROM were matched for gestational and maternal ages with the study cases.

Maternal prolactin concentrations, as measured by radioimmunoassay, were significantly lower in cases of PROM than in controls. Fetal serum prolactin concentrations were in the same range in PROM and control cases. The ratio of fetal to maternal prolactin concentrations was significantly higher in the cases of PROM.

Fetal and maternal prolactin concentrations are influenced by the same stimuli, but they are regulated independently. Prolactin is involved in osmotic and electrolyte regulation in the fetal compartment. A prolactin-induced shift in electrolyte balance may cause a change in the viscoelastic properties of the amniotic membrane that leads to PROM. Further studies should determine prolactin concentrations in the amniotic fluid, decidua, and membranes.

▶ [The authors of this report speculate that the observed increase in the ratio of fetal to maternal prolactin concentrations in patients with premature rupture of the membranes compared with controls might affect water and electrolyte movement through the membranes, altering their viscoelastic properties and predisposing them to rupture. This is an interesting thought, but much more study is needed. Is the etiology of membrane rupture at term the same as that in the preterm situation, or are these two separate entities?] ◀

(3–15) Acta Obstet. Gynecol. Scand. 62:37–38, 1983.

3-16 ***Bacteroides Fragilis, Streptococus intermedius,* and Group B Streptococci in Ascending Infection of Pregnancy: An Animal Experimental Study.** Infectious complications of mother and fetus associated with premature rupture of the membranes (PROM) previously have been believed to be secondary to PROM. However, there have been several reports of chorioamnionitis occurring despite unruptured membranes, and it has been suggested that some instances of PROM are preceded by occult intrauterine infection. G. Evaldson, A.-S. Malmborg, C. E. Nord, and K. Östensson used bacteriologic, histologic, and immunofluorescence methods to study the ascending spread of endocervically inoculated bacteria in 14 pregnant sheep. Eight ewes near term were exposed for 2 to 4 days to group B streptococci, *B. fragilis,* or *S. intermedius,* while the 6 other ewes, which were in midpregnancy, were exposed to one of the three bacteria for 30 days. Aerobic and anaerobic culture specimens were obtained from the cervix and amniotic fluid before inoculation. In addition to culture specimens, membrane and placental tissues were collected at the time of delivery by cesarean section.

Among the 3 near-term ewes inoculated with *B. fragilis,* all showed significant microbial infiltration of the membranes in specimens obtained near the internal cervical os, although only occasional bacteria could be found in the proximal samples in 2 ewes. Bacterial scores were significant in 1 of the 3 corresponding placentas. Both ewes with longtime exposure to *B. fragilis* showed significant bacterial invasion of both membranes and placentas. All 3 near-term and both midpregnancy ewes inoculated with *S. intermedius* exhibited significant invasion of the membranes, with no difference in bacterial scores between distal and proximal membrane specimens. The near-term animals showed heavy placental infiltration of *S. intermedius* in 2 of the 3 cases, whereas the 2 placentas of ewes inoculated at midpregnancy showed only occasional bacteria. All 4 animals inoculated with group B streptococci, 2 near-term and 2 midpregnancy ewes, exhibited significant bacterial invasion of the membranes, with no obvious difference between proximal and distal specimens. Significant bacterial infiltration of placental tissue was seen in 2 of these cases. In the entire study, the ascending infection was arrested within the membranes and placental structure, except in 1 ewe, inoculated with *S. intermedius,* in which the ascending infection was found to have reached the amniotic fluid.

The results confirm the hypothesis that endocervical bacteria in the indigenous microflora may produce ascending infection in pregnancy, reaching all levels of the birth canal and spreading to the products of conception. As *B. fragilis, S. intermedius,* and group B streptococci have been implicated in PROM, the findings of this study suggest an etiologic role of ascending infection in this complication of pregnancy.

▶ [This sheep study adds support to the contemporary view that ascending infection of the membranes (in one case involving the amniotic fluid) can occur in the absence

---

(3–16) Gynecol. Obstet. Invest. 15:230–241, April 1983.

of membrane rupture. In certain cases of threatened premature labor and PROM, bacterial infection is probably of etiologic importance, rather than a secondary phenomenon.] ◀

3–17 **Antepartum Prediction of Postmature Infant.** William F. Rayburn, Mary E. Motley, Laurence E. Stempel, and R. Michael Gendreau (Ohio State Univ.) conducted a prospective study of 147 strictly defined postdate (42 weeks or more) pregnancies to determine whether present antepartum methods of fetal assessment are useful in predicting postmaturity.

Spontaneous labor occurred in 123 of the 147 women (87%), and the average patient delivered at 43 weeks' gestation (range, 42 to 47 weeks). Incidence of postmaturity in the infants was 22% (32 of 147).

No condition in the obstetric history (including prior postdate pregnancy) or on clinical examination (including presence or absence of oligohydramnios, cervical dilation, or hypertension) was reliable in screening for postmaturity. All fetuses were active. Although the 3 fetal heart rate tests with abnormal results (nonreactive nonstress test followed by a suspicious or positive contraction stress test) involved postmature fetuses, this technique was not predictive of postmaturity in the remaining 29 affected infants. Fetal movement charting was not useful.

In 65 pregnancies, the single-voiding estrogen-creatinine (E-C) ratio was determined within 1 week before delivery. Mean ratio was 17 in women delivering a postmature infant and 28 in those delivering a term-appearing infant. Mean E-C ratio for all postdate pregnancies was 26. All the 12 women with an E-C ratio below 19 delivered a postmature infant. A normal E-C ratio was predictive of nonpostmaturity in 50 of 53 cases (94%).

Visible evidence of oligohydramnios on real-time ultrasound scanning was a sensitive indicator of postmaturity in 24 of 29 cases. Conversely, the presence of pockets or an adequate volume of amniotic fluid was very predictive of nonpostmaturity (110 of 118, 93%). The placenta was not clearly visible for grading purposes in 70 of 147 cases (48%).

In the expectant management of postdate pregnancies, urine E-C ratios should be monitored routinely to screen for fetal postmaturity. Real-time ultrasound studies also should be performed routinely to search for oligohydramnios. Any abnormal finding is an indication for delivery with optimal fetal monitoring and precautions against meconium aspiration.

▶ [Infants with the stigmas of postmaturity not surprisingly fared less well in labor than did "term-appearing" postdate infants. Oligohydramnios on ultrasound examination frequently was identified in the postmature pregnancies. Although estriol determinations have taken a backseat to antepartum heart rate testing for the past several years, this report suggests that low estriol values are helpful in predicting postmaturity. On our service, patients with favorable cervices are induced at 42 weeks' gestation. If the cervix is unfavorable, we institute fetal surveillance with both estriol determinations and fetal heart rate testing.] ◀

(3–17) Obstet. Gynecol. 60:148–153, August 1982.

3–18 **Management of Postterm Pregnancy in a Large Obstetric Population.** Sze-Ya Yeh and John A. Read (Univ. of Southern California, Los Angeles) describe the management protocol used in a clinic for patients with postterm pregnancy and the results of the protocol after 1 year. A practical management protocol to handle the large volume of postterm gestations at Los Angeles County-University of Southern California Medical Center was introduced and evaluated in 880 patients between March 1, 1979, and February 29, 1980. The protocol placed patients into two groups based on substantiated "good" or unsubstantiated "poor" obstetric dates. After clinical examinations, the primary screening test used was twice-weekly plasma unconjugated estriol (E_3) determinations. Antepartum testing of fetal heart rate in the form of nonstress tests was used initially in the group with good obstetric dates, and was subsequently done twice weekly only if the E_3 value was abnormal (less than 18 ng/ml in patients with good obstetric dates and less than 12 ng/ml in patients with poor obstetric dates).

Patients with good obstetric dates were delivered electively at more than 42 weeks' gestation if the cervix was favorable (Bishop score 9 or greater); otherwise, intervention occurred only in patients with abnormal test findings and a positive or suspicious contraction stress test, or with other medical indications. Only 8 perinatal losses (3 neonatal deaths and 5 stillbirths) occurred in 880 patients. Each of these patients received a follow-up examination; 3 had infants with severe congenital anomalies, and 5 deaths occurred in patients who did not comply with the protocol. Rate of cesarean section was 15.8%. A large number of macrosomic infants were observed in this study. There were 317 cases (36.7%) in which passage of meconium was noticed before or during labor, and 55 cases (6.3%) in which fetal distress was diagnosed clinically during labor. Postmaturity syndrome (dysmaturity in postterm gestation) occurred in 106 neonates (12.0%). When patients were grouped according to outcome of antepartum testing, a statistically higher incidence of fetal distress and low 1-minute Apgar scores occurred in the group with abnormal test results than in the group with normal test results.

Careful adherence to a well-defined protocol is a key factor in reduction of perinatal morbidity and mortality in postterm gestations. In the management of a large obstetric population, this protocol combines practical considerations with a sound testing plan, which emphasizes close observation, selective intervention, and intensification of antepartum and intrapartum surveillance when results of one or more tests are abnormal.

▶ [The primary screening tool used in this large series of postdate pregnancies at Los Angeles County Hospital was plasma unconjugated estriol measurement twice weekly. Only when the estriol concentration was low was heart rate monitoring involved. This approach is consistent with the findings of a report abstracted in the 1983 YEAR BOOK (pp. 34–35) in which urinary estrogen assays seemed more sensitive than cardiotocography in postdate pregnancy. In any event, it must be acknowledged that the rate of perinatal mortality in this study (9/1,000 overall, corrected for malformations to 7/1,000) is excellent.] ◀

(3–18) Obstet. Gynecol. 60:282–287, September 1982.

3–19 **Association Between Rates of Premature Delivery and Intrauterine Growth Retardation.** Because mothers of growth-retarded infants and those of prematurely born infants have some features in common and there are increased risks of congenital malformation and intellectual impairment in both groups of infants, these two states possibly may have a common cause. P. S. Spiers and S. Wacholder (Univ. of Washington) undertook to determine whether the proportions of premature infants and infants with intrauterine growth retardation in a given population are correlated. All live births occurring in Washington and North Carolina between 1968 and 1977 and between 1970 and 1974, respectively, were reviewed. A positive association was found in white births between the percentages of premature delivery and infants weighing less than 2,500 gm at birth. The lack of such correlation in blacks might be due to some fraction of small-at-term black infants being related to maternal age and gravidity in a different way from the rest.

It appears that a real correlation exists between the rates of premature delivery and growth retardation. Postnatal experience is a possible explanation for the increased risk of intellectual impairment in premature infants, but it cannot explain their increased risk of certain congenital malformations. If growth retardation increases the risk of congenital malformation, the association of premature delivery with both congenital and malformations and intellectual impairment could be explained by an increased likelihood for premature infants to experience growth retardation during early gestation. This hypothesis could be tested by studying mothers with a previous premature delivery and comparing the early growth characteristics of fetuses that are born prematurely with those of fetuses who go to term.

► [This study notes a significant correlation between preterm birth and fetal growth retardation, a not altogether unexpected finding in view of a number of common causes (e.g., fetal malformation and maternal hypertension, smoking, and malnutrition). The data base was birth certificates, and there is always some concern about the reliability of gestational age records from this source. Nevertheless, the high correlation coefficients (0.7 to 0.8) provide confidence in the relationship. Clinically, this means that a woman who experiences one complication is at increased risk for both in a subsequent pregnancy.] ◄

3–20 **Uteroplacental Blood Flow Index in Intrauterine Growth Retardation of Fetal or Maternal Origin.** L. Nylund, N.-O. Lunell, R. Lewander, and B. Sarby (Karolinska Inst., Stockholm) evaluated the maternal placental circulation in 56 women in the last trimester who were hospitalized because of complications of pregnancy, e.g., suspected fetal growth retardation or vaginal bleeding. Fetal growth retardation was diagnosed in 30 instances because of a birth weight below the tenth centile for sex and gestational age. Eleven of these women had preeclampsia. Six infants in the growth-retarded group were born with malformations. The uteroplacental blood flow index was calculated from the isotope accumulation curve after injection of 1 mCi of ^{113m}In-chloride. Counts were registered by a computer-linked

---

(3–19) Dev. Med. Child. Neurol. 24:808–816, December 1982.
(3–20) Br. J. Obstet. Gynaecol. 90:16–20, January 1983.

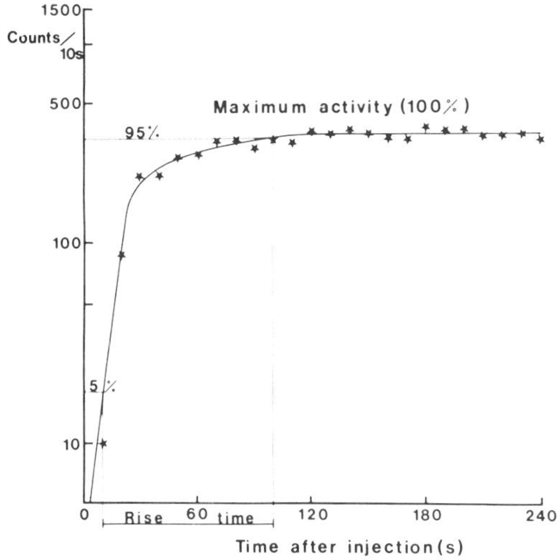

Fig 3–3.—Time-activity curve registered over placenta after intravenous injection of 1 mCi of ^{113m}In-chloride. (Courtesy of Nylund, L., et al.: Br. J. Obstet. Gynaecol. 90:16–20, January 1983.)

camera placed above the placenta for 10-second intervals over a 4-minute period. The method is illustrated in Figure 3–3.

The results are shown in the table. The median uteroplacental blood flow index was reduced by more than half in the group with intrauterine growth retardation. All patients in this group had a reduced index. Median placental weight was reduced significantly in the subgroup with fetal malformations, but no other differences were apparent. Even in the absence of preeclampsia the flow index was lower in growth-retarded pregnancies.

Overall, in this series, uteroplacental blood flow was reduced by more than 50% in women with intrauterine growth retardation, compared with findings in controls. The flow index was as low in women delivering infants with congenital malformations as in those with fetal growth retardation caused by maternal factors. Maternal placental blood flow may be regulated in part by the fetus. Changes in the

Uteroplacental Blood Flow Indices in Normal and Growth-Retarded Pregancies (IUGR)

		IUGR group	
	Control group	No malformation	With malformation
n	26	24	6
Rise time (s)	50(20–84)	65(30–185)**	85(30–105) NS
Maximum activity (counts/10s)	890(420–1540)	645(360–1350)**	864(204–1125) NS
Blood flow index (proportional to ml/s)	19·0(7·4–51·3)	8·3(2·1–21·4)***	9·0(4·1–37·5)*

Results are given as median (range).

Significance of difference: *$P < .05$; **$P < .01$; ***$P < .001$; NS, not significant (Mann-Whitney *U* test, comparison with controls).

(Courtesy of Nylund, L., et al.: Br. J. Obstet. Gynaecol. 90:16–20, January 1983.)

spiral arteries of the placental bed have been described in women with fetal growth retardation, even in the absence of hypertension.

▶ [Most intrauterine growth retardation is thought to be secondary to impaired uteroplacental blood flow. At times there is a primary placental cause (large infarct) or an intrinsic fetal cause (anomaly, often chromosomal, or chronic infection). One might have predicted normal blood flow indices in anomalous growth-retarded fetuses, i.e., the fetal problem might explain the growth retardation without the need to implicate diminished blood flow. Not so, in this small series. The decreased uteroplacental blood flow is probably a secondary phenomenon in these cases. This suggests that the fetus partly may regulate maternal blood flow to the placenta. Placental size is one possible mechanism.] ◀

3–21 **Use of Amniotic Fluid 3-Methyl Histidine to Creatinine Molar Ratio For Diagnosis of Intrauterine Growth Retardation.** Menachem Miodovnik, Justin P. Lavin, Zvi Gimmon, Jan Hill, Josef E. Fischer, and Tom P. Barden (Univ. of Cincinnati) observed that intrauterine growth retardation (IUGR) complicates 3%–7% of pregnancies in the United States and Canada. In extrauterine life, metabolic stress is characterized by breakdown of muscle protein, which produces amino acids for gluconeogenesis. Muscle contractile protein is unique among proteins because it has a methylated histidine component. Proteolysis of myosin results in release of 3-methyl histidine. In extrauterine life, the urinary 3-methyl histidine to creatinine molar ratio (3MH:CR) can indicate the degree of muscle protein breakdown in nutritionally deprived states. The 3MH:CR in amniotic fluid could serve as a diagnostic technique to identify IUGR.

Three groups of human amniotic fluid were studied. Group A consisted of amniotic fluids from pregnancies yielding IUGR fetuses whose birth weight was less than or equal to the 10th percentile for gestational age; group B consisted of fluid from pregnancies resulting in infants whose birth weight was greater than the 10th, but less than or equal to the 25th, percentile for gestational age; group C consisted of fluids from pregnancies resulting in infants whose birth weights were greater than the 25th percentile but less than or equal to the 75th percentile for gestational age. The mean 3MH:CR $\times 10^{-3}$ for groups A, B, and C, were 15.9 ± 1.9, 5.4 ± 0.8, and 6.2 ± 0.5, respectively. The mean 3MH:CR $\times 10^{-3}$ was statistically different between groups A and B and between groups A and C, but not statistically different between the two control groups. With use of the higher limit of the normal ratio of 8 for the 3MH:CR $\times 10^{-3}$, 13 of 15 neonates with IUGR were correctly identified, and 23 of 27 neonates were correctly identified as being of normal birth weight for gestation age (sensitivity, 86.7%; specificity, 85.2%; incidence of correct diagnosis, 85.7%). No consistent relationship was shown to exist between maternal serum and amniotic fluid levels of 3-methyl histidine. No statistically significant relationship was found between 3MH:CR $\times 10^{-3}$ and gestational age.

Amniotic fluid 3MH:CR ratio may prove helpful in establishing the antenatal diagnosis of IUGR, particularly in cases with uncertain gestational age.

(3–21) Obstet. Gynecol. 60:288–293, September 1982.

▶ [These results suggest that measurement of 3-methyl histidine (expressed as the creatinine molar ratio) may identify fetuses at risk for growth retardation. In 15 cases in which infant weight was below the 10th percentile for gestational age, amniotic fluid 3MH:CR values were significantly higher than with normally grown fetuses. The amino acid 3-methyl histidine comes from breakdown of muscle and is not reused in protein synthesis. Thus, it is not unexpected that high amniotic fluid levels would occur in conjunction with conditions (such as hypertensive vascular disease) that potentially limit provision of substrates to the fetus.] ◀

3–22 **Decreased Prostacyclin Production by Placental Cells in Culture From Pregnancies Complicated by Fetal Growth Retardation.** Reduced production of prostacyclin (PGI_2), a potent platelet antiaggregatory prostanoid, by maternal, fetal, or placental tissue may be a factor in the development of pregnancy-induced hypertension, with or without fetal growth retardation. M. Jogee, L. Myatt, and M. G. Elder (Hammersmith Hosp., London) compared PGI_2 production in placental cell cultures from human pregnancies complicated by fetal growth retardation with that in placental cultures from normal pregnancies of either matched gestation or at term.

Production of the metabolites 6-oxo-$PGF_{1\alpha}$ and 13,14-dihydro-6,15-dioxo-$PGF_{1\alpha}$ by placental cells from pregnancies complicated by fetal growth retardation was significantly lower than that by placental cells from normal pregnancies ($P < .001$). The addition of estradiol and progesterone, either alone or in combination, to cell cultures from pregnancies with fetal growth retardation produced significant increases in 6-oxo-$PGF_{1\alpha}$ over a 24-hour period ($P < .05$ to $P < .005$). These increases were similar to those observed in first-trimester placental cells when these steroids were added to cell cultures, but were surprisingly different from the effects in normal term placental cells, where progesterone alone exerted a slight, but significant, inhibitory effect and was antiestrogenic when added in combination with estradiol.

The finding that the cellular response to estrogen and progesterone of cells from pregnancies complicated by fetal growth retardation was similar to that of first-trimester placental cells implies that reduced PGI_2 production is not an irreversible change as a result of placental ischemia. It is concluded that decreased PGI_2 production by cells of trophoblastic origin may be an etiologic factor in thrombotic occlusion of the uteroplacental circulation, which impairs fetal growth.

▶ [The observed decreased placental production of the antiaggregatory and vasodilatory prostacyclin might be only an effect of, rather than a cause of, intrauterine growth retardation. The authors speculate on a causal role. Lower prostacyclin concentrations might result in increased platelet deposition within the uteroplacental circulation and diminished perfusion on that basis. Readers may recall that platelet lifespan reportedly is decreased in cases of fetal growth retardation (1981 YEAR BOOK, pp. 95–97).] ◀

3–23 **Anti-D Antibodies in D- and D^u-Positive Women: A Cause of Hemolytic Disease of the Newborn** is discussed by Charles A. White, Charles M. Stedman, and Sally Frank (New Orleans). The recent decline in Rh-induced hemolytic disease of the newborn should

---

(3–22) Br. J. Obstet. Gynaecol. 90:247–250, March 1983.
(3–23) Am. J. Obstet. Gynecol. 145:1069–1075, Apr. 15, 1983.

not lead to a complacent attitude. The persistence of other causative antigens makes it necessary for all obstetric patients to have antenatal antibody screening tests, regardless of their blood type. The relative incidence of hemolytic disease caused by sensitization to such irregular antibodies as Kell, Kidd, and Duffy is increasing. Five women had D-positive or D^u-positive blood and antenatal anti-D sensitization and neonates with hemolytic disease of varying severity. One infant had hydrocephalus secondary to intracranial hemorrhage.

Bloods that are D-positive and D^u-positive with anti-D lack part of the D mosaic and are considered to be "D variants," yet routinely are typed as Rh-positive. The anti-D antibody produced by D-positive and D^u-positive blood is indistinguishable from the ordinary variety of anti-D antibody. Anti-D hemolytic disease of the newborn in 12 infants born to D-positive women has been reported previously. There is some evidence supporting the administration of Rh immune globulin postpartum to all mothers with D^u blood who deliver infants with D-positive blood. The rarity with which they may become sensitized, however, negates the cost-benefit effectiveness of this approach. Nevertheless, women with D^u-positive blood should be screened throughout pregnancy with the same diligence as those with D-negative blood are screened.

▶ [This article calls attention to an unusual but potentially important situation in which a D- or D^u-positive individual has a genetic form of the antigen that is different enough to lead to antibody production when exposed to "normal" D or D^u. Thus, such a woman would test Rh-positive but could become sensitized and have an erythroblastotic fetus.] ◀

3–24 **Promethazine Hydrochloride Therapy in Severely Rh-Sensitized Pregnancies.** Allan G. Charles and Lewis S. Blumenthal (Chicago) treated 17 severely Rh-sensitized women with promethazine hydrochloride (Phenergan) in 18 pregnancies according to a protocol described by Gusdon et al. Severe Rh-sensitization was defined as presence of antibody titers high enough to cause fetal death and a history of fetal or neonatal loss or hemolytic disease of the newborn due to Rh-sensitization. A starting dose of 150 mg of promethazine hydrochloride per day was increased by 25 mg each day until a dose of 300 mg per day was reached. This dosage was maintained until intrauterine transfusion or until delivery.

Seventeen of 19 infants delivered were live born; 2 were stillborn. One died after a third intrauterine transfusion and the other had anomalies incompatible with life. Five infants were Rh-negative. In retrospect, promethazine therapy was unnecessary in 4 of these cases. Twelve live-born Rh-positive infants were treated with promethazine. After a comparison with past obstetric history, it is believed that such treatment produced a significant amelioration of the disease process in 10 of the 12.

Although dosages of promethazine used in this study were lower than those used by Gusdon, the present authors recommend its use for severely Rh-sensitized pregnancies in which there is significant risk of fetal loss. As with all drugs used during pregnancy, the au-

---

(3–24) Obstet. Gynecol. 60:627–630, November 1982.

thors recommend continued studies of the long-term effects of promethazine on surviving infants, because there is significant concern about the possibility of a global effect on the fetal immune system that may involve more than impaired phagocytosis.

▶ [This article was abstracted to remind the readership that promethazine hydrochloride is being used on an experimental basis in an attempt to ameliorate the effects of Rh sensitization. Although promethazine does have an effect on leukocyte function and phagocytosis, this enthusiastic report should be placed in perspective. "Severe sensitization" was defined on the basis of antibody titer. This is imprecise at best. There is no control group and treatment was not randomly assigned. Indeed, five infants were Rh-negative. There may be something to promethazine treatment, but better designed trials are needed before this sort of therapy is widely adopted.] ◀

3–25 **Intrauterine Fetal Transfusions: Winnipeg 1982.** John M. Bowman and Frank A. Manning (Winnipeg, Man.) reviewed trends in perinatal survival after fetal transfusion in Winnipeg since 1966. Survival in 21 cases in 1978–1980 was 52%, compared with 70% in 113 cases of transfusion in the preceding 12 years. The difference was attributed to narrowing of the side hole opening diameters of the epidural transfusion catheter, causing donor red blood cell hemolysis and hydrops fetalis. Catheter-induced hemolysis was directly responsible for 3 perinatal deaths and probably contributed to 2 others. Indications for intrauterine transfusion were unchanged, as was the transfusion volume formula. Catheter-induced red blood cell hemolysis was completely prevented by removing the catheter tip and side hole openings, and permitting red blood cell egress through the open end of the catheter. All but 2 of 24 infants given transfusions in 1980–1982 survived (table). Six of 8 hydropic fetuses given transfusions in this period survived.

Highly satisfactory perinatal salvage can be obtained after intrauterine red blood cell transfusion therapy with meticulous prenatal care, amniotic fluid transmittance measurements starting at 20.5

Intrauterine Fetal Transfusions (IUT), Intervals 1 and 2

	1 February 1978– June 1980	2 July 1980– June 1982
Gestation at first IUT—mean (range) wk	25.9 ($21\frac{6}{7}$–$33\frac{3}{7}$)	26.9 ($23\frac{5}{7}$–31)
Fetal transfusions	53	64
Fetuses	21	24
Survivors	11 (52%)	22 (92%)
Hydropic at IUT	7*	8†
Hydropic at first IUT	0	7
Hydropic survivors	3 (43%)	6 (75%)

*Catheter side hole-induced hemolysis, 4 (alive, 1).
†Catheter side hole-induced hemolysis, 1 (alive, 1).
(Courtesy of Bowman, J. M., and Manning, F. A.: Obstet. Gynecol. 61:203–209, February 1983. Reprinted with permission from The American College of Obstetricians and Gynecologists.)

(3–25) Obstet. Gynecol. 61:203–209, February 1983.

weeks' gestation, and transfusion under ultrasonic guidance, starting as early as 22.5 weeks' gestation if necessary. Intensive plasma exchange as an adjunct should be reserved for cases with a history of hydropic fetal death before 28 weeks' gestation. Intensive plasma exchange starting at 12–14 weeks' gestation offers the best chance of salvaging severely affected erythroblastotic fetuses that otherwise would become hydropic and die before 31 to 32 weeks' gestation.

▶ [This reads like a detective story. Doctor Bowman and his associates in Winnipeg certainly have had more experience with Rh sensitization and intrauterine transfusion than anyone else in the western hemisphere and perhaps in the world. They noticed in 1980 that they were losing fetuses they thought should survive transfusion. Systematic review of the technique indicated the reason—the holes in the catheter had been made smaller, causing hemolysis of the erythrocytes as they were injected. Correction of the problem led to subsequent statistics that are little short of astounding—92% salvage overall and 75% with hydrops.] ◀

3–26 **Incompetent Cervix During Pregnancy Diagnosed by Ultrasound.** Cervical incompetence is an important cause of late abortion. P. Vaalamo and A. Kivikoski (Lahti, Finland) used ultrasonography to examine 91 midtrimester patients for suspected cervical incompetence. The women were examined several times from the late first trimester up to 28 weeks' gestation. Thirteen patients had a history of premature delivery, 2 or more therapeutic first-trimester abortions, or 1 or more midtrimester abortions. Thirty-six patients experienced contractions in pregnancy, and 6 underwent cone biopsy. Picker grayscale ultrasound studies were carried out with a Foley catheter inserted against the external os and the balloon filled with water. A full-bladder technique was used.

Thirteen patients had findings of cervical incompetence, with detached membranes at the internal os bulging into a dilated cervical

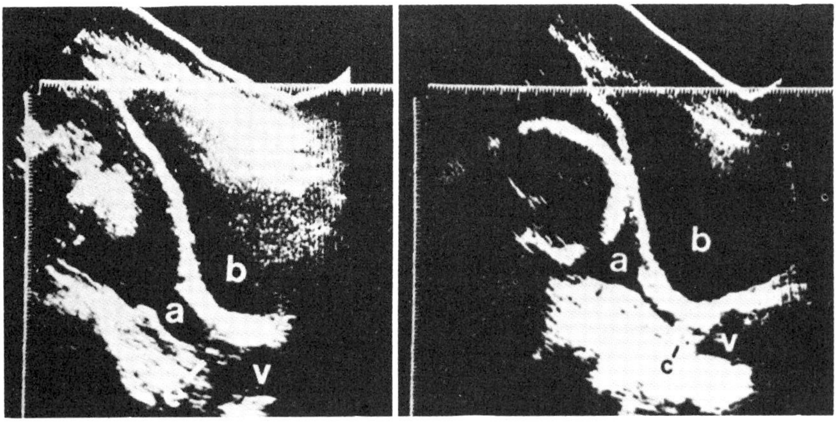

Fig 3–4 (left).—Cervix of patient at 25 weeks of pregnancy whose history included 3 incomplete pregnancies. Membranes with amniotic fluid *(a)* are seen to bulge into cervical canal; *b* = bladder; c = lower part of cervix; v = vagina.

Fig 3–5 (right).—Same patient as in Figure 3–4 at 26 weeks of pregnancy after McDonald's purse-string suture was performed; a = amniotic fluid; b = bladder; c = cervix; v = vagina.

(Courtesy of Vaalamo, P., and Kivikoski, A.: Acta Obstet. Gynaecol. Scand. 62:19–21, 1983.)

(3–26) Acta Obstet. Gynecol. Scand. 62:19–21, 1983.

canal. Seven patients had premature delivery or abortion previously, 4 had contractions during pregnancy, and 2 had undergone cone biopsy. The patients were operated on by the McDonald purse-string suture technique. One patient with premature membrane rupture gave birth at 35 weeks. In the other patients pregnancy was maintained beyond 37 weeks. The findings in 1 patient are shown in Figures 3–4 and 3–5.

Ultrasonography is a useful objective means of diagnosing cervical incompetence during pregnancy. Patients with a suggestive history or evidence of incompetence in the current pregnancy should be examined ultrasonically.

▶ [Figure 3–4 nicely demonstrates the membranes bulging into the upper cervix. The issue that needs to be settled involves the findings on physical examination in this situation. If the cervix is long and closed and if there is no ballooning of the lower uterine segment, then ultrasound may well have an important role in diagnosing cervical incompetence. If, however, suggestive findings on vaginal examination are already present when the ultrasound picture becomes abnormal, then what we have is another, although not necessarily better, means of making the diagnosis.] ◀

3–27 **Early Therapy for the Incompetent Cervix in Patients With Habitual Abortion.** Jonathan W. T. Ayers (Cleveland Clinic), Edwin P. Peterson and Rudi Ansbacher (Univ. of Michigan) evaluated data on 66 patients with a history of habitual abortion (3 or more spontaneous pregnancy losses) and report the results of therapy during the first trimester of pregnancy.

Fifty (76%) of the 66 patients did not have any of the characteristic endocrine, müllerian, or chromosomal abnormalities classically described as causes of habitual abortion. Of these 50 patients, 42 (84%) had significant widening (greater than 3 mm) of the uterine isthmus, as demonstrated by hysterosalpingography (Fig 3–6), as their only abnormality. First-trimester cervical effacement of 50% was present in 90% of these patients. Treatment consisted of progesterone therapy (25 mg vaginal suppositories twice daily) and modified McDonald cervical cerclage. The suppositories were discontinued at 16 weeks' gestation and Delalutin (250 mg weekly) was administered intramuscularly until 35 weeks' gestation. The cerclage was removed at 37 weeks.

Of the 42 patients, 6 (14%) had abnormal pregnancies and did not undergo cerclage: 2 presented at the first examination with a threatened abortion; 2 aborted prior to demonstrable cervical effacement; and cerclage was deferred in 2 because of inadequate growth patterns. Of the 36 patients whose treatment began in the first trimester of pregnancy, 35 (97%) had a successful term pregnancy. All but 4 had had first-trimester cervical effacement; 9 had declined progestin therapy. Six patients required adjunctive tocolysis for premature labor. There were also 8 placental abnormalities (24%), which included 3 cases of accessory lobes and 4 cases with major areas of infarction.

The results suggest that functional cervical incompetence may play a significant role in habitual abortion and that the habitual aborter may be defined clinically by a widened uterine isthmus on hystero-

---

(3–27) Fertil. Steril. 38:177–181, August 1982.

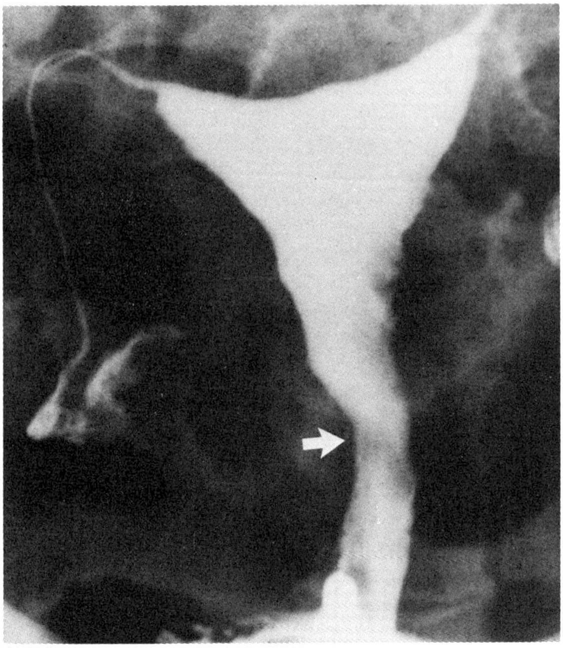

Fig 3–6.—Hysterosalpingography of 24-year-old habitual aborter. There is loss of isthmic integrity with "funneling" of lower segment to a 4.2-mm isthmus *(arrow)*. (Courtesy of Ayers, J. W. T., et al.: Fertil. Steril. 38:177–181, August 1982.)

salpingography and first-trimester cervical effacement. Early recognition and therapy for an incompetent cervix can interrupt the sequence of events leading to the loss of an otherwise normally developing fetus. Because of the increased perinatal morbidity in these patients, continuous antepartum assessment of fetoplacental integrity is necessary.

▶ [Although the etiology of habitual abortion in a particular patient may be identified, many times no "cause" is found and often the subsequent pregnancy is successful (see 1979 YEAR BOOK, pp. 430–431). In the present report, two thirds of the 141 previous pregnancy losses occurred in the first trimester (we don't know how the losses are distributed among the 36 patients). Excluding patients with "characteristic endocrine, müllerian, or chromosomal" causes, 84% of the others had widening of the uterine isthmus on hysterosalpingography (nicely demonstrated in Fig 3–7). Most of these patients manifested cervical "effacement" in the first trimester and underwent early (mode = 9–10 weeks) cerclage and progestin treatment. Do the excellent results reflect cerclage, the timing of the cerclage, progestin treatment, or the close individual attention of a concerned physician? As we have said before, despite the emotionally charged nature of the situation, controlled studies are required.] ◀

3–28 **Management of Antepartum Hemorrhage (Excluding Placenta Previa).** Ross Pagano, F. Douglas Adey, and Louis J. H. Butterfield believe there is a place for conservative management in cases of moderate antepartum hemorrhage (APH), as for mild bleeding. Review was made of the management of patients seen in a 3-year period

(3–28) Aust. N.Z. J. Obstet. Gynaecol. 23:20–24, February 1983.

PERINATAL MORTALITY

	Accidental haemorrhage		APH of unknown aetiology	
	No. of patients	Perinatal deaths	No. of patients	Perinatal deaths
Mild haemorrhage	53	5	94	6
Moderate and severe haemorrhage	45	18	7	0
Total	98	23(23.4%)	101	6(5.9%)

(Courtesy of Pagano, R., et al.: Aust. N. Z. J. Obstet. Gynaecol. 23:20–24, February 1983.)

at Royal Women's Hospital, Melbourne, with APH, defined as bleeding of 15 ml or more from the birth canal between 20 weeks' gestation and the onset of labor. All 98 women with accidental hemorrhage and 101 with APH of unknown cause included in the study had a normally implanted placenta.

Perinatal mortality was 23% in the group with accidental hemorrhage and 6% in the group with APH of unknown cause (table). All but 2 of 11 perinatal deaths in cases of mild APH, with bleeding of less than 200 ml and no generalized uterine tenderness or tenseness, were due to extreme prematurity (26 weeks or less). Fourteen of 18 perinatal deaths in the group with moderate to severe APH were not preventable. Two others were unavoidable because of coincidental prematurity and fetal abnormality, but 2 were avoidable. Four patients with moderately severe APH had immediate cesarean section because of fetal distress or previous cesarean section, and all 4 infants were healthy. Generalized uterine tenderness and tenseness were the most consistent features associated with imminent fetal compromise. Clotting abnormalities were infrequent in this series. There were no maternal deaths.

Perinatal mortality in cases of moderate APH in this series where the fetus was alive at admission was 10.5%. Two of the 4 deaths were due to congenital heart disease and 2 to intrauterine hypoxia. Active suppression of labor probably is warranted in cases of mild APH. In moderately severe cases where the fetus is alive and fetal distress is evident, immediate cesarean section is justified if the mother is in stable condition. Frank coagulation failure is rare in these cases. Intrapartum monitoring is not reliable in this setting when significant uterine tenderness is present.

▶ [Our personal experience is not consistent with the authors' finding that frank coagulation failure was not observed in the presence of a living fetus. We've seen it; the memory is indelible.

Generalized uterine tenderness and tenseness were often associated with poor outcomes in this series. The authors suggest cesarean section in this situation even if the monitor tracing doesn't indicate fetal distress. Again, we beg to differ; we think this will inflate the cesarean section rate without affecting the perinatal death rate.] ◀

3-29 **Fetomaternal Bleeding as a Cause for "Unexplained" Fetal Death.** Douglas W. Laube and Charles W. Schauberger (Univ. of Iowa) report data on a series of 29 antepartum fetal deaths that occurred during a 3-year period and without apparent cause. In 4 cases, spontaneous transplacental hemorrhage appeared to have been responsible for fetal death. Medical records of these were reviewed to identify factors that might have contributed to these deaths. Kleihauer-Betke staining of maternal blood smears was done either before or immediately after delivery in all cases of "unexplained" fetal death.

Of 119 fetal deaths studied, some potentially responsible factor or condition was identified in 90. The other 29 (24.4%) all occurred before labor and thus represented antepartum fetal deaths without apparent cause. Kleihauer-Betke staining of maternal blood was positive in 4 cases (13.8%) of unexplained fetal deaths. In all 4, the extent of fetomaternal hemorrhage was massive, amounting to 150 ml or more. Postmortem examination of the fetus, placenta, cord, and membranes in each case was unremarkable except for changes consistent with severe anemia.

CASE 1.—Woman, 23, had an uncomplicated pregnancy until 43 weeks' gestation. After a second oxytocin challenge, she was in labor and a normal-appearing female stillborn infant was delivered spontaneously. Kleihauer-Betke studies the next day showed 5% fetal cells in the maternal circulation, indicating a 216-ml fetomaternal transfusion.

CASE 2.—Woman, 25, a primigravida, was admitted in early labor when no fetal heart tones were heard. A 2,900-gm female stillborn infant was delivered by low forceps. Kleihauer-Betke tests before delivery showed that 6% of the red blood cells in the maternal circulation were of fetal origin.

CASE 3.—Woman, 28, was referred at 39 weeks' gestation with an intrauterine fetal death. Kleihauer-Betke tests showed 3.6% fetal cells in the maternal circulation.

CASE 4.—Woman, 26, a primigravida, had no detectable fetal heart tones at 40 weeks' gestation. A Kleihauer-Betke test before induction of labor showed that 5.3% of maternal circulating red blood cells were of fetal origin.

Massive transplacental hemorrhage has been identified in the European medical literature but has not received much attention in the American medical literature. The present data show transplacental hemorrhage to be present in 13.8% of unexplained fetal deaths, 3.4% of all fetal deaths, and 0.04% of all births. The principal conclusion of this study is that massive fetomaternal hemorrhage occurring without apparent cause or predisposing factors represents a significant cause of fetal deaths. The clinician should examine for this problem in those patients whose fetuses die in utero for no apparent reason.

▶ [This report serves as a useful reminder of a problem that is more common than generally is appreciated. Would the measurement of serum haptoglobin levels be helpful in diagnosis in instances of fetomaternal ABO incompatibility?] ◀

3-30 **Abdominal Pregnancy: Review of Current Management and Addition of 10 Cases.** Isaac Delke, Norma Perez Veridiano, and M.

(3-29) Obstet. Gynecol. 60:649-651, November 1982.
(3-30) Ibid., pp. 200-204, August 1982.

Leon Tancer (SUNY, Downstate Med. Center) discuss abdominal pregnancy based on the 10 cases seen in 1965 through 1981. Incidence was 1 per 7,095 deliveries on 1 per 70 ectopic pregnancies. The 10 women, all from low socioeconomic backgrounds, were aged 29 to 37 years (mean, 32 years). Nine had a history compatible with a tubal accident early in pregnancy. None met the criteria for primary abdominal pregnancy. In 5 patients, the condition was suspected and a diagnosis was made at 16 to 24 weeks' gestation, but in the other 5, diagnosis was much delayed. The perinatal mortality was 80%; 2 of the 3 infants born alive survived. All the mothers survived.

As with ectopic pregnancy, infertility (primary or secondary) is a significant antecedent historic fact in abdominal pregnancy. Other clues include lower abdominal pain, vaginal bleeding, cessation of fetal movement, vomiting late in pregnancy, abdominal tenderness, fetal malpresentation, and a closed and uneffaced cervix. An extremely helpful clinical clue is the absence of palpable uterine contractions after small doses of parenteral oxytocin or vaginal prostaglandin E_2. Management of intrauterine fetal death must be preceded by consideration of the presence of abdominal pregnancy.

When abdominal pregnancy is suspected, ultrasound is useful in confirming the diagnosis, but it also can give a false diagnosis of intrauterine pregnancy. In this series, ultrasound was confirmatory in 3 cases and in error in 2, and in none of the 5 cases was the chorionic plate of the placenta shown clearly. Further support for the diagnosis may be obtained by studying the waveform of the fetal movement pattern by using standard fetal monitoring equipment. Radiographic findings are variable; in this series, a flat-plate abdominal radiograph showed fetal malpresentation in 4 of 5 cases. Hysterography, done in 4 patients, was diagnostic in all.

Assessing fetal status and choosing the optimal time for delivery are also problems. The role of ultrasound, nonstress testing, and serial estriol determinations in the diagnosis and ongoing assessment of the potentially viable abdominal pregnancy needs more study. Patients deliberately have been allowed to proceed to near term and were delivered of a live fetus without additional maternal morbidity, but the risk in this course is the possibility of intraperitoneal hemorrhage. One report found the fetus to have a 25% chance of survival and a 10% chance of being normal. Thus, in general, immediate planned surgery with adequate compatible blood available is the proper management of abdominal pregnancy. If the blood supply of the placenta can be ligated safely, it can be removed in toto. Its partial removal, when its whole blood supply cannot be ligated, may result in massive hemorrhage and shock; in such cases, the placenta should be left in situ.

▶ [Perhaps we're according this rare problem too much attention (see 1983 YEAR BOOK, pp. 88–90), but the diagnosis is often missed, at times with serious consequences. Good points made in the present report include the frequent history of infertility in these patients and the advisability of considering the occurrence of an abdominal pregnancy when a patient presents with a dead fetus. Fetal death and fetal death in utero are not synonymous.] ◀

4. Antepartum Fetal Surveillance

4–1 **Comparison of Reliability of Estimated Date of Confinement Predicted by Crown-Rump Length and Biparietal Diameter.** Mazie M. Kopta, Retha R. May, and James P. Crane (Washington Univ.) compared the accuracy of estimated dates of confinement predicted by first-trimester crown-rump length (CRL) measurements and second-trimester biparietal diameter (BPD) measurements in a prospective study of 45 patients. Scans were made using a real-time unit in the first trimester and again at 20–24 weeks' gestation. Fetal BPD was measured using a gray-scale compound-contact scanner. Delivery information was available on 36 patients.

With 3 exceptions there were not more than 8 days' difference between the 2 estimated dates of confinement predicted for each patient, and in 75% the difference was 4 days or less. There was no significant difference between the two methods in ability to predict onset of labor and delivery. The mean error with the CRL technique was 7.7 days and with the BPD method, 7.65 days. The number of patients delivered before and after the predicted date of confinement was about the same with both techniques. The two methods were similar when the mean numbers of days by which the delivery date was either underestimated or overestimated were compared.

Both the CRL and the BPD methods have a role in obstetric sonography. It is important to be able to confirm viability and estimate gestational age in patients who bleed in the first trimester and also to have an accurate dating method in the second trimester. The second trimester is a better time to localize the placenta, estimate amniotic fluid volume, and exclude fetal anomalies. There is no definitive evidence that diagnostic ultrasound is teratogenic, but prospective controlled data on the long-term follow-up of prenatally exposed individuals are not available. Determination of gestational age in the second trimester offers the theoretical advantage of avoiding the most critical phase of embryogenesis.

▶ [Some have suggested that the first-trimester crown-rump length is a more reliable predictor of the estimated date of confinement than is the midpregnancy biparietal diameter. This carefully done study indicates that the two measurements perform equally well.] ◀

▶ ↓A vote for femur length is found in the following article. Read on. . . . ◀

4–2 **Ultrasonic Measurement of the Femur Length as an Index of Fetal Gestational Age.** Ming-Neng Yeh, Luis Bracero, Kevin B. Reilly, Louise Murtha, Michael Aboulafia, and Bruce A. Barron (Columbia Univ.) measured the fetal femur length with a linear-array, real-time ultrasound scanner in 145 uncomplicated gravid patients

(4–1) Am. J. Obstet. Gynecol. 145:562–565, Mar. 1, 1983.
(4–2) Ibid., 144:519–522, Nov. 1, 1982.

from 16 to 42 weeks' gestation. The data were analyzed by the method of least-squares linear regression. In each case, gestational age was documented by last menstrual period and correlated with ultrasonic biparietal diameter measurements within ± 1.5 weeks.

Results of the data analysis generated the following equation: $Y = -0.6809 + 0.2127X$, where Y = femur length (cm) and X = gestational age (weeks). In contrasting the results, the gestational age is the independent variable and the femur length is the dependent variable; thus, the standard deviation for each parameter estimate is smaller than that for the gestational age versus biparietal diameter or for dates by biparietal diameter versus fetal femur length. With the use of these data, the error in estimating gestational age given femur length at 25 to 35 weeks' gestation is less than 5 days. Outside these intervals, there is less precision in this measurement, with a range from 8 days at 15 weeks to 6 days at 40 weeks. The correlation coefficient of gestational age versus fetal femur length is statistically greater than that of the gestational age versus fetal biparietal diameter.

These results suggest that measurement of fetal femur length provides a more precise index of gestational age than does biparietal diameter. The authors propose that the ultrasonic measurement of fetal femur length is a sensitive and precise variable for estimation of fetal growth and development, especially after 27 weeks' gestation.

▶ [The normal range of biparietal diameters increases with advancing gestational age and by the time of the third trimester is sufficiently wide to limit severely the clinical usefulness of a single measurement. These results indicate that femur length, previously found to correlate with earlier gestational ages, is also of value in late pregnancy. The range seems narrower than that with biparietal diameter. If these findings are confirmed by others and if the technique proves relatively easy, the measurement of femur length may become the method of choice for estimating gestational age ultrasonically.] ◀

4–3 **Antenatal Biochemical Screening To Predict Low Birth Weight Infants.** D. R. Aickin, G. B. Duff, J. J. Evans, and M. Legge (Christchurch, New Zealand) examined the ability of various biochemical determinations to predict infants of low birth weight in a series of 608 consecutive pregnancies in which fetal gestational age was confirmed by ultrasound before 28 weeks' gestation. When indicated, a second ultrasound study was done 4 weeks later. Concentrations of urinary and plasma estriol, plasma progesterone, human placental lactogen, β_1-glycoprotein, and serum cystyl aminopeptidase were determined at intervals often enough to analyze changes over every week from 28 weeks' gestation to delivery. The data were analyzed to obtain 10th to 90th centile values for each test.

Groups with values under the lower centiles had higher proportions but smaller absolute numbers of low birth weight infants than did those under higher centiles. No test was superior to the others at all centiles and for all gestations. There usually was a marked increase in the proportion of correct predictions of low birth weight at cutoffs below the 30th centile. This was more evident near term than early

(4–3) Br. J. Obstet. Gynaecol. 90:129–133, February 1983.

in the third trimester. The urinary estriol level was more likely than the other tests to predict low birth weight infants at gestations before term. The β_1-glycoprotein level was less predictive than the other tests were in most instances. Correlation between test values was generally poor, although it usually was better for pregnancies resulting in low birth weight infants.

Biochemical screening of pregnant populations to identify groups at high risk for purposes of intensive fetal monitoring would appear to have limited potential. If screening is used, high-risk groups are best defined by practical rather than statistical criteria. Higher centile "cutoffs" can be used to define fetal risk if monitoring facilities are available and are well accepted by patients. Low centiles such as the 10th are best used when fetal monitoring methods are unavailable or are not well accepted.

▶ [This report indicates that none of the six biochemical markers studied effectively identified intrauterine growth retardation. At the 10th percentile of the tests, for example, 30% of the babies were small for gestation age (SGA). Not only were most babies in the lowest decile not SGA, but, using this cutoff, two thirds of SGA fetuses would not be identified. In our view, the diagnosis of intrauterine growth retardation is made *clinically* in a carefully dated pregnancy. Sensitivity? Not terrific, but if the lowest decile is considered SGA, remember that 1 in 10 newborns is so classified. Everybody can't play basketball! The adverse consequences of intrauterine growth retardation are greater the more restricted the definition is (e.g., lowest third percentile). The more restricted the definition, the easier is the clinical identification.] ◀

▶ ↓A simpler means of identifying the growth-retarded fetus is considered in the following article. Read on . . . . ◀

4–4 **Antenatal Screening by Measurement of Symphysis-Fundus Height.** John P. Calvert, Ernest E. Crean, Robert G. Newcombe, and James F. Pearson (Welsh Natl. School of Medicine, Cardiff) assessed the value of symphysis-fundus measurement as a screening procedure for intrauterine growth retardation in two groups of 6 patients, each measured six times by 6 different observers to document the reproducibility of this procedure.

Data was available from 381 pregnancies in nondiabetic mothers with confirmed dates. Figure 4–1 shows the normal curve derived from 1,775 observations of the 313 patients for whom the birth weight was between the 10th and 90th centiles. A chart of symphysis-fundus measurements derived from data from Cardiff, Wales, was found to be similar to others previously published; one measurement below the 10th centile identified 64% of pregnancies in which the eventual birth weight was below the 10th centile for gestational age. The table shows the results of testing of the ability of the Cardiff chart to detect those pregnancies with varying degrees of growth retardation using a variety of previously suggested criteria.

Measurement of the symphysis-fundus height provides a communicable way of expressing fundal height and an easy and inexpensive screening test for intrauterine growth retardation. Because no special skill is necessary, the procedure may be used with equal accuracy by all who care for the pregnant woman. A chart of symphysis-fundus

(4–4) Br. Med. J. 285:846–849, Sept. 25, 1982.

Results From Cardoff Chart Using Different Criteria Indicating Growth Retardation

Criteria used to indicate growth retardation	Results: Birth weight	Results: No predicted as: Retarded	Results: No predicted as: Not retarded	Predictive performance: Birth weight	Sensitivity*	Specificity†	False-positive rate
One value > 2 cm below mean, or three consecutive static or declining values (*Westin*[8])	< 5th centile (n = 25)	18	7	< 5th centile	72%	58%	89%
	5th–10th centile (n = 20)	16	4	< 10th centile	76%	60%	80%
	> 10th centile (n = 336)	133	203				
	All patients	167 (44%)	214 (56%)				
One value < 10th centile (Belizan *et al*[9])	< 5th centile	15	10	5th centile	60%	76%	85%
	5th–10th centile	14	6	10th centile	64%	79%	71%
	> 10th centile	71	265				
	All patients	100 (26%)	281 (74%)				
Two consecutive or three isolated values < 10th centile (Quaranta *et al*[10])	< 5th centile	9	16	< 5th centile	36%	92%	76%
	5th–10th centile	7	13	< 10th centile	36%	94%	57%
	> 10th centile	21	315				
	All patients	37 (10%)	344 (90%)				

*Sensitivity = proportion of low birth weight infants predicted to be retarded.
†Specificity = proportion of appropriately grown or large infants predicted not to be retarded.
(Courtesy of Calvert, J. P., et al.: Br. Med. J. 285:846–849, Sept. 25, 1982.)

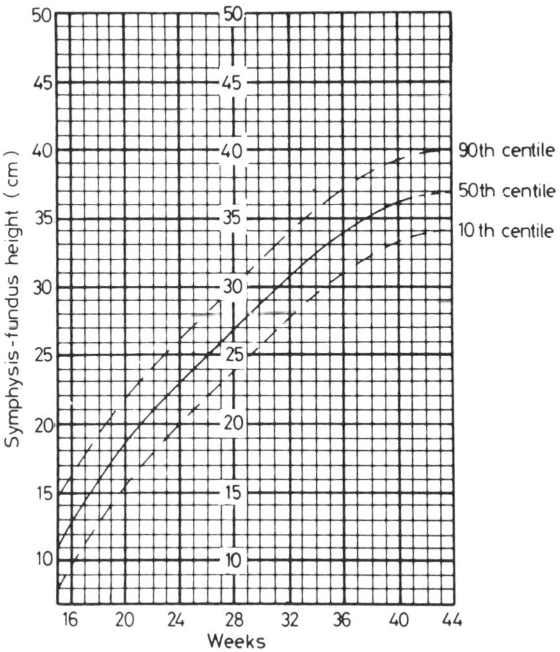

Fig 4–1.—Graph showing symphysis-fundus height based on data from Cardiff, Wales. (Courtesy of Calvert, J. P., et al.: Br. Med. J. 285:846–849, Sept. 25, 1982.)

heights would enhance communication among midwife, general practitioner, and hospital obstetrician.

▶ [The fundal height-weeks' gestation values reported here from Wales are virtually identical to those from Argentina reported by Belizan et al. (1979 YEAR BOOK, pp. 44–45). We agree with the authors of both reports that this simple determination is quite effective in identifying the fetus with intrauterine growth retardation and that it should be a routine part of antepartum care. The addition of abdominal girth measurement may improve the accuracy.] ◀

4–5 **Fetal Echocardiography: A Tool for Evaluation of In Utero Cardiac Arrhythmias and Monitoring of In Utero Therapy: Analysis of 71 Patients.** Charles S. Kleinman, Richard L. Donnerstein, C. Carl Jaffe, Greggory R. DeVore, Ellen M. Weinstein, Diana C. Lynch, Norman S. Talner, Richard L. Berkowitz, and John C. Hobbins (Yale Univ.) performed fetal echocardiography in 71 patients referred at 24 to 40 weeks' gestation for evaluation of cardiac rhythm disorders. After a two-dimensional echocardiographic analysis of fetal cardiac structure and gross study of the cardiac rhythm in real time, a simultaneous or sequential M-mode study, or both, were done to analyze the heart rate, atrioventricular contraction sequence, atrioventricular valve motion, and duration of postectopic pauses.

Satisfactory real-time and M-mode studies were obtained in all cases. Fifty-nine patients had documented rhythm disturbances at the time of echocardiography. Of 34 patients with isolated ectopic

---

(4–5) Am. J. Cardiol. 51:237–243, Jan. 15, 1983.

beats, 26 had resolution of the arrhythmia in later pregnancy, and 8 had resolution within 5 days of delivery. Six patients had mild sinus bradycardia, and 8 had frequent sinus pauses. All these patients had resolution of the arrhythmia during pregnancy. Eleven patients had sustained fetal arrhythmias. Several of them had associated nonimmune hydrops fetalis or structural heart disease, or both. Fetal or neonatal wastage occurred when there was congenital cardiac malformation or severe hydrops fetalis, or both. Supraventricular tachycardia was diagnosed in 3 fetuses, and echocardiography was used to monitor transplacental digoxin therapy in these cases.

Fetal echocardiography permits the noninvasive diagnosis of rhythm disorders in the fetus and is a means of monitoring responses to in utero treatment. Isolated ectopy is nearly always self-limited, but monitoring through pregnancy is warranted. Sustained arrhythmias have a more ominous prognosis, especially if associated with structural cardiac disease or fetal heart failure, or both. Supraventricular tachyarrhythmias associated with congestive heart failure can be controlled by transplacental digoxin therapy. Propranolol is reserved for use if digoxin alone is unsuccessful.

▶ [This experience is consistent with that reported in the literature. Isolated premature cardiac contractions in the fetus usually disappear by delivery or soon thereafter. The prognosis is variable in sustained arrhythmias and is worsened in the presence of associated structural heart disease or in utero congestive heart failure. The latter can be diagnosed by ultrasound (hydrops, hydramnios, effusions), as is illustrated by the following case. Read on . . . .] ◀

4–6 **Transplacental Cardioversion of Fetal Supraventricular Tachycardia With Procainamide.** Daniel A. Dumesic, Norman H. Silverman, Serge Tobias, and Mitchell S. Golbus (Univ. of California, San Francisco) report data on a case of fetal supraventricular tachycardia complicated by intrauterine congestive heart failure that was cardioverted temporarily several times by intravenous injection of procainamide after digoxin and propranolol had failed to alter the fetal heart rate.

Woman, 24, a primigravida, presented at 30 weeks' gestation for evaluation of fetal tachycardia. Class I diabetes complicated the pregnancy. A grade 2/6 systolic ejection murmur was heard. Fetal heart rate was 230 beats per minute. Fetal echocardiography showed no structural abnormalities, but a small pericardial effusion and minimal ascites were present. Fetal tachycardia persisted despite maternal digoxin therapy, and pleural effusions developed along with increasing ascitic fluid. Propranolol infusion led to no marked change in the arrhythmia. Normal sinus rhythm returned for 30 minutes after a 340-mg bolus dose of procainamide, and sinus rhythm persisted after another bolus and a maintenance infusion of 2 mg per minute. All serous effusions resolved, and the fetal heart rate fell to 130.

The patient was discharged receiving digoxin and sustained-release procainamide, but was seen at 33 weeks' gestation with recurrent fetal tachycardia, edema of the fetal scalp and body, and recurrent effusions. The arrhythmia was difficult to control even with large doses of procainamide, and cesarean section was carried out. Removal of ascitic fluid markedly improved the infant's ventilatory status. Digoxin therapy led to normal sinus rhythm. Exchange transfusion was necessary for hyperbilirubinemia. The supraven-

---

(4–6) N. Engl. J. Med. 307:1128–1131, Oct. 28, 1982.

tricular tachycardia was controlled with digoxin and propranolol. An ECG when the infant was aged 6 months showed normal sinus rhythm with a normal PR interval and normal voltages.

Procainamide treatment provided control of supraventricular fetal tachycardia in this case after digoxin and propranolol had failed. Procainamide is considered a standard treatment for supraventricular tachycardias after birth. In this case, the level of procainamide in neonatal serum was only one fourth that of the maternal level despite delivery 3 hours after the mother's last drug dose, suggesting that simple transplacental diffusion of procainamide may not occur.

▶ [Newberger and Keane, in an article abstracted in the 1981 YEAR BOOK (pp. 106–107), reviewed 37 reported cases of fetal supraventricular tachycardia. In published cases, as well as in our own experience, digitalis and propranolol administered to the pregnant woman have not been very effective. The case described above responded, albeit temporarily, to procainamide. Thus, it seems that with fetal tachycardia causing ultrasound evidence of congestive failure, procainamide may be the best drug to use until delivery, when the infant may be treated directly.] ◀

4–7 **Antepartum Fetal Heart Rate Testing in Preterm Pregnancy.** The nonstress test (NST) and the contraction stress test (CST) have had wide application to term pregnancies, but they have not often been used in management of preterm fetuses. Lawrence D. Devoe (Univ. of Chicago) studied 72 of 438 high-risk gravidas who received both tests between 25 and 34 weeks' gestation. All 72 delivered singleton infants before completion of their 34th week. On the basis of the last NST and CST preceding delivery, the 72 fetuses could be divided into reactive-negative and nonreactive-positive groups.

The nonreactive-positive fetuses experienced greater perinatal mortality and significantly higher rates of intrapartum fetal distress, neonatal depression, respiratory distress syndrome (RDS), intrauterine growth retardation, and cesarean section. Pulmonary complications in nonreactive-positive fetuses, regardless of the lecithin-sphingomyelin ratio, were significantly increased if intrapartum fetal distress had preceded delivery. Most neonatal deaths stemmed from RDS-related complications; more than 80% preceded the 31st week of gestation. Nearly 50% of perinatal deaths before the 30th week of gestation followed reactive NSTs. Overall, estriol values correctly predicted perinatal outcome in 73% of cases. A good perinatal outcome was predicted accurately in 80% of cases when both fetal heart rate tests and maternal estriol values were favorable. A poor outcome was correctly forecast in 95% of cases when both were unfavorable.

These data suggest that for clinical management of preterm pregnancy, fetal heart rate testing should be initiated after the 29th week; earlier, the test significance is less clear and infant survival less likely. Maternal estriol determinations are of little help in the management of nonreactive-positive fetuses. Rather, the care in these selected pregnancies should be temporized through the 30th week. When delivery is then elected, intrapartum fetal distress should be avoided through liberal use of cesarean section in the nonreactive-positive group. This policy will not prevent RDS in all nonreactive-

---

(4–7) Obstet. Gynecol. 60:431–436, October 1982.

positive cases but should decrease its severity and fatal sequelae by avoiding fetal distress.

▶ [When fetal surveillance tests should be initiated is an often-asked question. The answer depends on the experience of the specific unit with respect to survival at various gestational age-birth weight groupings. In this report from the University of Chicago, 9 of 11 neonatal deaths occurred in infants born prior to 31 weeks' gestation, apparently leading the author to recommend that cardiotocography not be initiated until after the 29th week. We do not hesitate to do heart rate testing as much as 2 weeks earlier than this if it seems indicated by the history of something else about the case; in the absence of such an indication (e.g., in a diabetic or chronic hypertensive patient who has not had a previous loss and whose fetus now seems normally grown), we would wait until 31 or 32 weeks' gestation.] ◀

4–8 **Randomized Controlled Trial of Nonstress Antepartum Cardiotocography.** Antepartum cardiotocography (CTG) is believed to improve perinatal outcome in the high-risk patient, especially by reducing the antepartum stillbirth rate. To evaluate CTG as a test of fetal well-being, Anna M. Flynn, John Kelly, Hugh Mansfield, Peter Needham, Maria O'Conor, and Osborn Viegas (Birmingham, England) conducted a prospective randomized controlled study of 569 nonstress CTGs performed on 300 patients, 258 of whom were considered to be at risk.

Four stillbirths and 3 neonatal deaths occurred. The CTG was nonreactive in 6 of these deaths and reactive in 1. The reactive CTG occurred in a patient aged 42 years whose infant died at age 2 days with trisomy 18. Of the 7 infants who died, 4 had a lethal congenital malformation and another had osteogenesis imperfecta. When the 18 mothers who had been sedated were excluded from the 39 with nonreactive CTGs, there was a 29% mortality for infants whose mothers had a nonreactive response. Nonreactive tracings were associated sig-

TABLE 1.—Effect on Management When Cardiotocographic Report Is Available

Management	Report available	Report withheld	P
No. of CTGs per patient (mean)	1·570	1·776	N.S.*
Following cardiotocography			
(1) Repeat antenatal clinic visits			
One visit	16	9	N.S.†
More than one visit	4	7	N.S.†
(2) Antenatal in-patient days	8·65	11·00	N.S.*
(3) Patients discharged from hospital before delivery	22	11	< 0·01
(4) Patients allowed to continue antenatal care as out-patients	19	8	< 0·01
Induction of labour (patients)	60	63	N.S.†
Induction of labour followed by			
Spontaneous labour	45	50	N.S.†
Forceps delivery	9	9	N.S.†
Caesarean section	6	4	N.S.†
Elective caesarean section	8	12	N.S.†

N.S. = not significant.
*Significance of difference by t test.
†Significance of difference by χ^2 test.
(Courtesy of Flynn, A. M., et al.: Br. J. Obstet. Gynaecol. 89:427–433, June 1982.)

(4–8) Br. J. Obstet. Gynaecol. 89:427–433, June 1982.

TABLE 2.—EFFECT ON OUTCOME WHEN CARDIOTOCOGRAPHIC REPORT IS AVAILABLE

Outcome	Report available	Report withheld	*P* (*t*-test)
Stillbirths	3 (1 L)	1	—
Neonatal deaths	1 (1 L)	2 (2 L)	—
Neonatal convulsions	1	2	—
Neonatal irritability	3	1	—
Mean Apgar score at 1 min	7·725	7·12	N.S.
Mean Apgar score at 5 min	8·972	8·904	N.S.

L = lethal congenital abnormality (preceding numbers indicate number of babies affected). N.S. = not significant.

(Courtesy of Flynn, A. M., et al.: Br. J. Obstet. Gynaecol. 89:427–433, June 1982.)

nificantly with stillbirths and neonatal deaths, intrauterine growth retardation, admission to the special care baby unit for conditions related to intrauterine hypoxia, and low 1- and 5-minute Apgar scores.

When the CTG report was made available to the attending clinician, significantly more patients were discharged from the hospital before delivery and significantly more patients were allowed to continue antenatal care as outpatients (Table 1). When the report was not made available, there were more antenatal inpatient days and more elective cesarean sections, although these differences were not statistically significant. The effect of the availability of the CTG reports did not significantly influence the occurrence of stillbirths and neonatal deaths, neonatal convulsions, neonatal irritability, or the mean 1- and 5-minute Apgar scores (Table 2).

The results indicate that nonstress CTG is a good predictor of stillbirth or neonatal death. Reassurance provided by a satisfactory CTG will influence the clinician to discharge patients from the hospital and maintain surveillance on an outpatient basis, an important cost-effectiveness consideration. Nonetheless, it is believed that CTG, viewed separately from other clinical data, may lead to unnecessary intervention.

▶ [The most interesting aspect of this article is that having to do with the randomized reporting or not reporting of results of nonstress tests. The only significant difference between the groups was a tendency for reporting to lead to hospital discharge and outpatient follow-up care. This is not surprising, for it is easy to imagine that the assurance provided by a reactive nonstress test reported in a high-risk patient would make the physician more likely to discharge her from the hospital than would be the case if this information were not available. The fact that differences in outcome were not significant may well reflect the relatively small sample size.] ◀

4–9 **The Value of Antenatal Cardiotocography in Management of High-Risk Pregnancy: Randomized Controlled Trial.** Nonstressed antinatal cardiotocography (CTG) is now widely accepted as a method of monitoring fetal health. Valerie A. Brown, R. S. Sawers, R. J. Parsons, Sheila L. B. Duncan, and I. D. Cooke (Sheffield, England) assessed the value of routine, regular antenatal CTG in the management of high-risk pregnancy in a prospective, randomized, and controlled study of 353 women. All patients had a weekly CTG

(4–9) Br. J. Obstet. Gynaecol. 89:716–722, September 1982.

trace during the last 6 weeks of pregnancy and, according to random allocation, the tracings were concealed from (group 1), or available to (group 2), the clinicians. Other methods of assessing fetal welfare were available to both groups.

Results show no significant difference between the groups in the mean gestational age at delivery nor in the incidence of elective delivery, either by induction of labor or planned cesarean section. There was no significant difference between the groups in the mean gestational age, birth weight, incidence of fetal heart rate abnormality in labor, and low Apgar score at 1 minute. Only 5 infants had a low Apgar score at 5 minutes; 4 were in group 2. Forty patients had a low score of equal to or less than 4 out of 6 for the last trace before delivery. In agreement with findings of other researchers, an association existed between a low-scoring trace and fetal heart rate abnormality in labor, neonatal complications, and low birth weight. These significant differences were found within both groups and, therefore, cannot be attributed to medical intervention following a revealed trace.

These study results do not support findings from other reports that show a significantly higher incidence of abnormal CTG traces with fetuses small for gestational age. Use of routine antenatal CTG on a regular basis, particularly if performed daily, makes heavy demands on patients, staff, and equipment. The technique may be valuable for a more highly selected group of patients for whom other methods of assessment are less appropriate.

▶ [This randomized trial of antepartum fetal heart rate testing has important limitations. The number of women (353) is small for a study of this type and over half of the "high-risk" subjects were deemed so only because the mothers were young or old or had low human placental lactogen levels. Furthermore, patients with nonreactive tracings were apparently not evaluated with oxytocin challenge tests.

A larger, admittedly not randomized or blinded, trial is reported in the following article.] ◀

4–10 **Prospective Multi-institutional Study of Antepartum Fetal Heart Rate Monitoring: I. Risk of Perinatal Mortality and Morbidity According to Antepartum Fetal Heart Rate Test Results.** To evaluate the risks of perinatal mortality and morbidity, Roger K. Freeman, Gerald Anderson, and Wendy Dorchester analyzed prospectively collected data for 18,517 antepartum fetal heart rate monitoring studies performed on 7,448 high-risk patients in 18 institutions in the United States between September 1976 and December 1980.

A total of 12,656 contraction stress tests (CSTs) and 5,861 nonstress tests (NSTs) were carried out. Both tests were performed in 1,167 patients, CSTs only were performed in 4,485, and NSTs only were performed in 1,796. Negative CSTs or reactive NSTs accounted for 83.9% of the test results, equivocal CSTs for 9.3%, and nonreactive NSTs or positive CSTs for 2.9%. Ranking of the tests from the least ominous result to the most ominous showed that 76.6% of the patients had either a negative CST or a reactive NST as the worst test result. In 15.2% of the patients the worst test result was an equivocal CST, in 6.1% it was a nonreactive NST or a positive CST (Table 1).

(4–10) Am. J. Obstet. Gynecol. 143:771–777, Aug. 1, 1982.

TABLE 1.—WORST TEST RESULT

Result	*No.*	*%*	
Unsatisfactory	152	2.0	
Negative CST	3,556	47.7	76.6%
Reactive NST	2,154	28.9	
Equivocal CST	1,133	15.2	
Nonreactive NST	245	3.3	6.1%
Reactive positive CST	137	1.8	
Nonreactive positive CST	71	1.0	
Total	7,448	100.0	

(Courtesy of Freeman, R. K., et al.: Am. J. Obstet. Gynecol. 143:771–777, Aug. 1, 1982.

The highest percentages of a nonreactive NST or a positive CST occurred in patients with Rh disease (12.9%), intrauterine growth retardation (IUGR) as the indication for testing (11.3%), insulin-dependent diabetes (10.3%), hypertension (7.6%), and postmaturity (3.8%) (Table 2). Correlations were investigated for the worst test result and IUGR, Apgar score of less than 7 at 5 minutes, late deceleration in labor, and total fetal distress. In patients with a negative CST as a worst result, differences were statistically significant in the nonreactive positive CST in all four categories, in the nonreactive NST in percentage of IUGR and percentage of low Apgar scores, and in the reactive positive CST for percentages of IUGR, late deceleration, and total fetal distress in labor. Patients with a reactive NST had significantly fewer late decelerations in labor than the negative CST group. When compared with negative CSTs, severe variable deceleration and prolonged deceleration did not differ significantly in any category of worst test result.

Perinatal mortality was initially 12.9 per 1,000 and fetal death rate was 3.2 per 1,000. Nonreactive NSTs, reactive and nonreactive positive CSTs, and unsatisfactory tests all were associated with significantly higher perinatal death rates than negative CSTs when ranked by worst test result. After exclusion of 55 perinatal deaths in which

TABLE 2.—REASON FOR TEST BY WORST TEST RESULT*

Reason for test	*No.*	*Uns. (%)*	*Neg. CST (%)*	*R NST (%)*	*E CST (%)*	*NR NST (%)*	*R Pos. CST (%)*	*NR Pos. CST (%)*	*NR NST and Pos. CST (%)*
Diabetes, Class A	736	2.4	33.9	49.7	9.4	2.7	1.5	0.4	4.6
Diabetes, Classes B to R	457	0.9	38.5	31.0	19.3	5.9	2.0	2.4	10.3
All diabetes	1193	1.9	36.0	42.9	13.3	4.0	1.7	1.2	6.9
Chronic hypertension	881	3.1	48.0	26.0	14.3	3.9	2.8	1.9	8.6
Preeclampsia	1310	1.9	39.9	36.8	13.3	4.0	1.9	1.4	7.3
Eclampsia	12	0.0	66.7	16.7	8.3	0.0	8.3	0.0	8.3
Other hypertension	271	0.0	53.8	22.5	18.1	1.5	3.0	1.1	5.6
All hypertension	2474	2.1	44.3	31.2	14.4	3.7	2.4	1.5	7.6
Previous stillbirth	326	0.6	35.2	35.2	19.6	4.9	2.1	2.1	9.1
IUGR	802	1.6	40.7	27.1	19.2	3.9	5.0	2.4	11.3
Postdates	3123	1.7	52.7	25.4	16.2	2.2	1.2	0.4	3.8
Rh disease	87	2.2	34.4	39.0	9.1	6.9	5.9	2.3	12.9
Cardiac disease	56	0.9	26.7	41.0	17.9	5.3	0.0	0.0	5.3

*Uns. = unsatisfactory; Neg. = negative; Pos. = positive; E = equivocal; R = reactive; NR = nonreactive.
(Courtesy of Freeman, R. K., et al.: Am. J. Obstet. Gynecol. 143:771–777, Aug. 1, 1982.)

TABLE 3.—CORRECTED PERINATAL MORTALITY BY WORST TEST RESULT

		Stillbirths									
		Antepartum deaths		Intrapartum deaths		Total		Neonatal deaths		Perinatal deaths	
Result	No.*	No.	No./1,000	No.	No./1,000	No.	No./1,000	No.	No./1,000	No.	No./1,000
Neg. CST	3,540	0	—	1	0.3	1	0.3	7	2.0	8	2.3
R NST	2,141	3	1.4	1	0.5	4	1.9	5	2.3	9	4.2
E CST	1,128	2	1.8	0	—	2	1.8	2	1.8	4	3.5
NR NST	236	4	17.0†	2	8.5	6	25.4†	0	—	6	25.4†
R Pos. CST	131	0	—	0	—	0	—	1	7.6	1	7.6
NR Pos. CST	68	5	73.5†	1	14.7†	6	88.2†	6	88.2†	12	176.5†
Unsatisfactory	149	0	—	0	—	0	—	1	6.7	1	6.7
Total	7,393	14	1.9	5	0.7	19	2.6	22	3.0	41	5.5

*Deaths excluded by correction are not included.
†$P < .5$ compared to negative CST group.
(Courtesy of Freeman, R. K., et al.: Am. J. Obstet. Gynecol. 143:771–777, Aug. 1, 1982.)

antepartum fetal heart rate monitoring could not have been expected to offer possible prevention of death, the perinatal death rate was corrected to 5.5 per 1,000 and the fetal death rate was corrected to 1.9 per 1,000. Then it was found that only nonreactive NST and nonreactive positive CST as worst test result were associated with significantly increased morbidity and mortality (Table 3).

When patients are ranked by worst test result, the presence of persistent late decelerations appeared to be an earlier warning sign of fetal deterioration than did the absence of reactivity.

▶ [This multi-institutional, nonblinded study should not be used to compare the merits of the NST vs. the CST, although it is likely that such comparisons will be made. The large numbers do demonstrate that both forms of antepartum fetal heart rate testing are effective in assessing fetal well-being. If all positive CSTs are considered together, the fetal death rate (30.2) is about that of the nonreactive NST group (25.4). Table 3 indicates the importance of the presence or absence of reactivity in those patients with positive CSTs. Although intervention for an abnormal test finding did not result in neonatal death, there were 16 nonfatal cases of respiratory distress syndrome in this situation.] ◀

▶ ↓A report comparing the NST and CST follows. Read on . . . . ◀

4–11 **Oxytocin-Stressed and Unstressed Cardiotocograms for Prediction of Fetal Compromise.** R. Homburg, M. Ben-David, and H. Zakut compared the results of unstressed and oxytocin-stressed cardiotocograms (CTG) recorded in 222 high-risk pregnancies within 48 hours of delivery with the occurrence of signs of fetal distress in labor and Apgar scores to assess the predictive value of these antepartum tests.

Persistent late decelerations of the fetal heart rate (FHR) during labor occurred in 39 patients (18%), and 18 infants (8%) had an Apgar score of less than 7 at 1 minute. Fourteen (56%) of the 25 patients with a nonreactive unstressed CTG exhibited a late deceleration pattern of the FHR during labor, compared with 35 (92%) of 38 patients with a positive or suspicious stressed CTG. Two (8%) of 25 patients with a nonreactive unstressed CTG and 12 (32%) of 38 patients with a positive or suspicious stressed CTG delivered infants with low Ap-

(4–11) Br. J. Obstet. Gynaecol. 89:516–519, July 1982.

gar scores at 1 minute. In cases in which the results of the unstressed and stressed CTGs were at variance, the stressed CTG, both when negative or positive/suspicious, seemed to predict the fetal condition more accurately than the unstressed CTG. When the Fisher's exact test was used, the predictive value of the stressed CTG was significantly better than the predictive value of the unstressed CTG with regard to a late deceleration pattern of the FHR in labor and to low Apgar scores.

It is concluded that the exclusion, or highly selective use, of the oxytocin-stressed CTG and reliance on the unstressed CTG for the antepartum evaluation of high-risk pregnancies sacrifices accuracy for convenience.

▶ [This comparison of NST and CST seems to indicate that the CST is both more specific and more sensitive than the NST. Greater specificity is no surprise, but enhanced sensitivity (i.e., CST identifying fetal jeopardy better than NST) certainly is. The authors caution that the common practice of using the NST primarily may be sacrificing accuracy for convenience. We don't believe so, but the question has been raised and more information is needed.] ◀

4–12 **External Physical Stimulation of Human Fetus During Episodes of Low Heart Rate Variation.** Shaking the fetus through the maternal abdomen during a nonreactive heart rate episode is a maneuver often used to determine whether the fetus is well, but no systematic studies have shown that a reactive heart rate can be produced in this way in the healthy fetus. G. H. A. Visser, H. J. Zeelenberg, J. I. P. de Vries, and G. S. Dawes undertook a controlled study of this maneuver in 10 healthy nulliparous women near term with normal pregnancies. The subsequent outcome was uneventful in all cases. Heart rate monitoring was combined with real-time scanning to assess body movements and fetal breathing. Recordings were made with the patient in bed, usually semirecumbent, over two or more 1-hour periods.

Two episodes of low variation were assessed in each fetus, one in association with external stimulation. No differences in duration of the nonreactive trace or heart rate variation, or in the incidence of breathing or body movements, were noted with and without stimulation. The lengths of time during which the fetal heart remained unreactive with and without shaking were nearly identical. The longest nonreactive episode without stimulation lasted for 35 minutes and that with stimulation, 34 minutes.

Shaking the fetus during a nonreactive heart rate episode appears to serve no useful purpose. It may lead to oxytocin stress testing with false positive reactions. It is best to continue monitoring until the heart rate pattern changes spontaneously. Episodes of low heart rate variation near term may last for 40 minutes, and only longer-lasting nonreactive traces should be considered suspicious. It is not the heart rate pattern itself, but the underlying fetal behavioral state that is properly said to be nonreactive.

▶ [If the fetal heart rate pattern is "nonreactive," it simply may mean the fetus is in a state of "quiet sleep." The not uncommon clinical practice of stimulating the fetus

---

(4–12) Am. J. Obstet. Gynecol. 145:579–584, Mar. 1, 1983.

to "awaken" him or her is not useful, according to these authors. Expectancy is the answer; the episodes of low variations don't generally last longer than 40 minutes. Richardson et al. reported similar findings (1982 YEAR BOOK, pp. 108–109).] ◀

4–13 **Perinatal Outcome in Absence of Antepartum Fetal Heart Rate Acceleration.** Kenneth J. Leveno, M. Lynne Williams, Ralph T. DePalma, and Peggy J. Whalley (Univ. of Texas Health Science Center, Dallas) examined the outcome of 27 pregnancies in which fetal heart rate acceleration due to movement was either absent or amounted to less than 10 beats per minute during an 80-minute antepartum recording period. Recordings were made with an electronic fetal monitor having a Doppler transducer. None of the women received medications known to sedate the fetus. Contraction stress tests were carried out immediately in most instances. All live-born infants were delivered by cesarean section without labor, performed under general anesthesia.

The most common primary pregnancy complications were preeclampsia with suspected fetal growth retardation in 13 patients and chronic hypertension in 8. In all, 20 women had preeclampsia as either a primary or secondary complication. All pregnancies had features consistent with uteroplacental insufficiency. Fetal growth retardation was present in 74%, oligohydramnios in 81%, fetal acidosis in 41%, meconium in 30%, and placental infarction in 93%. There were 4 fetal and 7 neonatal deaths, for a perinatal mortality of 41%. The condition at birth of the infants who died neonatally appeared to be so poor as to preclude survival. The surviving infants were chronologically older than the others, and most of them were delivered the same day that fetal heart rate acceleration was found to be deficient. Also, they usually were in good acid-base balance at birth. Only 3 of the 16 survivors had serious complications in the neonatal period.

An 80-minute fetal activity test that demonstrates acceleration to be absent or persistently less than 10 beats per minute in response to spontaneous movement indicates perinatal pathology. All fetuses with such test results had findings consistent with uteroplacental insufficiency. Only 16 of 27 fetuses in the present study survived, and 1 of them is neurologically damaged. Although mortality has improved with prompt intervention, some of these fetuses may be in such poor condition that they cannot survive the neonatal period.

▶ [The most common cause of the nonreactive nonstress test is a "sleeping" fetus (i.e., there is neither fetal heart rate acceleration nor fetal movement). This series describes a much more ominous circumstance in which the heart rate fails to accelerate in conjunction with fetal body movements perceived by the pregnant woman. This finding should prompt immediate intervention according to the authors of this report.] ◀

4–14 **Comparison of Antepartum Testing Schemes For the Management of Postdate Pregnancy.** Robert D. Eden, Robert Z. Gergely, Barry S. Schifrin, and Maclyn E. Wade (Univ. of Southern California, Los Angeles) analyzed the outcome of 583 postdate pregnancies managed prospectively by one of three antepartum testing schemes, each predicted on the nonstress test. In scheme 1, the con-

---

(4–13) Obstet. Gynecol. 61:347–355, March 1983.
(4–14) Am. J. Obstet. Gynecol. 144:683–692, Nov. 15, 1982.

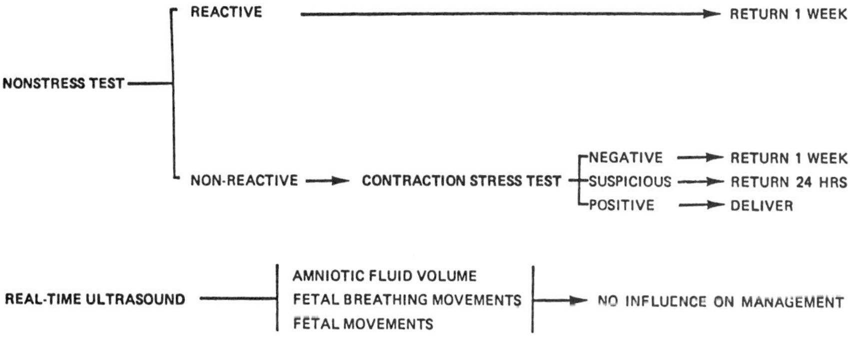

Fig 4–2.—Scheme 1 showing weekly nonstress test and contraction stress test protocol. (Courtesy of Eden, R. D., et al.: Am. J. Obstet. Gynecol. 144:683–692, Nov. 15, 1982.)

traction stress test was used for evaluation of the nonreactive nonstress test. In scheme 2, a modified biophysical profile was used to evaluate the nonreactive nonstress test and patients were tested semiweekly. In scheme 3, routine weekly ultrasound evaluation of volume of amniotic fluid was added to scheme 2. Only in scheme 3 was labor induced because of decreased volume of amniotic fluid or fetal cardiac decelerations irrespective of reactivity. Figures 4–2 and 4–3 show schemes 1 and 3, respectively.

Table 1 shows the comparison between perinatal morbidity and mortality according to testing schemes. Both parameters varied significantly according to scheme; incidence of neonatal resuscitation, meconium aspiration, and low 5-minute Apgar score was significantly higher in scheme 1 than in schemes 2 and 3. Table 2 compares schemes 1 and 3 according to the presence or absence of decelerations in fetal heart rate. The majority (86.4%) of fetuses with decelerations in fetal heart rate during the nonstress test showed these decelerations during labor.

Six perinatal deaths occurred in the entire series of 583 patients. Three deaths were related to congenital anomalies incompatible with life; the other 3 deaths occurred in patients with both reactive and nonreactive nonstress tests. One death occurred under scheme 1, the other 2 occurred under scheme 2.

Fig 4–3.—Scheme 3 showing semiweekly nonstress test and weekly amniotic fluid volume *(AFV)* determination plus real-time B-scanning *(RTBS)* protocol. (Courtesy of Eden, R. D., et al.: Am. J. Obstet. Gynecol. 144:683–692, Nov. 15, 1982.)

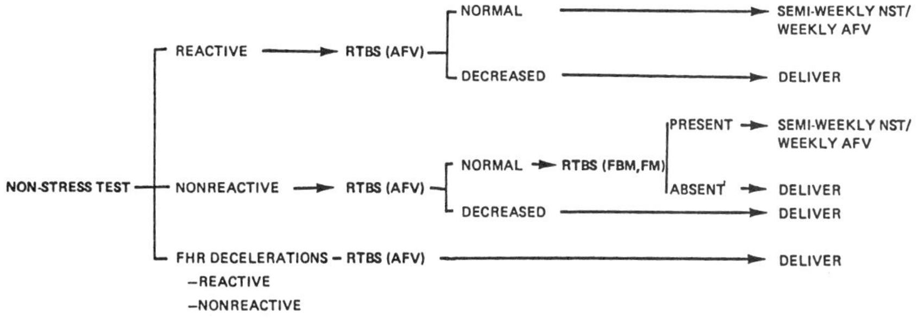

TABLE 1.—COMPARISON OF PERINATAL MORBIDITY AND MORTALITY ACCORDING TO TESTING SCHEMES

	Scheme 1	*Scheme 2*	*Scheme 3*
No. of patients	78	398	109
1-minute Apgar score <7 (%)	15.4	13.1	7.3
5-minute Apgar score <7 (%)	10.3*	2.3	0†
Resuscitation (%)	12.8*	10.1‡	0†
Macrosomia (%)	21.8	30.8	28.4
Postmaturity syndrome (%)	5.1	2.8	0
Meconium aspiration (%)	6.4*	1.3	0†
Morbidity (%)	25.6*	14.3‡	5.5†
Mortality rate (corrected)	12.8	5.0	0

*$P < .05$ between schemes 1 and 2.
†$P < .05$ between schemes 1 and 3.
‡$P < .05$ between schemes 2 and 3.
(Courtesy of Eden, R. D., et al.: Am. J. Obstet. Gynecol. 144:683–692, Nov. 15, 1982.)

Results of this study confirm the relationship among oligohydramnios, decelerations in fetal heart rate, and postmaturity syndrome. The evidence suggests that the reactive nonstress test is at least as good a predictor of immediate normal outcome as negative contraction stress tests and that prolongation of pregnancy in postdate pregnancy increases the risk of abnormal outcome. These results suggest a benefit from both semiweekly testing and liberalized criteria for intervention in these pregnancies.

▶ [Postdatism is the most frequent indication for antepartum fetal well-being testing in the United States. This report compares various testing strategies. In scheme 3 the nonstress test (NST) was performed twice a week and ultrasound weekly. Decelerations of 30 seconds in duration during the NST (whether reactive or nonreactive) and oligohydramnios were indications to effect delivery. The results in scheme 3 were excellent, but the rates of intervention (24%) and cesarean section (29%) were high and the immediate dollar costs must have been, too. Estriol determinations are con-

TABLE 2.—PERINATAL OUTCOME ACCORDING TO SCHEME AND PRESENCE OF DECELERATIONS IN FETAL HEART RATE

	Scheme 1		*Scheme 3*	
	FHR decelerations absent	*FHR decelerations present*	*FHR decelerations absent*	*FHR decelerations present*
No. of patients	68	10	97	12
Reactive NST (last test) (%)	88.2*	50.0	92.9*	58.3
Decreased amniotic fluid volume (%)	27.9*	80.0	14.4*	100.0
Meconium (%)	32.4*	80.0	17.6*	50.0
FHR abnormalities (%)	42.7*	90.0	30.9*	83.3
Fetal distress (%)	22.1	50.0	3.1*	25.0
Cesarean section (%)	10.3	20.0	27.8*	41.7
1-minute Apgar score <7 (%)	10.3*	50.0	5.1	25.0
5-minute Apgar score <7 (%)	5.9*	40.0	0	0†
Resuscitation (%)	8.8*	50.0	0	0†
Macrosomia	25.0	0	28.9	25.0
Postmaturity syndrome (%)	4.4	10.0	0	0
Meconium aspiration (%)	7.3	10.0	0	0
Morbidity (%)	20.6*	60.0	3.1*	25.0†

*Comparison of presence or absence of decelerations in fetal heart rate with each scheme, $P < .05$.
Comparison between decelerations in fetal heart rate of schemes 1 and 3, $P < .05$.
(Courtesy of Eden, R. D., et al.: Am. J. Obstet. Gynecol. 144:683–692, Nov. 15, 1982.)

sidered worthwhile by others in this situation (1983 YEAR BOOK, pp. 34–35), but were not used here. Fetal heart rate decelerations during the NST may reflect cord compression related to decreased amniotic fluid volume. The authors' opinion, that delivery should be effected in the postdate patient if decelerations are present on the NST, even if it is "reactive," is probably on target.] ◀

4–15 **Correlation of Ultrasonic Placental Grading and Fetal Pulmonary Maturation in 563 Pregnancies.** In a previous study it was suggested that the presence of a grade III placenta correlates 100% with a mature lecithin-sphingomyelin (L/S) ratio and may replace amniocentesis in confirming fetal lung maturity. C. R. Harman, F. A. Manning, E. Stearns, and I. Morrison (Univ. of Manitoba) tested this hypothesis by studying 563 pregnancies. All patients underwent amniocentesis and simultaneously had placental grading.

Six patients had grade 0 placentas; 158, grade I; 269, grade II; and 130, grade III. Nine of the 130 patients with grade III placentas had an L/S ratio less than 2.0. Correlations between placental grade and a mature L/S ratio were grade 0, 17%; grade I, 68%; grade II, 91%; and grade III, 93%. Biparietal diameter (BPD) was accurately determined in 235 patients. A BPD of greater than or equal to 9.0 cm correlated with an L/S ratio of greater than or equal to 2.0 in 79%, whereas a BPD of less than 9.0 cm was associated with a mature L/S ratio in 80%. Date of last normal menstrual period allowed assignment of gestational age with certainty in 402 patients. Placental grade was distributed as follows: grade 0, all less than 37 weeks' gestation; grade I, 71% less than 37 weeks; grade II, 75% greater than 37 weeks and grade III, 86% greater than 37 weeks.

The results of this study show that placental grading by ultrasound is not accurate enough to eliminate the need for amniocentesis. The presence of grade III placenta may offer assistance in specific instances, but in a large group of patients, it falsely predicted pulmonary maturity in 6.9%. The phospholipid profile of amniotic fluid remains the standard means of predicting fetal lung maturity in the authors' institution.

▶ [There is an association between the L/S ratio and the presence of phosphatidylglycerol and the "grade" of the placenta as determined by ultrasound. The authors of this report found that the association was not tight enough to permit one to regard a grade III placenta as uniformly indicating an L/S ratio ≥2.0. The L/S ratio and phosphatidylglycerol positive distributions did not differ between patients with grade II and grade III placentas. The ultrasonographic appearance of the placenta may play an adjunctive role in clinical decision-making, but it probably shouldn't replace amniotic fluid analysis.] ◀

4–16 **Amniotic Fluid Phosphatidylglycerol and the Lecithin/Sphingomyelin Ratio in Assessment of Fetal Lung Maturity.** M. J. Whittle, A. I. Wilson, C. R. Whitfield, R. D. Paton, and R. W. Logan (Glasgow) modified the standard technique to assess fetal lung maturity by estimating the lecithin-sphingomyelin (L/S) ratio. The modification included measuring only the amniotic fluid L/S ratio and noting the presence or absence of phosphatidylglycerol (PG). Quantitation of PG did not improve the predictive ability of the test. The

(4–15) Am. J. Obstet. Gynecol. 143:941–943, Aug. 15, 1982.
(4–16) Br. J. Obstet. Gynaecol. 89:727–732, September 1982.

AMNIOTIC FLUID LECITHIN-SPHINGOMYELIN (L/S) RATIO AND PHOSPHATIDYLGLYCEROL (PG) STATUS IN ALL SAMPLES COLLECTED WITHIN 72 HOURS OF DELIVERY AND INCIDENCE OF RESPIRATORY DISTRESS SYNDROME (RDS)

L/S ratio	No.	PG present	RDS (%)	PG absent	RDS (%)
⩾2·0	445	444	0	1	0
<2·0	116	88	3[a] (3·4)	28	24[b] (85·7)
Total	561	532	3 (0·6)	29	24 (82·8)

[a]Two babies died.
[b]Nine babies died.
(Courtesy of Whittle, M. J., et al.: Br. J. Obstet. Gynaecol. 89:727–732, September 1982.)

authors' preliminary report showed that, with an L/S ratio ≥2.0 and PG present, no baby developed neonatal respiratory distress syndrome (RDS) but 75% of babies were affected when the L/S ratio was <2.0 and PG was absent. When L/S ratio was <2.0 and PG was present, 9% of babies developed RDS.

In this series, 561 consecutive patients, from whom amniotic fluid had been collected within 72 hours of delivery, were studied. The table relates the findings in all amniotic fluids. With amniotic fluid PG alone, only 3 of 532 (0.6%) babies developed RDS when PG was present, compared with 24 of 29 (83%) babies (including 9 deaths) when it was absent. The predictive ability was improved by knowing the L/S ratio because in the presence of both PG and a mature L/S ratio (≥2.0), no baby developed RDS, whereas 3.4% of them did when the ratio was immature despite the presence of PG. The sensitivity of PG detection alone, in samples collected from the vagina, was 94%, and the specificity was 99.6%. Incorporating the L/S ratio raised sensitivity to 100% but specificity was reduced to 86%.

The authors recommend the results of the two tests be reported as one of four combinations: category I—PG present, L/S ratio ≥2.0, which indicates with virtual certainty that fetal lung maturation is complete and RDS will not develop; category II—PG present, L/S <2.0, which carries a slight but significant risk of RDS; category III—PG absent, L/S ratio ≥2.0, which may mean a risk of RDS; category IV—PG absent, L/S ratio <2.0, which indicates there is a substantial risk of RDS, and delivery should be postponed.

▶ [This is an update of the Glasgow experience with the L/S ratio and PG (cf. 1982 YEAR BOOK, pp. 128–129). In the experience of the authors, PG was present more often than the L/S was ≥2.0. The former helped them characterize the RDS risk in patients with immature L/S ratios, thereby reducing the number of "false immature" test results. As we have said before (probably too often in your view!), methodologic differences between laboratories preclude extrapolation. When utilizing amniotic fluid phopholipid determinations in assessing fetal lung maturity, each obstetric service must learn what the values reported from its laboratory signify.] ◀

5. Labor and Operative Obstetrics

5–1 **Improvement in Perinatal Mortality Rate Attributed To Spontaneous Preterm Labor Without Use of Tocolytic Agents.** There presently is wide agreement in Europe that suspected preterm labor should be managed with tocolytic therapy, usually β-sympathomimetic drugs, and this is likely to occur in the United States as well. Peter Boylan and Kieran O'Driscoll (Univ. College Dublin) undertook a review of the influence of spontaneous preterm labor on perinatal mortality over a 15-year period at a hospital in which tocolytic agents have never been used. The series included 104,892 infants. Perinatal mortality declined from 48.3 in 1966 to 16.7 in 1980. The rate of perinatal mortality associated with preterm birth fell from 24.8 to 9.8 during this period. The incidence of spontaneous preterm labor fell from 4.4% to 2.9% and that of low birth weight infants declined from 8% to 4%. There was an overall upward shift in socioeconomic status of mothers during the review period and also a shift toward younger mothers.

A progressive decrease in number of perinatal deaths attributed to spontaneous preterm labor was documented in this study. No tocolytic therapy was used. The authors believe that the current enthusiasm for the use of tocolytic agents should be tempered with caution until these drugs are shown to lead to a reduction in perinatal deaths from spontaneous preterm labor exceeding that which could result from natural causes. The progressive decline in perinatal deaths due to spontaneous preterm labor could result from the less frequent occurrence of spontaneous preterm labor or from improved neonatal care.

▶ [The authors conclude, "[C]urrent enthusiasm for tocolytic agents should be tempered with caution until they can be shown to produce a reduction in perinatal deaths, *from spontaneous preterm labor,* exceeding that which could result from natural causes." It's been recognized for a long time that tocolytic therapy is not going to be *the* answer to the problem of prematurity (*Am. J. Obstet. Gynecol.* 113:704, 1972). Clearly, demographic and socioeconomic influences are important, and medical and obstetric situations in which tocolysis isn't applicable or doesn't work are frequent. Nonetheless, tocolytic therapy is valuable in selected circumstances. It seems to us that the demonstration asked for above has been provided already (Merkatz, I. R., et al.: *Obstet. Gynecol.* 56:7, 1980).] ◀

5–2 **Effect of Tocolysis on Incidence of Low Birth Weight.** Although tocolytic therapy initially promised a reduction in low birth weight deliveries, no reduction has been documented in countries where tocolytic agents are used extensively. Nergesh A. Tejani and Uma L. Verma (SUNY at Stony Brook) examined the role of tocolysis in reducing the incidence of low birth weight in a series of 570 consecutive low birth weight deliveries made in 1980 and 1981. Tocolysis

---

(5–1) Am. J. Obstet. Gynecol. 145:781–783, Apr. 1, 1983.
(5–2) Obstet. Gynecol. 61:556–558, May 1983.

was attempted in only 2.5% of cases. Neonatal mortality in infants weighing over 2,000 gm was 6.4/1,000 live births. Of cases in which the neonates weighed 2,000 gm or less, about one-fifth had severe maternal or fetal problems and the mothers were delivered or allowed to proceed in labor. Nearly one-third had premature membrane rupture, chorioamnionitis, or both. Thirteen percent had third-trimester bleeding as a contraindication to tocolysis. Ten percent of fetuses were small for gestational age, and fetal death or anomaly occurred in 9% of cases. Tocolysis was attempted prospectively in 13.8% of patients in preterm labor, with a success rate of 82%. Ritodrine was used most frequently. If tocolysis had not been attempted in these cases, the incidence of a birth weight below 2,500 gm would have increased from 11.7% to 12.6% and that of a birth weight of 2,000 gm or less from 5.6% to 6.4%. Neither change was statistically significant.

Tocolytic therapy cannot be applied in most cases of preterm labor and cannot be expected to eliminate preterm births. More emphasis should be placed on the nontraumatic delivery of small neonates in the best possible state of oxygenation and acid-base balance. Tocolysis is definitely beneficial in individual cases of uncomplicated premature labor, but it has failed to solve the problem of low birth weight in the larger sense. A reduction in the overall rate of low birth weight was an unrealistic expectation from tocolytic therapy. The long-term effects of the use of β-mimetic agents remain unknown.

▶ [Tocolytic therapy is valuable in individual cases but, as indicated by this study, it cannot be expected to make much of a dent in the statistics relating to preterm birth. Perhaps one reason we like this article is one of its concluding statements: "Ten years ago Zlatnik astutely predicted that tocolysis had limited application." There is an old saying, "When I'm right, nobody remembers, but if I'm wrong, nobody forgets," a lament that doesn't apply in this case.] ◀

5–3 **Potassium and Glucose Concentrations Without Treatment During Ritodrine Tocolysis.** The catecholamine effects of ritodrine are thought to induce glycogenolysis, resulting in increases in plasma glucose and insulin concentrations and a rise in intracellular potassium concentration, with a consequent fall in plasma potassium concentration. David C. Young, Ali Toofanian, and Kenneth J. Leveno (Univ. of Texas, Dallas) examined these effects of ritodrine in 27 consecutive women treated for labor before 34 weeks' gestation. Ritodrine was infused in normal saline, and patients did not receive potassium supplementation or corticosteroids. Ritodrine was begun at the rate of 50 μg per minute and increased until contractions stopped or a maximum of 350 μg per minute was reached. The effective dose was continued for 24 hours after the cessation of uterine contractions. Ritodrine then was given orally in a dosage of 20 mg every 3 hours until 36 weeks' gestation.

Maternal side effects necessitated a reduction in the dosage of ritodrine in 3 cases and discontinuance of therapy in 2. A significant increase in serum glucose concentration and a fall in serum potassium concentration continued throughout ritodrine infusion. The

---

(5–3) Am. J. Obstet. Gynecol. 145:105–106, Jan. 1, 1983.

highest glucose value was 175 mg/dl, and the lowest potassium concentration was 2.3 mEq/L. No clinical problems were attributed to these changes. No significant changes were observed during oral ritodrine therapy.

Ritodrine infusion causes significant changes in maternal glucose and potassium concentrations, which resolve without active intervention. No untoward clinical events occurred in the women in this study, from whom potassium supplementation was withheld. Insulin therapy did not appear to be warranted. Glucose and potassium concentrations should be measured before ritodrine therapy and 3 and 6 hours after the start of treatment. Ritodrine-induced metabolic changes could be of clinical importance in women with diabetes, renal disease, or cardiac abnormalities.

▶ [Maximum changes in serum glucose and potassium levels were observed 3–6 hours after the initiation of ritodrine tocolysis. This would seem to be the appropriate time to draw a blood specimen. We don't routinely administer potassium to these patients. Benedetti, in the same issue of the "gray journal" in which this article appeared (*Am. J. Obstet. Gynecol.* 145:1, Jan. 1, 1983), nicely reviews the maternal complications, including myocardial ischemia and cardiac arrhythmia, that can occur with parenteral β-sympathomimetic therapy for premature labor. Close observation of the patients (mother and fetus) is essential when these drugs are used.] ◀

5–4 **Simple Estimated Fetal Weight Equation Based on Real-Time Ultrasound Measurements of Fetuses Less Than 34 Weeks' Gestation.** Accurate antenatal determination of fetal weight can be helpful in planning management when delivery of a preterm infant is anticipated. Gary R. Thurnau, Ralph K. Tamura, Rudy Sabbagha, O. Richard Depp, III, Alan Dyer, Ron Larkin, Timothy Lee, and Colby Laughlin attempted to develop a simple equation based on real-time ultrasonography that could be accurately applied to preterm or low birth weight infants. Real-time ultrasound measurements of fetal biparietal diameter (BPD) and abdominal circumference (AC) were obtained in 62 pregnant women within a week of premature delivery. The mean gestational age was 28.5 weeks, and the mean birth weight was 1,135 gm.

Computer analysis yielded the following regression equation: $EFW = (BPD \times AC \times 9.337) - 299$, where EFW is the predicted estimated fetal weight. The coefficient of correlation of EFW with actual birth weight was 0.957. Analysis of results in 19 prospective cases showed an absolute mean difference between EFWs and actual birth weights of within 7% of actual weight, or 70 gm/kg of actual birth weight. The standard deviation of the difference was 9.3%, or 93 gm/kg of actual birth weight.

This simple equation appears to be a clinically reliable, easily used means of estimating the weights of preterm or low birth weight infants of less than 2,500 gm. Further prospective testing is needed to determine the applicability of the equation to fetuses weighing less than 1,000 gm.

▶ [An important management decision that must be made in patients in premature labor is whether or not there should be intervention (i.e., cesarean section) for fetal distress. Is the fetus far enough along in gestation and large enough to have a decent

(5–4) Am. J. Obstet. Gynecol. 145:557–561, Mar. 1, 1983.

chance of survival? An accurate estimate of fetal weight is valuable in this situation. Because we do not do very well in our clinical estimates, various ultrasound formulas have been proposed. The preliminary results reported here look good; an advantage of the formula advocated by these authors is its simplicity.] ◀

5–5 **Prelabor Evaluation of Inducibility.** Aksel P. Lange, Niels J. Secher, Jes G. Westergaard, and Ib Skovgård prospectively studied the predictive value of the Bishop pelvic score on the duration of labor in 1,189 women, of whom 381 were admitted for stimulation of labor because of premature rupture of the membranes and 808 were admitted for induction of labor (by primary amniotomy in 337 and by other methods in 471 who had relatively unfavorable cervical conditions). All inductions were for medical or obstetric reasons. Induction of labor failed on the first day in 181 of the 471 women (38.4%) with an unfavorable cervix. All women were eventually delivered vaginally of one living infant in cephalic presentation.

The predictive value of the Bishop score and other factors regarding the duration of labor (time from induction to delivery) and inducibility of labor (latency period from commencement of treatment to establishment of labor) were evaluated by multiple regression analyses. Maternal age, gestational age, and fetal weight were not significantly related to duration of labor. Parity had a very constant and highly significant influence on duration of labor, whereas it had little effect on inducibility. The only factor significantly related to inducibility was the prelabor cervical condition. Of the five components of the Bishop score, dilatation was most important; it should be weighted at at least twice the value given it by Bishop.

The authors have proposed a new cervical score system for prelabor evaluation of inducibility. In contrast to the Bishop pelvic scoring system, the weight of cervix dilatation is doubled, consistency and position of the cervix are omitted, and station of the presenting fetal part and length of the cervix are unchanged. The new system is simple, accurate, and reproducible. It gives an almost straight-line correlation between scores and success rates. It is simpler than the Bishop system and easier to remember, making it more suitable for routine use.

The decisive factor as to whether labor is inducible or not is almost entirely the cervical condition, especially degree of dilatation. A closed cervix is the worst possible prognostic sign, regardless of most other factors. If primary amniotomy can be carried out, delivery is inducible inasmuch as all patients will give birth the same day. If primary amniotomy is not performed, nearly all will deliver the same day if the new score is 8 or above. If the score is 5 to 7, the success rate will be 75% or more. With a score of 4 or less, there will be a considerable failure rate.

▶ [The authors of this analysis of the components of the Bishop score reach similar conclusions to those reached by E. A. Friedman several years ago. Dilatation is the most important predictor of the ease of induction of labor. The station of the vertex and the effacement of the cervix are each about half as important as the dilatation. Once these three factors are considered, the consistency and position of the cervix don't add much information.] ◀

(5–5) Obstet. Gynecol. 60:137–147, August 1982.

5–6 ***Laminaria* for Preinduction Cervical Ripening.** Roger H. Gower, Jules Toraya, and Joseph M. Miller, Jr. (Med. Univ. of South Carolina) conducted a controlled, randomized double-blind study to test the safety and efficacy of *Laminaria japonica,* a popular cervical dilator in the middle of the 19th century, as a preinduction cervical ripening agent. A 2-day induction with amniotomy on day 2 was allowed. Forty-eight patients were studied, including 22 controls. All patients had a Bishop score of 5 or lower. Successful induction was defined as one that progressed to the active phase of labor.

In this high-risk group of patients fetal distress developed in 5, who consequently underwent cesarean section prior to entering the active phase of labor. These cases were removed from further statistical consideration, leaving 23 patients in the *Laminaria* group and 20 in the control group. *Laminaria* significantly improved the Bishop score from a mean of 3.0 before to 6.7 after insertion. The control group began with a Bishop score that was significantly more favorable than that of the *Laminaria* group (3.8 versus 3.0) and also underwent a small change toward favorability overnight (from a mean of 3.8 to 4.5). *Laminaria* was significantly better than placebo for ripening the cervix.

There was a high rate of successful induction in both groups: 91% for the *Laminaria* group and 90% for controls. There was no significant difference in the mean length of induction between the two groups. Endometritis occurred in 3 patients in the *Laminaria* group after cesarean section and in 3 patients in the control group, 2 after cesarean section and 1 after spontaneous vaginal delivery. There were no neonatal infections.

The authors conclude the chief benefit of *Laminaria* is its ability to dilate the cervix overnight and improve the Bishop score. In practice, this would facilitate amniotomy, especially with the extremely unfavorable cervix. This study also supports the safety of *Laminaria,* even in conjunction with a 2-day induction. However, the success rate reported by other researchers is not confirmed. Therefore, for a standard 2-day induction protocol, *Laminaria* offers no clear advantage.

5–7 **Efficacy and Safety of *Laminaria Digitata* for Preinduction Ripening of Cervix.** George M. Kazzi, Sidney F. Bottoms, and Mortimer G. Rosen (Cleveland) used *Laminaria* tents for cervical ripening in 25 women prior to induction carried out for obstetric indications such as preeclampsia or diabetes mellitus. Results were compared with those of 28 matched patients undergoing induction without the use of *Laminaria.* Only about half the patients in each group were at term. Patients delivered by cesarean section received prophylactic antibiotics after operation.

Laminaria tents appeared to be effective in reducing the duration of induction in women with a very unfavorable cervix. However, they did not reduce the incidence of cesarean births and they appeared to increase the incidence of endometritis (in both cesarean and vaginal deliveries), neonatal sepsis, and neonatal death (table). Of the 5 in-

---

(5–6) Obstet. Gynecol. 60:617–619, November 1982.
(5–7) Ibid., pp. 440–443, October 1982.

OUTCOME OF INDUCTION IN STUDY AND CONTROL GROUPS

	Study	Control	P
No. of patients	25	28	
Cesarean delivery	9	11	NS
Vaginal delivery	16	17	NS
Endometritis	15	3	<.05
Cesarean	9/9	3/11	<.005
Vaginal	6/16	0/17	<.001
Neonatal sepsis	5	0	<.05
Neonatal death	3	0	<.1

NS = not significant.
(Courtesy of Kazzi, G. M., et al.: Obstet. Gynecol. 60:440–443, October 1982. Reprinted with permission from The American College of Obstetricians and Gynecologists.)

fants with sepsis, 4 were less than 36 weeks' gestational age. These 4 had blood cultures showing group B β-hemolytic streptococci (3 cases) or *Enterobacter* organisms (1 case). The frequency of sepsis due to group B β-hemolytic streptococci was 16%, compared to a usual attack rate of such organisms of 0.1% to 0.2% of live births.

The reasons for the high rates of serious maternal and neonatal morbidity in this series, as compared with other reports showing the safety of *Laminaria,* are not known. The presence of a large number of preterm pregnancies in the present series may be a factor. Further research is needed to establish guidelines (such as avoiding the use of *Laminaria* in preterm pregnancies and assessing the cervix bacteriologically) and to document safety before considering *Laminaria* for widespread use.

▶ [*Laminaria* tents have been used on our service for some time to "ripen" the unfavorable cervix prior to induction. In fact, the original publication on the subject came from us (Cross and Pitkin: *Obstet. Gynecol.* 51:606, 1978). We found the preceding article by Gower et al. difficult to interpret. Although *Laminaria* tents did seem to increase cervical ripening, the "hours of induction" didn't differ between control and experimental groups. The 2-day induction format further complicates the issue.

We don't regard *Laminaria* tents as anything like a perfect answer to this difficult dilemma, but we've had little reason to question their safety. Thus, the report of Kazzi and colleagues noting an apparently high incidence of maternal and perinatal infection is alarming. The study is retrospective, with "controls" selected from a computerized data base. Nevertheless, the high rates of infections listed in the table can't and shouldn't be dismissed. Clearly, more study of the safety issue is needed.] ◀

5–8 **Use of Breast Stimulation To Ripen Cervix in Term Pregnancies.** John P. Elliott and James F. Flaherty (Letterman Army Med. Center, San Francisco) evaluated breast stimulation for "ripening" the cervix in 81 women at 39 weeks' gestation or later. All had uncomplicated prenatal courses and were at low risk of uteroplacental insufficiency. Study patients were asked to stimulate the breasts by gentle massage with a warm, moist cloth for 1 hour 3 times a day. After completing a blind randomized trial, 40 patients participated in a crossover trial with 3-day study periods. Patients avoided intercourse throughout the study period.

(5–8) Am. J. Obstet. Gynecol. 145:553–556, Mar. 1, 1983.

PATIENT CHARACTERISTICS AND OUTCOME OF COMBINED STUDY

Factor ± *SD*

Factor	*Breast-stimulated group*	*Control group*	*Level of significance*
No. of patients	42	36	—
Age (yr)	24.8 ± 5.2	24.5 ± 4.8	NS
Parity	0.7 ± 0.8	0.7 ± 1.0	NS
Initial Bishop score	5.1 ± 2.8	4.4 ± 2.5	NS
Gestational age (weeks)	40.0 ± 0.7	39.7 ± 0.7	NS
Birth weight (gm)	3,396 ± 403	3,522 ± 443	NS
Change in Bishop score	2.4 ± 1.7	0.35 ± 1.5	$p < 0.0001$
No. in labor	19/42 (45%)	2/36 (6%)	$p < 0.0001$

NS = not significant.
(Courtesy of Elliott, J. P., and Flaherty, J. F.: Am. J. Obstet. Gynecol. 145:553–556, Mar. 1, 1983.)

The mean change in Bishop score was significantly greater in study than in control patients. Eleven of 22 study patients and 1 of 16 controls entered labor during the 3-day trial period. Cervical dilatation, effacement, and station all progressed significantly more in breast-stimulated women. A significant difference favoring breast stimulation also was noted in the crossover trial. Five of 19 breast-stimulated patients and 1 of 9 controls entered labor. The combined results are given in the table. Of breast-stimulated patients, 45% went into labor during the trial, as did only 6% of controls.

Breast stimulation for 3 days was associated with onset of labor in 45% of these term patients. The Bishop score was increased by a mean of 2.4 points in patients not going into labor. The chance of labor and change in Bishop score were not related to state of the cervix at the start of the trial. The mechanism by which breast stimulation acts to enhance cervical dilatation and promote labor requires further study. The role of oxytocin or prostaglandins in the changes related to breast stimulation is unknown.

▶ [These results are somewhat surprising. Breast stimulation (3 hours per day for 3 days) was associated with the onset of labor in 45% of the patients and a significant improvement in Bishop score in the remainder. We would have guessed that more control patients would have labored during the 3-day study period. If breast stimulation is effective, it may act through oxytocin release. The authors don't comment on orgasm or genital stimulation in the study patients. We are certain to see others report their experience with this technique. If the efficacy of breast stimulation for this purpose is confirmed, a simple, inexpensive, and presumably safe tool will have been added to the obstetrician's armamentarium.] ◀

5–9 **Evidence for Local Effect of Intracervical Prostaglandin E_2 Gel.** In a recent study, intracervical application of 2.5 ml of prostaglandin E_2 (PGE_2) gel was found to stimulate myometrial activity. Axel Forman, Ulf Ulmsten, Jolán Bányai, Lars Wingerup, and Niels

(5–9) Am. J. Obstet. Gynecol. 143:756–760, Aug. 1, 1982.

Uldbjerg hypothesized that reduction in gel volume, together with an exact technique of application, might have a local priming effect on the cervix without enhancing myometrial contractions.

Studies were conducted in 8 primigravid women, aged 18 to 24 years, who were admitted to an outpatient clinic at 9 or 10 weeks' gestation for abortion by dilation and evacuation. Four randomly selected women received 0.5 mg of PGE_2 in 0.5 ml of viscous gel instilled strictly within the cervical canal by means of a 12-cm long catheter that had an outer diameter of 3 mm and two side holes near the tip. Gel deposition was started below the internal os and continued during slow withdrawal of the catheter. Gel did not flow into the vagina. The other 4 women received intravenous infusion of oxytocin, which was started with a bolus injection of 3 IU and continued at 120 mIU/minute. Evacuation was performed 6 hours after PGE_2 or oxytocin treatment was begun.

In patients treated with PGE_2, cervical dilation increased from 4.0 to 7.3 mm, and cervical consistency improved from 1.3 to 2.3 (on a 3-point scoring scale). At evacuation the final dilation was performed easily. There were no regular uterine contractions although a transient rise in tone and isolated contractions sometimes occurred. In patients treated with oxytocin, no improvement in cervical state occurred and subsequent dilation was more difficult in these patients. A rise in uterine tone of 10 to 45 mm Hg, with superimposed contractions of 5 to 15 mm Hg occurred, and uterine activity remained elevated throughout the recording period. Mean 15-minute integrated activity was 148 mm Hg for the oxytocin group and 21 mm Hg for the PGE_2 group.

Intracervical PGE_2 gel apparently has direct effects on the cervical tissues independent of uterine contractile activity. Myometrial stimulation induced by escape of gel into the extra-amniotic space can be avoided by adjusting the volume of gel and the technique of application to the dimensions of the cervix.

▶ [Whether the "ripening" effect of PGE_2 on the cervix is independent of uterine activity is an extremely important, yet unresolved, question. This present study involving a small number of pregnant women in the first trimester is consistent with the view that there is a direct effect unrelated to myometrial contractions. If this is true at term, one might avoid or minimize important risks associated with any oxytocic agent, namely, uterine hyperstimulation or uterine rupture. As we said above, however, the issue is not settled.] ◀

5–10 **Chronic Stimulation of Uterine Prostaglandin Synthesis During Cervical Ripening Before Onset of Labor.** Softening and increasing compliance of the cervix are essential for its efficient dilatation during labor, and prostaglandins have been implicated in this process because of their successful use in ripening the unfavorable cervix before labor is induced. There is, however, no evidence of a direct relation between cervical changes and prostaglandin synthesis in human pregnancy.

Marc J. N. C. Keirse, Michel Thiery, Walter Parewijck, and Murray D. Mitchell examined prostaglandin release at term during cervical

---

(5–10) Prostaglandins 25:671–682, May 1983.

CONCENTRATIONS OF PGFM IN MATERNAL PERIPHERAL CIRCULATION BEFORE AND AFTER EXTRA-AMNIOTIC INSERTION OF FOLEY CATHETER WITH OR WITHOUT TYLOSE GEL*

Interval after Foley insertion	PGFM levels (mean ± SEM) pg/ml (n=6)	% of initial values	Statistical difference (Wilcoxon) with pre-insertion values
before	91 ± 11	100 ± 0	-
5 min.	135 ± 19	154 ± 25	$P < 0.025$
6 hours	152 ± 20	179 ± 32	$P < 0.01$
12 hours	143 ± 32	169 ± 45	$0.05 < p < 0.1$

*PGFM = 13,14-dihydro-15-keto-$PGF2_{\alpha}$.
(Courtesy of Keirse, M. J. N. C., et al.: Prostaglandins 25:671–682, May 1983.)

ripening and independently of uterine activation in 6 normal primigravid women with uncomplicated pregnancies, who had elected to be induced at term. All were at 38–41 weeks' gestation and had Bishop scores of 3 or less. After a Foley catheter was inserted extra-amniotically, 3 women also received a nonmedicated methylhydroxyethyl cellulose suspension (Tylose) that was administered extra-amniotically in a dose of 0.5 gm, after which the catheter was either deflated and removed or left in place.

Prostaglandin concentrations in the maternal peripheral circulation of these women are shown in the table. Catheter insertion led to an acute elevation that persisted for at least 6 hours, and administration of Tylose gel caused a greater rise in prostaglandin concentration that lasted for 12 hours or longer. This effect was noted regardless of whether the catheter was removed or remained in place. The patient with the greatest response at 5 minutes exhibited the most marked cervical effect. Two patients not given Tylose who had no uterine contractility had the smallest elevations in prostaglandin levels.

Cervical ripening by nonpharmacologic means is associated with prolonged prostaglandin elevation in the maternal circulation. Lasting stimulation of intrauterine production of prostaglandin can be evoked at term, well before the onset of labor-like uterine activation. An increase in prostaglandin synthesis may cause not only uterine contractility, but also cervical ripening and possibly even rupture of the fetal membranes.

▶ [Assuming that blood levels of prostaglandin (PG) metabolites reflect PG release, these findings indicate that a mechanical means of cervical ripening causes prompt and sustained release of $PGF_{2\alpha}$. Because the cervix changed but patients did not enter labor, it would seem that the cervical effect resulted from direct PG action rather than secondary to uterine contractions. However, as we noted above, this point is far from settled.

In a related study, Manabe and colleagues (*Gynecol. Obstet. Invest.* 15:343, 1983) measured amniotic PGE and PGF levels before and after insertion of a rubber bougie into the cervix. The α-fetoprotein PG levels increased markedly, but sampling was not done until there had been enough labor to dilate the cervix to 3–4 cm, so it cannot be determined whether the increase bore a cause or effect relationship to uterine contractions.] ◀

5–11 **Impact of Sex Ratio on Onset and Management of Labor.** Marion H. Hall and Roy Carr-Hill (Univ. of Aberdeen) studied the sex ratio in a large series of births with special reference to whether or not labor was induced and then related the sex ratio to factors such as parity, birth weight, and mode of delivery.

Records of all 52,266 live singleton deliveries for the total population in Aberdeen City District between 1961 and 1979 were studied. When analysis was by gestational age, only the 41,456 in which this was certain were included. Among all the births during this time period, the overall sex ratio was 105.6 boys to 100 girls, and the variation according to parity was small. The previous observation that boys were more likely to be delivered at earlier gestation than girls was confirmed and was true of all parities. Births of boys were statistically less likely to be induced than births of girls, the sex ratio in all induced labors being 100.9 compared with 105.0 in spontaneous labors. Births of girls were more likely to be induced after term, partly because they were still undelivered. The overall sex ratio in cesarean sections was high—that is, more boys were delivered by cesarean section than girls. Birth weight analysis by gestation for spontaneous labors showed the sex ratio of 967 low birth weight babies was 92.2 while that of 871 large babies was 178.3. Boys were much more likely to be delivered by forceps or emergency cesarean section and less likely to be delivered spontaneously or by vaginal breech delivery (table). Analysis of fetal presentation at delivery for those delivered between 1976 to 1979 showed that breech presentation was more common in pregnancies with girls (4%) than with boys (3%).

The earlier delivery of boys did not seem to be due to induction or elective cesarean section and thus was unlikely to be due to any antenatal pathology. Cephalopelvic disproportion may occur more often with boys because of the greater weight of male babies, or the male fetal hormonal contribution to the progress of labor may be less effective than the female, thus resulting in maternal uterine dysfunction.

▶ [This immense data base permits some interesting observations. If the onset of labor is spontaneous, boy babies are delivered at earlier gestational ages than are girl babies. Is this due to differences in weight or to differences in fetal hormone production? If the latter pertains, is it an estrogen, a corticosteroid, or testosterone that is the key? Girl fetuses are more apt to be breeches and to have labor induced (presumably for postdatism).] ◀

Sex Ratio and Mode of Delivery in Breech Presentations (1976–1979 Cases)

Mode of delivery	No of births		Sex ratio (male per 100 female births)
	Boys	Girls	
Spontaneous	20 790	20 391	102·0
Forceps	3 825	3 005	127·3
Caesarean section	1 846	1 570	117·6
Breech	388	451	86·0
Total	26 849	25 417	105·6

(Courtesy of Hall, M. H., and Carr-Hill, R.: Br. Med. J. 285:401–403, Aug. 7, 1982.)

(5–11) Br. Med. J. 285:401–403, Aug. 7, 1982.

5–12 **The 24-Hour Rhythmicity of Birth: Population Study.** Many studies have suggested a 24-hour rhythmicity in both the onset and the culmination of spontaneous births, but most investigations have been based on relatively small or selected samples, or both. Eystein Glattre and Tor Bjerkedal (Univ. of Oslo) examined this question in over 617,000 births occurring in Norway between 1968 and 1977. The hourly incidence of various categories of births in pregnancies lasting 16 weeks or longer was determined. The curve for hourly incidence of births of spontaneous onset and parturition coincided closely with previous findings. When multiple births were excluded and first and later births in northern and southern Norway were examined, dissimilarities appeared between the respective 24-hour incidence curves. The rhythmicities of births with delivery intervention, induced births, and induced births with delivery intervention appeared to reflect the work activity rhythms of hospital staff.

The findings indicate that 24-hour variations in birth incidence have an underlying endogenous, circadian rhythmicity, possibly synchronized by the sun. Factors involved in the rhythmicity of spontaneous births probably act by initiating labor.

▶ [It is interesting that the plot of hourly incidence of spontaneous births in Norway strongly resembles one based on 10 independent studies from 1848 to 1960 (Kaiser, I. H., and Halberg, F.: *Ann. N.Y. Acad. Sci.* 98:1056, 1962). The authors think the night and morning peaks and early evening nadir reflect some regulator (? the sun) for the initiation of labor.] ◀

5–13 **Influence of the Moon on Deliveries.** It is claimed in folklore that there is an association between the number of deliveries and the phase of the moon. The full moon usually is thought to be related to the most deliveries in the United States. Frank R. Witter (Johns Hopkins School of Medicine) reviewed obstetric records over 12 consecutive lunar months, during which time there were 2,697 deliveries. Analysis of findings in the 77% of patients in spontaneous labor showed no significant relationship between deliveries and phase of the moon, nor was premature rupture of the membranes correlated significantly with the day of the lunar month. This study found no significant association between the day of the lunar month and number of deliveries, number of patients in active labor, or premature membrane rupture.

▶ [Say it ain't so, Doctor Witter. In Iowa City, over coffee, the full moon is often blamed for busy times in labor and delivery departments. This sophisticated analysis suggests that there is no relationship between the onset of labor and phases of the moon. That may be true in Baltimore, but . . .] ◀

5–14 **Outcome of Spontaneous Labor in Multigravidas.** D. M. F. Gibb, L. D. Cardozo, J. W. W. Studd, A. L. Magos, and D. J. Cooper (Dulwich Hosp., London) examined the outcome of 847 multigravid patients admitted in spontaneous labor, from a series of 2,000 consecutive labors. Labor was classified according to cervimetric pattern and response to oxytocin given according to a strict protocol with use of a nomogram and partogram. Patients were divided into six groups:

(5–12) Acta Obstet. Gynecol. Scand. 62:31–36, 1983.
(5–13) Am. J. Obstet. Gynecol. 145:637–639, Mar. 1, 1983.
(5–14) Br. J. Obstet. Gynaecol. 89:708–711, September 1982.

MULTIGRAVIDAS: LABOR DATA ACCORDING TO CERVIMETRIC PATTERN*

		Admission data				First stage (h)		Second stage (min)		Type of delivery (%)		
Group	n	Mean (cm)	Mean cervical dilatation (cm)	Mean head level (fifth)	Mean birth-weight (kg)	Mean	⩾12 (n)	Mean	⩾30 (n)	SVD	CS	INST
A	749	162	4·7	2·2	3·36	2·7	0	17	95	98·1	0·5	1·4
B	12	157	1·9	3·2	3·09	9·9	5	19	3	91·7	8·3	0
C	62	160	3·0	3·1	3·35	8·1	8	24	17	92·0	0	8·0
D	7	160	3·0	3·7	3·52	10·3	1	43	2	14·3	85·7	0
E	12	159	3·5	2·8	3·40	8·5	2	34	4	83·3	0	16·7
F	5	162	4·0	3·2	3·79	8·4	1	16	1	80·0	20·0	0
Total	847	161·7	4·5	2·3	3·36	3·4	17 (2%)	18	122 (14·4%)	96·6	1·4	2·0

*SVD, spontaneous vaginal delivery; CS, cesarian section; INST, instrumental.
(Courtesy of Gibb, D. M. F., et al.: Br. J. Obstet. Gynaecol. 89:708–711, September 1982.)

group A, normal labor; group B, prolonged latent phase; group C, primary dysfunctional labor, improved with oxytocin; group D, primary dysfunctional labor not improved with oxytocin; group E, secondary arrest improved with oxytocin; group F, secondary arrest not improved with oxytocin.

Obstetric data and neonatal outcome are shown in the table. Mean gestation was 39.3 weeks. Mean observed first stage was 3.4 hours and 17 patients (2%) labored for greater than 12 hours. Mean duration of the second stage was 18 minutes, with 122 patients having second stage of greater than 30 minutes. Augmentation was required in 98 patients (11.6%) and improved progress in 86. Average duration of stimulation was 3.3 hours and mean total dose of oxytocin was 1.89 units. Overall cesarean section rate was 1.4% and only 2% of patients had an instrumental delivery. Average birth weight was 3.36 kg; there were 5 stillbirths and 1 neonatal death. Normal patients of group A had a mean first stage of 2.7 hours with spontaneous vaginal delivery occurring in 98.1%. A prolonged latent phase occurred only in 12 patients (group B). Primary dysfunctional labor was the most frequent aberrant labor pattern; labor improved in 62 of these (group C). Six of 7 patients who were not improved (group D) required abdominal delivery. Secondary arrest occurred in 17 patients, and 12 of these improved with oxytocin (group E). Five patients in group F had a satisfactory outcome with 4 being delivered without instrumentation and 1 by cesarean section. Only group D showed an increased neonatal morbidity.

The authors conclude that oxytocin is effective in correcting abnormal labor in most multigravidas, but failure to improve progress requires close supervision and a prompt surgical response. They suggest that if no improvement in progress occurs after 3 hours of augmentation for either primary dysfunctional labor or secondary arrest, cesarean section should be performed.

▶ [This study quantitates what experienced obstetricians realize. Eighty-eight percent of these multigravid (presumably parous) women labored normally. Eighty-eight percent of the remainder responded to oxytocin stimulation with normal progress and vaginal delivery. The authors conclude that cesarean section should be performed if there is no progress after 3 hours of oxytocin augmentation in patients with primary dysfunctional labor or secondary arrest. We would opt for a somewhat shorter (e.g., 2-hour) interval. In addition, we would use oxytocin only if the contraction pattern was hypotonic and there was no apparent cephalopelvic disproportion.] ◀

5–15 **Oxytocin Augmentation of Dysfunctional Labor.** —*Part II. Uterine Activity Data.*—Joseph Seitchik and Maria Castillo (Univ. of Texas at San Antonio) reviewed intrauterine pressure data from oxytocin-treated patients in dysfunctional labor who were managed by a specific regimen with a computer-defined goal of uterine activity. All were nulliparas at 37 weeks' or more gestation. Oxytocin was begun at a rate of 1 mU/minute and increased by 1 mU/minute if necessary at intervals of not less than 30 minutes until "adequate contractility" occurred or up to 4 mU/minute. The dose was maintained at that level for 2 hours. The protocol was followed closely in 42 of 45 women.

No single parameter identified hypocontractile labor perfectly (Table 1). Only 1 patient achieved complete dilatation without meeting criteria for adequate contractility. The false positive diagnostic rate was 1 in 45. There were no significant differences between the computer-defined goal of activity and that associated with cervical dilatation if the dose used had time to achieve its maximum effect. Quantitation of uterine contractility was adequate for selecting an oxytocin dose associated with cervical dilatation in about 75% of the patients to within 1 mU/minute.

Quantitation of uterine contractility can identify hypocontractility and the need for oxytocin in patients with lack of progress in cervical dilatation. Most patients in dysfunctional labor respond with cervical dilatation of doses of oxytocin of 4 mU/minute or less. The rate of incrementation should not be less than 30–40 minutes/mU as a compromise between an unacceptably prolonged interval to effect a response and an excessive oxytocin dose, with the need for constant professional monitoring.

▶ [The clinical implications here are that low doses of oxytocin are usually sufficient to correct dysfunctional labor if given time and that it may take as long as 40–60 minutes from the initiation of a pharmacologic dose of oxytocin to the attainment of its maximal contractile effect. Low initial doses and slow rates of increase should

TABLE 1.—OXYTOCIN AUGMENTATION STUDY

	Preoxytocin (N = 45)		*At adequate contractility (N = 44)*		*At first cervical dilatation (N = 43)*	
Parameter	*Mean ± SD*	*Range*	*Mean ± SD*	*Range*	*Mean ± SD*	*Range*
Amplitude (mm Hg)	30.0 ± 8.5	16-51	39.9 ± 9.5	22-60	42.3 ± 12.6	23-77
Period (sec)	290 ± 109	135-745	169 ± 35	103-252	165 ± 37	108-274
Montevideo units	77 ± 27	25-132	152 ± 29	100-231	165 ± 56	94-395
Three-contraction score	4.7 ± 2.7	−1.5-9.5	10.1 ± 0.8	9-12	10.0 ± 1.3	7-12
Oxytocin (mU/min)	0		2.27 ± 1.06	1-4	2.77 ± 1.43	1-8

(Courtesy of Seitchif, J., and Castillo, M.: Am. J. Obstet. Gynecol. 145:526–529, Mar. 1, 1983.)

(5–15) Am. J. Obstet. Gynecol. 145:526–529, Mar. 1, 1983; 145:777–780, Apr. 1, 1983.

TABLE 2.—OXYTOCIN AUGMENTATION OF LABOR: DURATION (MINUTES) FROM INITIATION OF OXYTOCIN TO IDENTIFICATION OF COMPLETE DILATATION

	Protocol/computer	*Control*
All patients	186 ± 119	235 ± 167
Oxytocin never stopped/ reduced	179 ± 125	198 ± 131
Oxytocin stopped/reduced	235 ± 31	409 ± 217

(Courtesy of Seitchik, J., and Castillo, M.: Am. J. Obstet. Gynecol. 145:777–780, Apr. 1, 1983.)

TABLE 3.—OXYTOCIN AUGMENTATION OF LABOR: MINIMUM INCREMENT INTERVAL (MINUTES PER MILLIUNIT) DISTRIBUTION (PERCENT)

Patient group	*No. of patients*	*Interval* 10-19	20-29	30-39	≥40	*HC/TFD** (%)
Protocol/computer	28	4	21	61	14	11
Control	32	44	25	22	9	22
All	60	25	23	40	12	17

(Courtesy of Seitchik, J., and Castillo, M.: Am. J. Obstet. Gynecol. 145:777–780, Apr. 1, 1983.)

minimize hyperstimulation of the uterus and iatrogenic fetal distress on that basis. On our service, when labor is being stimulated with oxytocin we generally increase the infusion rate more rapidly than the authors of this study advocate. It sounds as though comparative clinical trials are in order.] ◀

Part III.—Multiparous patients.—Seitchik and Castillo evaluated a continuous intravenous oxytocin regimen that was effective previously in nulliparous patients with arrested dilatation resulting from uterine hypocontractility. It consists of an initial oxytocin dose of 1 mU/minute, incrementation at a rate not greater than 1 mU per 30 minutes, and maintenance of an oxytocin dose of 4 mU/minute, if reached, for at least 1 hour. The initial treatment goal is a computer-defined level of uterine contractility. The series included 34 multiparous patients in apparent spontaneous true labor with arrest in the first stage because of uterine hypocontractility. All eventually delivered vaginally. Results in the study patients were compared with those in 34 controls who received oxytocin without use of a computer. The two groups were clinically comparable.

Mean times from the start of oxytocin infusion to complete dilatation were not significantly different in the 2 patients groups (Table 2), but reducing or discontinuing oxytocin led to a delay in complete dilatation in the control group. The maximum dose of oxytocin administered was significantly greater in the control group. Minimal increment intervals were significantly shorter in the controls (Table 3). This is the chief determinant of the dose received at the first observation of cervical dilatation and the maximum dose. The mean doses of oxytocin required by multiparous and nulliparous patients at "adequate contractility" and at first cervical dilatation were not significantly different. The two groups differed only in the mean times from onset of oxytocin therapy to complete dilatation.

Quantitation of uterine contractility is a useful but imperfect means of identifying hypocontractility and guiding oxytocin therapy in multiparous patients. The risk of damage from hypercontractility is real, especially when the fetus has subnormal life support systems or the uterus is especially sensitive to oxytocin. The minimum effective dose of oxytocin should be administered. Optimal therapy can be achieved most often if the initial oxytocin doses are small and the rates of incrementation slow.

▶ [These results with parous patients are similar to those reported in Part II of this study in nulliparas. The message is the same. A low dose of oxytocin initially, coupled with relatively long intervals between increases in the rate of drug administration, was efficacious. Problems with hyperstimulation were less frequent than in control patients, although not to a statistically significant degree (this lack of statistical significance may be a reflection of the small numbers involved). Given the modest cervical dilatation at the start of oxytocin infusion, many of these patients were probably in the latent phase of labor. More study is needed before one can extrapolate these findings to induction of labor or to stimulation of labor in cases of secondary arrest of dilatation in the active phase.] ◀

5–16 **Influence of Oxytocin on Human Memory Processes: Validation by a Control Study.** An earlier report of an adverse effect of high doses of oxytocin on human memory included results of studies on women receiving oxytocin as part of treatment to induce second-trimester therapeutic abortion. These women served as their own controls. D. J. Kennett, M. C. Devlin, and B. M. Ferrier (McMaster Univ., Hamilton, Ont.) report a study of women who have been treated in all ways like the original group, except that these women did not receive oxytocin. Six women in the second trimester of pregnancy were admitted for induced therapeutic abortion. They were given word-pair recall and picture-matching tests before and 4 hours after the start of treatment with oxytocin. Six women in the control group were matched to women in the experimental group.

Results show that the performance of the women in the control group in a task of word recall did not deteriorate after 4 hours. Learning and immediate recall were not different in the experimental and control groups, which agreed with previous findings that oxytocin did not influence learning. However, later recall was different for the two groups. The experimental group performed less well after 4 hours of treatment with oxytocin than before treatment, whereas the control group performed as well or better after 4 hours of treatment without oxytocin. The difference between experimental and control groups is significant whether the number of words correctly matched (P = .008) or the number of words correctly recalled (P = .014) were compared.

The impairment in performance in memory tasks after several hours of infusion of high doses of oxytocin is due to the hormone itself and not to any other treatment-associated factor. This effect of oxy-

---

(5–16) Life Sci. 31:273–275, July 19, 1982.

tocin in human beings agrees with observations of amnesic effects of oxytocin in rats.

▶ [These findings are fascinating. What could be the mechanism by which oxytocin adversely affects memory?] ◀

5–17 **Intrapartum Fetal Heart Rate Monitoring: VIII. Atypical Variable Decelerations.** H.-B. Krebs, R. E. Petres, and L. J. Dunn (Med. College of Virginia) reviewed 1,996 fetal heart rate recordings to determine the prognostic significance of variable decelerations. Only singleton pregnancies of 34 or more gestational weeks were included. Atypical variable decelerations are shown in Figure 5–1. Variable decelerations were recorded in the first 30-minute segment of monitored labor in 12% of cases. The total incidence of variable decelerations in any 30-minute segment in the first stage of labor was 34%. Nearly 80% persisted into the second stage, and variable decelerations were present in 49% of tracings of the last 30-minute segment of monitored labor.

Severe variable decelerations were associated with low Apgar scores significantly more often than were mild or moderate changes. When atypical variable decelerations were excluded, no such difference was apparent (Table 1). Atypical features greatly aided in identification of variable decelerations later in labor as being prognosti-

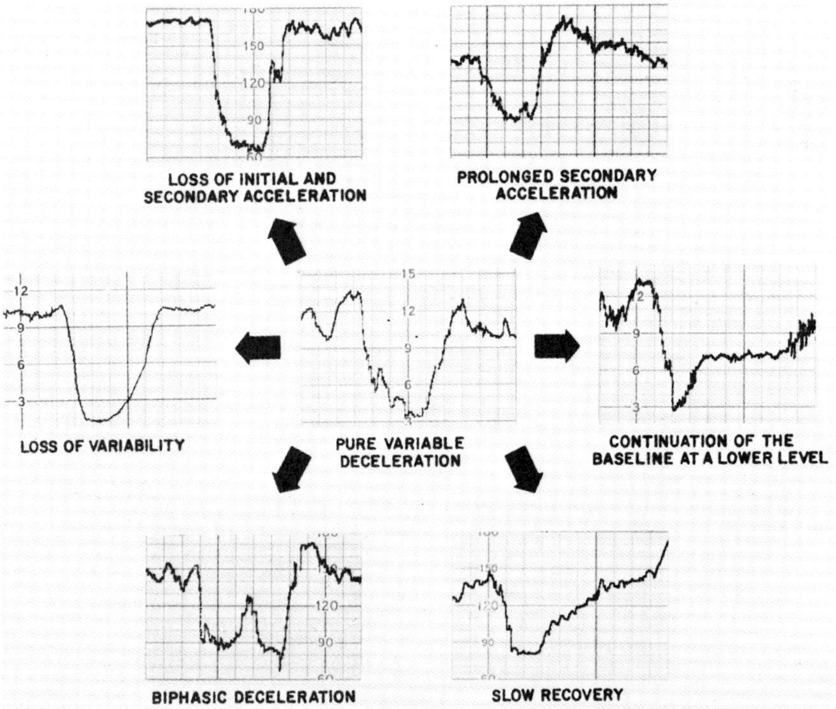

Fig 5–1.—Atypical variable decelerations. (Courtesy of Krebs, H.-B., et al.: Am. J. Obstet. Gynecol. 145:297–305, Feb. 1, 1983.)

(5–17) Am. J. Obstet. Gynecol. 145:297–305, Feb. 1, 1983.

TABLE 1.—PROGNOSIS OF PURE VARIABLE DECELERATIONS GRADED ACCORDING TO DURATION AND AMPLITUDE OF DECELERATION, EXCLUDING VARIABLE DECELERATIONS WITH ATYPIA (LAST 30 MINUTES OF MONITORING)

		One-minute Apgar score <7		*Five-minute Apgar score <7*	
Pure variable decelerations	*N*	*n*	*% of N*	*n*	*% of N*
Mild	267	41	15.3	8	3.0
Moderate	445	82	18.4	16	3.6
Severe	90	20	22.2	5	5.6
Test of homogeneity		$p > 0.1$		$p > 0.1$	

(Courtesy of Krebs, H.-B., et al.: Am. Obstet. Gynecol. 145:297–305, Feb. 1, 1983.)

TABLE 2.—PROGNOSIS OF ATYPICAL VARIABLE DECELERATIONS GRADED ACCORDING TO DURATION AND AMPLITUDE (LAST 30 MINUTES OF MONITORING)

		One-minute Apgar score <7		*Five-minute Apgar score <7*	
Atypical variable decelerations	*N*	*n*	*% of N*	*n*	*% of N*
Mild	20	9	45.0	2	10.0
Moderate	65	29	44.6	3	4.6
Severe	101	48	47.5	13	12.9
Test of homogeneity		$p > 0.1$		$p > 0.1$	

(Courtesy of Krebs, H.-B., et al.: Am. J. Obstet. Gynecol. 145:297–305, Feb. 1, 1983.)

cally unfavorable (Table 2). Atypical variable decelerations of any severity were frequently associated with fetal acidosis. Loss of initial acceleration was the most common atypical feature. Most tracings showed two or more atypical features at the same time. Other fetal heart rate abnormalities were associated with atypical variable decelerations in 84% of cases and with pure variable decelerations in 63%.

Variable decelerations in the fetal heart rate are probably innocuous so long as atypical features are absent. Atypical variable decelerations reflect significant fetal hypoxia and many be associated with a depressed infant at birth. Associated baseline fetal heart rate changes, reduced variability, or both indicate fetal acidosis in many instances and can predict a poor fetal outcome.

▶ [These authors previously have emphasized the importance of looking at all features of the monitor tracing and not just at the periodic changes (1980 YEAR BOOK, pp. 152–154). The present report puts variable decelerations in perspective. The traditional "mild, moderate, severe" based on depth and duration of deceleration aren't too helpful. The associated variability, reactivity, and pattern of recovery are more effective predictors of neonatal outcome.] ◀

5–18 **Intrapartum Fetal Monitoring in Preterm Deliveries: Prospective Study.** Magnus Westgren, Peter Holmquist, Nils W. Svenningsen, and Ingemar Ingemarsson (Univ. Hosp., Lund, Sweden) studied prospectively the relationship between fetal heart rate (FHR) changes and fetal acid-base status and evaluated the incidence of fetal asphyxia in 23 patients delivered at 28–33 weeks' gestation (group A) and in 38 patients delivered at 34–36 weeks' gestation (group B). Preterm labor was of unknown etiology in all cases and there were no additional maternal or fetal complications.

Bradycardia occurred in 2 patients in group B only. Tachycardia was seen in 18 patients in group A (78%) and 8 patients in group B (21%). About 50% of patients in group A with normal baseline FHR values or tachycardia had fetal acidosis, whereas fetal acidosis occurred only in group B patients who had an abnormal baseline FHR. Variability of FHR was normal in 10 group A patients (44%) and 24 group B patients (63%), but decreased variability or a silent pattern was seen in 13 group A patients (57%) and 11 group B patients (29%). A positive correlation with fetal acidosis was demonstrated among these patients in group B, but not those in group A. Increased variability or a saltatory pattern was seen in 3 patients in the 36th week; all 3 had a normal fetal pH.

No FHR decelerations occurred in 3 patients in group A (13%) and 12 patients in group B (32%) (Fig 5–2). Early decelerations were rare, occurring only at 35 to 36 weeks' gestation. Four patients in group A (17%) and 2 patients in group B (5%) exhibited late decelerations and except for 1 patient in group A, all had fetal acidosis. Variable decel-

Fig 5–2.—Periodic changes in fetal heart rate in group A and group B. Speckled area = fetal acidosis (pH < 7.25 at 5 cm or at full dilatation). (Courtesy of Westgren, M., et al.: Obstet. Gynecol. 60:99–106, July 1982. Reprinted with permission from The American College of Obstetricians and Gynecologists.)

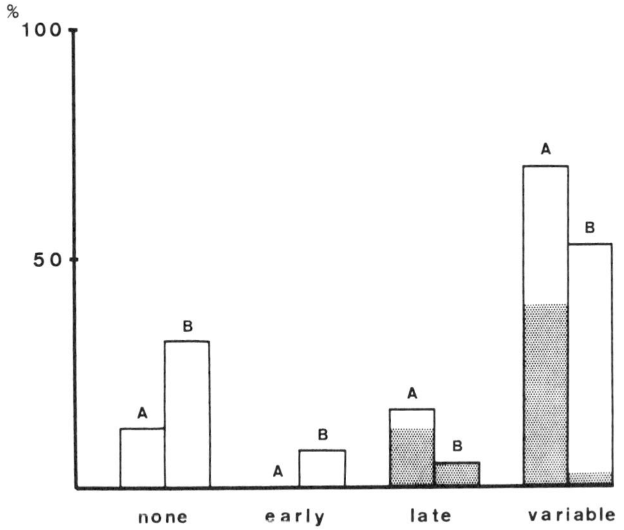

(5–18) Obstet. Gynecol. 60:99–106, July 1982.

erations occurred in 16 group A patients (70%) and 21 group B patients (55%). Three dominant types of variable FHR decelerations were observed, 1 of which had a duration of 10 to 40 seconds and a rapid recovery to baseline; the other 2 were more complex. In group A, 5 of 9 patients with a loss of 30 to 60 beats had a fetal scalp pH of less than 7.25, whereas only 1 of these patients in group B had fetal acidosis. Sporadic FHR accelerations showed a negative correlation to fetal acidosis in group B, but not in group A.

Fetal tachycardia and decreased variability occurred more often in patients treated with terbutaline, a β-receptor agonist for inhibition of preterm labor, than in untreated patients. No positive correlation between fetal acidosis and FHR changes was observed for the terbutaline-treated patients. There were 2 infant deaths during the neonatal period, both caused by idiopathic respiratory distress syndrome. Both had variable decelerations with an overshoot pattern during labor, but had normal pH values.

Fetal acidosis can occur frequently and rapidly among most infants during preterm labor. Thus, the obstetrician should consider gestational age and the administration of β-receptor stimulators when assessing the FHR pattern in preterm labor.

▶ [Preterm labor is one of the clear indications for electronic fetal monitoring, and this article tells why. The preterm fetus is more likely than the term fetus to develop a heart rate abnormality and, once developed, such an abnormality is more likely to be associated with acidosis. Thus, the premature fetus is less resistant to hypoxia, and this vulnerability increases with decreasing gestational age. The lower limit of gestational age at which fetal monitoring should be used will vary from unit to unit and from time to time, depending on neonatal prognosis at given gestational ages and birth weights. In the individual case, it is essential to make the decision about whether there should be intervention for fetal distress *before* the monitor is applied. We have seen a number of unfortunate instances in which this was not done (i.e., the monitor was inserted "routinely" because of preterm labor at a borderline gestational age), and then when fetal distress appeared there was a dilemma, with much discussion, argument, and consequent loss of potentially valuable time, about whether to perform a cesarean section. We feel strongly that it is implicit in the use of fetal monitoring that fetal distress will be acted upon. On our service, presently we will monitor at 27 completed weeks of gestation and beyond, but not earlier.] ◀

5–19 **Ten-Year Experience With Intrapartum Fetal Monitoring in Los Angeles County-University of Southern California Medical Center.** To evaluate the impact of intrapartum electronic fetal monitoring on obstetric practice and perinatal outcome, Sze-Ya Yeh, Fidelia Diaz, and Richard H. Paul reviewed deliveries performed at Los Angeles County-University of Southern California Medical Center from 1970 through 1979.

Of the 115,096 deliveries, 47,467 (41.3%) were monitored, with the monitoring rate being increased from 18% in 1970 to 74% in 1979 (Fig 5–3). The sharp increase in monitoring rate after 1976 was attributable to availability of additional equipment in the labor and delivery area. As the monitoring rate increased, perinatal mortality gradually decreased, with reduction in intrapartum and neonatal deaths contributing most to the decrease. The antepartum death rate remained relatively constant throughout the 10-year period.

(5–19) Am. J. Obstet. Gynecol. 143:496–500, July 1, 1982.

TABLE 1.—INTRAPARTUM FETAL DEATHS AT LAC-USC MEDICAL CENTER IN 1970–1979

	Monitored	*Unmonitored*
Total patients:	46,524	67,367
Fetal deaths	70	171
Rate per 1,000	1.5	2.5*
Birth weight >1,500 gm (uncorrected):		
Total patients	45,880	66,208
Fetal deaths	34	71
Rate per 1,000	0.7	1.1
Birth weight >1,500 gm (corrected):†		
Total patients	45,880	66,208
Fetal deaths	10	45
Rate per 1,000	0.2	0.7*

*$P < .005$ by chi-square tests.
†Exclusions: congenital malformations incompatible with life and traumatic deliveries.
(Courtesy of Yeh, S.-Y., et al.: Am. J. Obstet. Gynecol. 143:496–500, July 1, 1982.)

A total of 12,248 (10.6%) cesarean sections were performed; 8,623 (70.4%) were primary procedures. The total cesarean section rate increased from about 9% in the early 1970s to 12.5% in the late 1970s. However, in monitored patients, this rate decreased from 20% in 1970 to 11% in 1979, with an overall rate of 15%.

There were 70 intrapartum fetal deaths among 46,524 monitored patients (1.5/1,000) and 171 deaths among 67,367 nonmonitored patients (2.5/1,000) (Table 1). In the monitored group, there were 377 neonatal deaths among 46,454 live births (8.1/1,000), compared with 986 deaths among 67,196 nonmonitored live births (14.7/1,000) (Table

TABLE 2.—NEONATAL DEATHS AT LAC-USC MEDICAL CENTER

	Monitored	*Unmonitored*
Total live births	46,454	67,196
Total neonatal deaths	377	986
Rate per 1,000	8.1	14.7*
Birth weight >1,500 gm		
Live births	45,847	66,108
Neonatal deaths	162	307
Rate per 1,000	3.5	4.6†
Birth weight ≤1,500 gm		
Live births	607	1,088
Neonatal deaths	216	679
Rate per 1,000	356	624*

*$P < .001$ by chi-square tests.
†$P < .005$ by chi-square tests.
(Courtesy of Yeh, S. Y., et al.: Am. J. Obstet. Gynecol. 143:496–500, July 1, 1982.)

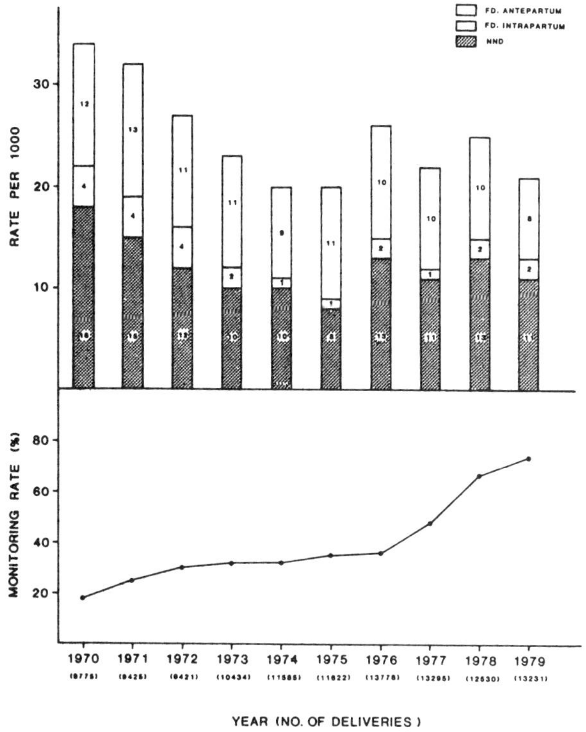

Fig 5–3.—Annual perinatal mortality *(bar graph)* and monitoring rate *(line graph)*. Numbers in parentheses below year indicate total number of deliveries. *FD,* fetal death; *NND,* neonatal death. (Courtesy of Yeh, S.-Y., et al.: Am. J. Obstet. Gynecol. 143:496–500, July 1, 1982.)

2). When these patients were grouped according to birth weight, neonatal mortality for nonmonitored patients remained consistently higher than that for monitored.

In this study most high-risk patients were included in the monitored group. The results suggest that intrapartum fetal monitoring improves perinatal outcome.

▶ [This article is particularly important because it comes from the institution that had "led the way" in electronic fetal heart rate monitoring. The data indicate that increasing usage of electronic fetal heart rate monitoring has been associated with a progressive decline in intrapartum and neonatal death rates, although the authors' statement, "The antepartum death rate remained relatively consistent throughout the 10-year period," does not seem to us to be supported by Figure 5–3. Is a fluctuation between 13 and 8 per 1,000 "relatively consistent"? Nonetheless, this report provides interesting and valuable information from an enormous data base.] ◀

5–20 **Fetal Heart Rate Response to Scalp Blood Sampling.** Steven L. Clark, Martin L. Gimovsky, and Frank C. Miller (Univ. of Southern California) note that fetal heart rate acceleration in response to various stimuli has long been considered a reliable sign of fetal well-being in both the intrapartum and antepartum periods. To define the correlation between fetal heart rate response and fetal blood pH

(5–20) Am. J. Obstet. Gynecol. 144:706–708, Nov. 15, 1982.

value, they analyzed 200 heart rate tracings of fetuses who had undergone scalp blood sampling in early labor. Data on fetal heart rate response to endoscope placement and scalp puncture and resultant scalp pH level were then analyzed.

Of the 200 tracings reviewed, 169 were judged to show an acceleration of fetal heart rate in response to scalp blood sampling, whereas 31 showed no such response. Of 144 fetuses with a scalp pH greater than 7.28, 142 reacted to sampling with acceleration, whereas no fetus whose scalp pH was less than 7.20 demonstrated such a response. Those fetuses with scalp pH of 7.21–7.28 showed a variable response. The differences among these three groups were statistically significant.

Fetal scalp blood sampling probably represents a painful stimulus that results in an immediate decrease in vagal tone and an increase in sympathetic response. The findings of this study appear to have clinical implications. Although direct confirmation of fetal acid-base status by scalp blood sampling is the diagnostic method of choice in the presence of a fetal heart rate pattern suggestive of hypoxia, scalp blood sampling may not be universally available or technically possible. In such cases, the results suggest that if an acceleration of fetal heart rate can be induced by tactile stimulation, the clinician may be reassured that fetal scalp pH is likely to be greater than 7.20, which represents a nonacidotic condition. A prospective study is currently under way to test this possibility.

▶ ["Routine" fetal scalp blood sampling was performed in these study subjects. In clinical practice this determination usually is done in response to an abnormal fetal heart rate pattern often in the presence of decelerations or bradycardia. In this situation, is it easy to label fetal heart rate changes as accelerations with confidence? If so, noninvasive, tactile scalp stimulation may have a role in assessing intrapartum fetal well-being.] ◀

5–21 **Ritodrine in the Management of Fetal Distress.** S. Sheybany, J. F. Murphy, D. Evans, R. G. Newcombe, and J. F. Pearson studied the potential value of a bolus injection of ritodrine in patients with fetal distress to determine if β_2-sympathomimetic drugs will reduce uterine activity and improve placental blood flow. A total of 47 patients with fetal distress in the first stage of labor was studied. Twenty-four were given ritodrine and 23 were controls. Pregnancies were all singleton cephalic presentations and of more than 37 weeks' gestation. Diagnosis of fetal distress was based mainly on the cardiotocogram pattern.

Changes in CTG pattern after ritodrine are shown in the table. Eight of 24 tracings were unsuitable for analysis because of incomplete recordings; the other 16 were used. The pattern had reverted to normal in 5 patients after ritodrine, was less ominous in 9, and remained unchanged in 2. After the decision to operate, uterine activity remained unchanged in controls. In those patients receiving ritodrine, uterine activity measured over 14.7 ± 6.3 (SD) minutes after injection was reduced to an average 22% of the preinjection value. Two patients given ritodrine who had had atropine premedicaton de-

---

(5–21) Br. J. Obstet. Gynaecol. 89:723–726, September 1982.

FETAL HEART RATE (FHR) PATTERNS BEFORE AND AFTER RITODRINE

FHR pattern before ritodrine ($n=16$)	FHR pattern after ritodrine ($n=16$)
Severe variable decelerations ($n=3$)	2 normal pattern 1 no change
Late decelerations (normal baseline; $n=5$)	3 normal pattern 1 simple tachycardia 1 complicated tachycardia
Complicated tachycardia ($n=8$)	7 simple tachycardia 1 no change

No alterations in FHR patterns were seen in the control group.
(Courtesy of Sheybany, S., et al.: Br. J. Obstet. Gynaecol. 89:723–726, September 1982.)

veloped pulse rates of 190 beats per minute that persisted for 15 minutes and did not fall below 100 beats per minute for 1 hour. The infants in the control group were more depressed as judged by the 1-minute Apgar score and the time required to establish regular respiration. Cord blood gases and acid-base values were similar in both groups. Neurobehavioral tests and tests of tone were made on days 4–7 inclusive, but no differences were found between the groups.

Although ritodrine consistently improved the cardiotocogram pattern, the resultant benefits for the infants were only marginal. The authors conclude that early detection of fetal distress followed by emergency cesarean section remains effective management. They believe, that the administration of ritodrine probably would not be worthwhile generally, but may be useful when cesarean section is unavoidably delayed.

▶ [The use of tocolysis in the treatment of fetal distress was considered in the 1979 YEAR BOOK (pp. 145–147). This controlled study suggests an improvement in fetal heart rate patterns and in Apgar scores, but not in cord blood gas values or neonatal course. It's too bad that a double-blind format was not used. The most important point here is that the combination of ritodrine and atropine resulted in worrisome maternal tachycardia and hypertension. The authors of this report conclude that tocolysis is not generally worthwhile in this situation, but suggest it might have a place when cesarean section is unavoidably delayed.] ◀

5–22 **Rotational Delivery of the Fetus: Kielland's Forceps and Two Other Methods Compared.** In modern obstetric practice, high forceps delivery has been replaced by cesarean section. However, whether delivery with Kielland's forceps is more dangerous than delivery by other means when rotation of the fetal head in midpelvis is required has not been adequately assessed. D. L. Healy, M. A. Quinn, and R. J. Pepperell (Royal Women's Hosp., Melbourne) compared re-

(5–22) Br. J. Obstet. Gynaecol. 89:501–506, July 1982.

trospectively the results of 552 cases in which Kielland's forceps were used for rotation and delivery, 95 cases in which other forceps were used, and 160 cases in which manual rotation and forceps were used.

The most common indication for expediting delivery was delay of the second stage of labor in the occipitoposterior position (50%). Delay of labor in a lateral position occurred in 27% of deliveries. In 21%, fetal distress was the primary indication for using Kielland's forceps. Fifty deliveries (9%) were from a position at the level of the ischial spines.

The most frequent maternal complications associated with the use of Kielland's forceps were vaginal and cervical lacerations and significant extensions of the episiotomy (15%). Postpartum hemorrhage occurred in 14% of the patients. Manual removal of the placenta was performed in 13% of deliveries. Incidence of maternal or fetal morbidity did not differ significantly among the three modes of delivery, regardless of whether the indication for delivery was a delayed second stage of labor or fetal distress. Incidence of vaginal and cervical lacerations and of primary postpartum hemorrhage was higher when the Kielland's forceps was used by junior staff rather than by senior staff, but there was no increase in fetal morbidity.

The absence of statistically significant differences in maternal or fetal complicatons when rotational delivery with Kielland's forceps was compared with rotation using other forcepts and with manual rotation and forceps delivery supports the view that maternal and fetal trauma during rotational delivery are implicit in the procedure itself and that there is no special risk from the use of Kielland's forceps.

▶ [This study compared three methods of midpelvic rotation and delivery—Kielland's forceps, other forceps, and manual rotation followed by forceps delivery—with respect to maternal and infant outcome. In essence, no differences were found, indicating that any dangers in vaginal delivery of midpelvic arrest are due to the condition or its general treatment rather than to any specific risk of the Kielland instrument. Of course, the larger question of whether there is any place in modern obstetrics for the midforceps operation is a knottier issue. It appears that many would answer that question in the negative. However, we are not among them.] ◀

5–23 **Large for Gestational Age Neonates: Anthropometric Reasons for Shoulder Dystocia** are discussed by Houchang D. Modanlou, Glen Komatsu, Wendy Dorchester, Roger K. Freeman, and Sogba K. Bosu. From 1960 to 1980, the mean birth weight for term-size neonates at Memorial Hospital Medical Center-Miller Children's Hospital of Long Beach, in California, increased from 3,381 to 3,458 gm despite increases in ethnic groups known to have smaller infants. The incidence of birth weights of greater than 4,000 gm increased from 7.0% to 10.7%.

Because of this marked increase a prospective study was designed to characterize the macrosomic neonate. Anthropometric studies were done in 202 newborn infants weighing more than 4,000 gm, in 100 newborns weighing 2,501 to 4,000 gm, and in 27 infants born to diabetic mothers.

(5–23) Obstet. Gynecol. 60:417–423, October 1982.

TABLE 1.—Comparison of Anthropometric Measurements of Newborn Infants With Birth Weights Greater Than 4,000 gm From Diabetic and Nondiabetic Mothers

Anthropometric measurements	Nondiabetic (*N* = 202)	Diabetic (*N* = 11)	*P*
Birth weight (g)*	4247 ± 471	4585 ± 522	<.025
Gestational age (wk)*	40.7 ± 1.3	38.6 ± 1.3	<.001
Length (cm)*	54.6 ± 2.8	54.9 ± 2.4	NS
Head circumference (cm)*	36.3 ± 1.2	36.2 ± 0.9	NS
Chest circumference (cm)*	36.2 ± 2.8	37.0 ± 1.6	NS
Shoulder circumference (cm)*	39.5 ± 1.6	43.5 ± 4.9	<.001
Shoulder–head (cm)*	3.2 ± 1.9	7.4 ± 4.5	<.001
Chest–head (cm)*	0.06 ± 1.6	0.8 ± 1.5	NS

NS = not significant.
*Mean ± 1 SD.
(Courtesy of Modanlou, H. D., et al.: Obstet. Gynecol. 60:417–434, October 1982. Reprinted with permission from The American College of Obstetricians and Gynecologists.)

Shoulder dystocia was experienced by 10 infants in the macrosomic group and by 2 in the control group. Neonates experiencing shoulder dystocia had significantly greater shoulder-to-head and chest-to-head disproportion than did macrosomic neonates delivered by cesarean section because of failed progress in labor or macrosomic infants delivered without shoulder dystocia. Macrosomic infants of diabetic mothers, despite having lower gestational age than macrosomic infants of nondiabetic mothers, had higher birth weights and their shoulder circumference and shoulder-to-head circumference differences were greater (Table 1). Normal-sized (2,500 to 4,000 gm) infants of diabetic mothers had a greater shoulder-to-head circumference difference, were shorter, and had smaller head circumference than normal-sized infants of nondiabetic mothers (Table 2).

Antenatal ultrasonic measurements should be obtained in fetuses

TABLE 2.—Comparison of Anthropometric Measurements of Newborn Infants With Birth Weights of 2,501–4,000 gm From Diabetic and Nondiabetic Mothers

Anthropometric measurements	Diabetic (*N* = 16)	Nondiabetic (*N* = 100)	*P*
Birth weight (g)*	3257 ± 372	3399 ± 363	NS
Gestational age (wk)*	37.7 ± 2.2	39.6 ± 3.9	NS
Length (cm)*	49.6 ± 3.1	51.7 ± 2.6	<.005
Head circumference (cm)*	33.4 ± 1.9	34.6 ± 1.3	<.005
Chest circumference (cm)*	32.9 ± 2.2	33.6 ± 1.8	NS
Shoulder circumference (cm)*	36.9 ± 2.6	36.5 ± 2.0	NS
Shoulder–head (cm)*	3.6 ± 2.8	1.7 ± 1.3	<.001
Chest–head (cm)*	−0.5 ± 2.6	−1.1 ± 1.5	NS

NS = not significant.
*Mean ± 1 DS.
(Courtesy of Modanlou, H. D., et al.: Obstet. Gynecol. 60:417–434, October 1982. Reprinted with permission from The American College of Obstetricians and Gynecologists.)

suspected to be macrosomic and in fetuses of any size in diabetic pregnancies. A chest-to-head circumference difference of 1.6 cm or a shoulder-to-head circumference difference of 4.8 cm should be considered as anthropometric disproportions indicating possible shoulder dystocia. If such disproportion is found, delivery by cesarean section would be necessary to obviate birth injury. If vaginal delivery is attempted, a physician experienced in the delivery of shoulder dystocia and anesthesia should be present.

► [There is no occurrence in obstetrics more frightening than the sudden realization that shoulder dystocia exists. Because the problem largely derives from its totally unexpected nature, some method of prenatal diagnosis would be of great value. This article reports anthropometric measurements in infants with and without shoulder dystocia. Hardly surprising is the finding that shoulder and chest diameters and shoulder-head differences were all greater when there had been shoulder dystocia. It is well known that infants of diabetic mothers are at risk for this complication, so the finding that they have larger shoulders than infants of nondiabetics comes as no shock either. The authors suggest that differences of 1.6 cm and 4.8 cm in ultrasonically measured circumferences of chest-to-head and shoulder-to-head, respectively, should alert one to the likelihood of shoulder dystocia.] ◄

5–24 **An Alternate Maneuver for Management of Shoulder Dystocia** is described by Bernard Gonik, C. Allen Stringer, and Berel Held (Univ. of Texas, Houston). Previously described maneuvers for shoulder dystocia involve manipulation of the infant to permit delivery of the shoulders through the pelvic outlet. The suggested methods include upward traction followed by downward traction with suprapubic pressure, corkscrew rotation of the shoulder girdle, delivery of the posterior arm, and cleidotomy. A liberal episiotomy is necessary before any of these maneuvers can be performed, and serious newborn morbidity is not infrequent. Asphyxia, seizures, brachial plexus palsies, and orthopedic injuries have been described. The authors evaluated the McRoberts maneuver, involving exaggerated flexion of the mother's legs to straighten the sacrum relative to the lumbar spine, leading to cephalad rotation of the pubic symphysis and a decreased angle of inclination.

Woman, 25, gravida 7, para 2, abortus 4, was hospitalized at term in early active labor. She was thought to have a macrosomic infant, despite absence of a history of diabetes and a normal postprandial blood sugar level. The first stage of labor lasted for 11 hours and the second stage, 82 minutes. A left mediolateral episiotomy was performed. Spontaneous delivery of the vertex in the occipitoanterior position was followed by retraction of the chin tightly against the perineum. After gentle downward traction failed to deliver the anterior shoulder, the McRoberts maneuver was carried out, with sharp flexion of the patient's legs against her abdomen. Additional mild traction was used to free the impacted shoulder. The 5,221-gm infant was without complications.

The pubic symphysis rotated superiorly by a distance of 8 cm in this patient when McRoberts' maneuver was applied, and the angle of inclination was reduced from 26 degrees to 10 degrees. Rotation of the pubic symphysis superiorly frees the impacted anterior shoulder without manipulation of the fetus.

(5–24) Am. J. Obstet. Gynecol. 145:882–884, Apr. 1, 1983.

▶ [Until reading this article, we were not aware of the McRoberts maneuver. Since, we've had one occasion to use it and it seemed to work like a charm. The extreme thigh flexion straightens the lumbosacral angle and rotates the pubic symphysis to a more cephalad position. In cases of shoulder dystocia, we need all the help we can get. It's nice to learn of another way to deal with this problem.] ◀

5–25 **Changed Prognosis of Breech-Presenting Low Birth Weight Infants.** Charles Cox, A. C. Kendall, and Marion Hommers compared the mortality and morbidity of low birth weight breech-presenting singleton infants born in the Coventry England, Maternity Hospital during 1973 and 1974 with those born during 1979 and 1980. During this period, changes in management have included an increase in the rate of cesarean sections and the continuing development of intensive care for newborns. Women in both groups were comparable for all variables.

In 1979 and 1980 there were considerably more deliveries by cesarean section, fewer stillbirths, and fewer neonatal deaths; neonatal mortality corrected for lethal abnormalities was 23.9% in 1973–1974 and 8.7% in 1979–1980. Among 10 infants ventilated during the later years, 5 died and only 1 survived as normal; no infants were ventilated earlier. Among 80 live-born infants in 1979–1980, 64 survived and 14 were abnormal. Expressed as a percentage of traced live births, the survival rate of normal babies was similar for the two periods, 63.1% and 64.1%. Expressed differently, in 1973–1974, 1 in 21.5 survivors was handicapped (including nonneurologic handicaps) and in 1979–1980, 1 in 4.6. The overall mortality and morbidity figures show that from 1973–1974 to 1979–1980, during which time the rate of cesarean sections increased from 19.1% to 42.2%, the stillbirth rate decreased from 24.7% to 11.1%. The handicap rate in survivors, however, increased from 4.7% to 21.9% for these two periods. The neurologic handicap rate was greater in those infants by cesarean section (25.8%) than in those delivered vaginally (12.1%).

Results of the study show that neonatal mortality has decreased, although the increased survival rate is accounted for by the survival of handicapped infants. The value of routine cesarean section in the absence of other obstetric pathologic conditions for low birth weight breech infants is unproved and may be deleterious to mother and baby.

▶ [This represents another chapter in the continuing controversy surrounding management of the preterm breech. Between 1973–1974 and 1979–1980, the cesarean rate more than doubled (19.1% or 42.2%) and modern neonatal intensive care was introduced. Presumably as a result of one or the other or both, the corrected neonatal mortality fell from 23.9% to 8.7%, but the handicap rate among survivors *increased* from 4.7% to 21.9%. The percentage of live-born infants who survived and were normal was virtually identical in the two periods. The implication seems to be that aggressive obstetric and pediatric management simply converts mortality to morbidity.

In an editorial on this subject, Frank Hytten (*Br. J. Obstet. Gynaecol.* 89:879, 1982) suggested that, rather than brain damage resulting from breech delivery, perhaps the baby presenting by the breech does so because it is already brain damaged. This point of view finds support in a study by Kitchen et al. (ibid., p. 887) of infants born at less than 29 weeks' gestation in which handicap varied with presentation (i.e., more likely with breech than with vertex) but *not* with modes of delivery.] ◀

(5–25) Br. J. Obstet. Gynecol. 89:881–886, November 1982.

5-26 **Randomized Management of Nonfrank Breech Presentation at Term: Preliminary Report.** Definite proof of the superiority of cesarean section in breech delivery is difficult to obtain, and some believe that too many cesarean section deliveries are performed. Martin L. Gimovsky, Roger L. Wallace, Barry S. Schifrin, and Richard H. Paul (Univ. of Southern California) undertook a prospective study comparing elective cesarean section with a selective management regimen for nonfrank breech presentations at term in 105 women. All had singleton pregnancies at 36–42 weeks' gestation, with an estimated fetal weight of 2–4 kg, a cervix less than 7 cm dilated, and no contraindications to labor. Seventy patients were randomized to a trial of labor and 35 to elective cesarean section.

There were 31 (44%) patients who gave birth vaginally after being randomized to a trial of labor. Four in the cesarean section group delivered vaginally before operation. Two patients in the trial of labor group who delivered vaginally required oxytocin. Delivery was usually by assisted breech technique with forceps to the aftercoming head. The average umbilicus to delivery time was 1 minute. Two infants had 5-minute Apgar scores below 7. There were 2 neonatal deaths, 1 of an infant with multiple anomalies. The most common cause of a "failed" trial of labor was inadequate pelvic size as seen on x-ray pelvimetry. Neonatal morbidity was comparable in the vaginal delivery and cesarean section groups. Maternal morbidity was significantly greater in the cesarean group. Two of 3 neonatal deaths were of infants having major anomalies. The third infant may have been inadequately resuscitated.

A selective managment protocol is a reasonable alternative to elective cesarean section for nonfrank breech presentations at term. About half of the patients permitted a trial of labor can be expected to deliver vaginally, with neonatal morbidity comparable to that associated with cesarean section delivery. Further emphasis on the management of labor and vaginal delivery in these patients will maximize the benefits of cesarean section in breech delivery.

► [Nearly all of the many reports of breech delivery are retrospective and therefore, as we have commented several times previously, of limited usefulness in assessing an intervention. The University of Southern California group has reported the only prospective randomized study, abstracted in the 1981 YEAR BOOK (p. 147), involving term frank breech. Now investigators from the same institution have carried out a similar study of term nonfrank breeches. The outcome of vaginal delivery under carefully controlled circumstances appears equivalent to that of routine cesarean section, with one possible exception. There was a neonatal death in the vaginal delivery group that could have been due to the delivery; however, a number of characteristics of the case suggest that it also might have been due to inadequate or inappropriate resuscitation. In any event, this study demonstrates that vaginal birth of the breech-presenting infant is reasonable. Older obstetricians will hardly find this astonishing.] ◄

5-27 **Effect of External Cephalic Version in Late Pregnancy on Breech Presentation and Cesarean Section Rate: A Controlled Trial.** The role of external cephalic version (ECV) in the management of breech presentation remains unclear. G. J. Hofmeyer (Univ. of the Witwatersrand, Johannesburg, South Africa) undertook a prospective

---

(5–26) Am. J. Obstet. Gynecol. 146:34–40, May 1, 1983.
(5–27) Br. J. Obstet. Gynaecol. 90:392–399, May 1983.

trial of ECV in 60 African patients with breech presentation after 36 weeks' gestation. Ultrasound study and an unstressed cardiotocogram were obtained before randomization. No analgesia was used. Supine hypotension was avoided by placing the patient in a steep lateral position, with the operator seated alongside. The breech was elevated from the pelvis with one hand and if version was incomplete, the head was manipulated downward with the other hand. For a forward somersault the patient was positioned with the fetal back upward; for a backward somersault the patient was positioned with the fetal back downward. When the head would be inaccessible behind the costal margin after elevation of the breech, the patient was placed supine and the head was manipulated forward and downward before elevation of the breech.

In all but 1 of 30 cases ECV was successful. Presentation was breech at delivery in 3% of the ECV group and in 67% of the control group of 30 cases. Respective cesarean section rates were 20% and 43%. In patients with frank breech presentation and in those with lateral or cornual placentas, ECV tended to be more difficult. Tocolysis was used in 7 cases. Cardiotocography showed fetal movements to be reduced after ECV. There were no perinatal deaths, and all infants had 5-minute Apgar scores above 7.

External cephalic version can be carried out safely in late pregnancy and can reduce the incidence of breech presentation at delivery, and probably that of cesarean section. Prerequisites include a recent ultrasound study and either a reactive unstressed cardiotocogram or a negative contraction stress test. Absolute contraindications to ECV include multiple pregnancy, antepartum bleeding, placenta previa, ruptured membranes, and severe fetal anomaly. Previous cesarean section is a relative contraindication, as are obesity, hypertension, impaired intrauterine growth, and an anterior placenta.

▶ [This randomized trial demonstrates again the efficacy of external cephalic version in breech presentation. External cephalic version, under tocolysis if necessary, after 36 weeks' gestation was almost completely effective in preventing breech delivery at term. The technique employed by this author is somewhat different than what we have used in that the patient assumes a lateral recumbent position (to eliminate caval compression) and version is first attempted by manipulating the breech only. The preferred technique was a forward somersault, for which the woman is positioned with the fetal back upward. The literature reviewed in the article covers 477 cases of external cephalic version without anesthesia, with no fetal deaths reported.] ◀

5–28 **Management of the Breech Second Twin.** The risk of vaginal delivery of breech infants is well-documented and is reflected in a high cesarean section rate for those infants. Among sets of twins delivered between 1970 and 1977, breech first twins were significantly more likely to be delivered by cesarean section than were vertex first twins. Breech second twins, however, did not have a cesarean section rate significantly higher than that of vertex second twins. Frances Kelsick and Howard Minkoff (SUNY Downstate Med. Center) evaluated whether less aggressive use of cesarean section for the second breech twin is justified.

Breech first twins delivered vaginally had a perinatal mortality

---

(5–28) Am. J. Obstet. Gynecol. 144:783–786, Dec. 1, 1982.

and incidence of low Apgar scores similar to those of breech second twins delivered vaginally. Cesarean section improved the outcome equally for breech first and second twins. There was a significantly higher perinatal mortality for breech infants born vaginally than for vertex infants. This difference disappeared among infants delivered by cesarean section, whether first or second twin. However, cesarean section failed to reduce the incidence of low Apgar scores; this failure may be secondary to the effects of anesthesia on 1-minute scores. There were no significant differences in outcome observed between primiparous and multiparous patients.

The data did not justify a less frequent use of cesarean section for breech second twins. Appropriate management of twins during labor should include determination of the presentation of the second twin and use of the same indications for cesarean section for both first and second twins in breech presentation.

▶ [The conclusion of this study—that a breech-presenting second twin should be managed the same way as a breech-presenting first twin—is predicated entirely on the assumption that the presentation of the second twin does not change during labor and delivery. This, in our judgment, is not a valid premise, for we have seen a number of instances in which the presentation of a second twin changes between the time an x-ray study or sonogram is done in early labor and the time the first twin is born. Moreover, the data in this study are confounded by small numbers and wide weight ranges in the groups. We believe that delivery of twins should be based on the presentation of the first twin, and presentation of the second (unless there is marked disparity in size) is of relatively little import.] ◀

5–29 **Comparative Safety of the Low Transverse Versus the Low Vertical Uterine Incision for Cesarean Delivery of Breech Infants** was investigated by Eva B. Schutterman and David A. Grimes (Atlanta). Complications were reviewed in 221 deliveries done by low transverse incision and 195 done by low vertical incision between 1977 and 1981. Most deliveries were done by the resident staff under faculty supervision. The two groups of patients had comparable clinical characteristics.

Perinatal mortalities were 41/1,000 births in the low transverse incision group and 92/1,000 in the low vertical group. The relative risk was little affected by standardization for the effects of primary versus repeat cesarean delivery, type of anesthesia, and physician experience. When controlled for infant weight and gestational age, however, the difference was no longer significant. Rates of complications were similar in the two groups. The rate of a 5-minute Apgar score of 6 or below was significantly lower for infants in the low transverse incision group when standardized for the effect of type of anesthesia. Rates of blood transfusion, extension of the uterine incision, and maternal fever were not significantly different in the two groups.

The low transverse and low vertical uterine incisions for cesarean section delivery of singleton breech infants are associated with comparable rates of short-term maternal and infant complications. The possibility of subsequent vaginal delivery may be the determining factor, and the low transverse uterine incision appears to have the advantage in this regard.

(5–29) Obstet. Gynecol. 61:593–597, May 1983.

▶ [These authors found little difference in short-term effects on either mother or infants of transverse and vertical lower uterine segment incisions for cesarean delivery of a breech-presenting infant. It generally is held that trial labor in a subsequent pregnancy should be limited to patients with a transverse incision, and so the authors, reasoning that there is no difference in present complications and a potential benefit in the future, suggest that the transverse incision should be used whenever possible. We agree, but we would object to any implication that it is always or nearly always possible. This study does not establish that the transverse incision is *always* better because it was retrospective and there was undoubtedly some selection (i.e., clinical judgment) involved in the "assignment" of vertical versus transverse incision. In some cases, typically the preterm breech or the transverse lie, the lower uterine segment is poorly developed so that a transverse incision either extends or is extended through the uterine vessels—and we have seen several such cases where hysterectomy was necessary.] ◀

5–30 **Urinary Tract Injury During Cesarean Section.** Scott M. Eisenkop, Robin Richman, Lawrence D. Platt, and Richard H. Paul (Los Angeles) reviewed data on 7,527 cesarean sections performed from July 1976 to October 1980 at Los Angeles County-University of Southern California Medical Center and found there were 52 cystotomies (23 because of accidental bladder injuries and 29 for diagnostic purposes). Seven patients had ureteral injuries. The rates for bladder and ureter injuries were 0.31% and 0.09%, respectively.

Bladder injury usually was due to surgical difficulty caused by scar tissue from previous operations and encountered during development of the bladder flap over the lower uterine segment (Table 1). Therefore, during repeat cesarean section, it is important to use meticulous sharp dissection to mobilize the bladder. If bladder dissection is difficult, integrity of the lower urinary tract should be evaluated, at the least, by distending the bladder with a dilute solution of methylene blue dye.

Ureteral injury usually was due to ureteral transection or ligation

TABLE 1.—FACTORS ASSOCIATED WITH BLADDER INJURY

	No. of patients
Displacement of bladder base during repeat cesarean section	8
Displacement of bladder base during primary cesarean section	2
Injury during uterine incision	3
Adherence of bladder to abdominal wall from previous cesarean section	2
Extraperitoneal cesarean section	2
Extensions through bladder and/or ureter	2
Distended bladder	1
Ruptured uterus	2
Unspecified	1

(Courtesy of Eisenkop, S. M.: et al.: Obstet. Gynecol. 60:591–596, November 1982. Reprinted with permission of The American College of Obstetricians and Gynecologists.)

(5–30) Obstet. Gynecol. 60:591–596, November 1982.

TABLE 2.—Evaluation of Ureteral Integrity

	Accidental cystotomy	Diagnostic cystotomy
Intravenous indigo carmine with bilateral ureteral efflux after cystotomy	7	23
Passage of ureteral catheters bilaterally	2	2
Intravenous indigo carmine with unilateral efflux: renal agenesis unilaterally	1	0
Intravenous indigo carmine with unilateral efflux: ureteral patency established with catheter	0	1
Intravenous indigo carmine with unilateral efflux: ureteral ligation	1	3

(Courtesy of Eisenkop, S. M., et al.: Obstet. Gynecol. 60:591–596, November 1982. Reprinted with permission of The American College of Obstetricians and Gynecologists.)

associated with extension of the uterine incision into the lower uterine segment or vagina, and to attempts to achieve hemostasis. Therefore, when obtaining hemostasis in a patient in whom the uterine incision has been extended, the possibility of ureteral injury must be suspected and steps taken to document patency.

Of the various methods available for evaluation of bladder and ureter integrity (Table 2), cystotomy with intravenous injection of a bolus (5 ml) of indigo carmine and observation of symmetric efflux at the ureteral orifices is advised. Retroperitoneal extravasation of blue liquid suggests a partial ureteral transection. If efflux is not symmetric, further investigation by retrograde catheterization is indicated. In women with known or suspected ureteral anomalies and suspected lower urinary tract injury, intraoperative intravenous pyelography is advisable. Cystotomy does not increase the morbidity associated with cesarean section. Prophylactic antibiotics are not justified merely because a cystotomy was performed.

For bladder closure, various two-layer techniques with chromic suture are used. The bladder mucosa should be incorporated in the deepest layer, as opposed to the use of a submucosal stitch, to avoid postoperative bleeding from the mucosal edges and to assure a more anatomical closure. Postoperatively, the bladder is decompressed for 10 days by using a suprapubic catheter. A defect from bladder entry during cesarean section, whether accidental or intentional, can be repaired without complication if recognized intraoperatively.

Management of ureteral injury is more complicated and must be individualized. If the tissue is not devitalized and ureteral continuity is clearly shown, crush injuries and ligations may be managed conservatively by catheterizing the ureter through the ureteral orifice, exteriorizing the catheter through the urethra or abdominal wall, and removing it 10 to 14 days later. If the ureter is transected or devitalized within 5 cm of the bladder, primary reimplantation is the treatment of choice. Injuries further removed from the bladder may be managed by reimplantation with a psoas muscle hitch or end-to-end anastomosis. Management of injury discovered after operation is more controversial.

▶ [This large series of patients with an uncommon complication of cesarean section confirms the tenet that intraoperative recognition of injury to the urinary tract with prompt repair is usually associated with an uncomplicated postoperative course. Instillation of methylene blue into the bladder is used to confirm the integrity of that organ. If ureteral injury is suspected, diagnostic cystotomy should be performed and indigo carmine injected intravenously. Efflux of the dye from the ureteral orifices is a welcome sign.] ◀

5–31 **Short-term Antibiotic Prophylaxis in High-Risk Patients Following Cesarean Section.** Although antibiotic prophylaxis can reduce postoperative febrile morbidity significantly, many obstetricians have been reluctant to use it for fear that bacterial resistance will develop. P. A. Hawrylyshyn, P. Bernstein, and F. R. Papsin (Univ. of Toronto) evaluated single-dose and triple-dose prophylactic regimens in 189 high-risk patients undergoing cesarean section in 1980 and 1981. Cefoxitin, a new cephamycin with a broad antibacterial spectrum, was used. All patients had ruptured membranes when in active labor before cesarean section. Infusions were given at cord clamping and 4 and 8 hours postoperatively. Patients received three 2-gm doses of cefoxitin, one dose of drug followed by two of placebo, or three placebo infusions.

Primary cesarean section was performed in 173 of the 182 evaluable patients. Only 11 patients required general anesthesia. Endometritis occurred in 29% of the placebo group, 9.4% of patients given one dose of cefoxitin, and 5% of those given three doses of cefoxitin. Multiple organisms were isolated in over 40% of cases of endometritis. A disproportionately high rate of infection caused by enterococci was found in the actively treated patients. The most common organism isolated in placebo cases was *Bacteroides*. No adverse drug reactions were observed. No patient had septicemia, but 4 placebo patients were considered to be seriously ill and were hospitalized for more than 12 days. Five of 9 placebo patients with a postoperative hemoglobin concentration of less than 10.5 gm/dl developed endometritis, compared with 3 of 10 patients given one dose of cefoxitin and none of 7 given three doses.

Three doses of cefoxitin provide effective, safe, short-term prophylaxis after cesarean section. The regimen can reduce the rate of postoperative endometritis to a rate comparable with that associated with vaginal delivery, but it is not a panacea. Prophylaxis is warranted only in patients at the highest risk of postoperative infectious complications.

▶ [One of the aims of this study was to determine how brief "short-term" prophylaxis can be. The endometritis rate was lower in the group receiving three doses of cefoxitin 4 hours apart than in the group receiving one dose at clamping of the cord only, but statistical significance was not achieved. This may be a function of sample size.

(5–31) Am. J. Obstet. Gynecol. 145:285–289, Feb. 1, 1983.

Our personal practice is to prescribe a three-dose course of ampicillin or cephalothin as prophylaxis. These drugs are still effective at our institution. The later-generation antibiotics do have broader spectra, but we don't think they have been demonstrated to be superior for this purpose. The older drugs offer a cost advantage.] ◀

5-32 **A Double-Blind, Randomized Comparison of Clindamycin-Gentamicin Versus Cefamandole for Treatment of Post-cesarean Section Endomyometritis** was carried out by R. S. Gibbs, J. D. Blanco, Y. S. Castaneda, and P. J. St. Clair (Univ. of Texas, San Antonio) studied in 198 patients during an 18-month period. Criteria for exclusion from the study were use of prophylactic antibiotics or allergy to drugs used and those for entry were uterine tenderness, oral temperature ≥ 101 F, and leukocytosis. Uterine specimens for culture were obtained via a single-lumen transcervical catheter. A total of 106 patients received clindamycin, 600 mg intravenously every 6 hours in 20 ml of diluent, and gentamicin, 80 mg for the first three doses, then 1 mg/kg of body weight intravenously every 8 hours in 10 ml of diluent; 92 patients received cefamandole, 2.0 gm intravenously every 6 hours in 20 ml of diluent, plus placebo, 10 ml.

Bacterial isolates from the two treatment groups were similar. Of 6 therapeutic failures in the clindamycin-gentamicin group, there were apparent explanations for 2 (pelvic mass and isolation of a resistant enterococcus); the other 4 cases had no apparent cause. All 6 patients had apparent responses to empiric addition of penicillin G. In 6 patients with diarrhea, this was stopped by withdrawal of clindamycin and empiric treatment with chloramphenicol; all 6 had shown clinical signs that infection was clearing before cessation of combination therapy. Of 13 therapeutic failures in the cefamandole-placebo group, 3 were explained as resistant isolates. In 1 case there was a pelvic mass with resistant isolate. No apparent causes were found for the other 9 therapeutic failures. All 13 patients had good response to penicillin. Of 11 patients in the clindamycin-gentamicin group with bacteremia, 7 were cured, 2 had a therapeutic failure, and 2 had a side effect failure. Of 7 patients in the cefamandole-placebo group with bacteremia, 6 were cured, and 1 had a failure. When side effect failures were excluded, there were more clinical cures in the clindamycin-gentamicin group.

Although the clindamycin-gentamicin regimen had fewer therapeutic failures, it had more side effect failures. Newer antibiotics eventually may prove more efficacious than cefamandole but with fewer side effects.

▶ [This well-designed and apparently well-executed clinical trial doesn't provide clear answers. Cefamandole, a second-generation cephalosporin, was associated with more therapeutic failures in the treatment of post-cesarean section endomyometritis than was the clindamycin-gentamicin combination (13 vs. 6), but there were fewer side effect failures (3 vs. 7). Both regimens performed well, as no patients died, developed septic phlebitis, or required reoperation for pelvic abscess. Newer penicillins and cephalosporins have improved anaerobic and gram-negative coverage so that single drugs probably will be effective in this situation, although they won't be inexpensive.

Our usual practice is to use prophylactic antibiotics at cesarean section unless the

---

(5-32) Am. J. Obstet. Gynecol. 144:261-267, Oct. 1, 1982.

membranes are intact and the patient has not labored. If a patient subsequently develops endomyometritis, we frequently treat with a single drug (ampicillin or cephalothin), adding gentamicin and clindamycin if we don't see a response in 24–48 hours. There are many ways to skin this cat.] ◀

5–33 **Correlation of Decrease in Perinatal Mortality and Increase in Cesarean Section Rates.** Kieran O'Driscoll and Michael Foley (Univ. College, Dublin) observed that during 1965 to 1980, when cesarean birth rates increased dramatically in centers across the United States from less than 5% to more than 15%, the number of infants born in the National Maternity Hospital, Dublin, was 108,987. Although the incidence of cesarean section remained virtually unchanged at 4.2%, 4.2%, 4.1%, and 4.8% in 1965, 1970, 1975, and 1980, respectively, perinatal mortality fell progressively from 42.1 to 36.5, 24.0, and 16.8 per 1,000 infants born who weighed 500 gm or more. These results do not support the contention that an increase in cesarean birth rates has contributed significantly to reduced perinatal mortality in recent years.

Figure 5–4 shows the cesarean birth rates per 100 deliveries in the United States and in Dublin from 1965 to 1980. Most studies of this subject lack any reliable information as to the possible outcome in terms of perinatal mortality had the cesarean birth rate been maintained at the previous level of 5%. The Dublin experience provides

Fig 5–4.—Cesarean birth rates per 100 deliveries *(solid lines)* and perinatal mortality per 1,000 deliveries *(broken lines)* in the United States according to Bottoms et al., 1980 *(circles)*, and in National Maternity Hospital, Dublin *(crosses)*. *(Open circle* indicates estimate based on survey of 64 hospitals throughout the United States.) (Courtesy of O'Driscoll, K., and Foley, M.: Obstet. Gynecol. 61:1–5, January 1983. Reprinted with permission from The American College of Obstetricians and Gynecologists.)

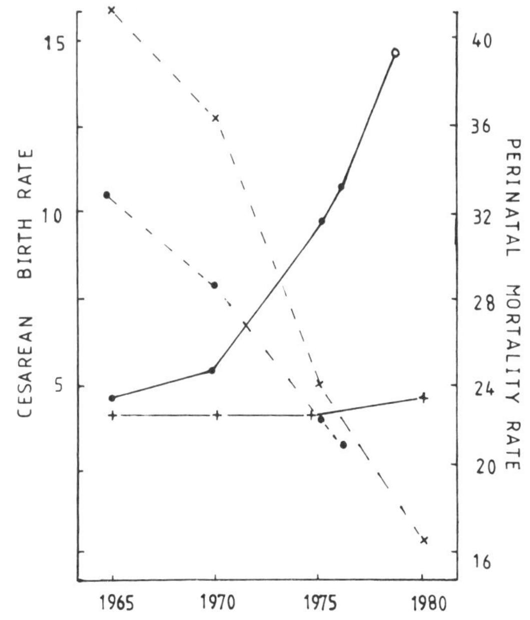

(5–33) Obstet. Gynecol. 61:1–5, January 1983.

FREQUENCIES OF CESAREAN DELIVERIES ACCORDING TO DIAGNOSTIC CATEGORIES*

Indication	United States[12]† (1978)	Dublin (1980)
Dystocia	4.7	0.7
Repeat Section	4.7	1.1
Breech	1.8	0.6
Fetal Distress	0.8	0.5
Others	3.2	1.9
Total	15.2	4.8

*Expressed as percentage of all births.
†United States figures calculated from National Institutes of Health Consensus Statement based on data from New York City; Dublin figures refer to National Maternity Hospital.
(Courtesy of O'Driscoll, K., and Foley, M.: Obstet. Gynecol. 61:1–5, January 1983. Reprinted with permission from The American College of Obstetricians and Gynecologists.)

such information. Among the 108,987 births during these 16 years in Dublin, 5,005 were cesarean (4.6%). Indications for primary cesarean section, expressed as a percentage of all births, were dystocia (0.7%), antepartum hemorrhage (0.7%), breech presentation (0.6%), fetal distress (0.5%), and others (1.2%). Twenty-two percent of the 246 breech presentations were delivered by cesarean section. In the United States, the largest number of primary cesarean sections are performed for abnormal labor (table). Not less than 5% of all babies born in the United States are delivered by repeat cesarean section, in contrast to Dublin's 1.1%. Three times as many cesarean sections are performed for breech presentation in the United States, 1.8% of all births compared with 0.6% in Dublin.

Caution must be used in comparing perinatal results taken from medical centers located on different continents. However, consideration of indications for primary cesarean section shows that the threefold difference in cesarean birth rate that now exists between Dublin and similar centers across the United States can be accounted for almost entirely by a different approach to management of labor in nulliparous women, compounded by rigid adherence to the precept, "Once a cesarean section, always a cesarean section."

▶ [It would be naive to assume that the tripling or quadrupling of the cesarean section rate has been responsible for the dramatic decline in perinatal mortality over the past decade or so, but most would feel that it surely has been one of the factors involved. This interesting report, however, must cause us to pause and wonder. Perinatal mortality has fallen at least as much in Dublin as it has in the United States, yet the cesarean section rate in Dublin has remained remarkably constant at slightly less than 5%. The principal difference between American and Irish practices lies in the frequency with which abdominal delivery is used for dystocia (alias failure to progress, cephalopelvic disproportion, etc.), with lesser influences due to repeat cesarean section and breech presentation.] ◀

5–34 **Vaginal Delivery After Cesarean Section: Experience in Private Practice.** Many reports over the past half century have attested

(5–34) JAMA 249:2935–2937, June 3, 1983.

to the safety of vaginal delivery after cesarean section in selected cases. Elliott Gellman, Martin S. Goldstein, Solomon Kaplan, and William J. Shapiro (Mt. Sinai Med. Center, New York) have, since 1971, offered the option of vaginal delivery to patients. Data on a total of 2,350 deliveries over a 10-year period were reviewed. Eighty-five women met predetermined safety criteria and were permitted a trial of labor. These criteria included previous low-segment transverse uterine incision, vertex presentation, ability to monitor labor closely with an obstetrician present, available emergency facilities, no administration of oxytocin, patient consent, and an ability to participate actively in labor. Fifty-five percent of patients having previous cesarean section were eligible for a trial of labor, but patient motivational factors eliminated 36 of these 121 patients.

Fifty-three women were followed through 85 pregnancies. Forty-four (80%) of the 53 were successful in their objective of vaginal delivery, with 14 having between 2 and 5 successful vaginal deliveries. The rate of vaginal delivery among the 85 labors was 89%. Indications for primary cesarean section were heavily weighted in favor of nonrecurrent indications. There was no maternal or fetal morbidity. No uterine ruptures were detected on postpartum evaluation or at the time of cesarean section.

These results support the 1980 report of the National Institute of Child Health and Human Development, which recommends that labor and vaginal delivery after cesarean section are not of high risk to the mother and fetus in properly selected cases. No special expertise or training is needed to monitor these labors. The approach of these authors is that there should be an indication for every repeat cesarean section that is performed. This approach requires an obstetric facility that can provide instant support in the face of complications.

▶ [The unusual thing here is that the authors are in private practice. To their credit, they apparently are willing to spend the time required to provide obstetric care to patients who desire an attempt at vaginal delivery after cesarean section. Most practitioners practice "Once a cesarean section, always a cesarean section." Convenience is probably a more important factor involved in reaching this decision than are the perceived risks of labor with a scarred uterus.] ◀

6. Obstetric Analgesia and Anesthesia

6–1 **Pain Relief During Delivery: Evaluation of Conventional Methods.** Peter Bundsen, Lars-Erik Peterson, and Urban Selstam (Univ. of Göteborg) evaluated the effect of conventional obstetric analgesia on 544 parturients and their newborn infants. The women's pain situation was evaluated with respect to both the effect of pain relief given and the total pain experience in the first and second stages of labor. Methods of obstetric analgesia used included nitrous oxide and oxygen, pethidine, diazepam, transcutaneous electric nerve stimulation and pudendal block (all of which were given by a midwife), paracervical block given by the obstetrician, and extradural analgesia (EDA) given by an anesthetist.

The mean age was 24 years for primiparas and 28 years for multiparas. Induced deliveries were less common among primiparas (13%) than among multiparas (23%). Half of the women experienced both low-back and abdominal pain in the first stage. The rate of vacuum extraction was the same as that for the whole year (7%). For primiparas with EDA the vacuum extraction rate was 31%, with the indication of prolonged second stage in 70%. Total duration of labor was

DEGREE OF PAIN RELIEF BY DIFFERENT ANALGESIC METHODS ON LOW-BACK AND/OR SUPRAPUBIC PAIN COMPARED WITH TOTAL PAIN EXPERIENCE IN FIRST STAGE*

		Total pain experience			
Method	Degree of pain relief	No/moderate pain	Severe pain	Very severe/almost unbearable pain	Total
EDA	Good	24	17	31	72
	Moderate	2	2	7	11
	No	2	0	7	9
	No answer	5	1	2	8
n = 58	Total	33	20	47	100
Pethidine + N_2O/O_2	Good	18	20	10	48
	Moderate	7	13	9	29
	No	2	3	8	13
	No answer	3	6	1	10
n = 204	Total	30	42	28	100
N_2O/O_2	Good	15	8	6	29
	Moderate	4	9	5	18
	No	4	2	2	8
	No answer	23	18	4	45
n = 135	Total	46	37	17	100

*Figures given indicate percent of women within each group.
(Courtesy of Bundsen, P., et al.: Acta Obstet. Gynecol. Scand. 61:289–297, 1982.)

(6–1) Acta Obstet. Gynecol. Scand. 61:289–297, 1982.

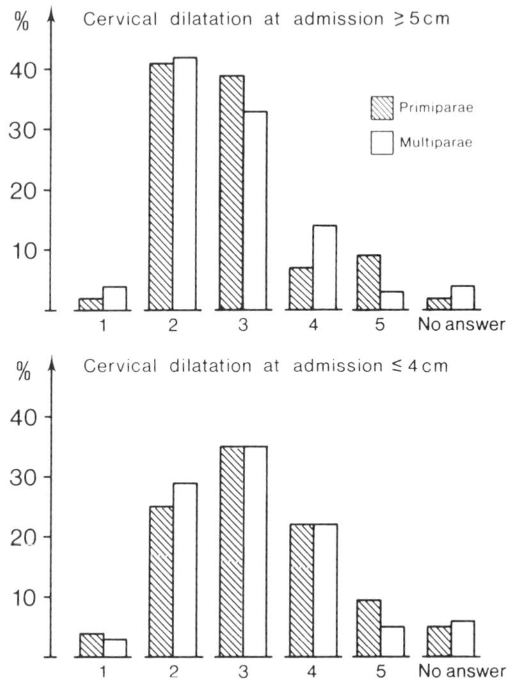

Fig 6–1.—Intensity of pain in first stage of labor in relation to cervical dilatation at admission (1 = no pain; 2 = moderate pain; 3 = severe pain; 4 = very severe pain; and 5 = almost unbearable pain). (Courtesy of Bundsen, P., et al.: Acta Obstet. Gynecol. Scand. 61:289–297, 1982.)

an average of 9.8 hours for all primiparas and 5.9 hours for all multiparas.

Sixty-four percent of all parturients graded their total pain experience in the first stage as severe to almost unbearable. Figure 6–1 presents the pain intensity ratings only for deliveries with spontaneous onset of labor. Duration of labor showed a positive correlation to total pain experience in the first stage. The first pain-relieving method was given at a mean cervical dilatation of 4.4 cm for all primiparas and 5.3 cm for all multiparas, compared with 3.0 cm for primiparas and 3.2 cm for multiparas who later had EDA. Most women received nitrous oxide and oxygen.

The degree of pain relief varied with the method, but nearly 20% of all parturients experienced good effect on low-back or suprapubic pain. The table records the most commonly used methods of pain relief, comparing these with total pain experience in the first stage. Eighty-five percent of primiparas and 71% of multiparas received pudendal block. Thirty-five percent of these women experienced no or moderate pain, whereas 65% reported severe to almost unbearable pain. No adverse effects on the newborn infants were seen, except for the well-known association between the drug-delivery interval and the slightly depressant effects of pethidine.

This study shows the pain-relieving methods used were insufficient for many parturients, but safe for mother and child. That parturients with a low degree of cervical dilatation at admission experienced the most intense pain may to some extent be due to the fact that they were immediately put to bed for electronic monitoring. It is, therefore, suggested that ambulant care be used more frequently.

▶ [Both a positive attitude toward an unmedicated childbirth and advanced cervical dilatation on admission were associated with a decreased "total pain experience" in the first stage of labor. Although epidural anesthesia provided good pain relief, it was used in patients whose total pain experience exceeded that of those using lesser analgesic techniques. This undoubtedly reflects the lack of random patient assignment to the options available. Those women with very painful labors eventually wound up with epidural anesthesia.] ◀

6–2 **Effectiveness of Pain Relief in Labor: Survey of 1,000 Mothers.** Barbara Morgan, C. J. Bulpitt, P. Clifton, and P. J. Lewis report data on the relative effectiveness of different methods of obstetric analgesia in a consecutive series of 1,000 women who had a vaginal delivery at Queen Charlotte's Maternity Hospital, London. The amount of pain experienced by these women during delivery of a live child was determined by interview within 48 hours of delivery. Patients had been encouraged to choose the method of analgesia they wished to receive. Patients requesting an epidural block were not initially given any other analgesia. Each woman was interviewed by a research midwife who had not met her before.

Mean age of the study population was 28 years. Social classes I and II accounted for 230 of the patients. Patients received one of the following categories of analgesia: 80 did not receive any analgesia, 128 received Entonox, 24 did not require any analgesia but required pudendal block for delivery, 120 received pethidine (meperidine), 88 received pethidine and Entonox, 423 received epidural analgesia alone, 38 received epidural analgesia plus Entonox, 47 received pethidine and epidural analgesia; and 52 received miscellaneous combinations. There were significantly more primiparas than multiparas in the groups that received an epidural block (64% versus 33%). Patients whose labor was induced were more likely to receive an epidural analgesic. Patients who had an epidural block had a significantly longer labor than those who did not. The proportion requiring assisted delivery was much greater among patients receiving epidural analgesia compared with those who did not (51% versus 6%). Patients receiving only epidural block had the lowest average pain score and the highest proportion of women claiming to have had no pain. About one third of all women experienced more pain than they had expected. Of the 1,000 women, only 536 chose the option that promised a painless labor. Those experiencing a pain-free labor included 12% of those who received pethidine alone, 12% of those who received Entonox alone, 59% of those who received epidural block alone, and 18% of those who received pethidine and Entonox.

The authors suggest that possibly the expectations of anesthetists are too high. A realistic expectation to encourage in antenatal patients is that modern methods can relieve, although not totally abol-

(6–2) Br. Med. J. 285:689–690, Sept. 11, 1982.

ish, pain in labor. The promise of a totally painless labor is probably unrealistic and may even be unwanted.

▶ [The interesting point here is not that epidural anesthesia was associated with the lowest "pain score," but, rather, that the proportion of patients who experienced more pain than they "expected" was virtually identical for each of the analgesic categories. As we have said before, the epidural block may be the Cadillac, but it seems that some would prefer walking or taking the bus.] ◀

6–3 **Maternal, Fetal, and Neonatal Responses After Epidural Anesthesia With Bupivacaine, 2-Chloroprocaine, or Lidocaine.** Therese K. Abboud, Swee Sim Khoo, Frank Miller, Thien Doan, and Eva H. Henriksen (Univ. of Southern California, Los Angeles) studied the effects of epidural analgesia on fetal heart rate, fetal heart rate variability, uterine activity, maternal blood pressure, newborn Apgar scores, neonatal acid-base status, and the early neonatal neurobehavioral status in 150 parturients during labor and delivery. The 50 patients in each group received 0.5% bupivacaine (group I), 2% 2-chloroprocaine (group II), or 1.5% lidocaine (group III). None of the three local anesthetics used had any significant effect on baseline fetal heart rate, beat-to-beat variability, or uterine activity. In cases in which monitoring of fetal heart rate was both technically satisfactory and continuous, late deceleration patterns were seen in 8 of 42, 0 of 34, and 3 of 47 of the fetuses in groups I, II, and III, respectively. The difference in incidence of late deceleration patterns between groups I and II was statistically significant. Early neonatal neurobehavioral status did not differ among the three groups of neonates, nor did any of the neonates in the three groups score lower than a control group of 20 neonates whose mothers did not receive any analgesia or medications for labor or delivery. The table presents the neonatal acid-base status of the three groups.

ACID-BASE AND BLOOD GAS DATA*

	Bupivacaine	2-Chloroprocaine	Lidocaine
Umbilical vein			
No.	32	34	38
pH	7.34 ± 0.01	7.32 ± 0.01	7.33 ± 0.01
P_{O_2} (torr)	30.9 ± 1.4	29.4 ± 1.2	29.0 ± 0.8
P_{CO_2} (torr)	35.7 ± 1.1	35.9 ± 1.0	36.5 ± 1.5
Base excess (meq/L)	6.5 ± 0.5	6.6 ± 0.5	6.2 ± 0.4
Umbilical artery			
No.	31	32	39
pH	7.26 ± 0.01	7.23 ± 0.02	7.25 ± 0.01
P_{O_2} (torr)	19.8 ± 0.9	19.0 ± 0.9	20.3 ± 0.8
P_{CO_2} (torr)	42.1 ± 1.8	47.1 ± 1.8	43.6 ± 1.8
Base excess (meq/L)	7.0 ± 0.8	7.0 ± 0.8	7.9 ± 0.6

*Values are means ± SE. No significant difference between groups by Student's *t* test.

(Courtesy of Abboud, T. K., et al.: Anesth. Analg. (Cleve.) 61:638–644, August 1982.)

(6–3) Anesth. Analg. (Cleve.) 61:638–644, August 1982.

The authors conclude that epidural anesthesia as administered in this study had no significant effect on the baseline fetal heart rate, uterine activity, or neurobehavioral status of the neonate. Bupivacaine is associated with a higher incidence of what appear to be transient abnormalities of fetal heart rate. In this study, only parturients with no medical or obstetric complications were included. In cases of compromised or borderline uteroplacental function, the lowest possible effective dosage of local anesthetics should be used for epidural anesthesia, and injections should be spaced adequately to avoid excessive increases in maternal and fetal blood levels of the local anesthetics.

▶ [This is a nice comparison study of three local anesthetic agents used in epidural anesthesia. All three get good marks. The late decelerations seen with bupivacaine were transient and were not associated with decreased cord blood pH values.] ◀

6–4 **Acid-Base Status of Diabetic Mothers and Their Infants Following Spinal Anesthesia For Cesarean Section.** Sanjay Datta, John L. Kitzmiller, J. Stephen Naulty, Gerard W. Ostheimer, and Jess B. Weiss (Harvard Med. School) evaluated acid-base status and Apgar scores in 10 rigidly controlled insulin-dependent diabetic mothers and in 10 healthy nondiabetic control women having spinal anesthesia for cesarean section. There were no significant differences between the groups in age, height, weight, or gestational age. Dextrose-free intravenous solutions were used for volume expansion in patients before induction of anesthesia, and hypotension was prevented in all cases by prompt treatment with ephedrine.

Two diabetic women were hospitalized 3 weeks before delivery for control of fasting blood glucose levels. Preoperatively, these levels were within normal limits in all the diabetic women. Systolic blood pressure did not exceed 130 torr in any woman within 24 hours of operation and none had systolic pressures of more than 30 torr from baseline levels during anesthesia. Total amount of ephedrine given varied from 10 to 30 mg and was not significantly different between the groups. There were no differences in the induction-delivery or uterine-incision delivery intervals between the groups. Acid-base status of women in both groups was normal at delivery. No significant differences were found in acid-base status or in blood gas tensions between infants in the control and in the diabetic groups. Only 1 infant in the diabetic group had an Apgar score of less than 7 at 1 minute.

Strict control of maternal diabetes, avoidance of dextrose-containing solutions for acute maternal volume expansion before anesthesia, and prompt treatment of any decrease of maternal blood pressure will maintain neonatal acid-base status at control levels during spinal anesthesia and will avoid the development of acidemia that may place the newborn at increased risk.

▶ [In contrast to earlier reports by these same authors, in the present study newborns delivered of diabetic women by cesarean section with the use of spinal anesthesia were in excellent condition at birth. The diabetes was well controlled, a glu-

---

(6–4) Anesth. Analg. (Cleve.) 61:662–665, August 1982.

cose-free solution (Ringer's lactate) was used for preblock hydration, and hypotension after the block was treated promptly with intravenously administered ephedrine.] ◀

6–5 **Prophylactic Intravenous Ephedrine Infusion During Spinal Anesthesia for Cesarean Section.** Hypotension occurs in up to 80% of women undergoing cesarean section with the use of spinal anesthesia. Several methods have been used to maintain maternal blood pressure, but each has potential disadvantages. Yoo G. Kang, Ezzat Abouleish, and Steve Caritis (Pittsburgh) sought to determine whether continuous intravenous infusion of ephedrine, titrated against maternal blood pressure, can maintain maternal blood pressure safely and effectively.

Ephedrine sulfate was administered to 44 healthy women undergoing elective repeat cesarean section with the use of spinal anesthesia. Twenty randomly selected patients received ephedrine infusion (0.01% solution, beginning with approximately 5 mg/minute) immediately after induction of spinal anesthesia to maintain maternal systolic blood pressure at 90% to 100% of baseline levels (mean dose of ephedrine, 31.6 mg). The other 24 women received 20 mg of ephedrine as an intravenous bolus and additional 10-mg injections, if necessary, when systolic blood pressure decreased to 80% of baseline values (mean dose of ephedrine, 26.8 mg).

In women given the infusion, systolic blood pressure did not change significantly from baseline levels, whereas it did in those given bolus injections (Fig 6–2). Neither reactive hypertension nor tachycardia occurred in women given the infusion. Nausea or vomiting, or both, occurred in 1 woman in the infusion group and in 9 in the injection group. Apgar scores, fetal blood gas tensions, and time for onset of rhythmic respiration were similar in the two groups.

Prophylactic ephedrine infusion is apparently safe and effective for maintenance of maternal blood pressure in healthy parturients undergoing cesarean section with the use of spinal anesthesia.

Fig 6–2.—Systolic blood pressures with prophylactic ephedrine infusion *(open circles)* and with therapeutic bolus injection of ephedrine *(solid circles)*.* *Asterisk,* significantly different from baseline value ($P < .001$). *Dagger,* significantly different from corresponding value during infusion of ephedrine ($P < .025$). (Courtesy of Kang, Y. G., et al.: Anesth. Analg. (Cleve.) 61:839–842, October 1982.)

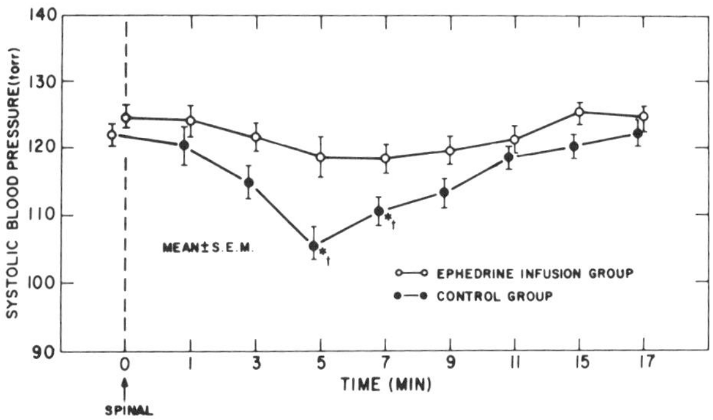

(6–5) Anesth. Analg. (Cleve.) 61:839–842, October 1982.

▶ [This study compared the effects of "prophylactic" intravenous ephedrine infusions and therapeutic bolus ephedrine injection in patients having spinal anesthesia for cesarean section. About 80% of the control subjects required ephedrine treatment. The results seem to favor the continuous prophylactic approach because this maintained the blood pressure in a much more nearly normal range.] ◀

6–6 **Epidural Morphine After Cesarean Section.** R. J. Binsted (Sydney) examined the effect of a single dose of epidurally administered morphine in controlling pain after elective cesarean section with the use of epidural anesthesia—bupivacaine, alone or with lidocaine—in 51 patients. Patients received 5 mg of morphine sulfate or a placebo solution via the epidural catheter 1 hour after operation. Pain was assessed by using a visual analogue scale. Papaveretum, 0.25 to 0.3 mg/kg, was injected intramuscularly every 4 hours on request.

Postoperative pain was significantly less in the morphine-treated patients than in the placebo group. Eight morphine-treated patients and 2 patients who received placebo required no narcotic analgesia after operation. Duration of analgesia until the first narcotic analgesic dose was significantly longer in the morphine-treated group, and significantly fewer doses of narcotic analgesic were necessary among this group. No serious respiratory depression was observed. More morphine-treated patients were nauseated and vomited, and more morphine-treated patients required catheterization of the bladder.

Epidural morphine injection significantly relieved pain after cesarean section in this study and reduced the need for parenteral narcotic administration. The only troublesome side effect of morphine treatment was pruritus. Large doses of antihistamines relieved pruritus in this setting.

▶ [The injection of small doses of morphine either extradurally or infradurally has been reported to be effective for analgesia in labor, abortion, and gynecologic surgery (see 1982 YEAR BOOK, pp. 177–179). This report describes epidural morphine administration 1 hour after cesarean section done with the use of epidural anesthesia. Patients who received morphine, in comparison with controls given placebo, had less pain and required less narcotic during the first 24 hours post partum. The principal side effect was itching, noted in 23%.

In a related study, Cohen and Woods (*Anesthesiology* 58:500, 1983) compared epidurally and intravenously administered morphine in patients after cesarean section. Those receiving epidural morphine administration had longer and better analgesia. Maternal interaction with the infants did not differ with respect to route of administration.] ◀

6–7 **Management of Headache Following Accidental Dural Puncture in Obstetric Patients.** Accidental dural taps will continue to occur as a complication of epidural anesthesia. Many of the treatments recommended are of dubious value. Peter Brownridge (Adelaide, Australia) reviewed the management of 58 obstetric patients with accidental dural puncture in 1975–1982. Trainee anesthetists had a relatively high accidental tap rate. Most incidents occurred during well-established labor. Forty-two patients had an epidural catheter successfully inserted. Conservative management in 19 cases included bed rest, systemic analgesics, high fluid intake and, in 3 instances, application of an abdominal binder. Twenty-five patients had

---

(6–6) Anesth. Intens. Care 11:130–134, May 1983.
(6–7) Ibid., pp. 4–15, February 1983.

epidural infusion of saline, and 12 received intermittent doses of saline or analgesia with bupivacaine or pethidine. A prophylactic blood patch was used in 2 instances initially, but nearly half the patients developed headache severe enough to receive 8–10 ml of autologous blood into the epidural space at the site of accidental puncture. This measure was completely successful in three fourths of the cases. A repeat blood patch was curative in 4 of 6 cases.

When accidental dural puncture occurs and time allows, the needle should be withdrawn and an epidural block should be done at a different interspace. Subarachnoid blockade may be considered if anesthesia is urgently needed. After delivery, either an epidural infusion of 1.5–2 L of fluid is given via a filter over 24 hours or 50-ml boluses of saline are injected at 4-hour intervals. If discomfort results, the epidural catheter is removed. The patient is advised to stay in bed in a comfortable lateral or semiprone position. Oral analgesia is liberally prescribed. If severe headache occurs, a blood patch is likely to cure it permanently within a few hours. Up to 20 ml of autologous blood is injected slowly under sterile conditions via a Tuohy needle at the site of the dural puncture. The patient is kept in bed for 6 hours after the procedure. A repeat patch can be considered if headache is not relieved or if it suddently returns after a period of relief. If the diagnosis is in doubt, a neurologic opinion is sought.

▶ [Postspinal headache is a fairly common problem when the dura is punctured inadvertently during a lumbar epidural puncture because of the large-bore needle used. This report outlines suggestions for management of such "wet taps." Performance of an epidural block at a different interspace permits an epidural infusion of saline post partum, either continuously or intermittently over the next 24 hours, and will decrease the incidence and severity of headache. For patients in whom symptoms develop despite this, epidural injection of 10–20 ml of autologous whole blood relieves symptoms promptly in 80%.] ◀

7. Genetics and Teratology

DRUG USE IN PREGNANCY

JENNIFER R. NIEBYL, M.D.
Associate Professor of Gynecology and Obstetrics and Director, Division of Maternal-Fetal Medicine, Johns Hopkins University School of Medicine

Behold, thou shalt conceive and bear a son
and now drink no wine nor strong drink,
neither eat any unclean thing.

(Judges 13:7.)

Caution with regard to dietary intake during pregnancy has been advised since ancient times. However, until recently the fetus has been thought to rest in a privileged site with little exposure to the environment experienced by the mother. The term "placental barrier" has been in widespread use, but is truly a contradiction because the placenta allows crossing of many drugs and dietary substances.

Lipid-soluble substances readily cross the placenta; water-soluble substances pass less well the greater their molecular weight. The degree to which a drug is bound to plasma protein also influences the amount of drug that is free to cross. Virtually all drugs cross the placenta to some degree, with the exception of large organic ions such as heparin and insulin that pass poorly or not at all.

Developmental defects in man may be the result of genetic, environmental, or unknown causes. Although approximately 25% are clearly genetic in origin, drug exposure accounts for probably only 2%–3% of birth defects. Approximately 65% of defects are of unknown etiology but may be from combinations of genetic and environmental factors.

The incidence of birth defects defined as major anomalies is approximately 2%–3%. A major anomaly usually is defined as one incompatible with life, such as anencephaly, or requiring major surgery for correction, such as cleft lip or congenital heart disease. If all minor malformations are included, such as extra digits, the rate is approximately 10%.

Teratogenesis

Variability and partial expression of teratogenic drug effects are observed, presumably related to dose, timing of exposure, host susceptibility, genetic differences, and interactions with other environmental agents.[1] Teratogens produce patterns of defects appropriate for the time in development at which they are administered. Single morphological abnormalities may not be specific for certain teratogenic agents. Early in gestation, a teratogenic agent will affect the organs that develop first, such as the heart, and later in the teratogenic period, such an agent may affect the palate, which closes approximately 10 weeks from the last menstrual period. In some situations, a drug or environmental agent may act in combination with a genetically susceptible host to produce a defect which in a nonsusceptible individual would not be expressed. Most teratogens exhibit a dose-response curve, and there may be a threshold below which the drug will not show an effect. Thus, patients should be managed with the least effective dose of a needed drug, and, theoretically, monitoring of blood levels would be helpful in minimizing the dose and possibly reducing teratogenicity.

The classic teratogenic period is from 17 days to 57 days after conception, that is, 31 days from menstruation to 71 days from menstruation in the human being (Fig 7–1). Prior to this period, i.e., around the time of conception and implantation, teratogenic agents have an all-or-none effect. Either the pregnancy does not survive or it survives intact and without any morphological defects. Also, beyond the classic teratogenic period, the internal organs and the brain are continuing to grow and develop, and environmental agents may influ-

Fig 7–1.—The classic teratogenic period in pregnancy. (Courtesy of J. R. Niebyl.)

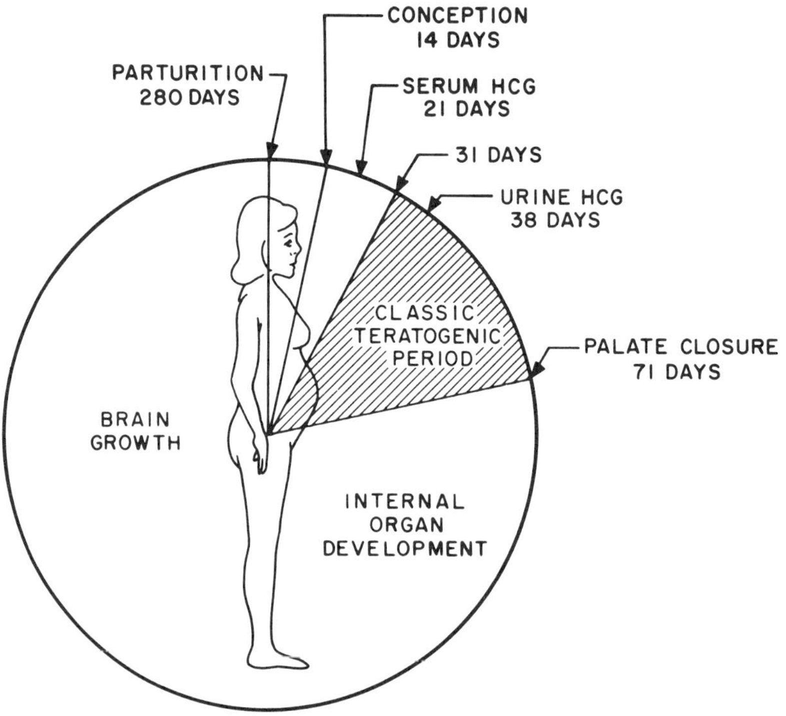

ence the organism at this time without apparent defects at birth. For example, the use of alcohol throughout the second and third trimesters may cause the fetal alcohol syndrome with developmental delays that may not be detected until later in life. Also, some of the anomalies caused by diethylstilbestrol were produced in the second trimester when the internal genitalia were developing, and these abnormalities usually were not recognized until after puberty.

One of the risks of drug exposure is that a woman may take a drug in early pregnancy before she recognizes that she is pregnant. Urine pregnancy tests are not usually positive until 10 days after the missed menses. With the current availability of serum assays for human chorionic gonadotropin (hCG) with sensitivity as early as 1 week after conception, if the possibility of pregnancy exists, serum hCG should be checked before a drug that may be teratogenic is prescribed.

Animal data do not correlate well with effects in man[2] as there is marked species specificity. The teratogenic period in the rat also represents a much greater proportion of the pregnancy than in the human being, approximately 10 of 21 days. For example, thalidomide, which was not teratogenic in mice and rats, was later found to be teratogenic in man. Conversely, corticosteroids have a marked ability to produce cleft lip in certain species of mice, but there is no evidence that corticosteroids have any teratogenic effect in human gestation.

Preoccupation with major anomalies has misled us into thinking some substances are safe, when, in fact, they may cause less obvious developmental problems, some of which do not become apparent until long after the perinatal period. Concern is now being directed toward behavioral teratogenesis, that is, abnormality in the development of behavioral patterns, intelligence, or learning processes. Some evidence suggests that exposure to hormones prenatally may contribute to abnormal behavioral development, such as homosexuality.[3] Clearly, although a drug has not been shown to cause any overt defects, this is not a guarantee that covert abnormalities will not be discovered in later years.

If a teratogenic event occurs with low frequency, many thousands of cases may be needed to identify a small risk and only certain patients may be genetically susceptible. Thus, although there may be no evidence that a drug is teratogenic, this does not mean that it cannot fall into this category. Caution therefore is advised with respect to taking any drugs in pregnancy.

Specific drug use in pregnancy will be reviewed in two categories: (1) teratogenic effects of drug use in the first trimester and (2) perinatal effects of drugs used throughout pregnancy and around the time of delivery.

Known Teratogens

Only a relatively few drugs are known teratogens. Thalidomide causes a typical bilateral limb reduction defect, and androgenic steroids have been documented to cause masculinization of the female fetus.[4] Diethylstilbestrol causes characteristic adenosis of the cervix and vagina and upper genital tract anomalies. Aminopterin, a folic acid antagonist that was used as an attempted abortifacient, caused multiple anomalies in the offspring who survived. Tetracycline has been shown to cause tooth discoloration, and iodide salts cause goiter. Oral anticoagulants of the warfarin type have been shown to cause nasal hypoplasia and bony stippling. In addition, many other drugs may be associated with birth defects, but a cause-and-effect relationship has not been clearly established.

Estrogens and Progestins

Various birth defects have been attributed to oral contraceptives and other female hormones given in the first trimester of pregnancy. In a prospective interview of 11,468 pregnant women, 432 were exposed to estrogens or progestagens in early pregnancy.[5] Malformations occurred in 10.9% (47) of the exposed and 7.7% of the nonexposed infants, a statistically significant difference ($P < .02$). In this study, however, all defects were combined and the drugs also were not divided as to the specific types of estrogens or progestagens.

Neural tube defects were once reported to be associated with ingestion of progestational agents in early pregnancy, but subsequent investigations have not confirmed this. In retrospective studies, limb reduction defects and a syndrome of multiple congenital anomalies (VACTERL—vertebral, anal, cardiac, tracheoesophageal, renal, and limb) were associated with ingestion of these hormones in early pregnancy. These findings have not been confirmed in prospective studies. The data are most supportive, however, of the risk of cardiac defects after first-trimester exposure. In the Collaborative Perinatal Project, 1,042 women were exposed to some female hormone during early pregnancy and 278 specifically took oral contraceptives.[6] In the 49,240 patients not exposed to any female hormone, the rate of cardiovascular defects was 7.8/1,000. In the group exposed to a female hormone, the rate was 18.2/1,000, and in the group exposed to oral contraceptives, the rate was 21.5/1,000 ($P < .05$). Thus, the risk of cardiovascular defects was increased twofold to threefold in patients exposed to these hormones in early pregnancy. However, as approximately 98% of the time the infant showed no evidence of adverse effect, a conservative approach should be taken to patient counseling. These data also should be placed in perspective by comparison with the incidence of 2%–3% of all major malformations in the general population. Nevertheless, it is important to inform a patient that there may be a risk to the fetus of continuing oral contraception after a missed period, especially if there is a possibility of pregnancy, for example, if the patient missed taking pills or is receiving a very low-dose formulation. Prior to the prescription of progestational agents for induction of withdrawal bleeding, serum hCG should be assayed if the patient is not using satisfactory contraception.

The natural hormone progesterone should be distinguished from the synthetic derivatives, the progestational agents, or progestins.[7] In the Collaborative Perinatal Project, there was no evidence for teratogenicity in 162 infants exposed to 17α-hydroxyprogesterone caproate (Delalutin) or in 253 exposed to progesterone.[8] In the study by Johnson et al.[9] of 43 infants exposed in early pregnancy, no risk was noted. In one study, however, evidence was presented suggesting that 17α-hydroxyprogesterone caproate may produce hypospadias if given prior to the 16th week of pregnancy.[10] Thus, for the prevention of premature labor, administraton of the drug usually is started after 16 weeks of pregnancy.

ANTICONVULSANTS

Epileptic women taking anticonvulsants during pregnancy have approximately double the risk of fetal malformations as that in the general population.[11] As the general risk is 2% to 3%, the risk of major fetal malformations in epileptic women taking anticonvulsants is about 5%, especially cleft lip, with or without cleft palate, and congenital heart disease. It recently has been recognized that valproic acid carries approximately a 1% risk of neural tube defects.[12] In addition, the offspring of epileptic women have approximately five times the general risk of epilepsy (making this 2% to 3%), but less than 10% have the fetal hydantoin syndrome.

Whenever a drug is claimed to be a teratogen, the issue always can be raised of whether the drug is a teratogen or the disease for which the drug was prescribed in some way contributed to the defect. Women with a convulsive disorder, even when they take no anticonvulsant drug, have an increased risk of birth defects in their offspring, and this information has been used to claim that it is the epilepsy rather than the drug that contributes to the birth defect.[13] Of the infants of 305 women in the Collaborative Perinatal Project who had a convulsive disorder, 10.5% had a birth defect. Among offspring of women who took phenytoin (Dilantin) daily, 11.8% had an abnormality; among offspring of women who took phenytoin sporadically from months 1 through 4, 7.1%; and among offspring of women who took phenytoin only after 4 months of pregnancy, 9%. A malformation occurred in 11.3% of the offspring of women who had a convulsive disorder and took no phenytoin at all. This contrasted with the total fetal malformation rate of 6.4% for the control women who did not have a convulsive disorder and therefore did not take any antiepileptic drugs.

With respect to major malformations, the data also showed an increased risk for epileptics not taking phenytoin. The issue is not resolved, as patients who take more drugs during pregnancy usually have more severe convulsive disorders than those who do not take any anticonvulsants. However, there is no evidence that the number of seizures a patient has during pregnancy influences the risk of birth defects.

Possible causes of malformations in epileptic women on anticonvulsants include the disease itself, a genetic predisposition to epilepsy and malformations, genetic differences in drug metabolism, the specific drugs themselves, and deficiency states, such as decreased serum concentrations of folate, induced by drugs. Phenytoin causes decreased absorption of folate and a lowering of the serum folate concentration, which has been implicated in birth defects.

The fetal hydantoin syndrome consists of microcephaly, growth deficiency, developmental delays, mental retardation, and dysmorphic craniofacial features. These defects also are found in other syndromes, such as fetal alcohol syndrome, but the characteristic unique to the fetal hydantoin syndrome appears to be hypoplasia of the nails and distal phalanges.

Some women may have taken anticonvulsant drugs for a long period without reevaluation of the need for continuation of the drug. It recently has been shown that if the patient with idiopathic epilepsy has been seizure-free for 4 years and has a normal EEG, a trial of withdrawal of the drug prior to pregnancy may be safe.[14] Also, if the patient has not been taking her dosage regularly, a low blood level may demonstrate her lack of compliance and lack of need for the drug.

If the patient is pregnant already, most authorities agree that the benefits of therapy outweigh the risks of discontinuation of the drug at that point. The blood level of drug should be monitored—if possible, monthly—in order to assure a therapeutic level but minimize dosage. Neonatologists need to be aware that the patient is taking phenytoin because this can affect clotting factors in the newborn.

Minor Tranquilizers

Conflicting reports of the possible teratogenicity of the various tranquilizers including meprobamate (Miltown) and chlordiazepoxide (Librium) have appeared, but in prospective studies no teratogenicity has been noted.[15] In one retrospective study,[16] exposure to diazepam (Valium) in the first trimester of pregnancy was four times more frequent among mothers of children with cleft lip, but this was not confirmed in other studies. Weighing against the teratogenicity of diazepam is the fact that billions of dollars worth of the drug have been sold in the United States in the past 10 years mainly to women of reproductive age, and yet the rate of cleft lip with or without cleft palate has been entirely stable. However, in most clinical situations, the risk-benefit ratio does not justify the use of the drug in early pregnancy. Perinatal maternal administration of diazepam has been associated with hypotonia, hypothermia, and respiratory depression in the infant.

Lithium

In two studies of lithium in which 263 infants were exposed in the first trimester of pregnancy, 19, or 7%, had cardiovascular malformations.[17] Half of the malformations were Ebstein's anomaly, which occurs in only 1 of 20,000 infants in the nonexposed population. No increased mental or physical abnormalities were noted in 60 exposed and apparently unaffected infants followed to age 5, compared to those in unexposed siblings.

Perinatal effects of lithium have been noted, including hypotonia, lethargy, and poor feeding in the infant, which may also occur when lithium passes through the breast milk. Also, complications similar to those seen in adults receiving lithium have been found in newborns, including goiter and hypothyroidism, and nephrogenic diabetes insipidus. Thus, the elimination of lithium as drug therapy in pregnant women is recommended to avoid fetal exposure, and lithium therapy is a relative contraindication to nursing, as the drug may cross through the breast milk and achieve significant blood levels in the infant.

Antiemetics

Remedies suggested to reduce nausea and vomiting in pregnant women without pharmacologic intervention include eating crackers before getting out of bed in the morning, getting up very slowly, omitting iron tablets, eating frequent small meals, and snacking on protein foods at night. Faced with a self-limited condition occurring at the time of organogenesis, the clinician is well advised to avoid the use of medications whenever possible and to encourage these supportive measures. When a clinician feels compelled to resort to pharmacologic measures, the attempt should be made to use relatively small amounts of those drugs that in the most appropriate studies have been found to be efficacious and unassociated with fetal malformations.

Bendectin

Bendectin contains 10 mg of doxylamine and 10 mg of pyridoxine (vitamin B_6). It was the drug of choice for nausea and vomiting in pregnancy. Although there was no evidence of teratogenicity with this drug, the cost of defense of law suits alleging adverse effects led the company to cease production in June 1983. As the incidence of congenital malformations in the general population is 2% to 3% and approximately 10% of women take antinauseants in the first trimester of pregnancy, it is not surprising that sporadic cases of malformation were reported in infants exposed to Bendectin in early pregnancy. Teratogenicity was claimed in some case-controlled retrospective studies. However, this was not confirmed in large prospective controlled trials.

In 1,169 patients who took doxylamine succinate in the Collaborative Perinatal Project,[8] no evidence of teratogenicity was noted. Mean birth weight, perinatal mortality, and IQ scores of children at age 4 also were similar in the exposed and control groups. In another 628 patients taking Bendectin in the Kaiser Health Plan, there again was no evidence of teratogenicity.[18] Likewise, no increase in the incidence of major defects was found in offspring of 2,298 women treated with Bendectin in England compared with offspring of control patients.

Thus, in a total of approximately 6,300 women studied whose infants were exposed to Bendectin in utero, no increase in the incidence of birth defects compared with that in controls has been noted.

Vitamin B_6 alone is available over the counter in 25-mg capsules and can be tried initially, although it is less effective this way than in combination with doxylamine. Several prenatal vitamin preparations also contain at least 10 mg of vitamin B_6.

Unisom contains 25 mg of doxylamine and is a scored tablet that provides 12.5 mg if broken in half, close to the 10 mg in Bendectin. Thus, a combination similar to Bendectin can be created with medications currently available over the counter. The physician faces a problem, however, as Unisom is labeled "not for use in pregnancy," as its manufacturer has not invested in all that is necessary for FDA approval for use of a drug during pregnancy.

Meclizine (Bonine, Antivert)

The Bendectin story has historical precedent in the saga of meclizine (Antivert, Bonine). After the United States Army, Navy, and Air Force Motion Sickness Team reported in 1956 that meclizine was the drug of choice in preventing motion sickness during long sea voyages, that drug also gained wide acceptance for treatment of nausea and vomiting of pregnancy. Uncontrolled studies reported complete or partial relief of symptoms in over 90% of patients and mild side effects (drowsiness) in 4%. In a small, randomized placebo-controlled study, meclizine gave significantly better results than placebo.[19] The addition of pyridoxine failed to improved the results with meclizine alone. Thus, meclizine was accepted as an efficacious agent for treating the nausea and vomiting of pregnancy.

After the thalidomide tragedy in 1956, the use of drugs at the time of organogenesis came under close scrutiny. Sporadic reports began to appear of congenital anomalies in infants born to mothers who had taken meclizine. However, no adequate control group was available, and the results were inconclusive and contradictory.

Despite these inadequacies of the available information, the Swedish National Board of Health withdrew meclizine from public sale in Sweden and warned doctors not to prescribe the drug for women in the early months of pregnancy. In addition, the Epidemic Observation Unit of the College of General Practitioners in England warned physicians of the "mounting evidence against the safety of meclizine."

After studies in rats demonstrated a teratogenic effect of cyclizine (an antihistaminic that approaches meclizine in its efficacy), congenital malformations were induced in the offspring of pregnant Sprague-Dawley rats by the administration of large doses of meclizine. However, the meaning of these results for man was questioned because the doses used were 25 to 50 times the recommended dose in human patients, and the possibility of species-specificity of effect had not been ruled out.

Prospective clinical studies have provided no evidence that meclizine is teratogenic in man. In 1,014 patients in the Collaborative Perinatal Project[8] and an additional 613 patients from the Kaiser Health Plan,[18] no teratogenic risk was found.

DIPHENHYDRAMINE (BENADRYL)

In 595 patients treated with diphenhydramine in the Collaborative Perinatal Project,[8] no increased teratogenic risk was observed. However, in patients treated with dimenhydrinate (Dramamine) a 29% failure rate and a significant incidence of side effects, especially drowsiness, have been reported.[20]

TRIMETHOBENZAMIDE (TIGAN)

Trimethobenzamide, an antinauseant that is not classified as either an antihistaminic or a phenothiazine, has been used to control nausea and vomiting in pregnancy. The data, collected on small numbers of patients, are conflicting. In the Kaiser Health Plan study,[18] 193 patients were exposed to trimethobenzamide and there was a suggestion of an excess of congenital anomalies ($P < .05$); however, no concentration of specific anomalies was observed in these children and some of the mothers took other drugs as well. In 340 patients in the Collaborative Perinatal Project,[8] no evidence for an association between this drug and malformations was found.

PHENOTHIAZINES

Because of the potential for severe side effects, the phenothiazines have not been used routinely in the treatment of mild or moderate nausea and vomiting. Instead, they have been reserved for the treatment of hyperemesis gravidarum. Chlorpromazine has been shown to be effective in hyperemesis gravidarum; the most important side effect is drowsiness.

Teratogenicity does not appear to be a problem with the phenothiazines when they are evaluated as a group. In the Kaiser Health Plan Study,[18] 976 patients were treated and in the Collaborative Perinatal Project,[8] 1,309 patients; no evidence of association was found in either study between these drugs and malformations. However, a suspicion of association between phenothiazines and cardiovascular malformations was noted, but it was of borderline significance and in the context of multiple comparisons was of doubtful import. When the phenothiazines were looked at individually, chlorpromazine (Thorazine) seemed to be associated with an increased risk of malformations ($P < .01$) in offspring of 141 exposed mothers. No increased risk of malformations was found in infants of 58 mothers exposed to promethazine (Phenergan) and in 48 mothers exposed to proclorperazine (Compazine).

EMETROL

Emetrol is a phosphorated carbohydrate solution containing balanced amounts of levulose (fructose) and dextrose (glucose) and orthophosphoric acid with a controlled hydrogen ion concentration. It relieves nausea and vomiting by local action on the wall of the hyperactive gastrointestinal tract. It reduces smooth muscle contractions in direct proportion to the amount used and is relatively free from toxicity or side effects. Recommended dosage in pregnancy is 1 to 2 tablespoons on arising, repeated every 3 hours or whenever nausea threatens.

Antibiotics and Anti-infective Agents

Antibiotics are used widely during pregnancy. As pregnant patients are particularly susceptible to vaginal yeast infections, prophylaxis with antifungal agents may be advisable during the course of therapy.

Penicillin derivatives including penicillin and ampicillin are apparently safe in pregnancy, as are erythromycin and the cephalosporins. Ampicillin decreases urinary estriol excretion due to its effect on the bowel flora, decreasing the enterohepatic circulation.[21] Mandelamine decreases urinary estriol excretion due to its breakdown product, formaldehyde, having a direct chemical interference in the urine.[22] Sulfonamides have not been associated with any particular risk except when given in the third trimester of pregnancy, when they may compete with bilirubin for albumin-binding sites and contribute to an increased risk of kernicterus in the newborn.

THE TETRACYCLINES

In 341 infants exposed to tetracycline in the first trimester, no teratogenic effect was observed.[8] However, the tetracyclines bind to developing enamel to cause discoloration of the teeth. The drug affects deciduous teeth in the infant if exposure occurs between approximately 26 weeks of gestation and age 6 months, but only affects the permanent teeth if given in childhood at about age 6 months to 5 years. In addition, the tetracyclines deposit in developing osseous sites and cause an inhibition of bone growth.[23] A 40% inhibition of fibular growth was demonstrated in fetuses of patients who subsequently underwent termination of pregnancy, but the effect was reversible when the drug was stopped.

AMINOGLYCOSIDES

No teratogenic effects were observed among 135 infants exposed to streptomycin in the first trimester.[8] However, transplacental passage has been demonstrated, and a rate of ototoxicity of 3%–11% in children of mothers who received prolonged streptomycin treatment for tuberculosis during pregnancy has been reported. Although the hearing loss appears to be dose related and has not been reported with other aminoglycosides, these agents should be avoided if possible during pregnancy. In cases in which the agents are required for serious infections, their use should be restricted to as short a time as possible and maternal serum levels should be monitored.

Other Antituberculosis Drugs

There is no evidence of teratogenic effects of INH, para-aminosalicylic acid rifampin, or ethambutol. In one report, ethionamide was associated with central nervous system anomalies in 7 of 23 infants exposed to the drug in utero.

Metronidazole (Flagyl)

Studies of small numbers of infants have failed to show any significant increase in the incidence of congenital defects among the newborns of mothers treated with metronidazole during early or late pregnancy. In one study,[24] 4 of 55 infants exposed in early gestation had a variety of minor defects, and in the Collaborative Perinatal Project,[8] 2 of 31 infants were abnormal, close to the expected incidence.

Controversy regarding the use of metronidazole during pregnancy was stirred when metronidazole was shown to be mutagenic in bacteria by the Ames test, which correlates with carcinogenicity in animals. Thus, if metronidazole is used during pregnancy, there is the theoretical potential for transplacental carcinogenicity. However, this has not been reported to date, and metronidazole remains the only effective drug for trichomoniasis. With the theoretical risks uncertain, it should only be given for clear-cut indications and in the minimal dose, which is the single-dose 2-gm regimen.[25]

The Warfarin Derivatives

Coumadin has been associated with chondrodysplasia punctata, similar to the Conradi-Hunerman syndrome. This syndrome includes nasal hypoplasia, bone stippling on x-ray studies, ophthalmologic abnormalities, including bilateral optic atrophy, and mental retardation. Even with its use only beyond the first trimester, the ophthalmologic abnormalities and mental retardation may occur.[26] Fetal and maternal hemorrhage also have been reported in pregnant women receiving Coumadin, although the incidence can be lowered with careful control of the prothrombin time. The alternative drug, heparin, does not cross the placenta, as it is a large molecule with a strong negative charge. As heparin does not have an adverse effect on the fetus when given in pregnancy, this should be the drug of choice for patients requiring anticoagulation. Teaching patients how to administer heparin subcutaneously or even with an intravenous heparin lock should be no more difficult than teaching patients how to self-administer insulin for diabetes.[27]

Thyroid and Antithyroid Drugs

Propylthiouracil (PTU) and methimazole (Tapazole) both cross the placenta and cause some degree of fetal goiter. However, the thyroid hormones triiodothyronine and thyroxine cross the placenta poorly, so that fetal hypothyroidism produced by antithyroid drugs cannot be corrected satisfactorily by administration of the thyroid hormones to the mother. Thus, the goal of such therapy during pregnancy is to keep the mother slightly hyperthyroid to minimize fetal drug exposure. As methimazole has been associated with scalp defects in the infants[28] and a higher incidence of side effects, PTU is the drug of choice.

In addition, iodide such as is found in a saturated solution of potassium iodide expectorant (SSKI) crosses the placenta and may cause very large fetal goiter, enough to produce respiratory obstruction in the newborn.[29] Thus, before a patient is advised that it is satisfactory to continue taking a cough medicine, it should be ascertained that it is not SSKI.

Iodine-131 administered for thyroid ablation or for diagnostic studies is not concentrated by the fetal thyroid until after 12 weeks' gestation.[29] Thus, with inadvertent exposures, which are usually around the time of missed menses, there is no specific risk to the fetal thyroid.

Propranolol (Inderal) is a β-adrenergic blocking agent in widespread use for a variety of indications. Although theoretically there might be increased uterine contractility in association with administration of this drug, this has not been reported. No evidence of teratogenicity has been noted to date. One review of 12 cases suggested an increased risk of intrauterine growth retardation,[30] but this has not been confirmed in other studies. Bradycardia has been reported in the newborn as a direct effect of a dose of the drug given to the mother within 2 hours before the birth of the infant.[30]

Studies from Scotland suggest improved outcome with the use of β-adrenergic blocking agents to treat chronic hypertension during pregnancy and do not suggest any of the adverse effects reported in isolated cases in the United States.[31]

Mild Analgesics

Aspirin

There is no evidence of any teratogenic effect of aspirin in human beings.[8] However, aspirin does have significant perinatal effects, as it inhibits prostaglandin synthesis. Uterine contractility is decreased and patients taking aspirin have a delayed onset and longer duration of labor and an increased risk of going postdates.[32] Aspirin also causes decreased platelet aggregation, which can result in an increased risk of bleeding before as well as at delivery.[32] Platelet dysfunction has been noted in newborns as long as a week after ingestion of aspirin by the mother.[33]

Prostaglandins are involved in multiple organ systems in the fetus, and as aspirin works by inhibition of prostaglandin synthetase, multiple organs may be affected by chronic aspirin use. Of note, prostaglandins mediate the neonatal closure of the ductus arteriosus, and one case has been reported in which ingestion of aspirin by the mother near the time of delivery presumably was related to closure of the ductus arteriosus in utero.[34]

PHENACETIN

There is no evidence of teratogenicity of phenacetin. However, because of nephrotoxic potential and possible methemoglobinemia in the newborn, this drug is not recommended in pregnancy. In fact, the FDA recently has withdrawn its approval for phenacetin, and it is expected to be removed from the market.

ACETAMINOPHEN

Acetaminophen (Tylenol, Datril) also has shown no evidence of teratogenicity. With acetaminophen, inhibition of prostaglandin synthesis is reversible; therefore, once the drug has cleared, platelet aggregation returns to normal. The bleeding time is not prolonged with acetominophen, in contrast to aspirin,[35] and the drug is not toxic to the newborn.

DARVON

Much less is known about propoxyphene (Darvon) with respect to pregnancy. It is an acceptable alternative mild analgesic with no known teratogenicity. However, it should not be used for trivial indications, as it has the potential for narcotic addiction. Evidence of risk in late pregnancy comes from two case reports of infants of mothers who were addicted to propoxyphene and had typical narcotic withdrawal in the neonatal period.

CODEINE

Little information is available about codeine in pregnancy. The Collaborative Perinatal Project suggested that there might be a slightly increased relative risk of malformations in 563 codeine users.[8] Because there is an alternative drug that is as effective as codeine and for which there is not even a suggestion of a risk of teratogenicity, that is, propoxyphene, it makes sense to choose this rather than codeine as a mild analgesic, if an agent of the narcotic type is indicated. Also, codeine can cause addiction and newborn withdrawal symptoms if used perinatally.

Few pains during pregnancy justify the use of a mild analgesic. Pregnant patients should be encouraged to use nonpharmacologic remedies, such as local heat and rest. If a mild analgesic or antipyretic agent seems appropriate, acetaminophen is the drug of choice.

Smoking

Smoking has been associated with a decreased birth weight as well as an increased prematurity rate.[36] The spontaneous abortion rate is up to twice that in nonsmokers, and abortions associated with maternal smoking tend to have a conceptus with a normal karyotype and to occur later than those of a conceptus with chromosomal aberrations.[37] The increased perinatal mortality associated with smoking is partly attributable to an increased risk of abruptio placenta and placenta previa, as well as premature and prolonged rupture of membranes. Risks of complications and of the associated perinatal loss increase with the number of cigarettes smoked. Discontinuation of smoking during pregnancy can reduce the risk of complications and of perinatal mortality, especially in women at high risk for other reasons. There is also a positive association between smoking and sudden infant death syndrome. In these studies, it is not possible to distinguish between apparent effects of maternal smoking during pregnancy and smoking after pregnancy, but both may play a role in increasing the risk of sudden infant death.

Alcohol

The fetal alcohol syndrome has been reported in offspring of alcoholic mothers and includes the features of gross physical retardation with onset occurring prenatally and continuing after birth.[38] Central nervous system dysfunction, including mental retardation and microcephaly, as well as minor ocular, facial, skeletal, and other anomalies, such as micrognathia, have all been described.

In one study,[39] 23 chronically alcoholic women were matched with 46 controls and the pregnancy outcomes of the two groups were compared. Perinatal deaths were about 8 times more frequent, and growth retardation, microcephaly, and IQ below 80 occurred considerably more often, in offspring of the alcoholic mothers than in those of the controls. Overall outcome was abnormal in 43% of the offspring of the alcoholic mothers compared with 2% of the offspring of the controls.

One study[40] addressed the risks of smaller amounts of alcohol. Among infants of abstinent or rare drinkers, 9% were categorized as having some abnormality; among infants of moderate drinkers, 14%; and among infants of heavy drinkers (average daily intake of 3 oz of 100-proof liquor or more), 32%. Overall, including anomalies, growth retardation, and an abnormal neurologic examination, 71% of the children of heavy drinkers were abnormal, which was twice the frequency found in the moderate and rarely drinking groups. In this study, it appeared that an increased frequency of abnormality was not found until 45 ml of ethanol daily (equivalent to three drinks daily) was exceeded. Heavy drinking remains a major risk to the fetus, but reduction of alcohol intake even in midpregnancy can benefit the newborn. An occasional drink during pregnancy carries no known risk, but at best represents "empty calories."

A number of confounding factors must be considered and controlled for before ethanol alone can be incriminated. Maternal malnutrition, particularly folate deficiency, which is frequent in heavy drinkers, affects fetal development, as might hypoglycemia induced by alcohol. The use of other drugs, particularly barbiturates, central nervous system depressants, and cigarettes, is highly correlated with heavy drinking, and these agents also may affect the fetus.

Narcotic Addiction

Menstrual abnormalities, especially amenorrhea, are common in heroin abusers, although they are not associated with the use of methadone. Heroin or methadone metabolites in urine may make pregnancy tests falsely positive and confuse dating of a pregnancy. The goal of methadone maintenance is to bring the patient to an intake of approximately 20–40 mg per day. The dosage should be individualized at a level sufficient to minimize the use of supplemental illicit drugs because they represent a greater risk to the fetus than the higher dosages of methadone required by some patients. Manipulation of the dosage in women maintained on methadone should be avoided in the last trimester because of an association with increased fetal complications, as the fetus may withdraw in utero.[41] As management of narcotic addiction during pregnancy requires a host of social, nutritional, educational, and psychiatric interventions, these patients are best managed in specialized programs.

The infant of the narcotic addict is at increased risk of abortion, prematurity, and intrauterine growth retardation. Withdrawal should be watched for carefully in the neonatal period.

Caffeine

There is no evidence of a teratogenic effect of caffeine in human beings. In the Collaborative Perinatal Project,[8] congenital defects in offspring of 5,773 women taking caffeine in pregnancy, usually in a fixed-dose analgesic medication, were not increased. There is conflicting evidence as to whether heavy ingestion of caffeine is associated with increased complications during pregnancy. Two studies suggested that greater than 7 to 8 cups of coffee per day were associated with low birth weight infants, spontaneous abortions, prematurity and stillbirths.[42, 43] However, these studies were not controlled for the use of tobacco and alcohol, making interpretation difficult. In one study controlled for smoking, other habits, demographic characteristics, and medical history, no relationship was found between low birth weight or short gestation and heavy coffee consumption. Also, there was no excess of malformations among coffee drinkers.[44]

Occupational Exposures

Drug exposure during pregnancy also may be due to one of many possible environmental causes. An early study suggested a risk involved in exposure to anesthetic gases in an operating room environment.[45] Of 159 nurses studied between 1966 and 1970, 67 worked in an operating room and 92 were general duty nurses. The miscarriage rate was 29.7% in the operating room nurses, compared with 8.6% in the general duty nurses. Similar figures were obtained when female physicians working with anesthetic agents were compared to general duty physicians, suggesting a possible abortifacient effect of exposure to trace anesthetic gases. This led to the installation of scavenging systems in most operating rooms in the 1970s, and working in such environments currently involves trivial exposure. However, pregnant personnel should ascertain that the environment in which they are working does contain such a scavenging system to assure negligible risk.

Conclusion

Many medical conditions during pregnancy are best treated initially with nonpharmacologic remedies. Before a drug is used in pregnancy, the indication should be clear and the risk-benefit ratio should justify the use of the drug. If possible, therapy should be postponed until after the first trimester. In addition, patients should be cautioned about the risks of "social" drug use, such as smoking and alcohol, during pregnancy.

References

1. Wilson J. G., Fraser F. C. (eds.): *Handbook of Teratology*. New York, Plenum Publishing Corp., 1979.
2. Blake D. A.: Requirements and limitations in reproductive and teratogenic risk assessment. In Niebyl J. R. (ed.): *Drug Use in Pregnancy*. Philadelphia, Lea & Febiger, 1982.
3. Meyer-Bahlburg H. F. L., Ehrhardt A. A.: Sex hormone administration during pregnancy: Behavioral sequelae in the offspring. In Youngs D. D., Ehrhardt A. A. (eds.): *Psychosomatic Obstetrics and Gynecology*. New York, Appleton-Century Crofts, 1980.
4. Wilkins L.: Masculinization of female fetus due to use of orally given progestins. *JAMA* 172:1028, 1960.
5. Harlap S., Prywes R., Davies A. M.: Birth defects and oestrogens and progesterones in pregnancy. *Lancet* 1:682, Mar. 22, 1975.
6. Heinonen O. P., Slone D., Monson R. R., et al.: Cardiovascular birth defects and antenatal exposure to female sex hormones. *N. Engl. J. Med.* 296:67, 1977.
7. Chez R. A.: Proceedings of the symposium "Progesterone, Progestins, and Fetal Development." *Fertil. Steril.* 30:16, 1978.
8. Heinonen O. P., Slone S., Shapiro S.: *Birth Defects and Drugs in Pregnancy*. Publishing Sciences Group, Inc., Littleton, Mass., 1977.
9. Johnson J. W. C., Austin K. L., Jones G. S., et al.: Efficacy of 17α-hydroxyprogesterone caproate in the prevention of premature labor. *N. Engl. J. Med.* 293:675, 1975.
10. Aarskog D.: Maternal progestins as a possible cause of hypospadias. *N. Engl. J. Med.* 300:75, 1979.
11. Speidel B. D., Meadow S. R.: Maternal epilepsy and abnormalities of the fetus and newborn. *Lancet* 2:839, 1972.

12. Robert E., Guibaud P.: Maternal valproic acid and congenital neural tube defects. *Lancet* 2:937, 1982.
13. Shapiro S., Hartz S. C., Siskind V., et al.: Anticonvulsants and parental epilepsy in the development of birth defects. *Lancet* 1:272, 1976.
14. Emerson R., D'Souza B. J., Vining E. P., et al.: Stopping medication in children with epilepsy. *N. Engl. J. Med.* 304:1125, 1981.
15. Hartz S. C., Heinonen O. P., Shapiro S., et al.: Antenatal exposure to meprobamate and chlordiazepoxide in relation to malformations, mental development, and childhood mortality. *N. Engl. J. Med.* 292:726, 1975.
16. Safra M. J., Oakley G. P.: Association between cleft lip with or without cleft palate and prenatal exposure to diazepam. *Lancet* 2:478, 1975.
17. Weinstein M. R., Goldfield M. D.: Cardiovascular malformations with lithium use during pregnancy. *Am. J. Psychol.* 132:529, 1975.
18. Milkovich L., Van Den Berg B. J.: An evaluation of the teratogenicity of certain antinauseant drugs. *Am. J. Obstet. Gynecol.* 125:244, 1976.
19. Diggory P. L. C., Tomkinson J. S.: Nausea and vomiting in pregnancy: A trial of meclozine dihydrochloride with and without pyridoxine. *Lancet* 2:370, 1962.
20. Cartwright E. W.: Dramamine in nausea and vomiting of pregnancy. *West. J. Surg. Obstet. Gynecol.* 59:216, 1951.
21. Willman K., Pulkkinen M. O.: Reduced maternal plasma and urinary estriol during ampicillin treatment. *Am. J. Obstet. Gynecol.* 109:893, 1971.
22. Eraz J., Hausknecht R.: Diminished urinary estriol due to Mandelamine administration during pregnancy. *Am. J. Obstet. Gynecol.* 109:924, 1969.
23. Cohlan S. Q., Bevelander G., Tiamsic T.: Growth inhibition of prematures receiving tetracycline. *Am. J. Dis. Child.* 105:453, 1963.
24. Peterson W. F., Stauch J. E., Ryder C. D.: Metronidazole in pregnancy. *Am. J. Obstet. Gynecol.* 94:343, 1966.
25. Dykers J. R.: Single-dose metronidazole for trichomonal vaginitis. *N. Engl. J. Med.* 293:23, 1975.
26. Hill R. M., Stern L.: Drugs in pregnancy: Effects on the fetus and newborn. *Drugs* 17:182, 1979.
27. Goldberg E.: Anticoagulants in pregnancy. In Neibyl J. R. (ed.): *Drug Use in Pregnancy*. Philadelphia, Lea & Febiger, 1982, p. 60.
28. Mujtaba Q., Burrow G. N.: Treatment of hyperthyroidism in pregnancy with propylthiouracil and methimazole. *Obstet. Gynecol.* 46:282, 1975.
29. Burrow G. N.: Thyroid diseases. In Burrow G. N., Ferris T. F. (eds.): *Medical Complications During Pregnancy*. Philadelphia, W. B. Saunders Co., 1982.
30. Pruyn S. C., Phelan J. P., Buchanan G. C.: Long-term propranolol therapy in pregnancy: Maternal and fetal outcome. *Am. J. Obstet. Gynecol.* 135:485, 1979.
31. Rubin P. C., Clark D. M., Sumner D. J.: Placebo-controlled trial of atenolol in treatment of pregnancy-associated hypertension. *Lancet* 1:431, 1983.
32. Collins E., Turner G.: Salicylates and pregnancy. *Lancet* 2:1494, 1973.
33. Corby D. G., Schulman I.: The effects of antenatal drug administration on aggregation of platelets of newborn infants. *J. Pediatr.* 75:74, 1969.
34. Areilla R. A., Thilenius O. B., Ranniger K.: Congestive heart failure from suspected ductal closure in utero. *J. Pediatr.* 75:74, 1969.
35. Waltman T., Tricomi V., Tavakoli F. M.: Effect of aspirin on bleeding time during elective abortion. *Obstet. Gynecol.* 48:108, 1976.
36. Meyer M. B.: Smoking and pregnancy. In Niebyl J. R. (ed.): *Drug Use in Pregnancy*. Philadelphia, Lea & Febiger, 1982.

37. Alberman E., Creasy M., Elliott M., et al.: Maternal factors associated with fetal chromosomal anomalies in spontaneous abortions. *J. Obstet. Gynecol.* 83:621, 1976.
38. Jones K. L., Smith D. W., Ulleland C. N., et al.: Patterns of malformation in offspring of chronic alcoholic mothers. *Lancet* 2:1267, 1973.
39. Jones K. L., Smith D. W., Streissguth A. P., et al.: Outcome of offspring of chronic alcoholic women. *Lancet* 2:1076, 1974.
40. Ouellette E. M., Rosett H. L., Rosman N. P., et al.: Adverse effects on offspring of maternal alcohol abuse during pregnancy. *N. Engl. J. Med.* 297:528, 1977.
41. Finnegan L. P., Chappel J. N., Kreeb M. J., et al.: Narcotic addiction in pregnancy. In Niebyl J. R. (ed.): *Drug Use in Pregnancy.* Philadelphia, Lea & Febiger, 1982.
42. Mau G., Netter P.: Kaffee-und alkoholkonsum-risikofaktoren in der schwangerschaft? *Geburtshilfe Fraunheilkd.* 34:1018, 1974.
43. Van den Berg B. J.: Epidemiologic observations of prematurity: Effects of tobacco, coffee and alcohol. In Reed D. M., Stanley F. J. (eds.): *The Epidemiology of Prematurity.* Baltimore, Urban and Schwarzenberg, 1977.
44. Linn S., Schoenbaum S. C., Monson R. R., et al.: No association between coffee consumption and adverse outcomes of pregnancy. *N. Engl. J. Med.* 306:141, 1982.
45. Occupational Disease Among Operating Room Personnel: A National Study: Report of an Ad Hoc Committee on the Effect of Trace Anesthetics on the Health of Operating Room Personnel, American Society of Anesthesiologists. *Anesthesiology* 41:321, 1974.

7–1 **Direct-Vision Chorion Biopsy and Chromosome-Specific DNA Probes for Determination of Fetal Sex in First-Trimester Prenatal Diagnosis.** Prenatal diagnosis in the first trimester would reduce the waiting period substantially and make possible earlier, safer abortions. Molecular hybridization can identify DNA sequences specific to the Y chromosome in male fetuses. J. R. Gosden, A. R. Mitchell, C. M. Gosden, C. H. Rodeck, and J. M. Morsman purified DNA from single chorionic villi and used it to determine fetal sex. The results were confirmed by chromosomal preparations from cultures of chorionic villus biopsy specimens obtained at the same time and of the conceptus. Chorionic biopsies were done in patients undergoing terminations at 6 to 13 weeks' gestation. Single villi were obtained transcervically under direct vision with ultrasonic guidance. A 2.2-mm endoscope was used.

The results of restriction endonuclease analysis for Y chromosome-specific DNA in biopsy specimens from 13 patients were confirmed by fetal karyotype analysis of cultures of biopsy specimens and of the products of conception in all instances. Prenatal sex determination by the former method took 3 to 4 days. As little as 1 μg of DNA may be adequate where a repeated sequence is sought, as in the Y-specific sequence. A conspicuous band in the autoradiograph at 3.4 kb is found in males. All 13 conceptuses had 46 chromosomes with a 46 XX or 46 XY karyotype. There were no Y chromosome variants with large or small heterochromatic regions.

(7–1) Lancet 2:1416–1419, Dec. 25, 1982.

Prenatal sex determination by molecular analysis of DNA from chorionic biopsy specimens is reliable when done in the first trimester of pregnancy. The method is not subject to the same errors as is F-body identification. Anxious parents will welcome the opportunity for early prenatal diagnosis. Chorionic biopsy can be done as early as at 6 weeks' gestation, and it is unlikely to cause the postural deformities and other fetal problems associated with amniocentesis and aspiration of fluid.

▶ [Restriction enzyme analysis of DNA permitted the correct ascertainment of fetal sex in all 13 cases reported here. The striking aspect of all this is that single chorionic villi were biopsied with the aid of ultrasound and a fetoscope. Biopsy specimens were taken of extraplacental villi (destined to become the chorion laeve) adjacent to the implantation site. Old et al. (*Lancet* 2:1413, 1982), using a slightly different biopsy technique, were able to diagnose hemoglobinopathies on tissue also obtained in the first trimester. Obtaining diagnostic samples so early in pregnancy offers advantages over current practice, but the safety of this approach concerning the continuation of pregnancy has not yet been established.] ◀

7-2 **Improved Detection of the Sickle Mutation by DNA Analysis: Application to Prenatal Diagnosis.** Stuart H. Orkin, Peter F. R. Little, Haig H. Kazazian, Jr., and Corinne D. Boehm observed that a fetal loss of about 5% currently can be attributed to invasive procedures for prenatal diagnosis of sickle cell anemia and thalassemia syndromes. An attempt was made to develop a safer diagnostic approach in the examination of amniotic cell DNA for a specific genetic trait. Detection of abnormal conditions of hemoglobin that result from point mutations in DNA, however, required a more specific assay. Direct identification of mutant genes in DNA was possible through the specificity of restriction enzymes. In a new assay, fragments 1.1 and 1.3 kb from β^A- and β^S-genes, respectively, were generated that were ideally suited for restriction-enzyme mapping and applicable to prenatal diagnosis of sickle cell anemia.

TECHNIQUE.—A recombinant DNA containing the β-globin gene and its flanking regions within a miniplasmid was digested with the restriction enzymes MstII and HpaI, either separately or in combination, and electrophoresis was performed. Fragments of DNA were stained by ethidium bromide. This method of direct detection of sickle cell mutation is based on the knowledge that the restriction enzyme MstII cleaves a sequence (CCTNAGG) that is a subset of DdeI sites (CTNAG). The normal gene is β^A; β^S is the sickle cell gene.

For prenatal diagnosis of sickle cell anemia, the MstII assay can readily identify all genotypes (AA, AS, and SS).

Two cases illustrate the usefulness of this assay. In the first case, a couple with no previous children showed paternal DNA with the more common AS pattern; maternal DNA had a common DNA pattern. Fetal DNA had a 13.0 kb/13.0 kb HpaI pattern, strongly suggesting (about 95%) sickle cell disease. In the second case, a couple with a child who had sickle cell trait showed paternal β^S-gene in the fetus but neither the AS or SS genotypes could be distinguished. The MstII assay showed the fetus to be AS. These results agreed with a fetal blood study.

(7–2) N. Engl. J. Med. 307:32–36, July 1, 1982.

This assay for the β^S-gene uses restriction enzyme MstII and is both direct and sensitive. No modification of standard gene-mapping procedures and no extensive family studies to establish linkage of DNA polymorphisms with the β^S-gene are required. This assay allows all cases at risk to be analyzed with a single, straightforward test.

▶ [Restriction enzyme identification of mutant genes in DNA represents an enormous scientific advance with practical application to prenatal genetic diagnosis. The use of this technology in the diagnosis of sickle cell anemia was considered in the 1983 YEAR BOOK (pp. 189–190). The present report concerns a different restriction enzyme that apparently offers advantages over that described previously. The test is sensitive enough that uncultured amniotic cells can be studied. The AS and SS genotypes can be distinguished.] ◀

7-3 **Prenatal Diagnosis Using DNA Polymorphisms: Report on 95 Pregnancies at Risk for Sickle Cell Disease or β-thalassemia.** Most fetuses at risk for sickle cell anemia and most at risk for β-thalassemia can be diagnosed using DNA polymorphisms in the region of the β-globin gene. Corinne D. Boehm, Stylianos E. Antonarakis, John A. Phillips, III, Gail Stetten, and Haig H. Kazazian, Jr. (Johns Hopkins Univ.) attempted to make a prenatal diagnosis by analyzing restriction site polymorphisms in amniocyte DNA in 57 pregnancies in which the fetus was at risk of sickle cell anemia, 32 with a risk of β-thalassemia, and 6 with a risk of other β-hemoglobinopathies. Ten highly polymorphic restriction sites were recognized in the β-globin gene region at the time of the study.

A diagnosis was made solely by analyzing DNA polymorphisms in cells recovered by amniocentesis in 82 (86%) patients. Diagnosis was completed by fetoscopy and fetal blood study in 6 other patients. Prenatal diagnosis was correct in all 78 infants available for confirmation to date, including 55 at risk for sickling disease and 23 for β-thalassemia.

Analysis of DNA polymorphisms can be useful in the prenatal diagnosis of genetic disorders in which the basic defect cannot be detected directly. Although many single-gene disorders may, like the β-thalassemias, be heterogeneous and not directly detectable by DNA restriction analysis, a safe, accurate prenatal test theoretically can be developed for any of these disorders given a cloned DNA sequence close to the affected gene. With such a sequence, restriction-site polymorphisms should be identifiable, allowing prenatal diagnosis by amniocentesis for most couples at risk.

▶ [Dr. Roger A. Williamson of the University of Iowa reviewed this article at our request and commented as follows: "This report highlights the remarkable advances in prenatal diagnosis that have occurred from the introduction of modern molecular genetics to the field. One need only reflect on the history of the prenatal diagnosis of sickle cell anemia to appreciate how far this technology has come in a few short years. The first such diagnoses required obtaining fetal blood by fetoscopy or placental aspiration for determination of globin-chain synthesis; rates of fetal loss approximated 5% with these procedures. The next advance involved analysis of a polymorphism or polymorphisms closely linked to the β-globin gene, as detailed in this study, for both sickle cell disease and β-thalassemia. Any nucleated cell can yield DNA for this type of analysis, so a routine genetic amniocentesis can be performed. However, family studies are required and a prenatal diagnosis by these means is not possible for all couples at risk. In addition, there are potential sources of error, and fetoscopy is necessary for definitive diagnosis in some cases. Currently, sickle cell disease can

(7–3) N. Engl. J. Med. 308:1054–1058, May 5, 1983.

be detected directly by use of a restriction endonuclease that 'recognizes' the mutant β-globin allele, obviating all the aforementioned difficulties. These testing strategies may, as the authors suggest, provide a means to detect many other single gene disorders not presently amenable to prenatal diagnosis."] ◀

7–4 **Dispermic Origin and Clinical Outcome of Three Complete Hydatidiform Moles With 46 XY Karyotype.** U. Surti, A. E. Szulman, and S. O'Brien report 3 new cases of hydatidiform mole with a 46 XY karyotype originating by dispermy, which was established through studies of cytogenetic and polymorphic biochemical markers. Histologic examination of all 3 specimens showed typical complete moles. Lymphocytes from peripheral blood of both parents and tissues from the moles were grown in appropriate short-term cultures for chromosome analyses and comparisons of Q banding.

Exclusive paternal origin of the 3 moles was established by data obtained in all 3 cases. The biologically most plausible mechanisms to be considered are fertilization by a single sperm produced by paternal first or second meiotic nondivision and dispermy. Nondisjunction at the first meiotic division results in the presence of both homologues of all paternal chromosomes; all paternal heterozygous markers also will be present in the mole. Nondisjunction at the second meiotic division results in complete duplication of one paternal haploid set with two copies derived from one of the two paternal homologues; the presence of heterologous sex chromosomes in XY moles eliminates such a possibility.

In the first case, both homologues of maternal chromosome 15 had markers different from those in the father. Neither of the maternal chromosomes 15 was in the mole, whereas both molar homologues 15 were referable to the father. At the same time, the father was heterozygous for glyoxalase, whereas the mole was homozygous for that enzyme. In the second case, chromosomes 3 and 14 were inherited exclusively from the father and were homozygous in the mole and heterozygous in the father. In the third case, the mole inherited both chromosomes 15 from the father; maternal chromosome 15 was absent, whereas only one of the paternal homologues of chromosomes 13, 15, and 21 was inherited in duplicate.

Levels of human chorionic gonadotropin spontaneously decreased to normal within a short time, indicating a benign course in these 3 cases. Of a total of 18 cases reported to date, postoperative clinical information was available for 10 patients. Two of these 10 patients had a malignant course with lung metastases. Establishment of the magnitude of the risk of malignancy for hydatidiform mole with a 46 XY karyotype is theoretically and clinically important.

▶ [It is now well-established that the chromosomes in hydatidiform moles are exclusively of paternal origin. Most often the pattern is 46 XX, resulting from fertilization of an "empty egg" with a 23 X sperm that then duplicates itself. The much less common 46 XY mole, according to this report, results from fertilization of an "empty egg" with two sperms, one 23 X and the other 23 Y.] ◀

7–5 **Are Spermicides Teratogenic?** James L. Mills, Ernest E. Harley, George F. Reed, and Heinz W. Berendes (Natl. Inst. of Health) note

---

(7–4) Am. J. Obstet. Gynecol. 144:84–87, Sept. 1, 1982.
(7–5) JAMA 248:2148–2151, Nov. 5, 1982.

that recent evidence suggests that spermicides could be teratogenic. Pregnant women provided data at their first prenatal visit on spermicide and other contraceptive exposures in each of the preceding 12 months. All pregnant women seen in one facility between 1974 and 1977 were requested to complete a prenatal questionnaire at their initial visit. The women were classified into two groups: those who had used spermicides and those who had used other contraceptive methods (oral contraceptives, condom alone, diaphragm alone, intrauterine device, or the rhythm method). These groups were further divided into those who had used contraceptives only before the last menstrual period and those exposed after the last menstrual period. The effects of strength and active ingredients were examined.

A total of 34,660 women participated in the study. Of these, 3,146 had used spermicides before their last menstrual period but not after; 2,282 were exposed to spermicides after their last menstrual period; 13,148 had used other forms of birth control before their last menstrual period only; and 2,831 were exposed after their last menstrual period. Among women who had practiced contraception before the last menstrual period but not after, the malformation rate in offspring of spermicide users was no higher than in those of users of other methods. The same was true for women who continued to practice contraception after the last menstrual period. When malformations were examined by organ system and by individual defect, spermicide exposure again was not associated with an increased risk. Comparing spermicides by active ingredient with other methods of contraception revealed no increased risk of malformations for any compound. Controlling for age, time in pregnancy at which exposure data were collected, concentration of spermicides used, and other possible confounding factors did not alter the results.

No association was shown between spermicide use around the time of conception and congenital anomalies. A woman who thinks she might be pregnant should have a pregnancy test before continuing the use of contraceptives. The data indicate, however, that accidental exposure to spermicides after conception is probably not teratogenic.

▶ [A study abstracted in the 1982 YEAR BOOK (pp. 206–207) found an association between vaginal spermicide usage (or, more accurately, having a prescription for a spermicide filled within 10 months of conception) and congenital disorders (limb reduction defects, neoplasms, and Down's syndrome). These results were not confirmed in a subsequent report (1983 YEAR BOOK, p. 183). The present report, utilizing recall at the first prenatal visit, also found no teratogenic action. We are more inclined to believe the negative results.] ◀

7–6 **Valproic Acid and Fetal Abnormality.** Infants born to epileptic mothers have an increased rate of abnormalities, some of which may be attributed to the teratogenic effects of anticonvulsants. Valproic acid and carbamazepine have been suggested for use in this setting in preference to phenytoin and phenobarbital. C. J. Bailey, R. W. Pool, E. M. E. Poskitt, and F. Harris (Liverpool) report 2 cases that call this recommendation into question with respect to valproic acid. An infant with finger-like thumbs, one of them triphalangeal, a ru-

---

(7–6) Br. Med. J. 286:190, Jan. 15, 1983.

dimentary extra digit in one hand, and a cleft foot with syndactyly was born to a mother with idiopathic epilepsy who took 400 mg of valproic acid twice daily during pregnancy and had a serum concentration of 340 mg/L at 35 weeks' gestation. The only other medication was dextropropoxyphene with paracetamol. The infant also had bilateral renal hypoplasia. An infant with micrognathia, bilateral undescended testes, glandular hypospadias, skeletal anomalies, and valvular aortic stenosis was born to a woman with idiopathic epilepsy who took 600 mg of valproic acid three times daily and had serum concentrations as high as 540 mg/L. A previous pregnancy had ended in spontaneous abortion at 8 weeks; valproic acid also had been used in this pregnancy.

Both women took valproic acid throughout pregnancy. Facial, digital, and skeletal abnormalities and developmental delay have been described in infants born after pregnancies in which valproic acid was the sole drug used. Four of 33 such pregnancies resulted in infants with congenital malformations, and 4 others resulted in spontaneous abortion. These and the present cases indicate that valproic acid may be hazardous when used during pregnancy.

▶ [These two cases do not establish valproic acid as a teratogen in human beings, but they certainly cause concern. Neural tube defects also have been reported in association with this anticonvulsant.] ◀

7–7 **Spontaneous Abortions in Hospital Staff Engaged in Sterilizing Instruments With Chemical Agents.** K. Hemminki, P. Mutanen, I. Saloniemi, M.-L. Niemi, and H. Vainio (Inst. of Occupational Health, Helsinki) analyzed spontaneous abortions in hospital sterilizing staff. Data obtained from a postal questionnaire and a hospital discharge register were used. The study included all sterilizing staff employed in Finnish hospitals in 1980; controls were nursing auxiliaries. Chemicals specifically studied included ethylene oxide, glutaraldehyde, and formaldehyde.

When the decade of reported pregnancy was studied in relation to frequency of spontaneous abortions to detect any differences in recall or reporting of spontaneous abortions, the frequency of spontaneous abortions was higher in the pregnancies of women exposed to sterilizing agents. The crude rate of spontaneous abortions was 11.3% for sterilizing staff and 10.6% for controls. When pregnancies of sterilizing staff were analyzed according to employment at time of conception, the rate was 16.7% for the exposed and 6.0% for nonexposed women. Exposure to ethylene oxide during early pregnancy appeared to be correlated with an increase in adjusted rate of spontaneous abortions from 7.8% to 16.1%. Exposure to glutaraldehyde increased the crude rate but not the adjusted rate. Similar increases were seen when either agent was used in combination with others. Exposure to formaldehyde did not correlate with an increase in spontaneous abortions. When data on pregnancies of sterilizing staff and controls obtained from hospital discharge registers were analyzed, the rate of spontaneous abortions was 14.2% for the exposed and 9.9% for the nonexposed staff. Controls had a rate of 9.2%.

(7–7) Br. Med. J. 285:1461–1463, Nov. 20, 1982.

These results suggest that exposure to ethylene oxide in early pregnancy may increase the risk of spontaneous abortion. Glutaraldehyde also may be not absolutely safe, but it appears to be less potent. Confirmation of these results is urgently needed so that staff involved in sterilizing procedures can be protected.

7-8 **Gastrointestinal Atresia and Maternal Occupation During Pregnancy.** This study originated in observations in cohort studies that women who work in laboratories during pregnancy may be at increased risk of having an infant with gastrointestinal (GI) atresia. Anders Ericson, Bengt Källén, Olav Meirik, and Peter Westerholm conducted a case-control study of 201 women who had infants with GI atresia and 402 women with infants without that malformation matched for age, parity, and time of year of delivery. Maternal occupation during pregnancy was ascertained by interviews or mailed inquiries and only referred to type of occupation; no efforts were made to obtain detailed information on occupational exposure. Occupation of nonresponders was checked using census data.

In the case-control study, laboratory work (occupations where chemical exposure is probable, e.g., hairdressers, pharmacists, plastics industry workers, or possible, e.g., laboratory workers, unspecified industrial workers) was reported to occur more often among case mothers than among controls. The actual exposure necessary for embryonic damage is not known. The excess risk is probably not great, and the contribution of laboratory work in the etiology of GI atresia is obviously small; laboratory work is a relatively rare occupation among pregnant women. If a fivefold increase in risk is accepted, the absolute risk for a woman in this occupation having an infant with GI atresia is less than 1:200, and only about 3% of the GI atresia cases are due to that maternal occupation.

▶ [This report and the preceding one, both from Scandinavia, concern potential adverse effects of the workplace on pregnancy. The first suggests that exposure to ethylene oxide, but not to glutaraldehyde or formaldehyde, is associated with an increased risk of spontaneous abortion. The second indicates that a "laboratory" occupation during pregnancy may be associated with gastrointestinal atresia in the newborn. "Laboratory" occupation doesn't identify what agent(s) might be teratogenic. These studies are interesting, but must be regarded as preliminary. The authors of the second study point out that even if there is a fivefold increase in risk of gastrointestinal atresia associated with laboratory work in Sweden, only 3% of these anomalies are explainable on the basis of occupation. Obviously, identification of a specific teratogen might alter these figures.] ◀

7-9 **Consequences of Confirmed Maternal Rubella at Successive Stages of Pregnancy.** Elizabeth Miller, John E. Craddock-Watson, and Thomas M. Pollock prospectively followed 1,016 women who had confirmed rubella infection during pregnancy. Sixty-six percent of the women were multiparous, and 95% had a rash.

Of the 966 women for whom the outcome of pregnancy was known, 523 (54%) had therapeutic abortions and 36 (4%) had spontaneous abortions. Among the 407 pregnancies that continued, there were 9 (2%) stillbirths, about twice the expected number (4 of the 9 had se-

(7-8) J. Occupat. Med. 24:515-518, July 1982.
(7-9) Lancet 2:781-784, Oct. 9, 1982.

TABLE 1.—CONGENITAL INFECTION RATES AFTER SYMPTOMATIC AND ASYMPTOMATIC RUBELLA AT SUCCESSIVE STAGES OF PREGNANCY

Stage of pregnancy (wk)	No. of infants tested	Seropositive
Symptomatic rubella:		
<11	10	9 (*90%*)
11–12	6	4 (*67%*)
13–14	18	12 (*67%*)
15–16	36	17 (*47%*)
17–18	33	13 (*39%*)
19–22	59	20 (*34%*)
23–26	32	8 (*25%*)
27–30	31	11 (*35%*)
31–36	25	15 (*60%*)
>36	8	8 (*100%*)
Total	258	117 (*45%*)
Asymptomatic rubella:		
<13	5	..
13–18	5	..
31–36	1	..
Total	11	..

(Courtesy of Miller, E., et al.: Lancet 2:781–784, Oct. 9, 1982.)

vere abnormalities and 5 had no abnormalities), and 5 (1%) neonatal deaths, about the expected number.

Of the surviving infants, 307 were followed to the age of 2 years. Infection was diagnosed in 117 of the 269 infants tested serologically (43% of all infants tested, 45% of those whose mothers had a rash). The frequency of congenital infection was more than 80% when maternal rubella with a rash occurred during the first 12 weeks of pregnancy; it fell to 25% by the end of the second trimester, and rose again in the last month (Table 1). No infant whose mother had symptomless rubella was infected.

In the 273 children (102 seropositive, 133 seronegative, and 38 not

TABLE 2.—DEFECTS FOUND AT FOLLOW-UP IN INFANTS INFECTED WITH RUBELLA AT SUCCESSIVE STAGES OF PREGNANCY

		Seropositive infants			Overall
Stage of pregnancy (wk)	No. followed up	Heart and other defect	Deafness alone	% with defect	risk* of rubella defect (%)
<11	9	5	4	100	90
11–12	4	0	2	50	33
13–14	12	0	2	17	11
15–16	14	0	7	50	24
17–18	10	0	0	..	..
>18	53	0	0	..	..
Total	102	5	15	20	..

Overall risk = % seropositive with defects × % infants infected.
*Estimated from congenital infection rate after symptomatic rubella at different stages of pregnancy (see Table 1).
(Courtesy of Miller, E., et al.: Lancet 2:781–784, Oct. 9, 1982.)

TABLE 3.—COMPARISON OF BIRTH WEIGHTS OF SEROPOSITIVE AND SERONEGATIVE INFANTS

Stage of pregnancy (wk)	No.	No. below 10th percentile	Mean birth-weight (kg)
Seropositive:			
<13	13	8 (*62%*)	2·69*
13–16	29	8 (*28%*)	3·11*
17–20	22	5 (*23%*)	3·15*
21–28	20	2 (*10%*)	3·38
29–36	19	4 (*21%*)	3·14*
>36	8	1 (*13%*)	3·38
Total	111	28 (*25%*)	3·14*
Total seronegative	148	12 (*8%*)	3·38

Birth weights not available for 6 seropositive and 4 seronegative infants.
Mean weights exclude 3 infants born more than 3 weeks prematurely.
*Difference with respect to seronegative group significant at 5% level or lower with t test.
(Courtesy of Miller, E., et al.: Lancet 2:781–784, Oct. 9, 1982.)

tested serologically) followed clinically, defects consistent with congenital rubella were found in 20, all of whom were seropositive (Table 2). Five exposed during the first 8 weeks had congenital heart defects reported at birth, and 15 exposed between 8 and 16 weeks had bilateral sensorineural deafness, usually severe, as their sole defect. No defects attributable to rubella were found in children infected after 16 weeks. Other defects reported at follow-up occurred with equal incidence (12%) in the seropositive and seronegative groups.

Birth weight below the 10th percentile was found in 25% of seropositive infants compared with 8% of seronegative infants, the excess being most striking in those exposed during the first trimester (Table 3). Intrauterine growth retardation was the sole manifestation of congenital infection in some infants exposed during the first 16 weeks. Deafness was found in many children of normal birth weight. Two mothers had records of previous vaccination against rubella.

▶ [This article provides an excellent summary of the results of rubella infection during pregnancy. During the first trimester there is a very high likelihood of fetal involvement, mainly in the form of malformations such as congenital heart defects and deafness. Fetal disease with maternal infection during the second trimester is less likely but the risk increases again during late gestation, where manifestations such as fetal growth retardation may be observed.] ◀

7-10 **Smoking and the Occurrence of Congenital Malformations and Spontaneous Abortions: Multivariate Analysis.** Smoking is well known to affect the developing embryo adversely, but most studies of abortion have been uncontrolled for confounding factors, and some studies have failed to confirm an increased risk of congenital anomalies. Kari Hemminki, Pertti Mutanen, and Irma Saloniemi (Helsinki) undertook a multivariate analysis of retrospective data on major malformations in about 3,300 affected children, reported between 1967 and 1977, to detect any relation between tobacco use and malformations. Many possible confounding variables were taken into

(7–10) Am. J. Obstet. Gynecol. 145:61–66, Jan. 1, 1983.

account in analyzing the data from the Finnish Register of Congenital Malformation.

The odds ratios for infants of smokers being born with central nervous system, oral cleft, and musculoskeletal malformations were 1.25, 1.25, and 0.75, respectively. None of the findings was significant. Thirteen possibly confounding variables were controlled for. A questionnaire study of hospital personnel indicated that smokers of over ten cigarettes daily had more spontaneous abortions than nonsmokers, but the differences were not significant. The data were controlled for age, parity, and coffee and alcohol consumption.

Moderate smoking during pregnancy appears not to have any substantial effect on the risk of major structural malformations in offspring, but it may have a slight effect on spontaneous abortions, especially if women smoke more than ten cigarettes a day.

▶ [The results of studies considering the relationship between cigarette smoking and congenital malformations have not been consistent (cf. 1981 YEAR BOOK, pp. 185–186). The present report based on the extensive data of the Finnish Register of Congenital Malformations indicates that smoking is not teratogenic.] ◀

7–11 **Patterns of Alcohol Consumption and Fetal Development.** An association between alcohol abuse during gestation and abnormal fetal development has long been recognized, but the effects of consumption of moderate amounts of alcohol during pregnancy are unclear. Henry L. Rosett, Lyn Weiner, Austin Lee, Barry Zuckerman, Elizabeth Dooling, and Edgar Oppenheimer (Boston Univ.) examined the relation of drinking patterns to fetal outcome in 469 mother-infant pairs. Differential effects of heavy drinking in early and late gestation were evaluated by separate analysis of neonates born to women who reduced their alcohol consumption before the third trimester. Heavy drinking was reported by 9% of the women, moderate drinking by 35%, and rare drinking or none by 56%. The median daily alcohol use reported by heavy drinkers was 15-fold greater than that reported by moderate drinkers. Sixteen of the 43 heavy drinkers abstained or significantly reduced their alcohol consumption to below heavy levels before the third trimester.

One third of the variance in birth weight was attributable to gestational age. The offspring of heavy drinkers had the lowest birth weight, length, and head circumference. There were no differences between offspring in the moderate-drinking and abstinent or rarely drinking groups. Growth retardation was most prevalent among infants of women who used alcohol heavily throughout pregnancy, whether or not they smoked cigarettes, marihuana, or both. Abnormalities were also more frequent in neonates whose mothers drank heavily throughout pregnancy. Infants born to drinkers who reduced their consumption had more abnormalities than those in the moderate and abstaining groups, but they did not differ in growth. The frequency of abnormalities did not differ in the reduced drinking and heavy drinking groups.

Heavy alcohol consumption throughout pregnancy is associated with a spectrum of adverse fetal effects, the most marked being the

---

(7–11) Obstet. Gynecol. 61:539–546, May 1983.

fetal alcohol syndrome. Fetal maldevelopment has not been associated with moderate alcohol consumption in pregnancy. Infants of heavy drinkers who reduce their consumption before the third trimester appear to develop normally, but they do have an increase in abnormalities. The findings suggest that identification and treatment of heavy drinking are essential components of prenatal care.

▶ [This study demonstrates a fetal growth-retarding and teratogenic effect of heavy alcohol consumption (defined as consumption of at least 22.5 oz of absolute alcohol per month and at least 2.5 oz on some occasions) during gestation. The results are particularly meaningful because of measures taken to separate confounding variables such as smoking, ethnicity, education, prepregnancy weight, and weight gain. Lesser degrees of alcohol consumption did not seem to cause any adverse fetal effects.] ◀

7–12 **Maternal Alcohol, Tobacco, and Cannabis Consumption and the Outcome of Pregnancy.** G. T. Gibson, P. A. Baghurst, and D. P. Colley (Adelaide, Australia) sought associations between maternal use of alcohol, tobacco, and cannabis and adverse outcomes of pregnancy in a prospective study of 7,301 births. About 25% of women reported they did not use alcohol, and only 1.5% drank more than 30 gm a day. Forty percent of the women smoked; 18% smoked more than 15 cigarettes a day. Only 5.4% of women admitted they used cannabis; only 0.5% used it more than once a week. Women who drank more tended to smoke more as well. More than 90% of cannabis users also used alcohol or tobacco, or both, during their pregnancies.

Maternal age and use of cannabis were significantly associated with prematurity. The association with use of cannabis was very significant and was independent of all other factors, including maternal age. There was little evidence that the use of other psychoactive drugs was directly responsible for the excess of premature births among users of cannabis. Low birth weight was strongly associated with increasing use of tobacco. Intrauterine growth retardation was associated with use of tobacco, but not significantly with use of cannabis. No association was apparent between congenital anomalies and the use of alcohol, tobacco, or cannabis. Perinatal mortality increased with high maternal age and, to a much lesser extent, with low maternal age. There was a suggestion of an association with use of cannabis. Substance use could not be related to low 1-minute Apgar scores.

Regular use of cannabis is significantly associated with preterm labor and its adverse sequelae and is probably associated with intrauterine growth retardation. A possible association with an increase in congenital abnormalities deserves further study, although no such association was noted in the present study. It has been suggested that use of cannabis may inhibit placental development.

▶ [Heavy cannabis use during pregnancy was independently associated with premature delivery in this large study population. Although 25% (9 of 36) of heavy users delivered prematurely, it is curious that those who reported using cannabis no more than once per week during pregnancy had a premature delivery rate no higher than nonusers (5%).] ◀

(7–12) Aust. N. Z. J. Obstet. Gynaecol. 23:15–19, February 1983.

7-13 **Comparison of Drinking and Smoking Patterns During Pregnancy Over a Six-Year Interval.** Ann Pytkowicz Streissguth, Betty L. Darby, Helen M. Barr, James R. Smith, and Donald C. Martin (Univ. of Washington) examined changes in the drinking and smoking habits of pregnant women in Seattle after the first American health advisory concerning the fetal alcohol syndrome. Cohorts of pregnant women were interviewed before the sixth month of pregnancy in 1974–1975 and in 1980–1981. The earlier sample included 1,529 women and the later one, 1,413 women. The women were chiefly white, married, and middle-class, although fairly broad demographic categories were represented.

The proportion of women reporting any alcohol use around the time of the first prenatal visit declined from 81% to 42% over the 6-year study interval, and the proportion of smokers fell from 25% to 22%. Binge drinking and heavier drinking declined in the interval, but among drinkers there was no reduction in the proportion of women who reported heavier drinking. A 50% reduction in heavy smokers was noted in the later survey, and there was an important decrease in the use of heavy-nicotine cigarettes.

Alcohol use by pregnant women appears to have declined substantially after recognition of the fetal alcohol syndrome. Older and highly educated women had the most pronounced reductions in drinking. Smoking during pregnancy also decreased significantly during this period. The relative constancy in the proportions of "heavier" drinkers and binge drinkers suggests the need for more attention to the earlier phase of pregnancy, around the time of conception, in advising women who are planning pregnancy. The earliest stage of embryologic and fetal development may be the most critical with respect to vulnerability to alcohol and other teratogens. Although many women clearly can reduce their use of alcohol during pregnancy, more attention must be given to those who drink at higher levels and for whom alcohol may be addictive.

▶ [These findings suggest that use of both alcohol and tobacco by pregnant women in Seattle has declined substantially over a 6-year period in the late 1970s. The adverse effects of smoking and drinking during gestaton certainly have been widely publicized, and this is presumably the reason for decreased usage. It is doubtful if there is a pregnant woman in the United States who is unaware of the harm associated with alcohol and tobacco, and therein lies the rub in interpreting data based on self-reporting at the first prenatal visit. Denial, conscious or unconscious, of a practice the women knows to be harmful to her unborn child may well be responsible for the decline in reported usage.] ◀

7-14 **Estimates of Birth Prevalence Rates of Spina Bifida in the United States From Computer-Generated Maps.** Frank Greenberg, Levy M. James, and Godfrey P. Oakley, Jr. (Centers for Disease Control, Atlanta) developed a computer-generated mapping procedure for estimating geographic and race-specific birth prevalence rates of open spina bifida. The estimates are based on birth certificate data adjusted for underascertainment. Data for 1973–1977 were obtained from the National Center for Health Statistics from all but four

---

(7–13) Am. J. Obstet. Gynecol. 145:716–724, Mar. 15, 1983.
(7–14) Ibid., pp. 570–573, Mar. 1, 1983.

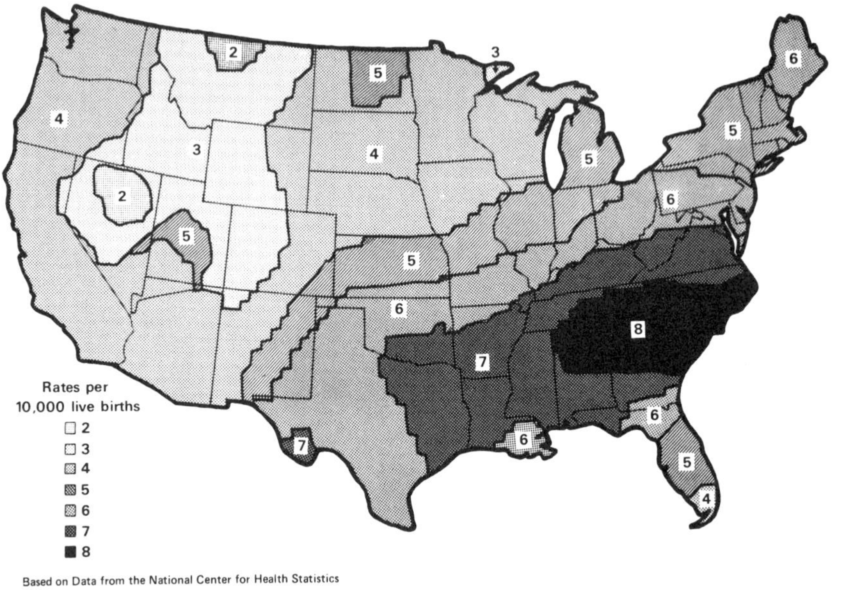

Fig 7–2—Estimated birth prevalence rates of spina bifida in white infants born in the United States based on computer-generated maps. (Courtesy of Greenberg, F., et al.: Am. J. Obstet. Gynecol. 145:570–573, Mar. 1, 1983.)

states. For both white and black births, there was a general decrease in the rate of spina bifida from east to west (Figs 7–2 and 7–3). Rates ranged from less than 1/10,000 for blacks in the Rocky Mountain states and the Pacific Northwest to 8/10,000 total births for whites in Southern Appalachia.

These maps are expected to prove useful in program planning and as an aid in interpreting maternal serum α-fetoprotein levels to detect neural tube defects. Because many more anencephalic infants are born dead, it would be much more difficult to generate similar maps for anencephaly prevalence.

▶ [As we have noted previously, the cost-risk-benefit considerations concerning maternal serum α-fetoprotein screening for open neural tube defects in areas of low prevalence are enormoulsy complex (cf. 1981 YEAR BOOK, pp. 177–178). These prevalence rate maps are based on birth certificate data and may therefore contain inaccuracies; however, they should be of some help to those making decisions about screening programs in specific states or regions.] ◀

7–15 **Screening for Fetal Malformations Using Ultrasound and Measurements of α-Fetoprotein in Maternal Serum.** P. H. Persson, S. Kullander, G. Gennser, L. Grennert, and C. B. Laurell (Univ. of Lund, Malmö, Sweden) reviewed experience in screening for neural tube defects by fetal ultrasonography and maternal serum α-fetoprotein (AFP) measurement. In a 44-month period, 10,147 pregnancies were screened. The first ultrasound study is done at 17 weeks' gestation, at which time blood is sampled for AFP measurement if the fetal biparietal diameter is 35–49 mm. The serum AFP concentration,

(7–15) Br. Med. J. 286:747–749, Mar. 5, 1983.

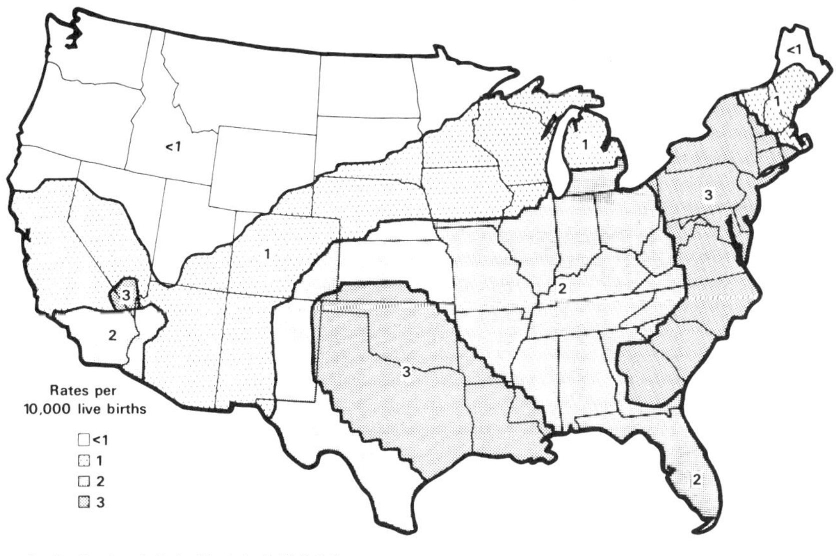

Fig 7–3.—Estimated birth prevalence rates of spina bifida in black infants born in the United States based on computer-generated maps. (Courtesy of Greenberg, F., et al.: Am. J. Obstet. Gynecol. 145:570–573, Mar. 1, 1983.)

measured at weekly intervals by countercurrent immunoelectrophoresis, was determined in 8,610 women.

There were 5 fetuses with open spina bifida, 3 with encephalocele, and 1 each with anencephalus and omphalocele in this series, 8 of which were detected by screening. The efficacy of the various methods is shown in Tables 1 and 2. Malformations occurred in 6.7% of fetuses when the serum AFP level was more than 100 μg/L. Nine of 117 women with elevated levels of serum AFP had amniotic fluid AFP values of more than 3 times the median. In 3 of these, primary ultrasound study disclosed a fetal malformation, and in 4, repeated focused ultrasound study did so. Six fetuses had neural tube defects and 1 had an omphalocele. The other 2 women delivered normal infants at term. All but 1 of the 9 fetal defects were visualized by careful ultrasound scanning, but 6 were not detected until an elevated maternal

TABLE 1.—EFFICIENCY OF TESTS USED IN SCREENING FOR NEURAL TUBE DEFECTS (FIGURES REPRESENT NUMBERS OF WOMEN TESTED)

	Serum α-fetoprotein	Ultrasound	Amniotic fluid α-fetoprotein*	Combined tests
True positive	8	4	7	8
False positive	112	0	2	0
True negative	8488	10 137	106	10 137
False negative	2	6	2	2
Total	8610	10 147	117	10 147

*Measured only in women having raised serum concentrations (>100 μg/L).
(Courtesy of Persson, P. H., et al.: Br. Med. J. 286:747–749, Mar. 5, 1983.)

TABLE 2.—SENSITIVITY, SPECIFICITY, AND PREDICTIVE VALUES OF THE FOUR DIFFERENT METHODS USED TO DETECT FETAL MALFORMATIONS (NEURAL TUBE DEFECTS AND OMPHALOCELE)

	Serum α-fetoprotein (%)	Ultrasound (%)	Amniotic fluid α-fetoprotein (%)	Combined tests (%)
Sensitivity (true positive/true positive + false negative)	80·00	40·00	77·8	80·00
Specificity (true negative/true negative + false positive)	98·70	100·00	98·1	100·00
Predictive value of positive test (true positive/true positive + false positive)	6·70	100·00	77·8	100·00
Predictive value of negative test (true negative/true negative + false negative)	99·98	99·94	98·1	99·98

(Courtesy of Persson, P. H., et al.: Br. Med. J. 286:747–749, Mar. 5, 1983.)

serum AFP level was found. Of the 107 women with elevated levels of serum AFP but no indication of fetal malformation on ultrasound study, 25% had spontaneous abortions previously, compared with 12% of the other women. Complications of pregnancy were more frequent in women having increased serum AFP values.

Determination of the serum AFP concentration should not be used to screen for neural tube defects in a low-risk population unless adequate ultrasound facilities are available. When the serum AFP level is elevated, focused ultrasound study may replace amniocentesis in many cases, but ultrasonography alone will not detect all small neural tube defects. Negative findings on AFP and ultrasound studies have very high predictive value. False results of AFP determination are avoided by reliably estimating gestational age and using semiquantitative analysis. The short interval between an elevated serum AFP level and subsequent evaluation minimizes anxiety.

▶ [This study of AFP screening comes from Sweden, which has an incidence of neural tube defects similar to that in the United States (approximately 1 per 1,000) and lower than that in the United Kingdom. The authors feel that in a low-risk population, both serum AFP and ultrasound screening are necessary to detect fetuses with neural tube defects. The addition of ultrasound adds greatly to the cost and would certainly reverse any favorable cost-benefit ratio, if indeed such exists for AFP screening of low-risk populations.] ◀

7–16 **Prenatal Ultrasonographic Diagnosis of Spina Bifida: Timing of Examination.** Ultrasonography and amniocentesis generally are done at about 16–18 weeks' gestation in pregnancies at risk for fetal neural tube defects; however, the timing of ultrasonography is a key factor in diagnosis. David Toms and B. St. J. Brown describe data on a fetus in which lumbar spina bifida was not conclusively demonstrated at 16 weeks' gestation, but was established at 20½ weeks.

Woman, 26, gravida 2, para 2, with gestational diabetes in her second pregnancy, had a biparietal diameter measurement indicating a 16-week ges-

(7–16) J. Can. Assoc. Radiol. 33:276–278, December 1982.

tation on initial ultrasonography 18½ weeks after the last menses, following pill withdrawal. A minimal focal area of divergence was noted in the upper lumbar spinal canal diameters that was not confirmed by observaton in other planes. The lower fetal extremities moved normally. Repeat study 4½ weeks later showed gross spina bifida of the upper lumbar region. A third study done at 22 weeks confirmed the previous findings and showed no evidence of hydrocephalus. A therapeutic abortion was performed. Radiography of the abortus showed an open myelomeningocele in the upper lumbar region. Subsequently, an amniotic fluid α-fetoprotein measurement on a specimen taken at 20½ weeks was reported as elevated.

Continued anatomical evoluton of spina bifida can occur in the second trimester of pregnancy, although the anomaly is established in the first trimester. It is suggested that, if there is any reason to suspect a neural tube defect, detailed ultrasonographic examination of the entire vertebral column be carried out at about 20 weeks' gestation if the diagnosis is not made earlier.

▶ [This report indicates that, on occasion, spina bifida may not be apparent on ultrasound examination at 16 weeks' gestation, but can be identified a few weeks later. Repeat scanning in suspected cases is indicated.] ◀

7–17 **Reproductive Outcome Following Amniocentesis for Genetic Indications.** Midtrimester amniocentesis for the antenatal diagnosis of genetic abnormalities is now standard care for women at special risk because of age or previous reproductive history, but the nature of the risk inherent in the procedure itself is controversial. Richard P. Porreco, Philip E. Young, Robert Resnik, Larry Cousins, Oliver W. Jones, Terri Richards, Colleen Kernahan, and Melinda Matson reviewed the outcome of 2,300 completed pregnancies in such women who underwent amniocentesis since 1971 at the University of California, San Diego, and of 331 pregnancies in women older than age 35 years who declined amniocentesis for genetic indications. (The latter group was seen at the Kaiser-Permanente Medical Center, San Diego.)

In the study group there were 63 total losses (2.84%). The bulk of them (2.07%) occurred between the time of amniocentesis and 28 weeks' gestation. Anterior placentation was associated with a twofold increase in losses when compared to posterior placentation (3.06% vs. 1.57%). Significantly more losses (4.76%) occurred in patients with unknown placentation than in those in whom placental location was assessed sonographically. When the details of the losses were investigated, a minimum estimate for the risk of a procedure-related fetal death was in the range of 0.6% to 0.9%.

Among the 700 women who had amniocentesis during 1980 there was only 1 loss within 7 days of the procedure. If this reflects a true decrease in procedure-related fetal deaths, it suggests that responsibility lies with use of small (20- and 22-gauge) needles or increased awareness on the part of the operator of the potential hazards of an anterior placenta, or both.

Among the 331 women in the control group, 6 losses (1.81%) occurred, which was not significantly different from the study group.

(7–17) Am. J. Obstet. Gynecol. 143:653–660, July 15, 1982.

Only 1 loss (0.30%) occurred between 16 and 28 weeks' gestation, compared with a loss of 2.07% in the same interval in the study group. The absolute difference in total losses between the study and control groups is consistent with the estimated procedure-related loss of 0.6% to 0.9%.

Midtrimester amniocentesis is relatively safe in light of the important information to be gained, but there is an inherent procedure-related risk that may be higher with anterior placentation. The use of static and real-time sonography provides data that may be important in achieving a safe amniocentesis and in assessing the possible problems that may arise immediately after the procedure.

▶ [This is a large series of genetic amniocenteses from a single institution (actually, the amniocenteses were done at multiple institutions and the fluid analysis was done at one place). From the data, it appears that the procedure-related fetal loss rate is less than 1% overall and somewhat higher with anterior than with posterior placentation. This is one of the few studies that seems to indicate improved outcome with ultrasound guidance.] ◀

7–18 **Midtrimester Amniocentesis: Analysis of 923 Cases With Neonatal Follow-up.** Midtrimester amniocentesis is used widely to diagnose fetal chromosomal abnormalities, neural tube defects, and various metabolic disorders. Dwight P. Cruikshank, Michael W. Varner, Jean E. Cruikshank, Stanley S. Grant, and Elizabeth Donnelly reviewed the results of 923 midtrimester amniocenteses done for genetic diagnosis at one institution between 1977 and 1980. Serious chromosome abnormalities were identified in 20 fetuses and less serious ones in 6. A maternal age of 35 or older was associated with a 2% risk of fetal trisomy 21 and 3% risk of any major chromosomal abnormality. The respective rates for women aged 40 or older were 4.8% and 7.2%. Neural tube defects were found in 0.15% of studies done because of maternal age and in 3.4% of those done because of a previous affected child.

Spontaneous abortion followed amniocentesis in 18 patients, or 2% of those followed up; however, the risk was only 0.2%–1.4%, as 6 cases clearly were unrelated to the procedure. Spontaneous abortion was disproportionately frequent in women aged 35 years or younger. The presence of mahogany-colored or green amniotic fluid was associated with a fetal loss rate of 29%. Unexplained rises in the maternal serum α-fetoprotein level were associated with a 38% risk of a low birth weight infant. Neonatal respiratory problems occurred in 2.5% of infants, an incidence that does not seem excessive. The only neonatal complications associated with amniocentesis were lower extremity orthopedic abnormalities, present in 2.3% of infants followed up. The most common condition was metatarsus adductus. Hip dislocation and clubfoot also were observed.

These findings confirm what others have demonstrated about the efficacy and safety of midtrimester genetic amniocentesis. An increased risk of orthopedic abnormalities in offspring also was confirmed. The mechanism of amniocentesis as the cause of these abnormalities is unclear, but a transient reduction in amniotic fluid volume

---

(7–18) Am. J. Obstet. Gynecol. 146:204–211, May 15, 1983.

with resultant crowding at a critical phase of gestation may be responsible.

▶ [Do the neonatal orthopedic problems reported here relate to the advanced maternal age of the population or to the amniocentesis procedure itself? The authors speculate that a transient diminution in amniotic fluid volume with resultant crowding might be involved.] ◀

7-19 **Management of the Fetus With Congenital Hydronephrosis.** Urinary tract dilatation in the fetus presents a diagnostic and therapeutic challenge. Michael R. Harrison, Mitchell S. Golbus, Roy A. Filly, Don K. Nakayama, Peter W. Callen, Alfred A. de Lorimier, and Hedvig Hricak (Univ. of California, San Francisco) review their experience in the management of 26 fetuses with sonographically demonstrated dilation of the urinary tract followed for a total of 206 weeks of gestation.

There were 8 fetuses with unilateral hydronephrosis. Because normal amniotic fluid volume indicated good function of the normal contralateral kidney, all 8 were followed without intervention and delivered near term and all are well after postnatal surgical correction. Three cases of bilateral hydronephrosis had resolved spontaneously by the time of delivery. Another 8 fetuses had bilateral hydronephrosis and evidence of poor function. Three of these fetuses were not treated and died soon after birth with small lungs and dysplastic kidneys, 3 underwent diagnostic intervention that demonstrated irreversible disease and allowed the pregnancy to be terminated, and 2 had obstruction that was corrected successfully in utero, but renal damage was too severe and precluded survival at birth. Early decompression was performed in 7 fetuses with bilateral hydronephrosis and equivocal function. Four of these fetuses were delivered early and the defect was corrected surgically; 1 has renal failure and the other 3 are well. The remaining 3 fetuses had the obstruction relieved in utero by percutaneous placement of a catheter shunt; 1 had multiple anomalies and died and the other 2 are well.

It is concluded that perinatal management of the fetus with a dilated urinary tract is improved by serial sonographic observation. Indications for diagostic or therapeutic intervention depend on the type and severity of obstruction and the time in gestation at which the obstruction is discovered. Although most fetuses will not require treatment before birth, a few may benefit from early decompression, either in utero or ex utero.

▶ [The San Francisco group is the team with the most experience in managing fetal urinary obstruction, and this report is an update of their experience as of mid-1982. It does appear that decompression of the renal pelvic in utero has a small but definite place.

In a related report, Vallancien and associates (*Urology* 20:647, 1982) described a case in which bilateral hydronephrosis due to ureteropelvic junction stenosis was treated by percutaneous nephrosotomy in utero at 31 weeks' gestational age.] ◀

-20 **Nature of Structural Defects Associated With Velamentous and Marginal Insertion of Umbilical Cord.** Previous studies have established an increased occurrence of structural fetal defects in as-

(7-19) J. Pediatr. Surg. 17:728-742, December 1982.
(7-20) Am. J. Obstet. Gynecol. 146:191-193, May 15, 1983.

sociation with velamentous and marginal umbilical cord insertions. Luther K. Robinson, Kenneth L. Jones, and Kurt Benirschke (Univ. of California at San Diego) attempted to confirm these associations in a study of 4,677 consecutive placentas. Marginal insertion of the umbilical cord was found in 8.5% and a velamentous insertion in 1.5%. Data were available on 384 infants whose cord was marginally inserted and 70 whose cord had a velamentous insertion. Structural defects occurred in 5.2% of infants with a marginal cord insertion and in 8.6% of those with a velamentous insertion. Malformations predominated in those with marginal cord insertion, and deformations predominated in the infants with a velamentous cord insertion. Four stillbirths, including a set of monozygotic twins, occurred in fetuses with a velamentous cord insertion, and 1 stillbirth was associated with a marginal insertion. None of these fetuses had structural defects.

This study confirmed an increased incidence of structural fetal defects in association with both marginal and velamentous umbilical cord insertions into the placenta. Most of the defects were the result of deformation of a normally formed part. These findings, and the observation of a disproportionate number of twins with a velamentous cord insertion, suggest that competition for space at the implantation site leads to both a velamentous cord insertion and associated structural fetal defects. Deformational defects are caused by intrauterine molding; the pressure causing molding usually is extrinsic, secondary to fetal crowding. A recognition that velamentous cord insertion in some instances is secondary to mechanical factors that force the bulk of placental tissue laterally should lead clinicians to evaluate mothers carefully for uterine malformation or myoma, which may influence subsequent pregnancies.

▶ [A previous report (1979 Year Book, p. 93) indicated that velamentous insertion of the umbilical cord was without clinical significance, except as a requisite for vasa previa. The current study suggests an association with fetal deformations (cf. 1980 Year Book, p. 212). The authors hypothesize that both the velamentous insertion and the deformation have the same underlying mechanism, i.e., crowding and "competition" for intrauterine space.] ◀

7–21 **Amniotic Band Syndrome** is discussed by John W. Seeds, Robert C. Cefalo, and William N. P. Herbert (Univ. of North Carolina). In this syndrome, there is random occurrence of fetal malformations associated with fibrous bands that appear to entangle or entrap various fetal parts, leading to deformation, malformation, or disruption deformities that do not occur together in any other genetic or chromosomal context. The spectrum of malformations (table) almost always includes constriction ring defects of the extremities. Craniofacial defects occur in about one third of the cases. Visceral manifestations are infrequent. Multiple anomalies are found in about three fourths of the cases. The obstetric characteristics of pregnancies that result in delivery of affected infants are usually unremarkable, and amniotic fluid volume is usually normal.

Amniotic band syndrome occurs in from 1:1,200 to 1:15,000 live

---

(7–21) Am. J. Obstet. Gynecol. 144:243–248, Oct. 1, 1982.

ABNORMALITIES ASSOCIATED WITH AMNIOTIC BAND SYNDROME

1. Limb defects, multiple, asymmetric:
   - Constriction rings of limbs or digits
   - Amputation of limbs or digits
   - Pseudosyndactyly
   - Abnormal dermal ridge patterns
   - Simian creases
   - Clubbed feet
2. Craniofacial defects:
   - Encephalocele, multiple, asymmetric
   - Anencephaly
   - Facial clefting—lip, palate
     - Embryologically appropriate
     - Embryologically inappropriate
   - Severe nasal deformity
   - Asymmetric microphthalmia
   - Incomplete or absent cranial calcification
3. Visceral defects:
   - Gastroschisis
   - Omphalocele

(Courtesy of Seeds, J. W., et al.: Am. J. Obstet. Gynecol. 144:243–248, Oct. 1, 1982.)

births. The sex ratio is equal, there is no racial predisposition, all cases are sporadic, parental ages are within normal range, no consanguinity is found, and there is no consistent association with prenatal maternal trauma or exposure to drugs or radiation.

Ultrasonography and radiography can demonstrate some severe defects prenatally, but frequently even neonatal diagnosis is difficult, being accomplished accurately in only 29% to 50% of cases in the absence of specialized genetic consultation. Etiology of the syndrome remains unclear, but the view of Torpin (1965) that it results from extra-amniotic, intrachorionic entanglement with mesodermic strands seems best able to explain the broad spectrum of clinical features.

Misdiagnoses of 2 of every 3 cases results in inaccurate and greatly exaggerated recurrence risk counseling. Accurate neonatal diagosis requires detailed and precise examination of every infant born with multiple birth defects. The multiple and asymmetric annular constrictions or congenital amputations of extremities or digits associated with the syndrome are pathognomonic and can almost always be identified if carefully sought. These bands are clues to the pathogenesis of the more severe cranofacial and visceral anomalies that may be seen. Anyone involved in the delivery of any infant manifesting elements of this unusual combination of defects should seek specialized consultation in the pursuit of accurate diagnosis and genetic counseling.

▶ [This is a nice review of a condition that is more common than is generally realized. The importance of making the diagnosis lies in the fact the risk of recurrence is minimal.] ◀

7–22 **Familial Congenital Amputations.** P. C. Etches A. R. Stewart, and E. J. Ives (Univ. of Alberta, Edmonton) report the familial recurrence of the so-called amniotic band disruption complex or sequence.

Woman, 23, primigravida, was delivered of a male infant by cesarean section at 27 weeks' gestation after 96 hours of ruptured membranes. Pregnancy had been without complication until this time. At delivery, the infant had congenital amputations of the right first and second toes, but was otherwise normal. The infant left the hospital at age 3½ months. The mother had a similar congenital defect affecting the first 3 toes of the right foot; she had weighed 2.8 kg at birth. Further inquiry into the family history revealed the mother's great aunt (sister of her maternal grandfather) had 3 fingers missing from one hand. The mother also had one male paternal first cousin whose middle toe on one foot comprised only a small lump of tissue. All other members of the mother's family were normal and the infant's father had no family history for this defect.

The commonly held theories for the genesis of ring constrictions and amputations of the extremities are interruption of normal morphogenesis, crowding of fetal parts, or disruption of previously differentiated structures brought about by rupture of the amniotic membrane, followed by formation of amniotic bands. This latter accident would be expected to be sporadic, and would have no familial connection. Other mechanisms, such as Streeter's defective germ plasm hypothesis, occasionally may play a role in cases similar to the present one and in those previously reported.

▶ [Although amniotic bands usually account for congenital amputations and limb constrictions (1982 YEAR BOOK, pp. 211–212, and preceding article), the case reported here suggests that at least some of these may be on a familial, presumably genetic, basis. Therefore although the risk of recurrence is very low in this situation, it is not zero.] ◀

7–23 **Effects of Acetylsalicylic Acid Ingestion on Maternal and Neonatal Hemostasis** were studied by Marie J. Stuart, Steven J. Gross, Haim Elrad, and Janet E. Graeber (SUNY, Upstate Med. Center) in 58 pairs of mothers and their infants. Data on direct and indirect aspirin ingestion were obtained by questioning women admitted at term in labor about their use, during the previous 10 days, of more than 100 nonproprietary drug preparations that contain acetylsalicylic acid. A positive or negative history of aspirin ingestion was verified by in vitro evaluation of platelet malondialdehyde formation, a technique that also allowed accurate estimation of the timing of previous aspirin ingestion.

Of the 58 mothers, 34 had not ingested aspirin in the 10 days before delivery (group 1), 10 had ingested 5–10 gm of aspirin within 5 days before delivery (group 2), 7 had ingested 5–15 gm of aspirin 6–10 days before delivery (group 3), and 7 had ingested no aspirin in the 10 days before delivery but did not receive it within 12 hours after delivery (group 4).

Aspirin ingestion within 5 days of delivery was associated with a marked increase in the incidence of hemostatic abnormalities in both mothers and infants (table). Six of these 10 mothers had an abnormal

---

(7–22) J. Pediatr. 101:448–449, September 1982.
(7–23) N. Engl. J. Med. 307:909–912, Oct. 7, 1982.

INCIDENCE OF HEMOSTATIC ABNORMALITIES IN MATERNAL-NEONATAL PAIRS

GROUP NO.	MOTHERS	NEONATES
	number of subjects (%)	
1 (34 pairs)	1/34 (3)	1/34 (3)
2 (10 pairs)	6/10 (60)*	9/10 (90)*
3 (7 pairs)	0/7 (0)	0/7 (0)
4 (7 pairs)	4/7 (57)*	0/7 (0)

*Values statistically different from those in group 1 controls.

(Courtesy of Stuart, M. J., et al.: N. Engl. J. Med. 307:909–912, Oct. 7, 1982.)

fall in hemoglobin level post partum; 4 of the 6 also had direct evidence of abnormal blood loss. Neonatal manifestations of hemostatic abnormalities include a profusion of petechiae over the presenting part in 4 infants, cephalhematoma in 1, subconjunctival hemorrhage in 1, bleeding from the circumcision site in 1, and microscopic hematuria in 2. Of the 7 women who received aspirin soon after delivery, 4 had a marked fall in hemoglobin level, which was associated with considerable post partum uterine bleeding in 2.

The type of hemostatic abnormality observed in affected neonates (mucosal and superficial bleeding) is characteristic of a platelet or capillary defect and occurred with greater frequency than in their mothers, suggesting that neonates may be more susceptible to the effects of aspirin than their mothers. Use of aspirin is best avoided during pregnancy and delivery. If ingestion has occurred within 5 days of delivery, the neonate should be evaluated carefully for the presence of clinical bleeding.

▶ [These results seem to indicate that aspirin ingestion within 5 days of delivery leads to impaired hemostasis in both mother and infant. Accordingly, the authors advise avoidance of aspirin during pregnancy. While the types of bleeding abnormality observed were, for the most part, not especially serious (e.g., petechiae over the presenting part), the fact that they occurred at all is significant. Earlier reports of hemostatic effects of aspirin in pregnancy have relied on memory to determine ingestion and have focused on laboratory effects; the improved methodology used in this study makes the conclusions all the more meaningful.] ◀

8. The Puerperium

8-1 **1981 Milk Feeding Patterns in the United States During First 12 Months of Life.** Gilbert A. Martinez and David A. Dodd (Ross Labs., Columbus, Ohio) reviewed responses to questionnaires sent between 1955 and 1981 to a nationally representative sample of mothers regarding their use of various milks to feed infants in the first 6 months of life. In 1981, questionnaires were sent to more than 51,000 new mothers, and a 55% response rate was obtained. A bimonthly telephone survey was initiated in 1980 to assess milk use by infants aged 8–12 months. More than 9,100 calls were made during 1981, and a 78% response rate was obtained.

An increasing incidence of breast-feeding was evident from 1971 through 1981 at all infant ages, particularly in older infants. Breast-feeding in the hospital more than doubled during this interval. Breast-feeding became more prevalent in all demographic subgroups (Table

TABLE 1.—PERCENTAGE OF INFANTS BREAST-FEEDING IN THE HOSPITAL BY SELECTED MATERNAL DEMOGRAPHIC CHARACTERISTICS*

	1971	1981	ARG 1971–1981
Parity			
Primiparous	28.1	62.4†	8.3
Multiparous	21.9	53.0†	9.2
Type of medical care			
Pediatrician	26.3	58.0†	8.2
General practitioner	22.0	57.8†	10.1
Education			
Grade and high school	19.4	50.8†	10.1
College	42.1	74.0†	5.8
Employment‡			
Not employed	. . .	59.5	. . .
Employed	. . .	50.9	. . .
Income			
<$7,000	22.3	38.8†	5.7
$7,000–$14,999	26.7	54.0†	7.3
≥$15,000	§	62.9	§
Total (all infants)	24.7	57.6	8.8

*Abbreviation: ARG = annual rate of gain.
†Trend significant, $P < .01$.
‡Refers to employment status at time of survey, i.e., when infants were 6 months of age. Employed represents mothers with full-time employment. Data are for three quarters of 1981.
§Income classification stopped at > $10,000. Statistical tests were performed on categories $7,000–$9,000.
(Courtesy of Martinez, G. A., and Dodd, D. A.: Pediatrics 71:166–170, February 1983; copyright 1983, American Academy of Pediatrics.)

(8–1) Pediatrics 71:166–170, February 1983.

TABLE 2.—PERCENTAGE OF INFANTS BREAST-FED BY MATERNAL EMPLOYMENT STATUS, 1981*

	Infant Age			
	In Hospital	2 mo	4 mo	6 mo
Full-time employment				
Breast-fed alone	45.1	24.8	8.5	3.6
Breast-fed with bottle	5.8	8.3	8.3	6.6
Total	50.9	33.1	16.8	10.1
Milk, bottle supplementation as % of total	11.4	25.1	49.4	65.4
% still breast-feeding among those breast-feeding in hospital	100.0	65.0	33.0	19.8
Not employed				
Breast-fed alone	53.4	41.1	30.8	22.9
Breast-fed with bottle	6.1	6.4	6.5	6.9
Total	59.5	47.4	37.3	29.8
Milk, bottle supplementation as % of total	10.3	13.5	17.4	23.2
% still breast-feeding among those breast-feeding in hospital	100.0	79.7	62.7	50.1

*Employment status was not elicited in second quarter of 1981. Data represent first, third, and fourth quarters only. Some totals do not add due to rounding.

(Courtesy of Martinez, G. A., and Dodd, D. A.: Pediatrics 71:166–170, February 1983; copyright 1983, American Academy of Pediatrics.)

1). Breast-feeding at age 6 months was most prevalent among mothers with some college education, those not employed at the time of the survey, and those with higher family incomes. Similar patterns were found in the telephone survey for feeding of infants aged 1 year. Feeding patterns are related to maternal employment status in Table 2.

Breast-feeding has continued to increase uninterruptedly since 1971, and the duration of breast-feeding, measured at age 6 months, has continued to increase at a faster rate than has the incidence of breast-feeding in the hospital. The chief discriminatory variables appear to be education and maternal employment, but breast-feeding is increasing in all demographic groups and at all levels of education and income.

▶ [Everyone dealing with mothers and infants knows that breast-feeding has increased dramatically over the past decade. This report, based on a scientific sampling study done by one of the major infant formula companies, indicates that the increase has been across all demographic categories. In 1981, 57.6% of infants were nursing on hospital discharge, and the persistence of nursing correlated with employment status—at 6 months, 10.2% in full-time employed mothers and 29.8% in those not employed outside the home.] ◀

8–2 **Vitamin D of Human Milk: Identification of Biologically Active Forms.** Human milk generally is considered a poor source of vitamin D, making it unclear why infants who are breast-fed do not develop vitamin D deficiency. Lorraine E. Reeve, Russell W. Chesney, and Hector F. DeLuca (Univ. of Wisconsin, Madison) determined the total amount of vitamin D activity in human milk and the compounds responsible for it in samples from 3 health subjects of normal vitamin

(8–2) Am. J. Clin. Nutr. 36:122–126, July 1982.

D status in midlactation. Their vitamin D intakes were 400 to 800 IU daily. Activity of vitamin D was assessed by measuring stimulation of intestinal calcium transport in the vitamin D-deficient rat.

Human milk was found to contain vitamin D activity of 40–50 IU/L. Both 24,25-dihydroxyvitamin D and 1,25-dihydroxyvitamin D were below the limits of detection, and 1 L of human milk would be expected to contain less than 21 and 0.6 ng, respectively. Vitamin D itself was found to be the chief form present; the sample analyzed contained 338 ng of vitamin D_2 and 41 ng of vitamin D_3 per L. The metabolite 25-hydroxyvitamin D_3 was present at a concentration of 163 ng/L, and it accounts for biologic activity of about 33 IU/L, or three fourths of the total vitamin D activity estimated from the calcium transport assay.

Human milk contains vitamin D activity of up to 50 IU/L, three fourths of it attributable to 25-hydroxyvitamin D_3. Along with vitamin D_2 and vitamin D_3, over 90% of total activity is accounted for. The findings fail to indicate that vitamin D-sulfate or other unknown metabolites of vitamin D provide significant activity in human milk. Although milk apparently can provide calcium and phosphorus to the rat neonate in usable form without vitamin D being present, vitamin D becomes progressively more important with aging, emphasizing the importance of vitamin D supplementation in older breast-fed infants.

▶ [The content and bioactivity of vitamin D in milk have been quite controversial. Traditional assay systems have indicated that vitamin D levels are low in milk, yet rickets in breast-fed infants is quite rare. However, this latter point may be subject to reevaluation in view of recent suggestions that nutritional rickets in breast-fed infants is being seen with increasing frequency in the case of unusual maternal diets (see 1981 YEAR BOOK, pp. 215–216). To further fuel the controversy, there has been the question of a water-soluble form, vitamin D sulfate, which was claimed in an article abstracted in the 1978 YEAR BOOK (p. 211) to be the reason. The study described above comes from the laboratory of Hector DeLuca, surely "Mister Vitamin D," and it indicates that total vitamin D activity in human milk (1) is low (40–50 IU/L) but not as low as formerly thought, (2) reflects for the most part vitamin D_3 and its 25-hydroxylated form, and (3) contains no significant contribution from vitamin D sulfate.] ◀

8–3 **Effect of Maternal Nutritional Status on Immunologic Substances in Human Colostrum and Milk.** It is recognized now that increased resistance to disease in suckling newborn infants is due, at least in part, to passive protection by antimicrobial substances in human milk, including lysozyme, lactoferrin, complement components, immunoglobulins, and specific antibodies. Maternal diet and nutritional status influence both the quantity and the quality of milk. Reynaldo Miranda, Nancy G. Saravia, Ruben Ackerman, Neva Murphy, Stephen Berman, and David N. McMurray examined the effects of maternal nutritional status and lactation interval on various substances in the colostrum and milk of Colombian women, including antibodies against the common pediatric pathogen respiratory syncytial virus (RSV). Twenty-three women were evaluated in the first 2 months of lactation. Eleven were malnourished.

Malnutrition was characterized by lower weight-height ratio, creatinine-height index, and total serum protein, serum albumin, and

(8–3) Am. J. Clin. Nutr. 37:632–640, April 1983.

serum IgG and IgA values. Colostrum from malnourished mothers contained one-third the normal concentration of IgG and less than half the normal concentration of albumin. Significant reductions in IgA and C4 also were found, but there were no abnormalities in colostral values for lysozyme, C3, or IgM. Antibody titers of RSV in milk were not influenced by maternal nutritional status. The differences between the two groups tended to disappear when mature milk was assessed, as the nutritional status of the malnourished mothers improved in the first several weeks after delivery. Birth weights were slightly lower in the malnourished group.

It tentatively is concluded that the protective qualities of colostrum and milk may be influenced significantly by maternal nutritional status. The findings are highly suggestive of a detrimental effect of maternal malnutrition on some protective substances in colostrum and transitional milk.

▶ [The quantity and nutritional quality of milk produced seem to be maintained across a wide range of maternal diets, and only with quite poor maternal nutritional status are there effects on the nutritional indices of milk. Of course, milk serves functions in addition to nutrition, notably, some immunologic protection against infections. This study by Miranda et al. indicates that this latter function is also subject to dietary influences. Colostral protein levels from malnourished women were only one third of those from normal women, and C4 complement, IgA, and IgG values also were reduced. The effects of maternal malnutrition tended to lessen with the transition to mature milk, reflecting either an improvement in maternal nutritional status or an adaptaion by the mother to her "deprived" state.] ◀

8–4 **Bone Mineral Status of Lactating Mothers of Different Ages.** Gary M. Chan, Patricia Slater, Nonie Ronald, Charles C. Roberts, M. Rita Thomas, David Folland, and Richard Jackson (Univ. of Utah, Salt Lake City) studied the effect of age on bone mineralization in 48 healthy white lactating mothers. Twelve were aged 16–18 years, 24 were aged 19–30 (mean age, 24), and 12 were aged 31–35 (mean age, 33). All exclusively breast-fed their infants and took a daily multivitamin that contained 400 IU of vitamin D and 200 mg of calcium.

Blood samples taken at 2 and at 16 weeks post partum showed no differences among the three age groups in serum calcium, phosphorus, and 25-hydroxyvitamin D values. At 16 weeks, alkaline phosphatase values were lower in the group aged 19–30, compared to the

Bone Mineral Content of Lactating Mothers

Age (yr)	*2 Weeks post partum*	*16 Weeks post partum*	*Paired t**
≤18	1.049 ± 0.088†	0.895 ± 0.051	<0.05
19 to 30	0.965 ± 0.030	0.964 ± 0.028	NS
>31	0.960 ± 0.024	0.974 ± 0.022	NS

NS = not significant.
*Two weeks vs. 16 weeks.
†Grams per cm; mean ± SE.
(Courtesy of Chan, G. M., et al.: Am. J. Obstet. Gynecol. 144:438–441, Oct. 15, 1982.)

(8–4) Am. J. Obstet. Gynecol. 144:438–441, Oct. 15, 1982.

other two groups. Bone mineral content, measured by photon absorptiometry, was similar in the three groups at 2 weeks post partum. However, between the 2 and 16 weeks, bone mineral content decreased by about 15% in the youngest age group (table).

Dietary studies showed similar intakes of total energy, protein, fat, carbohydrate, calcium, and phosphorus in mothers aged 16–18 and in those aged 19–30. However, the recommended dietary allowance for calcium or phosphorus was met by only 1 of 7 lactating mothers aged 16–18, compared with 6 or 7 aged 19–30.

Young lactating mothers (≤18 years of age) are at risk for bone demineralization because of low dietary intake of calcium and phosphorus. Female adolescents are known to require more calcium and phosphorus than adult women. Young lactating mothers should be counseled about the need for adequate intake of calcium and phosphorus.

▶ [Lactation potentially represents a considerable drain on maternal calcium stores. Because the calcium content of human milk averages 30 mg/dl, a daily production of 1 L means a loss of 300 mg per day. Calcium absorption from the gut is limited, so not many nursing women are able to meet this need from the diet and therefore call on bone mineral stores. Previous reports have been mixed with respect to the effect of lactation on maternal bone. This study indicates that bone mineral content is lost in patients aged 18 or younger but not in older mothers, suggesting that adolescents merit careful attention to calcium and vitamin D intake. It is unfortunate that concentrations of calcitonin were not measured, because this hormone might play a role in maintaining the skeleton, and levels have been reported to correlate positively with age.

In another study by this same group of investigators (*J. Pediatr.* 101:567, 1982), bone mineral content of adolescent lactating mothers was found to decrease, presumably due to low calcium-phosphate intake; in contrast, the bone of older mothers and nonlactating controls remained constant.] ◀

8–5 **Phenytoin Excretion in Human Breast Milk and Plasma Levels in Nursed Infants.** The increase in breast-feeding has raised concern about the passage of various drugs into breast milk. Bengt Steen, Anders Rane, Gudmar Lönnerholm, Olle Falk, Carl-Eric Elwin, and Folke Sjöqvist examined the transfer of phenytoin into breast milk in 6 epileptic mothers who nursed their infants. All had received a constant dosage of phenytoin long enough for a steady state to be established. Mean plasma phenytoin concentrations in the mothers were 12.8 to 78.5 μmole/L. Milk concentrations were considerably lower, with a mean milk-plasma concentration ratio of 0.13. Only 2 infants had detectable phenytoin, with plasma concentrations of 0.72 and 0.46 μmole/L, respectively. Only 1 infant had measurable 4-hydroxyphenytoin, at a concentration of 0.44 μmole/L. Correlation between mean plasma and milk phenytoin concentrations was 0.97. Correlation between the area under the curve for the plasma phenytoin concentration and the mean milk concentration was 0.99.

The body weight-related dose of phenytoin secreted into breast milk is less than 5% of the dose to infants and small children. The findings do not argue against breast-feeding during phenytoin therapy. None of the infants in this study had signs of phenytoin toxicity. Only 2 of the 6 infants had measurable, extremely low plasma concentrations

(8–5) Ther. Drug Monit. 4:331–334, December 1982.

of the drug, but it is possible that even small concentrations of phenytoin exert subtle effects in the newborn infant.

▶ [As good pharmacologic data are acquired concerning the passage of drugs from mother to infant in breast milk, a general picture of reassurance emerges. Oral anticoagulants and antithyroid drugs, which previously were considered dangerous, are no longer regarded as absolute contraindications to breast-feeding. The information reported here suggests that one should not discourage the epileptic woman taking phenytoin from breast-feeding.] ◀

8–6 **Role of Antenatal Estrogen in Postpartum Human Lactogenesis: Evidence From Estrogen-Deficient Pregnancies.** Postpartum lactogenesis requires the concerted efforts of several hormones, including estrogen, progesterone, and prolactin (PRL). R. H. Martin and R. E. Oakey (Univ. of Leeds) report a study of 5 women with severe antepartum estrogen deficiency (in 4 due to placental steroid sulfatase deficiency and in 1 due to an unknown cause) and low levels of PRL in peripheral plasma during delivery and in the puerperium. These women were unable to establish lactogenesis, which was assessed by plasma α-lactalbumin concentrations on the fourth day postpartum. The role of estrogen was specifically examined in postpartum lactogenesis.

Before delivery, estrogen production, assessed by urinary estrogen excretion or plasma estradiol concentrations, was subnormal for the appropriate period of gestation in all patients. Values were, however, much greater than those of nonpregnant women. Progesterone levels were within normal range. The PRL values in the estrogen-deficient women were much higher than those in nonpregnant women. Values of PRL during the first 10 days after delivery remained below normal or, in the 3 patients attempting breast-feeding, did not exceed 3,200 μ/L. Despite attempts to establish breast-feeding, PRL secretion remained depressed, equivalent to that in normal women who bottle-feed their infants. At delivery, plasma α-lactalbumin concentrations in the estrogen-deficient women were within the range for normal pregnant women; the levels remained low on the fourth day post partum, which indicated failure to establish lactogenesis.

Failure to establish lactogenesis and lactation can now be recognized as a common feature of pregnancies complicated by placental steroid sulfatase deficiency. This study demonstrates the failure of estrogen-deficient women to establish lactogenesis post partum. Antenatal estrogen possibly has an additional effect, directed toward breast tissue, and is required to permit initiation of α-lactalbumin synthesis in response to PRL.

▶ [Placental sulfatase deficiency is associated with male newborns, low estriol levels, the failure to develop effective labor, and, according to this report, the frequent failure to establish lactogenesis. Estrogen levels during pregnancy are, of course, low in this situation. Prolactin levels are also, both prior to delivery and in the early puerperium. In addition, the breasts are not subjected to the normally occurring estrogen withdrawal after delivery. Would a prolactin secretion-stimulating agent be clinically useful in this situation (cf. 1982 Year Book, pp. 222–223, and the following articles)?] ◀

(8–6) Clin. Endocrinol. (Oxf.) 17:403–408, October 1982.

8–7 **Sulpiride Improves Inadequate Lactation.** O. Ylikorkala, A. Kauppila, S. Kivinen, and L. Viinikka (Univ. of Helsinki) note that 20%–40% of mothers willing to breast-feed suffer from inadequate lactation. They tested sulpiride, a potent prolactin-releasing drug, in patients with insufficient lactation. Twenty-eight newly delivered mothers with inadequate lactation volunteered for a placebo-controlled, double-blind trial of sulpiride, 50 mg three times daily for 4 weeks. Treatment was allocated at random, and serum prolactin concentrations and yields of breast milk were measured before and serially during the trial. Of 26 women completing the study, 14 took sulpiride and 12, placebo.

The table shows no difference between the two treatment groups before the trial, but Figure 8–1 demonstrates the sulpiride treatment was accompanied by persistent rises in serum prolactin concentrations. In 13 of 14 women given sulpiride, daily milk yields increased by 90–730 ml. In the other patient, the daily milk yield decreased despite a substantial rise in serum prolactin. In 3 of 12 women given placebo, milk secretion increased, but it fell in all others. Of those completing the trial, 11 sulpiride and 3 placebo patients rated their respective treatment as effective. During sulpiride treatment, 1 woman complained of headache and 2 of tiredness. No side effects occurred in the placebo group.

This study is believed to be the first to show that sulpiride improves established lactational deficiency, apparently by increasing prolactin secretion. The effect of sulpiride on breast milk resulted in 4 infants

Fig 8–1.—Mean (± SE) serum prolactin concentrations and changes in daily milk yields in 14 mothers receiving sulpiride *(solid circles)*, and 12 receiving placebo *(open circles)*. *Asterisk, P* < .001. (Courtesy of Ylikorkala, O., et al.: Br. Med. J. 285:249–251, July 24, 1982.)

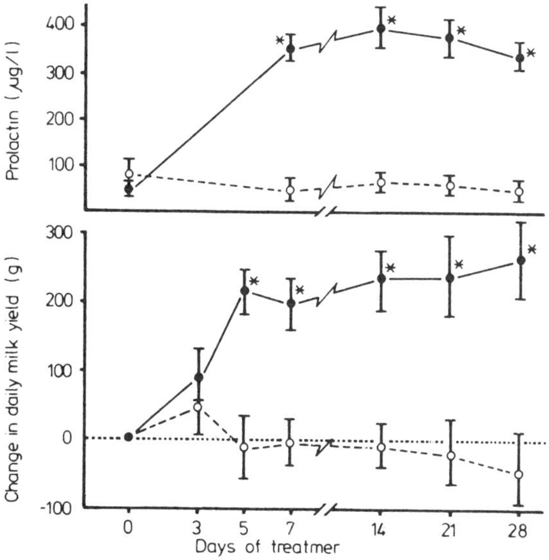

(8–7) Br. Med. J. 285:249–251, July 24, 1982.

CLINICAL DETAILS OF STUDY POPULATION AT START OF TRAIL*

	Group allocated to sulpiride	Group allocated to placebo
No of women	14	14
Age (years)	29·7 ± 1·3	29·1 ± 1·5
Parity	1·4 (1-5)	1·4 (1-4)
Height of nipples (mm) ..	8·9 ± 0·6	8·6 ± 0·7
Infants' weight (g)	5097 ± 505	4909 ± 266
Milk yield (ml/kg/day)	76·4 ± 47 (0-110)	72·3 ± 56 (0-105)
Days from delivery to entry to study	62·1 ± 12·1 (14-100)	55·6 ± 9·5 (18-120)
Duration of use of supplementary feeds (days)	22·3 ± 6·7 (3-49)	33·1 ± 9·1 (2-45)
Supplementary feeds (ml) ..	498 ± 88	434 ± 68
No of breast feeds/day	5·3 ± 0·3 (4-7)	5·3 ± 0·3 (4-7)

*Mean ± SE, with ranges in parentheses.
(Courtesy of Ylikorkala, O., et al.: Br. Med. J. 285:249–251, July 24, 1982.)

no longer needing supplementary feeds. Sulpiride is secreted in the breast milk, but with an average daily intake of 700 ml of milk, an infant would receive less than 1 mg sulpiride daily. Such a small amount would be very unlikely to stimulate prolactin release or have other central or peripheral actions in the infant.

8–8 **Effect of Sulpiride on Poor Puerperal Lactation.** Toshihiro Aono, Tadaatsu Aki, Koji Koike, and Keiichi Kurachi (Osaka, Japan) assessed the lactation-promoting effect of sulpiride in primiparous and multiparous mothers with poor lactation in the early puerperium. Forty-two primiparous and 54 multiparous women whose total yield of milk did not exceed 50 ml for the first 3 postpartum days were treated with sulpiride or placebo for 4 days from the third postpartum day. Sulpiride was given orally in 50 mg doses twice a day to 20 primiparous and 28 multiparous mothers. The other 22 primiparous and 26 multiparous mothers were given placebo according to the same schedule. Age range of these women was 21 to 35 years.

Results showed that sulpiride augmented the mean daily yield of milk to 111.4 ml, 224.5 ml, and 325.8 ml on the third, fourth, and fifth postpartum days, respectively. Volume of milk on the fourth and fifth days was significantly higher in the sulpiride-treated group than in the control group. Mean total yield of milk for the third to fifth postpartum days was 441.2 ml for the control group and 661.5 ml (a 49.9% increase) for the sulpiride-treated group. The proportion of mothers with poor secretion of milk was lower in the sulpiride-treated group than in the control group. The sulpiride-induced increase in PRL levels on the third and fifth postpartum days compared to that of the control group was statistically significant.

A follow-up study of breast-feeding routine was performed 1 month after delivery in 20 control and 20 sulpiride-treated primiparous women and in 25 control and 28 sulpiride-treated multiparous women. Among primiparous women, the rate of complete breast-feeding was 55% in the sulpiride-treated group and 30% in the control group. However, in multiparous women, the percentages of complete breast-feeding were similar for the two groups.

(8–8) Am. J. Obstet. Gynecol. 143:927–932, Aug. 15, 1982.

The authors conclude that poor initiation of puerperal lactation in primiparous mothers can be treated effectively with orally administered sulpiride.

▶ [An article abstracted in the 1982 YEAR BOOK (pp. 222–223) indicated that a dopamine antagonist, metoclopramide, could stimulate milk production. The two reports, one from Europe and the other from Asia, presented here indicate that sulpiride, another dopamine antagonist, may have clinical value in assisting lactation. Ylikorkala and associates found both prolactin levels and milk yields to increase dramatically with sulpiride administration in patients who had experienced lactational inadequacy. Aono and colleagues also found that sulpiride given for 4 days from the third postpartum day increased milk production substantially in treated primiparas. The safety of this sort of treatment hasn't been established as far as the newborn is concerned, but given the strong patient and medical interest in successful breast-feeding, we're sure to see dopamine antagonists used in this situation. Metoclopramide is available in the United States; sulpiride is not.] ◀

8–9 **Fertility Regulation in Nursing Women: III. Short-Term Influence of Low-Dose Combined Oral Contraceptive Upon Lactation and Infant Growth.** Previous studies of the effects of hormonal contraceptives on lactation report conflicting results. S. Díaz, O. Peralta, G. Juez, C. Herreros, M. E. Casado, A. M. Salvatierra, P. Miranda, E. Durán, and H. B. Croxatto (Santiago, Chile) examined the short-term effects on a low-dose combined oral contraceptive preparation containing 0.03 mg of ethinyl estradiol and 0.15 mg of levonorgestrel on lactation and infant growth. Treatment began 30–35 days post partum. Controls received either an oral or an injected placebo. All women in the study had a normal postpartum course and were fully nursing a month after delivery. Pills were taken daily for 3 weeks, followed by a 1-week pillfree interval.

The series included 291 women. Two discontinued oral contraception because of perceived decline in milk production. Fewer oral contraceptive users were exclusively breast-feeding by 90 days post partum (Table 1). Infants in the oral contraceptive group weighed less than those in both control groups (Table 2). Infants in all groups had similar daily weight increments in the first month of life. The effect of oral contraceptive use was evident when findings in both sexes were analyzed separately. Infant growth was similar in the two control groups.

TABLE 1.—DISTRIBUTION OF PATIENTS BY TYPE OF NURSING AND TREATEMENT AT DAY 91 POST PARTUM

Treatment	Exclusive Breast-feeding		Prescription of supplement: Medical		Maternal	
	N	%	N	%	N	%
OC	79*	80.6	10	10.2	9	9.2
IP	95	92.2	6	5.8	2	2.0
OP	69	92.0	3	4.0	3	4.0

*Oral contraceptive (OC) vs. injected placebo (IP): $P < .025$.
Oral contraceptive vs. oral placebo (OP): $P < .05$.
(Courtesy of Diaz, S., et al.: Contraception 27:1–10, January 1983.)

(8–9) Contraception 27:1–10, January 1983.

TABLE 2.—AVERAGE WEIGHT OF EXCLUSIVELY BREAST-FED INFANTS ACCORDING TO TREATMENT AND TO AGE

AGE (day)	BODY WEIGHT (g) Treatment OC			IP			OP		
X ± SD	N	X	± SD	N	X	± SD	N	X	± SD
0	103	3288	± 289	109	3297	± 289	79	3290	± 284
31 ± 2	103	4222	± 413	109	4259	± 411	79	4254	± 402
61 ± 2	91	5199	± 510*	98	5366	± 554	74	5380	± 551
91 ± 2	78	6011	± 588*	93	6220	± 605	67	6250	± 709

*Oral contraceptives (OC) = injective placebo (IP): $P < .05$.
Oral contraceptives = oral placebo (OP): $P < .05$.
(Courtesy of Diaz, S., et al.: Contraception 27:1–10, January 1983.)

This low-dose combined oral contraceptive had negative effects on both lactation and infant growth when instituted 30 days post partum. These effects seriously limit the use of low-dose oral contraceptives in lactating women in the first postpartum months. The adverse effects might be more important in populations not under study or without close medical supervision. Oral contraception should be used in nursing women only after alternatives have been carefully considered; close observation of the infant's growth rate is necessary.

▶ [Reports in the older literature demonstrating an adverse effect on lactation by oral contraceptives used relatively high-dose agents. In this study, the estrogen content was 30 μg, and oral contraceptives were not instituted until lactation was well established. Nonetheless, there was a definite (small but statistically significant) effect on nursing success and infant growth over the next 60 days.

In a companion study, the same investigative group (Croxatto, H. B., et al.: *Contraception* 27:13, 1983) studied longer-term effects. Again, oral contraceptive use was associated with lower success rates and lighter infants at age 10 months than was the use of intrauterine devices. In yet another study, the same authors (ibid., p. 27) withheld initiation of oral contraceptive use until 90 days, but even with this modification there was still modest inhibition. The lactation-inhibitory effect of even ultra-low-dose oral contraceptives seems clearly established; whether or not this is of practical significance remains to be seen.] ◀

8–10 **Left-Side Preference for Holding and Carrying Newborn Infants: Parental Holding and Carrying During First Week of Life.** About 80% of all newly delivered mothers hold their infants to the left of the body midline, the proportion decreasing with separation in the neonatal period. Peter de Château (Karolinska Inst., Stockholm) examined the infant holding and carrying behavior of 66 newly delivered first-time and second-time healthy mothers, the 66 fathers of the same infants, 43 other fathers with children older than age 1 year, and 41 men without children of their own. All participants were aged 20–35 years and were right-handed. The infant was held to the left by 80% of new mothers and 84% of the fathers. Mother-father pairs held the infant on the same side of the body in

(8–10) J. Nerv. Ment. Dis. 171:241–245, April 1983.

most instances. Fathers with older children behaved as the new parents did, but men without children of their own showed a significantly less left-side preference in holding. No significant differences were found for carrying the infant.

Both mothers and fathers exhibit a distinct preference for holding their infants to the left of the body midline, whereas men without children of their own do not show such a marked left-side preference. It may be that the maternal heartbeat has a soothing effect on the infant and can reduce anxiety in the infant and mother. Right-sided holding increases in separated mothers and is related to great prenatal and postnatal anxiety. Adjustment to the parental role, sensitivity to the infant's needs, and the ability to meet these needs may be less cognitive functions than emotional, empathic ones. If men are less well prepared than women in these respects, as their behavior indirectly indicates, more effort might be made to activate and promote their feelings.

▶ [These findings that both mothers and fathers tend to hold babies to the left are fascinating. The study involved only right-handed individuals, but literature is cited to indicate that the tendency is independent of handedness.] ◀

9. The Newborn

9–1 **Measurement of Motor Nerve Conduction Velocity: Precise Method of Estimating Maturity in Newborn.** Knowledge of the maturity of newborn infants can be important in both management and interpretation of hospital statistics. K. Goeschen, M. Pluta, J. Rothe, and E. Saling (Free Univ. of Berlin) measured the motor nerve conduction velocity (NCV) of the ulnar nerve 548 times in 523 infants in order to estimate maturity. The nerve was stimulated transcutaneously at the elbow and wrist with supramaximal square wave current; the action potential was recorded at the abductor digiti minimi muscle. Measurements were made on the right arm, with the infant under a heating lamp or in an incubator. Maturity also was estimated by the Farr system. The study group included 78 singleton infants small for gestational age, 26 infants large for gestational age, and 40 twins. Twenty-five infants were restudied after 4–14 days.

Centiles of NCV during gestation are shown in Figure 9–1. The

Fig 9–1.—The 10th *(10 P)*, 50th *(M)*, and 90th *(90 P)* centiles of 379 measurements of nerve conduction velocity *(NCV)* in normal singleton infants of 33–43 weeks' gestation. (Courtesy of Goeschen, K., et al.: Br. J. Obstet. Gynaecol. 90:61–68, January 1983.)

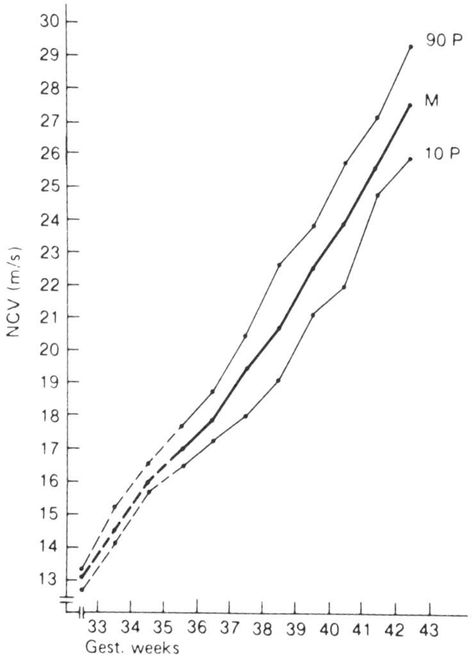

(9–1) Br. J. Obstet. Gynaecol. 90:61–68, January 1983.

median rose nearly linearly from week 33 to week 44 at a rate of 1.6 m/second per week. The tenth and ninetieth centiles remained close; the greatest deviation from the median was 1 week. The calculated correlation coefficient was .946. Testing for a second time showed a course similar to that of intrauterine maturation. The Farr system falsely exaggerated gestational age in immature children. Small singleton infants had a distribution of NCV values similar to that in controls. Close correlation beween corresponding twin and singleton values also was noted. Values were closely similar in twin pairs having large differences in weight.

Measurements of NCV are readily learned and the results are reproducible and fairly objective. Even infants with neurologic or traumatic damage or malformations in the central nervous system can be assessed in this way. A close positive correlation with gestational age is obtained, independent of body weight and length, so that undergrown mature infants and well-grown premature infants can be distinguished. Extrauterine maturation also can be evaluated by the NCV method. However, the apparatus needed, while highly reliable, is expensive. The method is not applicable to infants close to death or those with a low body temperature.

▶ [Nerve conduction velocities were correlated more highly with gestational age than was a score based on physical characteristics of the neonate. This technique might be of value for research purposes, but the expense of the equipment argues against its routine clinical use.] ◀

9–2 **Scalp Abscess: Benign and Infrequent Complication of Fetal Monitoring.** Leandro Cordero, Craig W. Anderson, and Frederick P. Zuspan (Ohio State Univ.) discuss the occurrence of scalp abscess as a complication to implantation of a fetal scalp electrode for internal monitoring. The lesions typically begin as small, indurated masses that soon fluctuate and suppurate. They appear from 1 day to 3 weeks after the start of monitoring, usually within 3–4 days. Abscesses usually are single. Most patients have little evidence of generalized disease. Scalp abscesses have been reported in 0.3% to 0.8% of infants on whom clip scalp electrodes were used, but this may well be an underestimate. Okada et al. reported lesions in 4.5% of infants on whom spiral fetal heart rate electrodes were used, but instances of localized cellulitis were probably also included. Apart from skin puncture, tissue compression and local trauma may contribute to scalp abscess formation. The most common aerobic isolates reported are *Streptococcus* groups A, B, and D and *Streptococcus epidermidis*.

Most scalp abscesses are localized, benign, and self-limited, but sepsis, major cellulitis, and osteomyelitis may develop. Reported morbidity is shown in the table. The only death occurred in a premature infant with overwhelming *Escherichia coli* septicemia. Several cases of herpes simplex virus infection in an area of scalp electrode implantation in infants have been reported. Seven of 9 infants described had generalized infection; all but 2 survived. Herpes simplex virus type 2 was present in all infants but 1. The maternal history was consistent with genital herpes in half of the women.

(9–2) Am. J. Obstet. Gynecol. 146:126–130, May 15, 1983.

NEONATAL MORBIDITY AND MORTALITY ASSOCIATED WITH SCALP ABSCESS*

Abscesses	No.	No. dead
Localized	140†	0
With associated complications		
Osteomyelitis	3	0
Cellulitis	1	0
Septicemia	4	1
Total	148	1

*Excluding herpes simplex infections.
†Included are four unpublished reports from the authors' institution.
(Courtesy of Cordero, L., et al.: Am. J. Obstet. Gynecol. 146:126–130, May 15, 1983.)

Scalp abscess is an infrequent, usually benign complication of monitoring electrode implantation. Local treatment usually suffices, but parenteral antibiotic therapy may be required. The benefits of electronic fetal heart rate monitoring, even when invasive, far outweigh the risks from scalp abscess formation.

▶ [At times, practitioners of obstetrics use the possibility of neonatal scalp infection as a reason to utilize the less helpful external, rather than internal, fetal heart rate monitoring in labor. Not surprisingly, this excuse is heard less often from obstetricians who practice in hospitals where resident physicians or nurses are permitted to apply the electrodes. Although scalp abscesses occasionally represent serious problems, this review of the published experience with these lesions suggests we should be careful not to overestimate their significance.] ◀

9–3 **Naloxone Reverses Neonatal Depression Caused by Fetal Asphyxia.** Endogenous opiates appear to play a role in the ventilatory response of neonates to asphyxia or hypoxia. Victor Chernick and Randy J. Craig (Univ. of Manitoba) postulated that endogenous opiates might be implicated in neonatal depression seen after intrauterine asphyxia.

On day 30 of pregnancy (full term is 31 days) rabbits were given naloxone (1 mg/kg) or saline intravenously. Five minutes later, each doe was placed in a 2-L chamber into which flowed nitrogen with 7% CO_2 at the rate of 20 L/minute. Within 3 or 4 minutes, the animal died. Eight minutes after being placed in the chamber, the uterus of each doe was exposed by laparotomy. At 10 minutes the fetuses were delivered by cesarean section. All fetuses in the control and treated groups survived the asphyxial insult. An observer who did not know which pups had been exposed to naloxone examined all neonates for respiration, color, muscle tone, response to stimulation, and general activity. For each parameter, 2, 1, or 0 points were scored, giving a maximum score of 10 for a normal, healthy pup.

Pups (27) whose mothers had received naloxone had significantly higher scores 1, 3, 5, 10, and 15 minutes after birth than did pups (24) whose mothers received saline. At 30 minutes of age, pups whose

(9–3) Science 216:1252–1253, June 11, 1982.

mothers were treated with naloxone had a slightly higher score than those whose mothers received saline, but the difference was not statistically significant. In a control experiment, pregnant does were placed in a chamber with air instead of the anoxic mixture. They were removed 10 minutes later and killed. All fetuses (controls and naloxone-exposed animals) had normal scores that did not change with time.

The present study suggests that poor condition of neonates asphyxiated in utero is due at least in part to the release of endogenous opiates. The data also indicate that naloxone might be effective in resuscitating neonates that have suffered asphyxia during delivery. However, these conclusions must be tempered with recent information suggesting that naloxone may not be as selective an antagonist of endogenous opiates as previously thought.

▶ [We have criticized our residents at times for what we considered to be indiscriminate use of naloxone in the delivery room. Depressed newborns were given the drug in circumstances in which narcotic-induced depression seemed unlikely. Perhaps our residents were right—again! This interesting rabbit study suggests that endogenous opiates may be reponsible for the neonatal depression after intrauterine asphyxia. Obviously, controlled clinical studies in human subjects are required before this sort of "treatment" should be advocated.] ◀

9–4 **Relationship of Apgar Score to Neurologic Handicap: Survey of Clinicians.** The association of various clinical indicators of peripartum asphyxia with neurologic impairment in childhood has justified a wide range of obstetric interventions in labor. Nigel Paneth and Harold E. Fox (New York) undertook a survey of 93 obstetricians and 79 other health professionals to determine their perceptions of the strength of the relation between indicators of perinatal asphyxia and later brain function. They were asked to estimate the likelihood of a normal outcome in infants surviving a 5-minute Apgar score of 3 or below, a clinical indicator of moderately severe perinatal asphyxia. Data from the United States Collabortive Perinatal Project indicated incidences of mental retardation and cerebral palsy of 3.9% and 5.1%, respectively, under these conditions.

The mean estimate of the proportion of infants who would achieve normal intelligence was 56%. Results were similar with respect to cerebral palsy; respondents estimated on average that 62% of infants would be free from the condition. Pediatricians generally were most pessimistic, whereas nurses and midwives were most optimistic. Physicians in private practice tended to give slightly lower estimates for the likelihood of normalcy than did those in academic medicine.

If indicators of moderate to severe perinatal asphyxia are perceived as having an extremely ominous prognosis, concerned obstetricians likely will attempt to intervene to prevent them. Although the recent marked rise in cesarean sections in the United States does not seem to be attributable chiefly to interventions for fetal distress, some interventions are conditioned by a fear of labor asphyxia and subsequent neonatal depression. Some interventions may be predicated on unrealistic fears of the handicapping potential of clinically defined

(9–4) Obstet. Gynecol. 61:547–550, May 1983.

perinatal asphyxia, which are undoubtedly reinforced by the prevailing legal climate. A more realistic appraisal of these relations by both the medical and the legal professions might help reduce the rate of increase in surgical interventions in labor.

▶ [Kenneth Niswander, in an excellent special article in the 1983 YEAR BOOK (pp. 107–125), reviewed the complex relationship between perinatal asphyxia and subsequent development. One of his points was that many believe the prognostic import of the low Apgar score to be much more ominous than it actually is, a situation confirmed by this survey. Whereas the likelihood of significant neurologic impairment, such as mental retardation or cerebral palsy, is only about 5% in survivors who had a 5-minute Apgar score of 3 or less, obstetricians, pediatricians, nurses, and midwives generally thought it to be 10 times as great. The subjects of this survey represent a select sample (attendees at a postgraduate course on labor management or pediatric grand rounds), but it seems unlikely the results would be any better, and they might be even worse, with a truly random sample of clinicians.] ◀

9–5 **Neonatal Seizures: I. Correlation of Prenatal and Perinatal Events With Outcomes.** Kenton R. Holden, E. David Mellits, and John M. Freeman (Johns Hopkins Univ., Baltimore) reviewed the cases of 277 infants with neonatal seizures from the National Collaborative Perinatal Project. The project provided 7-year to 8-year follow-up in approximately 54,000 pregnancies in 12 urban, university-affiliated hospitals. Care was taken not to classify apnea spells by themselves as seizures.

The observed frequency of neonatal seizures was 0.5% in the study population. Of these 277 infants, 245 were coded as having had definite seizures and 32 were coded as suspect. Race and sex distribution of infants was similar to the NCPP population as a whole, with a slight excess of males in the neonatal seizure population (NSP). Maternal age ranged from 13 to 43 years. There was a significant excess of small babies and early births among the infants who had neonatal seizures. Of the 258 infants with neonatal seizures whose 1-minute Apgar score was known, 59% had scores of 6 or less (compared with 19% in the NCPP), and 31% had scores of 3 or less (compared with 5.6% of the NCPP infants). Of the 277 infants with seizures, 96 (34.8%) died. Of the 181 survivors, most followed-up to age 7 years,

NEUROLOGIC SEQUELAE OF CHILDREN FROM NEONATAL SEIZURE POPULATION

	Cerebral Palsy (CP)* Only [n(%)]	Mental Retardation (MR)† Only [n(%)]	Seizures‡ Only [n(%)]	Seizures and CP [n(%)]	Seizures and MR [n(%)]	CP and MR [n(%)]	Seizures, CP and MR [n(%)]	None [n(%)]
All subjects (N = 277)	6 (2%)	10 (4%)	22 (8%)	12 (4%)	7 (3%)	8 (3%)	6 (2%)	206§ (74%)
Subjects alive at age 7 yr (N = 181)	4 (2%)	10 (6%)	17 (9%)	3 (2%)	7 (4%)	8 (4%)	6 (3%)	126 (70%)

*Moderate or severe CP at age 7 years (11 additional patients died with moderate or severe CP between ages 1 and 7 years).

†Full-scale IQ <70 at age 7 years in 165 of 181 tested and includes comments on institutionalized children with IQ too low to be tested.

‡Epilepsy and potential epilepsy at age 7 years.

§Includes 80 infants who died.

(Courtesy of Holden, K. R., et al.: Pediatrics 70:165–176, August 1982. Copyright American Academy of Pediatrics 1982.)

(9–5) Pediatrics 70:165–176, August 1982.

70% were normal. Thirteen percent had cerebral palsy, 19% had an IQ of less than 70, and 20% had epilepsy. Thirteen percent of survivors had a combination of mental retardation, cerebral palsy, or epilepsy. A low Apgar score, the need for resuscitation after 5 minutes of age, low birth weight, and early onset of seizures or prolonged seizures correlated with adverse outcome. Outcomes for all infants with neonatal seizures are summarized in the table. Despite the great increase in adverse outcomes in children with neonatal seizures, most children who survived did well.

▶ [Seizures in the neonatal period often reflect asphyxia and are associated with neonatal death and with later problems in a substantial minority (30%) of cases. Low 5-minute Apgar scores in this situation are predictive of death, cerebral palsy, and mental retardation. The 5-minute Apgar score in part reflects the quality of neonatal resuscitation. All who practice obstetrics should be skilled in this activity. Because these babies were delivered a quarter of a century ago, the results reported above may differ from those that are achieved with contemporary neonatal care.] ◀

9–6 **Hyaline Membrane Disease Treated With Bovine Surfactant.** J. A. Smyth, I. L. Metcalfe, P. Duffty, F. Possmayer, M. H. Bryan, and G. Enhorning report the use of bovine surfactant suspension in 6 preterm infants with established hyaline membrane disease who required ventilation. All were referred to The Hospital for Sick Children, Toronto. The infants, all in severe respiratory failure, were treated at a median age of 15 hours with a single intratracheal bolus of surfactant. All the preparations used had a high adsorption rate and low surface tension. After instillation of 8 ml over about 1 minute, the infant was held in different positions and was ventilated manually for 1 minute with 100% oxygen.

Arterial oxygenation improved dramatically after instillation of surfactant, despite a deliberate reduction in mean airway pressure in most cases. The degree of change in the alveolar-arterial Po_2 ratio was variable. The need for respiratory support was not eliminated by surfactant administration. Chest films showed improvement in all infants 2 to 4 hours after treatment, but deterioration was noted within 24 hours. Four patients had evidence on ultrasonographic study of intracranial bleeding at age 2 to 4 days. Two of the 5 infants followed for up to 18 months have delayed motor development. Three of the infants are free of respiratory problems.

A single intratracheal treatment with bovine surfactant suspension can improve arterial oxygenation in infants with respiratory failure due to hyaline membrane disease. The present infants probably had extensive morphological changes at the time of treatment that were not likely to be reversed by surfactant administration. These cases and the results of animal studies indicate that early treatment is necessary in order to obtain maximal benefit from administration of surfactant. Prophylactic administration before the first breath is a possibility.

9–7 **Isolation of Human Surfactant From Amniotic Fluid and Pilot Study of Its Efficacy in Respiratory Distress Syndrome.** Natural surfactant holds more promise in the treatment of respira-

---

(9–6) Pediatrics 71:913–917, June 1983.
(9–7) Ibid., pp. 473–482, April 1983.

IMMEDIATE EFFECTS OF SURFACTANT SUPPLEMENTATION*

	A Immediately Before Surfactant	B 5 Min After Surfactant	C 1 Hr After Surfactant
Pa_{O_2} (mm Hg)	69 ± 11	239 ± 19[a]	73 ± 13
Pa_{CO_2}	50 ± 3	48 ± 1	44 ± 2[b]
pH	7.26 ± 0.04	7.26 ± 0.03	7.32 ± 0.02
Fi_{O_2}	0.94 ± 0.03	0.95 ± 0.03	0.49 ± 0.03[a]
MAP (cm H_2O)	10.3 ± 1.1	10.2 ± 1.2	9.5 ± 0.7[c]

*Abbreviations: Fi_{O_2} = fraction of inspired oxygen; MAP = mean airway pressure; Pa_{O_2} = arterial oxygen pressure; Pa_{CO_2} = partial pressure of CO_2 in blood.

[a]$P < .001$ as compared with A.

[b]$P < .025$ as compared with A.

[c]$P < .05$ as compared with A.

(Courtesy of Hallman, M., et al.: Pediatrics 71:473–482, April 1983. Copyright American Academy of Pediatrics 1983.)

tory distress syndrome (RDS) than does artificial surfactant. Mikko Hallman, T. Allen Merritt, Howard Schneider, Benita L. Epstein, Frank Mannino, David K. Edwards, and Louis Gluck (Univ. of California at San Diego) describe the isolation of human surfactant from term amniotic fluid and its evaluation in infants with RDS. Surfactants were isolated with the use of sterile techniques from individual amniotic fluids at elective cesarean section in term gestations. The surfactant isolated was physically comparable to animal surfactants. An average of 1.6 L of amniotic fluid from 5 cesarean section deliveries was needed to treat 1 infant. Surfactant was given to infants weighing less than 1,250 gm at birth with a clinical and radiologic diagnosis of RDS who required mechanical ventilation and an inspired oxygen fraction of 0.8 or greater. Surfactant suspension was administered intratracheally in saline in a dose corresponding to 70 μmoles of surfactant lipid phosphorus, or 60 mg of dry natural surfactant, per kg. The infant then was ventilated by hand for about a minute while being turned.

The 5 infants treated had a mean birth weight of 974 gm. Treatment was given a mean of 6 hours after birth. The immediate effects of surfactant administration are shown in the table. In 4 infants, respiratory distress stabilized for 8–15 hours after surfactant supplementation. Distress then recurred, but the course was rather mild and the infants required no or only minimal ventilation after age 7–20 days. One infant improved only transiently and required supplemental oxygen and mechanical ventilation for 2 weeks. Treated infants required less oxygen and lower ventilator pressures than did conventionally treated infants with RDS. No side effects from surfactant administration were observed.

These results are encouraging, but the most suitable surfactant and the optimal means of administration remain to be established. Further study is needed to rule out immunologic effects, to determine whether treatment interferes with the development of endogenous surfactant, and to determine whether treatment will increase shunting in infants with a patent ductus.

▶ [The results of this study and the preceding one are encouraging about something specific with which to treat hyaline membrane disease. Smyth and colleagues describe intratracheal administration of bovine surfactant suspension to infants with respiratory distress syndrome at age 8 to 23 hours that led to dramatic, albeit temporary, improvement in oxygenation. Theoretically, it would seem that the earlier therapy of this type is initiated, the better. However, the earliest case was the one with the least improvement in oxygenation and also the only one with permanent sequelae (i.e., bronchopulmonary dysplasia).

The use of amniotic fluid surfactant, described by Hallman et al., is more appealing because it lessens concerns about immunologic problems and also is probably more available than bovine. The outcome in a small series was good. We're sure to hear more of this.] ◀

9–8 **Furosemide Promotes Patent Ductus Arteriosus in Premature Infants With the Respiratory Distress Syndrome.** Patent ductus arteriosus is a frequent complication in premature infants with respiratory distress syndrome. Experimental evidence indicates that furosemide is a stimulator of renal synthesis of prostaglandin E_2, which is a potent dilator of the ductus arteriosus. In contrast, chlorothiazide, another diuretic, does not seem to influence renal prostaglandin E production or cause vascular changes. Thomas P. Green, Theodore R. Thompson, Dana E. Johnson, and James E. Lock (Univ. of Minnesota, Minneapolis) assessed the effect of furosemide use on the incidence of patent ductus arteriosus in 33 premature infants with respiratory distress syndrome. Another 33 premature infants with respiratory distress syndrome received chlorothiazide as a control drug.

The diuretics were first administered between the second and third days of life. Of the 33 pairs of treated patients, 5 had equal clinical scores for patent ductus arteriosus; in 22 pairs the furosemide-treated patients had the higher score and in 6 pairs the chlorothiazide-treated patients had the higher score. Twenty-two of the 33 patients treated with furosemide had a characteristic ductal murmur on at least 1 day, compared with 13 of the 33 infants in the chlorothiazide group ($P < .05$). Findings of a patent ductus arteriosus persisting for 2 or more consecutive days were present in 18 of the furosemide-treated infants but in only 8 of the infants treated with chlorothiazide ($P < .02$). Eleven of the 22 furosemide-treated patients and 7 of the 13 chlorothiazide-treated patients with patent ductus arteriosus required ductal ligation ($P > 0.2$). Six infants, all from the furosemide group, who did not have evidence of a patent ductus during the study were later found to have one ($P < .01$). Overall survival was 76% in infants treated with furosemide and 61% in those treated with chlorothiazide ($P > .2$). After the initial dose of both drugs, small (less than twofold) increases in the urinary excretion of prostaglandin E were observed. However, after the fifth day of life, prostaglandin E excretion tripled after administration of furosemide, but did not increase after chlorothiazide administration.

It is concluded that furosemide increases the incidence of patent

(9–8) N. Engl. J. Med. 308:743–748, Mar. 31, 1983.

ductus arteriosus in premature infants with respiratory distress syndrome, most likely through a prostaglandin-mediated process. The results also do not support a role for the wider use of chlorothiazide in infants with respiratory distress syndrome, as data suggesting an improvement in morbidity or mortality were lacking.

▶ [Infants with respiratory distress syndrome are often given diuretics because of a suspected component of cardiac failure. In this prospective study, furosemide was compared with chlorothiazide, and clinically diagnosed patent ductus was more frequent with the former drug than with the latter, presumably reflecting a prostaglandin-stimulating action.] ◀

9–9 **Isolation of *Trichomonas vaginalis* From the Respiratory Tract of Infants With Respiratory Disease.** The finding of *Trichomonas* organisms in the human respiratory tract appears to be rare, and previous cases have been associated with lung disease in adults with chronic or debilitating conditions. Leroy C. McLaren, Larry E. Davis, George R. Healy, and Charles G. James report data on two cases of respiratory tract infection in infants, possibly due to *T. vaginalis*. Both infants were delivered vaginally by mothers known to have had previous episodes of *T. vaginalis* infection. Although *T. vaginalis* was present in inoculated cell cultures, bacterial and viral cultures of tracheal aspirates and nasopharyngeal specimens were negative. Both infants were initially intubated for respiratory distress, and *Trichomonas* was isolated during intubation in one case and afterward in the other. The former infant was treated with metronidazole. Both infants have been well.

Occasionally, newborn infants of mothers infected by *T. vaginalis* have acquired urinary tract or vaginal *T. vaginalis* infection. The present report is believed the first to show isolation of this organism from the respiratory tract of infants. Both infants had clinical evidence of pneumonitis without a recognized bacterial or viral cause. Although vaginal infections by *T. vaginalis* occur in up to one-fourth of pregnant women, infection in neonates after vaginal delivery appears to be uncommon. The possibility of *T. vaginalis* infection of the mouth or respiratory tract of an infant should, however, be kept in mind.

▶ [The number of infants born through *Trichomonas*-infested birth canals must be enormous, yet this is apparently the first report of pneumonia apparently due to *T. vaginalis*.] ◀

9–10 **Respiratory Distress Following Elective Repeat Cesarean Section.** It is widely held that most of the respiratory distress subsequent to elective cesarean section is due to hyaline membrane disease (HMD) secondary to iatrogenic delivery of a premature infant and that serious respiratory distress in an infant delivered by elective cesarean section without labor suggests poor prenatal care, which may have medicolegal implications. Richard L. Schreiner, Dennis C. Stevens, Wilbur L. Smith, James A. Lemons, Alan M. Golichowski, and Lillie M. Padilla (Indianapolis) suggest this is not so.

A review of 2,080 admissions over 30 months to the newborn inten-

---

(9–9) Pediatrics 71:888–890, June 1983.
(9–10) Am. J. Obstet. Gynecol. 143:689–692, July 1, 1982.

sive care unit of James Whitcomb Riley Hospital for Children showed 47 infants hospitalized because of respiratory distress after elective repeat cesarean section. Excluded were cesarean sections performed for medical reasons and pregnancies complicated by diabetes or rH incompatibility. Mean birth weight of the 47 was 2,930 gm (range, 2,090 to 4,082 gm), obstetric estimate of gestational age was 39.5 weeks (range, 36 to 40 weeks), and neonatal estimate of gestational age was 36.5 weeks (range, 34 to 40 weeks). Fourteen deliveries were at term. Mean difference in gestational age between obstetric and neonatal examination was 2.6 weeks.

All 47 infants required more than 40% oxygen; 30 required continuous positive airway pressure; and 18 required use of a respirator. Pneumothorax developed in 15 infants, pneumopericardium in 1, and bronchopulmonary dysplasia in 1; 1 infant died of bilateral pneumothoraces. Findings on chest films and the clinical course were consistent with HMD in 17 infants, respiratory distress syndrome type II in 24, and persistent fetal circulation in 3 (chest films were not available in 3 cases). Six of the 14 term infants and 8 of the 18 infants who required intermittent positive pressure ventilation had HMD.

This study confirms previous reports of significant respiratory morbidity associated with elective repeat cesarean section. However, the findings that many of these infants are, in fact, not premature and that much of the respiratory distress is not secondary to HMD suggest that respiratory distress in these infants is secondary to the mode of delivery rather than to prematurity. Thus, cases of respiratory distress subsequent to elective cesarean section are not suggestive of poor prenatal care and, therefore, not examples of medical negligence.

► [This paper makes a very important point—the respiratory distress syndrome is a *syndrome* that may be due to many basic causes and it is not always due to hyaline membrane disease of prematurity. Actually, in this series of cases of severe respiratory distress syndrome in infants born by elective repeat cesarean section, less than half the infants had hyaline membrane disease.] ◄

9–11 **Does Phenobarbital Prevent Periventricular Hemorrhage in Very Low Birth Weight Babies? A Controlled Trial.** Periventricular hemorrhage (PVH) occurs in 40%–50% of very low birth weight infants. M. E. I. Morgan, R. F. Massey, and R. W. I. Cooke (Liverpool Univ.) investigated the use of prophylactic phenobarbital on a prospective basis in a group of at-risk infants. Sixty infants who weighed less than 1,250 gm at birth, plus all infants weighing 1,250 to 1,500 gm who required artificial ventilation in the first 24 hours after birth were admitted to the trial. Phenobarbital (20 mg/kg administered intramuscularly) was given to alternate eligible infants after hospital admission, at a median time of 2 hours after birth (range 1–22 hours). In neonates, this loading dose will produce therapeutic anticonvulsant levels within 4 hours. Serum half-life of phenobarbital in this population varies from 37–133 hours. Periventricular hemorrhage was detected by real-time ultrasound scanning performed on

---

(9–11) Pediatrics 70:186–189, August 1982.

all infants daily or more frequently during the first 5 days and at least once thereafter.

Results showed that among 60 infants in the trial, 30 received phenobarbital. Serum phenobarbital levels were measured after 24 hours in 26 infants. In 24 infants, mean drug level attained was 17.2 μg/ml; in 2 infants the levels barely rose, which suggested faulty administration of the drug. More infants in the untreated group than in the treated group were born outside of the hospital, and more infants had an initially low Apgar score, although these differences did not have statistical significance (χ^2). No difference in the frequency of pneumothorax, hypercapnia, or acidosis occurred between groups; these factors were recognized as high-risk in the development of PVH. Survival rate was not significantly different in the two groups, nor was the number of intraventricular hemorrhages detected (14 treated, 16 untreated) or their distribution. When considering only those 16 infants whose measured levels of phenobarbital were known to be within the therapeutic anticonvulsant range, PVH occurred in 9. This incidence of 56% is not different from that in the untreated infants (53%).

Only a multicenter-controlled trial can establish whether barbiturates are valuable in the prevention of PVH. Since results of this study and others show no evidence of reduction of major PVH in surviving treated infants, it may be relevant to consider, instead, the use of drugs with direct capillary wall-stabilizing actions. These, together with other measures to stabilize fluctuating blood pressure and cerebral blood flow, may reduce the incidence of PVH.

▶ [Intraventricular hemorrhage is an important problem in small premature infants. An article abstracted last year (1983 YEAR BOOK, pp. 221–222) suggested that phenobarbital given prophylactically helped protect newborns against this adverse occurrence. Not so, according to the present study. We're sure to read of others' experience concerning phenobarbital in this situation.] ◀

9–12 **Congenital Neurosyphilis: A Reappraisal.** Neurosyphilis is one of the major hazards of syphilis. Congenital syphilis is well known to the pediatrician, but cases of congenital neurosyphilis are not so common. To investigate the presence and incidence of neurosyphilis in cases of congenital syphilis, J. C. Marcus (Coronation Hosp., Johannesburg) studied 20 infants with a diagnosis of congenital syphilis as determined by a positive serum fluorescent-treponemal-antibody-absorbed immunoglobulin M (FTA-IgM) test.

Eleven of the infants had clinical disease and 3 had nonspecific illnesses, though their x-ray studies were highly suggestive of syphilis. The remaining 6 were asymptomatic neonates whose mothers were known to have positive VDRL tests. There were no neurologic abnormalities and none of the infants had any clinical evidence of neurosyphilis. Four infants died. Based on the results of cerebrospinal fluid (CSF) studies, only 2 infants could be unequivocally diagnosed as having absolute evidence of neurosyphilis, with pleocytosis and positive IgM tests. A third infant had CSF findings that were most likely abnormal and was considered to have neurosyphilis. Two other in-

---

(9–12) Neuropediatrics 13:195–199, November 1982.

fants had strongly positive IgG tests, but cells were absent, protein levels were normal, and IgM and VDRL tests were negative. These 2 infants were not thought to have local disease, but diffusion of IgG into the CSF, which was compatible with their great prematurity.

In this series, the incidence of neurosyphilis was much lower than previously reported by others. The reasons for this low incidence and problems in the diagnosis of neurosyphilis are discussed.

▶ [The 10%–15% incidence of neurosyphilis in cases of congenital syphilis reported here is lower than the older literature would suggest. It seems likely that the explanation lies in the greater specificity of the newer tests.] ◀

9–13 **Comparison of Breast, Cow, and Soy Feedings in Prevention of Onset of Allergic Disease: A 15-Year Prospective Study.** It has been reported that the feeding of cow's milk may enhance the development of atopy in predisposed infants, but most such studies cover follow-up periods of only 1 to 4 years. Frank L. Gruskay (Yale Univ.) followed up a group of 908 newborns to age 15 years to determine whether food ingested during the first months of life is related to development of atopy in the offspring of allergic families.

Each of 328 children with a positive family history of major allergic diseases (i.e., atopic dermatitis, asthma, and allergic rhinitis) was assigned to one of three groups according to the feeding preference of the parents: 48 were fed breast milk (for at least 4 months in 75% of the subjects), 79 were fed soy-based formula, and 201 were fed cow's milk formula. All 328 had egg, citrus, tomato, wheat, chocolate, nuts, and fish restrictions and avoided inhalant allergens. These children were compared with a control group of 580 children without family history of allergy who were given standard feeding advice.

In infants with a positive family history, allergic disease occurred with equal frequency in those who received cow's milk formula and those who were given soy formula, with 53% of these children showing symptoms when followed for 15 years. In sharp contrast, allergic disease developed in only 28% of breast-fed children. These differences did not become statistically significant until the subjects were followed beyond the first 3 years of life. There was a threefold increase in clinically apparent atopic disease in offspring of allergic families when compared to controls, but only a twofold increase if the infant was breast-fed. Among infants with a positive family history, the incidence of atopic dermatitis was not significantly influenced by the type of feeding.

These findings support the hypothesis that breast-feeding for at least 3 months and delay of exposure to common food and environmental allergens may reduce the frequency of allergic disease in the offspring of allergic families. Substitution of soy formula for cow's milk for the prevention of allergic disease does not seem to have any advantage.

▶ [Whether breast-feeding helps protect against the development of allergic disease in childhood is an unsettled issue. This study with follow-up until 15 years of age suggests that it does. The IgA in colostrum and breast milk may inhibit antigen absorption by the neonate. Soy formulas were not associated with a lower incidence of atopy than cow's milk formulas.] ◀

(9–13) Clin. Pediatr. 21:486–491, August 1982.

9–14 **Routine Neonatal Circumcision: Gap Between Contemporary Policy and Practice.** Circumcision is the most common pediatric surgical procedure performed in the United States. The rate of neonatal circumcision approaches 90% in many parts of the United States, raising questions of whether deep-seated cultural, religious, and psychosocial factors dominate parental decision-making and of whether physicians have a significant role in the decision. Martin T. Stein, Myron Marx, Steven L. Taggart, and Robert A. Bass (Univ. of California at San Diego) examined attitudes toward circumcision and personal factors related to decision-making in 103 parents of male infants and 92 randomly selected primary care physicians.

Two thirds of the physicians who responded favored circumcision, 7% opposed it, and the rest were neutral. Most pediatricians were neutral, whereas family and general practitioners were likely to favor the procedure. More than two thirds of respondents usually counseled prospective parents about routine neonatal circumcision. Nearly 90% of physicians performed routine circumcision at the request of parents. Fewer than half of the physicians were aware that the newborn infant's foreskin is typically not fully retractable. Some were unaware that hypospadias and epispadias contraindicate routine neonatal circumcision. Of the 103 parents surveyed, 90 reported that their infant was circumcised. Two thirds received information on routine circumcision from a physician. Only 5% reported that the physician's attitude toward circumcision was negative. Decisions to circumcise the infant were related to the father's perceived circumcision status and a parental belief that there are valid medical indications for circumcision. Only 12 parents reported that a physician influenced their decision. The decision-making process was not difficult for most parents.

The American Academy of Pediatrics has concluded that routine neonatal circumcision is a procedure grounded in medical myths. Cultural, social, and historical factors appear to be dominant for physicians and parents. Although the final decision remains with the parents, more informed, objective counseling of parents by primary care physicians is necessary.

▶ [The finding reported here that is most consistent with our own experience is the limited influence physicians have on couples' decisions concerning neonatal circumcision. Parents make these decisions on psychosocial and cultural grounds, even when aware of contemporary medical opinion. In the United States, in 80+% of cases the decision is to have the operation performed. More on the subject follows. . . .] ◀

9–15 **Parental Information and Circumcision in Highly Motivated Couples With Higher Education.** Parents are not adequately informed about the benefits and risks of circumcision. Previous reports indicate that special counseling of clinic patients makes no difference in the incidence of the procedure. Alfredo J. Herrera, Beverly Cochran, Anne Herrera, and Barbara Wallace (St. Agnes Hosp., Baltimore) tried to determine whether counseling highly motivated couples of higher socioeconomic status and educational level makes a

(9–14) J. Fam. Pract. 15:47–53, July 1982.
(9–15) Pediatrics 71:233–234, February 1983.

difference in the performance of circumcision. Part of a Lamaze group was assigned to receive special counseling about circumcision at about the seventh month of pregnancy, and the parents were encouraged to discuss the issue with physicians. The control group was not given this special counseling. The incidence of circumcision was 84% in the counseled group and 87% in the controls.

This study of a highly educated and motivated group found no influence of counseling about circumcision on the performance of the procedure. It is not easy to change attitudes toward an established custom, but it is hoped that counseling on the benefits and risks of circumcision will lead to increased public awareness and questioning by parents and physicians of whether circumcision is necessary for all male neonates.

▶ [No one would argue that consent to an operative procedure, particularly when there is little or no medical indication for it, should be fully informed. However, in the case of neonatal circumcision this study indicates that the amount of information the parents are given has no relationship with whether they have the procedure done. Essentially the same results were found by Maisels and associates (*Pediatrics* 71:453, 1983): when parents were given written information indicating that there are no valid medical indications for circumcision, 21 of 23 elected the operation, whereas without written information it was chosen by 27 of 28, an insignificant difference. Circumcision of the newborn seems to be regarded as desirable by most parents in our culture, and to change this attitude, if such a change is worthwhile, is not easy.

This seems to be a popular area of study. Rand and colleagues (*Obstet. Gynecol.* 62:64, 1983) also attempted to see if an educational intervention would decrease newborn circumcision at the Johns Hopkins Hospital. They found a statistically significant drop, from 94 to 72%, but most mothers still wanted their sons circumcised despite the educational intervention.] ◀

9–16 **Neonatal Mortality Risk in Relation to Birth Weight and Gestational Age: Update.** Beverly L. Koops, Linda J. Morgan, and Frederick C. Battaglia reviewed neonatal mortality risks in relation to birth weight and gestational age in a series of 14,413 live births and 252 neonatal deaths occurring at the University of Colorado Health Sciences Center between 1974 and 1980. All infants of over 20 weeks'

TABLE 1.—NEONATAL MORTALITY BY BIRTH WEIGHT FOR ALL INBORN INFANTS AT UNIVERSITY HOSPITAL, 1974 TO 1980

Birth weight (gm)	*Live births*	*Neonatal deaths*	*Mortality (%)*
≥4,000	650	0	0
3,500-3,999	2,660	4	0.2
3,000-3,499	5,314	8	0.2
2,500-2,999	3,593	18	0.5
2,000-2,499	1,148	12	1.0
1,500-1,999	489	23	4.7
1,000-1,499	348	57	16.4
500-999	190	109	57.4
<500	21	21	100.0

(Courtesy of Koops, B. L., et al.: J. Pediatr. 101:969–977, December 1982.)

(9–16) J. Pediatr. 101:969–977, December 1982.

TABLE 2.—NEONATAL MORTALITY BY GESTATIONAL AGE FOR ALL INBORN INFANTS AT UNIVERSITY HOSPITAL, 1974 TO 1980

Gestational age (wk)	*Live births*	*Neonatal deaths*	*Mortality (%)*
≥ 42	888	4	0.4
38-41	10,722	22	0.2
35-37	1,738	11	0.6
32-34	570	37	6.5
29-31	263	41	15.6
26-28	157	70	45.0
< 26	75	67	89.0

(Courtesy of Koops, B. L., et al.: J. Pediatr. 101:969–977, December 1982.)

postmenstrual gestational age with a heart beat at birth were included. The results are given in Tables 1 and 2. Based on birth weight alone, neonatal mortality was 0.47% for infants weighing over 2,500 gm. Based on gestational age alone, mortality was 0.28% for infants over 34 weeks' gestational age. Neonatal mortality trends over time

Fig 9–2.—Plot of neonatal mortality risk at 50% birth weight versus gestational age; comparison of data from 1958 to 1969 and 1974 to 1980. (Courtesy of Koops, B. L., et al.: J. Pediatr. 101:969–977, December 1982.)

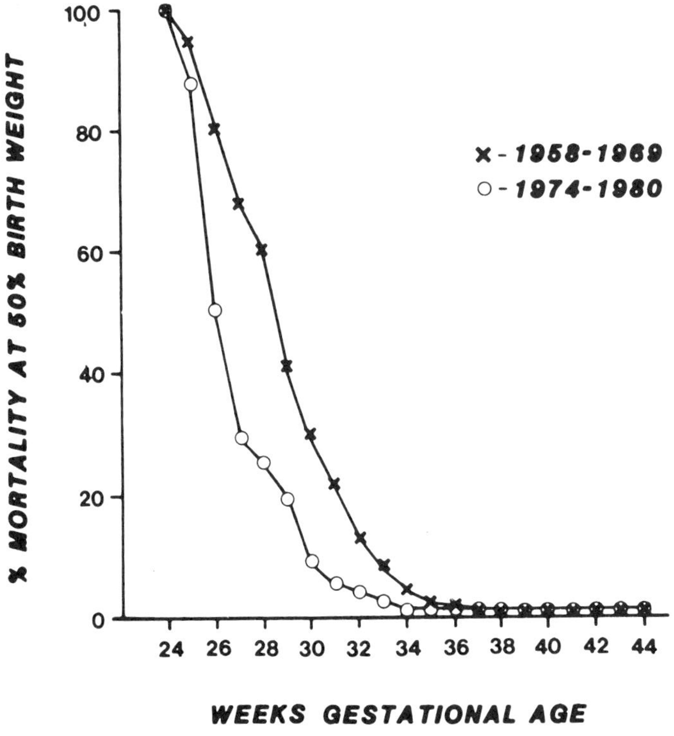

in relation to both birth weight and gestational age are shown in Figure 9–2.

Comparison with other perinatal centers indicates considerable similarity in neonatal survival rates, suggesting that continuing communication between obstetric perinatologists and neonatologists is an important factor in reducing neonatal mortality, rather than specific new therapeutic procedures instituted at any individual clinical center. Improved management of diabetic pregnancies and better recognition of potential problems with large for gestatonal age infants have contributed to the decline in neonatal mortality.

▶ [This is an update of the well-known and widely used Colorado grid of neonatal mortality risk for infants born alive at various birth weight-gestational age groupings. It demonstrates the improvement in outcome over a 15- to 20-year period. Data such as these are absolutely crucial in making obstetric decisions, such as whom to monitor and at what duration of pregnancy to intervene. An important caveat is that these figures really pertain only to the University of Colorado and there are some limitations in applying them to other populations, other altitudes, and other perinatal care capabilities.] ◀

9–17 **Outcome of Very Low Birth Weight Infants Born at a Perinatal Center.** The cost of supporting extremely immature infants is enormous. Elizabeth M. Hoskins, Elizabeth Elliot, Andrew T. Shennan, Martin B. Skidmore, and Eileen Keith (Women's College Hosp., Toronto) examined the outcome in a series of 106 infants, with birth weights of 1,000 gm and below, born at a perinatal center in 1979 and 1980. Eighty-three infants were born to women transferred to the center because of antenatal problems. The most common obstetric problem was premature labor, with or without premature membrane rupture. Twenty-six infants were small for gestational age. Neonatal resuscitation was aggressive.

Mean gestational age was 26.4 weeks, and mean birth weight was

TABLE 1.—FACTORS AFFECTING SURVIVAL*

	Died *(N = 34)*	*Survived* *(N = 72)*	*p*
Gestational age (wk)	25.2 ± 2.2	27 ± 2	<0.001
Birth weight (gm)	731 ± 138	835 ± 101	<0.001
Small for gestational age	3 (8.8%)	23 (32%)	<0.02
Betamethasone >36 hour	7 (20%)	34 (47%)	<0.02
Hyaline membrane disease	16 (47%)	15 (21%)	<0.02-<0.01
Seizures	14 (41%)	2 (2.7%)	<0.00001
Clinical intraventricular hemorrhage	17 (50%)	5 (7%)	<0.00001

*Values represent mean ± 1 SD.

(Courtesy of Hoskins, E. M., et al.: Am. J. Obstet. Gynecol. 145:135–140, Jan. 15, 1983.)

(9–17) Am. J. Obstet. Gynecol. 145:135–140, Jan. 15, 1983.

TABLE 2.—OUTCOME ACCORDING TO WEIGHT

Birth weight (gm)	*No.*	*Mean gestational age (wk)*	*Survival (%)*	*Handicap (%)*
751-1,000	67	27.5	79	6
≤750	39	25.3	49	32

(Courtesy of Hoskins, E. M., et al.: Am. J. Obstet. Gynecol. 145:135–140, Jan. 15, 1983.)

801 gm. Seventy-two infants (68%) survived. All but 7 of the 34 deaths occurred in the first 3 days. The factors significantly related to survival included increased birth weight and gestational age, antepartum corticosteroid therapy, and the absence of hyaline membrane disease, seizures, and clinical evidence of intraventricular hemorrhage (Table 1). One surviving infant died later of sudden infant death syndrome. The most common general health problem in survivors was recurrent middle ear infection. Growth was satisfactory. Significant neurologic or developmental handicap was observed in 13% of the 69 infants studied. Infants weighing less than 750 gm at delivery did much less well than heavier infants (Table 2).

The outcome of infants weighing 750 to 1,000 gm at delivery at a perinatal center certainly justifies the financial and emotional expenditures involved. The outcome for lighter infants is substantially poorer, but fewer such infants have been followed, and the obstetric approach in these cases was less consistent. The most significant factor in mortality and neurologic morbidity has been clinical evidence of intraventricular hemorrhage, and an improved understanding of the factors related to this condition may permit therapeutic changes that will decrease morbidity and mortality in very low birth weight infants.

► [This report is representative of several demonstrating the efficacy of contemporary intensive perinatal care of infants weighing less than 1 kg at birth. The overall survival was 68%, with a clear break at 750 gm (79% survival, with a 6% incidence of handicap at weights above 750 gm; 49% survival with a 32% incidence of handicap at lighter weights). The handicap figures probably should be regarded as minimum in view of the short duration of follow-up.] ◄

9–18 **Newborn Intensive Care and Neonatal Mortality in Low Birth Weight Infants: A Population Study.** Nigel Paneth, John L. Kiely, Sylvan Wallenstein, Michele Marcus, Jean Pakter, and Mervyn Susser (Columbia Univ.) conducted a study to test the hypothesis that differences in mortality across three levels of newborn intensive care, in a setting in which the levels could be specified in detail, varied systematically as a function of that care. Level 1 comprised care solely for normal or mildly ill newborns; level 2, care for more complicated pregnancies and neonatal illness, with referral of newborns to other hospitals if mechanical ventilation, surgery, or other complex procedures were required; and level 3, care at regional centers accepting referrals and providing the entire spectrum of medical surgical services for newborn infants.

(9–18) N. Engl. J. Med. 307:149–155, July 15, 1982.

Mortality of low birth weight infants (501–2,250 gm) born between 1976 and 1978 in hospitals providing one of the three levels of care in New York City was examined. Among 13,560 singleton low birth weight infants, the adjusted neonatal mortality for level 3 hospitals was 128.5 per 1,000 live births—significantly lower than the rates for both level 2 (168.1) and level 1 units (163.0). The association of level of care with mortality could not be accounted for by differences among groups in social or demographic status, in prenatal care, or in medical complications of pregnancy.

Birth at a level 3 center lowers neonatal mortality in low birth weight infants. However, only 34% of the patients in this study were born in such units. This study has implications for the policy of regionalizing perinatal care in urban areas. Unequal mortality risks among hospital levels point to inequities in the distribution of effective newborn care, even in the presence of an efficient municipal system of interhospital transport of infants. The data suggest some of the excessive mortality in level 2 units might be avoided if these units made more extensive use of the transfer system to refer infants promptly for level 3 care. Current knowledge does not extend to the effects of newborn intensive care on subsequent development and neurologic impairment.

▶ [This article was reviewed by Dr. Herman A. Hein, of the University of Iowa, who commented:

"Paneth and associates provide convincing evidence that low birth weight (LBW) infants (501–2,250 gm) have lower mortality rates when born in hospitals capable of providing tertiary-level newborn intensive care. This information is important because it represents objective proof of the effectiveness of newborn intensive care. However, an equally important implication of this study is the value of stratification of care based on risk status of obstetric patients. In the years 1976 to 1978, distressingly large numbers of LBW infants were born in level I and level II hospitals in New York. In a truly regionalized, stratified system of perinatal health care, careful screening and referral of high-risk gravidas should clearly skew the 'risk' population to the higher levels of care. Effective systems of regionalized perinatal health care require a practical partnership of obstetric and pediatric disciplines working in concert to insure that each gravida and neonate receives care appropriate to his or her needs."] ◀

9–19 **Decline in Neonatal Mortality, 1968 to 1977: Better Babies or Better Care?** Neonatal mortality began declining rapidly in the United States in the mid-1960s at the same time as many programs aimed at improving maternal health and the timing of pregnancies, as well as new methods of care for newborn infants, were introduced. Richard J. David and Earl Siegel reviewed neonatal mortality trends in North Carolina from 1968 to 1977 in order to determine to what degree the decrease in mortality is attributable to better risk characteristics in the newborn infant population. There were 894,911 live births and 13,497 neonatal deaths in the state during the 10-year study period.

Decade-average neonatal mortality was 13.2/1,000 for whites and 19.3/1,000 for nonwhites. A trend toward higher birth weights and longer gestations was noted, mostly among whites. An overall 19% reduction in low birth weight was observed. Birth weight-specific mortality improved substantially, especially in infants weighing

(9–19) Pediatrics 71:531–540, April 1983.

1,000–2,500 gm in the last 5 years of the review period. Application of a neonatal risk matrix model indicated that 34% of the decline in neonatal mortality during the study period was attributable to changes in the birth weight and gestational age makeup of the newborn population. This "better babies" factor was more prominent earlier in the study period and in the white population. The model predicted 44% of the improvement in neonatal mortality for whites and 9% of that for nonwhites.

Neonatal mortality was reduced in the past decade both through a lower proportion of premature births and the provision of better care for small and ill newborn infants. The racial disparity in neonatal mortality has widened, however, reflecting a less marked shift toward "better babies" in the nonwhite population. This problem could be addressed by increasing primary prevention programs designed to reduce prematurity rates among infants of low-income women. Improved perinatal medical care explains most of the improvement in neonatal mortality. The capacity for neonatal intensive care should be maintained or increased as needed to keep pace with the rate of delivery of premature infants. This alone, however, will not close the racial gap in newborn mortality.

▶ [The report serves as a reminder that when one is looking at neonatal mortality rates, one must consider both birth weight-specific mortality and birth weight distribution. Both recently have been improving in the United States. The former reflects better intrapartum obstetric care and improved neonatal care. The latter is harder to pin down. Demographic shifts, family-planning services, the availability of abortion, and obstetric interventions to prevent premature birth probably all play a role.] ◀

9–20 **Mortality in Infants Discharged From a Neonatal Intensive Care Unit.** Modern neonatal intensive care generally has been associated with improved neonatal survival and decreased morbidity, but little is known of mortality among infants discharged from these units. Clifford J. Sells, Terrence E. Neff, Forrest C. Bennett, and Nancy M. Robinson (Univ. of Washington) report a 3-year retrospective study of mortality among 1,123 infants discharged from a neonatal intensive care unit between 1976 and 1979. The mortality over 3 years was 3.8%. A large majority of deaths occurred before age 1 year. Sudden infant death syndrome accounted for 28% of deaths, congenital heart disease for 25%, and chronic pulmonary disease for 16%. Trauma, infection, and chromosomal disorders each accounted for 5% of deaths. Postdischarge mortality remained stable as infant mortality in the unit declined from 26.5% to 16.3%.

It appears that declining mortality among infants treated in neonatal intensive care units is not necessarily reflected in improved postdischarge mortality rates. The vast majority of postdischarge deaths are, at present, not preventable. Mortality from sudden infant death syndrome in this series occurred at a rate eight times that in the general population. The possibility that black infants may be at an increased risk of this cause of death deserves further study. Postdischarge deaths, especially those due to sudden infant death syndrome, are underrepresented in very low birth weight infants and

---

(9–20) Am. J. Dis. Child. 137:44–47, January 1983.

overrepresented in larger low birth weight infants. This suggests that at least some of the factors responsible for sudden infant death syndrome in low birth weight infants may differ from those responsible for low birth weight itself. It is encouraging that improved inpatient survival has not resulted in low birth weight infants being salvaged only to die later of chronic lung disease.

▶ [It seems particularly tragic to have a survivor of neonatal intensive care die after discharge from the neonatal intensive care unit. This report indicates that the likelihood of such an event occurring is remaining constant in the face of declining neonatal mortality prior to discharge. The postneonatal death rate in this series was 2.9%, a figure seven times that of the general population, implying some type of "fragility" in neonatal intensive care unit graduates that persisted through the first year or two of life. The most common cause was sudden infant death syndrome, followed closely by congenital heart disease and chronic lung disease.] ◀

9–21 **Support After Perinatal Death: A Study of Support and Counseling After Perinatal Bereavement.** Few systematic studies have been performed of family reactions to perinatal death. G. C. Forrest, E. Standish, and J. D. Baum (Univ. of Oxford, England) monitored the results of counseling offered to parents whose infants died perinatally and compared these parents with parents who did not receive counseling. Fifty unselected mothers of stillborn infants or of infants dying neonatally, all after 28 weeks' gestation, were included in the study and were randomized to receive planned support or routine hospital care. These women were followed up 6 and 14 months after the infant's death. The study parents were initially seen within 48 hours after the infant's death, and further counseling was offered by a family psychiatrist until the mourning process was well-established and the parents were well-supported in their respective neighborhoods. Most couples were adequately treated in 2 to 6 weeks.

Two of 16 evaluable mothers in the supported group and 10 of 19 in the control group showed evidence of psychiatric disorder after 6 months. The groups did not significantly differ after 14 months, when 80% of all women had recovered from psychiatric symptoms. Symptoms after 6 months were more frequent in socially isolated women and in those whose marital relationships lacked intimacy. Pregnancy within 6 months was associated with more frequent psychiatric symptoms in the unsupported group. The duration of bereavement after the infant's death was appreciably shorter in the supported group.

Supportive counseling after a perinatal death appears to benefit the parents and reduce the period of bereavement. Parents should have an opportunity to discuss what went wrong and also concerns about future pregnancies with medical staff. Results in this study suggest that the parents should wait a few months before attempting to conceive.

▶ [This well-designed clinical trial attests to the value of ongoing supportive counseling of parents who have suffered perinatal losses. A 6- to 8- week period usually was sufficient. The authors suggest that couples should wait at least 6 months before conceiving again.] ◀

9–22 **Death of a Newborn Twin: Analysis of a Parental Bereavement.** The death of a newborn twin in an intensive care nursery con-

(9–21) Br. Med. J. 285:1475–1479, Nov. 20, 1982.
(9–22) Pediatrics 70:587–591, October 1982.

fronts parents with both the loss of an infant and the anxiety of having a second infant receiving neonatal intensive care. Ann L. Wilson, Lawrence J. Fenton, Dennis C. Stevens, and Douglas J. Soule (Univ. of South Dakota) examined the responses of eight families who lost a singleton newborn infant and eight who lost a twin infant. Mean gestational age of the infants in both groups was 31 weeks. The questionnaire survey was carried out a mean of 15 months after the loss. A depression symptom inventory was embedded in the questionnaire.

Mothers had significantly more depressive symptoms than fathers. All symptoms declined markedly over time. There was no significant difference between the two parent groups in this respect. Family, friends, and hospital staff frequently underemphasized the death of the twin infant, assuming that parental grief would be minimized by the surviving twin, but the presence of a living twin did not at all lessen the grieving process. All the mothers of twins are initially told that they should feel fortunate to have a living infant. All continued to think about what life would have been like had both twins lived. At 15 months, all but one of the mothers thought about the dead twin when looking at the living one.

Staff should recognize that parents of surviving twins experience bereavement that includes symptoms of depression, and that this may impair their ability to become intimately involved with the surviving twin. They should not be told how fortunate they should feel to have a living infant; the surviving infant should not substitute for the parents' loss. Referral to individual counseling or a self-help group may be appropriate. It also may be helpful to offer ongoing discussions of parental reactions to the surviving twin.

▶ [Most would predict that the sense of bereavement after a neonatal death is greater in the mother than in the father, tends to heal in both with the passage of time, and is less where the death is of a twin as opposed to a singleton newborn. This study confirms the first two, but not the last of the predictions. Thus, it is probably inappropriate to minimize the loss of a twin by telling the parents how lucky they are to have one surviving baby. Instead, we should offer them the same types of support we'd provide for all parents who have experienced a neonatal death.] ◀

PART TWO

GYNECOLOGY

10. Operative Gynecology

10–1 **Abdominal Wound Closure: Randomized Prospective Study of 571 Patients Comparing Continuous vs. Interrupted Suture Techniques** is described by Peter C. Richards, Charles M. Balch, and Joaquin S. Aldrete (Univ. of Alabama). The patients (mean age, 50.4 years), had undergone operations encompassing the entire spectrum of abdominal procedures. Most were elective, and most cases of major abdominal trauma and heavy contamination were excluded. The incisions, all of which were greater than 5 cm in length, were stratified as to type of wound: clean, clean-contaminated, or contaminated.

The peritoneum was not closed as a separate layer. In vertical incisions, the continuous technique consisted of starting a strand of 0 polypropylene suture at each end of the incision (with the knots placed under the fascia), running each suture toward the other, and tying the strands in the middle of the incision. The interrupted technique consisted of placing 0 polyglycolic acid sutures using the Smead-Jones far-far, near-near suture technique. With both techniques, sutures were placed at least 1.5 cm from the fascial edge and 1.0 cm apart.

In oblique or transverse incisions, the continuous technique consisted of two layers. The deep layer (including the peritoneum and posterior rectus fascial sheet, transversalis muscle layer, and internal oblique musculoaponeurotic layer) was closed with one continuous 0 polypropylene suture as above. The superficial layer (incorporating the anterior rectus fascia and external oblique muscle) was closed with another continuous 0 polypropylene suture. The interrupted technique was that described by Smead-Jones using 0 polyglycolic acid sutures.

With both methods of closure, the sutures were pulled or tied with the fascial edges well approximated but not crushed together. Management of subcutaneous tissue and skin was left to the preference of each surgeon.

In midline incisions, the overall dehiscence rate was 2.0% for the continuous group and 0.9% for the interrupted group ($P = 0.503$). Ventral hernias formed in 2.0% of the continuous group and in 0.5% of the interrupted group (not significant). The type of wound had no influence on results. In oblique incisions, dehiscence occurred in 0% of wounds closed by the continuous method and in 2% of wounds closed by the interrupted method, not a significant difference at the $P = 0.05$ level. Incisional hernias developed in 5 of the patients and was independent of the method of closure.

Dehiscence was more likely related to improper surgical technique

(10–1) Ann. Surg. 197:238–243, February 1983.

or to infection than to method of closure. An abdominal incision could be closed with a continuous suture in about half the time required for placing interrupted sutures (20 vs. 40 minutes). Therefore, continuous closure is preferred because it is more expedient than interrupted closure without increasing the incidence of wound disruption.

▶ [This is a nice prospective study with random assignment to treatment groups. Continuous closure was associated with a slightly, but not statistically significantly, higher rate of wound disruption. Its advantage was that it was faster. Technical errors were thought responsible for five of the eight dehiscences. Sutures were placed too close to the fascial edge or were tied too tightly. The authors make the point in their discussion, "Proper surgical technique is the critical factor in any wound closure and the method of closure is only as effective as it is used."] ◀

10–2 **Abdominal Wound Closure Using a Nonabsorbable Single-Layer Technique.** Gynecologic laparotomies are followed by evisceration in up to 0.7% of cases, with mortality in up to 45% of instances. A single-layer mass closure is theoretically advantageous. John H. Shepherd, Denis Cavanagh, Daniel Riggs, Hora Praphat, and B. J. Wisniewski (Univ. of South Florida) evaluated a continuous, one-layer abdominal closure that uses no. 2 polypropylene suture in 200 unselected, consecutive gynecologic oncology patients undergoing laparotomy through an extended lower midline incision in a 1-year period. All were high-risk patients, and 82% had gynecologic malignancies. Preoperative radiotherapy had been given to 22.5% of patients. Another 18% of patients were obese, and 15% had had bowel operations. The suture technique is illustrated in Figures 10–1 and 10–2.

The patients were followed for 2 years. No eviscerations occurred, but 16 patients had some superficial wound breakdown to fascia, as-

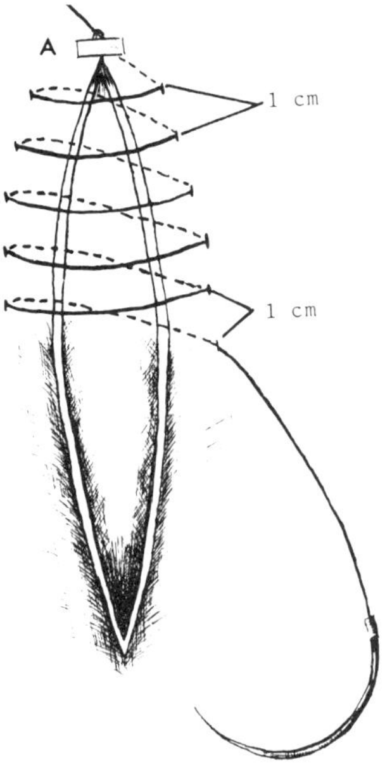

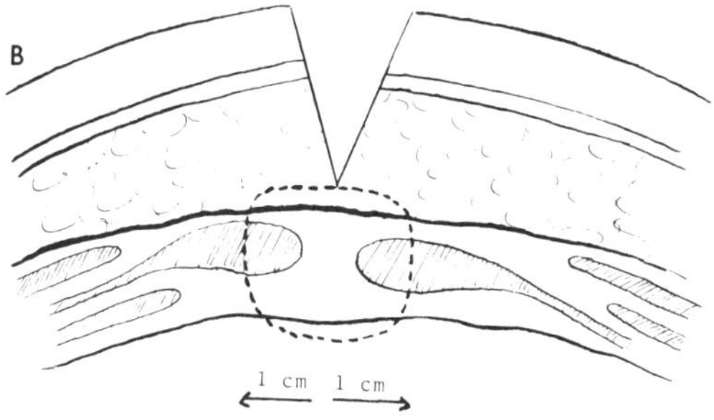

Fig 10–1 (left).—Number 2 polypropylene suture is fixed at apex of incision with five knots and metal hemostatic clip. Suture is carried through fascia, muscles, and peritoneum, taking 1-cm bites laterally and placing bites 1 cm apart throughout length of incision.

Fig 10–2 (above).—Coronal view of anterior abdominal wall showing bulk closure of fascia, muscles, and peritoneum, with each bite of continuous no. 2 polypropylene suture being placed 1 cm lateral to medial edge of these tissues.

(Courtesy of Shepherd, J. H., et al.: Obstet. Gynecol. 61:248–252, February 1983. Reprinted with permission from The American College of Obstetricians and Gynecologists.)

(10–2) Obstet. Gynecol. 61:248–252, February 1983.

sociated with wound hematoma formation and infection, and 5 of them required resuturing. Ten patients developed ventral hernias, 3 after an initial wound hematoma and superficial breakdown. The overall rate of minor wound complications was 14.5%. Five hernias were incisional and 5, paraincisional; 1 of each type required repair. One patient underwent exploration to remove a knot in the wound and another to exclude causes of discomfort other than thinning of the abdominal wall musculature.

This method of abdominal wound closure, using a monofilament, nonabsorbable, continuous suture, is a simple and successful technique. Morbidity has been low in patients at high risk of postoperative dehiscence. No eviscerations occurred in this series, and the rate of incisional hernia was low. The method would seem to be preferable to standard layered closure, especially in high-risk patients.

▶ [Every surgeon worth his (or her) salt has deeply held convictions about wound closure. The technique described here is a relatively gross one, in contrast to the meticulous layer-by-layer closure attributed to Halstead. Emotionally, we tend to favor the "Halsteadian" approach, yet it is hard to argue with these results. In what everyone must accept as a high-risk group (vertical incision, malignancy, etc.), there was no dehiscence and only a 5% incidence of hernia. Nevertheless, we would still like to see a prospective randomized comparison.] ◀

10–3 **Iatrogenic Femoral Neuropathy Subsequent to Abdominal Hysterectomy: Incidence and Prevention.** Henning Kvist-Poulsen and John Borel (Odense Univ. Hosp.) conducted a prospective study of femoral neuropathy in 147 patients undergoing elective total abdominal hysterectomy. The femoral nerve is the largest branch of the lumbar plexus. It runs obliquely within the substance of the psoas major muscle and leaves the muscle at the lower lateral border. Symptoms and signs indicating femoral neuropathy include numbness of the anteromedial aspect of the thigh and leg, instability of the knee during walking, pain localized to the anterior aspect of the hip joint area, inability to raise the leg straight off the bed, decreased or absent sensations of touch and pain over the anteromedial aspect of the thigh and leg, and decreased or absent patellar reflex. Diagnosis of femoral neuropathy was made on the basis of at least one subjective symptom and one objective sign.

Seventeen of the 147 patients met the criteria for diagnosis of femoral neuropathy, for an overall incidence of 11.6%. The incidence associated with the use of the large Balfour self-retaining retractor was significantly higher than that with use of other self-retaining retractors. The type of incision used was of no importance. A vertical midline incision was used in 9 cases and a Pfannenstiel incision in 8. The incidence of femoral neuropathy was 10.7% and 12.7%, respectively, for these two types of incisions. The 17 cases of femoral neuropathy occurred in a total of 107 operations, performed by 9 surgeons; thus, inexperience does not seem to have been a factor. Time consumed during surgery, patient weight, and length of hospital stay did not influence the incidence of this condition. Symptoms were bilateral in 5 patients and unilateral in 12. Mean duration of subjective symp-

(10–3) Obstet. Gynecol. 60:516–520, October 1982.

toms of injury was 19.6 days. Several patients also noticed temporary difficulty in climbing stairs and walking uphill.

Knowledge of this problem is mandatory for prevention. Although any type of retractor may cause this neurologic complication, one must be especially careful if a self-retaining retractor with large lateral blades is selected. The relationship of the lateral retractor blade to the psoas muscle should be determined repeatedly during the operation. In prolonged operations, frequent release of the pressure of the retractor seems advisable.

▶ [Nearly 12% of abdominal hysterectomy patients had evidence of femoral nerve injury in this study. The culprit was the deep-bladed self-retaining retractor. Surgeons are notoriously resistant to change, but this article has made us more careful in using the Balfour retractor.] ◀

10–4 **Colposcopy, Conization, and Hysterectomy Practices: Current Perspective.** Colposcopy recently has become the preferred method of investigating women with abnormal Papanicolaou smears. J. L. Benedet, G. H. Anderson, M. L. Simpson, and D. Shaw (Vancouver, B.C.) studied the impact of a diagnostic colposcopy service on conization and hysterectomy practices by reviewing the records of all 2,249 women admitted to Vancouver General Hospital for cervical conization or hysterectomy for cervical intraepithelial neoplasia, on the basis of either biopsy specimen or abnormal Papanicolaou smear, in 1971 (before the colposcopic era) and in 1976 through 1980 (after colposcopy had become well established).

Of the 2,249 patients, 1,075 had cone biopsies. The total number of cone biopsies per year increased in the 5 years after introduction of colposcopy, but the number and percentage of those performed for diagnostic, as opposed to therapeutic, purposes decreased, showing that conization was often used as a therapeutic modality. As colposcopy became more widely used, the percentage of patients who had diagnostic conization without prior colposcopy study decreased steadily from 52% in 1976 to 3% in 1980.

Since 1955 there has been a progressive increase in the number of cases of cervical carcinoma in situ detected in the general population and a doubling of the disease rate in women aged 20 to 29 years, with most cases now in women aged 25 to 29. This change in disease rates for young women coincided with establishment of the colposcopy program and probably reflects diagnosis of disease at its onset and, to a smaller extent, a change in philosophy concerning management of patients with cytology suggestive of mild to moderate dysplasia. Colposcopy showed that many of these women had severe dysplasia or carcinoma in situ, and they were treated rather than simply followed up with repeat smears. With the advent of colposcopy, the proportion of women with negative pathology or minimal lesions on cone biopsy markedly decreased; conversely, severe dysplasia or carcinoma in situ (CIN III) was found in 79% of patients in 1971 and in 91% of those seen in 1980.

Twenty-five percent of conization specimens reviewed showed dysplasia or carcinoma in situ extending to excision margins. There were

---

(10–4) Obstet. Gynecol. 60:539–545, November 1982.

no appreciable differences between diagnostic and therapeutic cones and the respective rates of incomplete excision. In the 318 women who proceeded from colposcopy to hysterectomy without intervening conization, no major degree of difference was found between the colposcopic evaluation and biopsy results and the final pathology noted on the hysterectomy specimen. An additional 856 women were treated with cryotherapy or laser surgery. Thus, 1,174 patients proceeded to definitive treatment without intervening conization.

With judicious use of colposcopy, the number of diagnostic cone biopsies can be reduced greatly, particularly in younger women, but therapeutic conization will continue to be required for many patients. In women with abnormal cervical cytology, colposcopy permits safe and accurate assessment of the nature and extent of lesions and provides a greater choice among the various treatment options available. It also aids in determining the size and shape of cone required.

Further therapy is advised in women whose lesions display carcinoma in situ at the resection margins, deep glandular extension, poor differentiation, or high mitotic activity. Hysterectomy is still recommended for women who do not wish to maintain fertility. In young women or those with lesions of lesser severity, close follow-up with cytology, colposcopy, and endocervical curettage is recommended, with further surgery if abnormal epithelium is again detected. Cytologic and colposcopic follow-up after conization may be more difficult and less precise. Whenever colposcopy indicates a significantly lesser lesion than that suggested by the cytology report, cone biopsy must be performed.

Therapeutic conization is advised for large lesions covering most of the ectocervix and extending close to the vaginal fornices, lesions with appreciable endocervical extension, lesions with deep glandular involvement on the colposcopic biopsy, patients unreliable for follow-up, patient preference, and cervixes with distorted surfaces or other anatomical configurations that preclude good cryoprobe contact.

▶ [This article serves as a nice summary of the changes in management of patients with abnormal Papanicolaou smears over the past decade. The incidence of abnormal histology at the cone margins (25%) is similar to that reported by others, but most of these patients have negative subsequent cytology in the absence of further therapy. It is noteworthy that the ectocervical margin was the one involved half of the time. Use of the colposcope in the operating room should result in free ectocervical margins.] ◀

10-5 **Treatment of Prolapsed Submucous Fibroids.** Prolapsed submucous fibroids are not uncommon. Patients present with a vaginal mass that is often necrotic and infected. P. Riley (Durban, South Africa) retrospectively studied data on 41 such patients.

The average parity of patients with vaginal fibroids was 4.4; the average number of years since the last delivery was 11. Presenting symptoms included abnormal vaginal bleeding (88%), lower abdominal pain (44%), abnormal vaginal discharge (44%), sensation of "something coming down" (15%), and symptoms probably relating to anemia (e.g., headache, dizziness; 12%).

(10–5) S. Afr. Med. J. 62:22–24, July 3, 1982.

Vaginal myomectomy was done in 28 patients and total abdominal hysterectomy in 13. Postoperative morbidity was slightly higher in patients with hysterectomy, but it was comparable to that for patients with hysterectomy for unprolapsed fibroids.

Tumors attached to the interior of the uterus by a stalk and expelled into the vagina may produce inversion of the uterus. If this is overlooked, the result can be disastrous because, in dividing what is regarded as the pedicle of the polyps, the surgeon cuts across the fundus of the uterus and opens into the peritoneal cavity. Before any such polyp is removed, the length of the uterine cavity should always be tested by a sound (Jeffcoate, 1975). If any doubt exists, the myoma should be "shelled out" of its capsule. When hysterectomy is believed to be in the patient's interest, initial vaginal myomectomy reduces the risk of spill of infected material into the peritoneal cavity.

▶ [This article describes a large experience with an unusual, but by no means rare, problem. Consistent with our personal experience, the author reports that vaginal myomectomy was apparently technically easy to perform and did not lead to troublesome operative or postoperative bleeding. Hysterectomy for prolapsed fibroids was not associated with a higher incidence of postoperative fever or a longer length of stay than was hysterectomy for unprolapsed fibroids, but the incidence of fever was high and the length of stay long in both groups. Because of concerns regarding infection, our personal choice is to perform a vaginal myomectomy. Hysterectomy, if indicated, is best done several weeks later.] ◀

10–6 **Postmyomectomy Evaluation of Uterine Scar: A New Hysterographic Method.** Hysterectomy is the most commonly performed operation for the treatment of myomas. However, myomectomy is preferred in younger patients who want to preserve their fertility. As about 50% of patients who undergo myomectomy will become pregnant, the presence of a uterine scar poses the clinical dilemma of cesarean section versus vaginal delivery. Yoram Beyth and Gonen Ohel (Hadassah Univ. Hosp., Jerusalem) describe a new hysterographic method for the evaluation of the postmyomectomy uterine wall.

TECHNIQUE.—After an intramural or submucosal myoma is removed, the myometrium is closed in several layers. Before the serosa is sutured, 5-mm tantalum clips are applied under the serosa, one to each end of the incision and one or two clips along the incision (Fig 10–3). The serosa is then closed, with the clips left embedded in the uterine wall. Three to 6 months after the procedure, hysterography is performed with appropriate views; a lateral view is preferable in cases in which the myoma was enucleated from either the anterior or posterior wall, whereas an anterolateral or posterolateral myoma requires an oblique view. The tantalum clips serve as markers, localizing the areas of scarring to be studied. Because the clips are located directly beneath the serosa and are of known size, they also serve as a built-in scale for measuring both the length of the scar and the thickness of the uterine wall at this site. The tantalum clips do not interfere with the healing process nor are they associated with any deleterious effects.

It is concluded that the subserous placement of tantalum clips may assist in decisions regarding future obstetric management of vaginal delivery or cesarean section.

▶ [The choice of route of delivery after myomectomy should be individualized. Although some have considered entry into the endometrial cavity as the critical deter-

---

(10–6) Fertil. Steril. 39:564–565, April 1983.

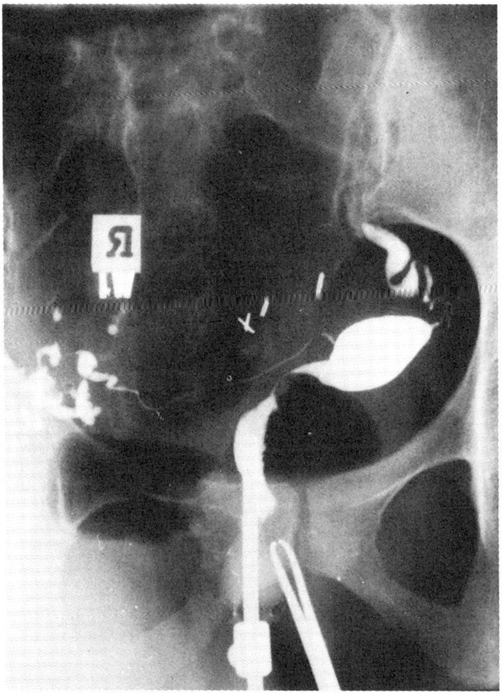

Fig 10–3.—Hysterography of a patient aged 29. Oblique view after removal of a 9 × 8-cm intramural myoma. Four tantalum clips are located along the incision in subserous layer of the uterus. (Courtesy of Beyth, Y., and Ohel, G.: Fertil. Steril. 39:564–565, April 1983.)

minant, we have relied more on the extent of dissection of the uterine wall. The technique described above may prove useful. Certainly in the case illustrated, one would not be too worried about uterine rupture in labor.] ◀

10–7 **Impairment of Tissue Defenses by Vasoconstrictors in Vaginal Hysterectomies.** Vasoconstrictors are used routinely to reduce blood loss during vaginal surgery. Gary T. England, Hugh W. Randall, and William L. Graves (Emory Univ.) examined the effects of this practice in a study of 100 patients having elective vaginal hysterectomy who received a dilute 1:200,000 epinephrine solution and 100 who received a normal saline placebo. The solutions were injected circumferentially around the cervix at the cervicovaginal junction before hysterectomy. The vaginal cuff was left open. All patients received antibiotics perioperatively. The epidemiologic data and indications for surgery were comparable in the two groups.

Vaginal cuff infections developed more often in epinephrine-treated patients (Table 1). The relative risk of cuff infection was 5.5 in epinephrine-treated patients, whether cuff cellulitis or cuff abscess was considered. All infected patients responded to conservative management, but the infections increased the mean hospital stay by about 3½ days. Surgical blood loss was not significantly less in the epineph-

(10–7) Obstet. Gynecol. 61:271–274, March 1983.

TABLE 1.—Percentage of Patients With Vaginal Cuff Infections

	Saline (N = 100)	Epinephrine (N = 100)	Relative risk
Total cuff infections	2	11	5.5*
Cuff cellulitis	1	6	6.0†
Cuff abscess	1	5	5.0†

*$P < .01$.
†$P < .05$.
(Courtesy of England, G. T., et al.: Obstet. Gynecol. 61:271–274, March 1983. Reprinted with permission from The American College of Obstetricians and Gynecologists.)

TABLE 2.—Surgical Blood Loss

	Saline (N = 100)	Epinephrine (N = 100)
Mean estimated blood loss	310 ml	280 ml
No. of patients requiring transfusions	4	5
Mean change in hematocrit	−5.1%	−4.8%

(Courtesy of England, G. T., et al.: Obstet. Gynecol. 61:271–274, March 1983. Reprinted with permission from The American College of Obstetricians and Gynecologists.)

rine-treated patients (Table 2). The mean venous hematocrit value declined by 5.1% in the control group and by 4.8% in the epinephrine-treated patients.

The use of epinephrine as a vasoconstrictor for vaginal hysterectomy significantly predisposed the surgical site to infection in this study and did not significantly reduce operative blood loss. It is suggested that a locally infected vasoconstrictor not be used during this operation.

▶ [A number of clinicians, including ourselves from time to time, inject a dilute solution of a vasoconstrictor into the cervix or the base of the broad ligament, or both, with the aim of reducing blood loss with vaginal hysterectomy. This nice clinical study casts considerable doubt on such a practice. The incidence of vaginal cuff infection was substantially higher (11% vs. 2%) when dilute epinephrine had been used, presumably reflecting tissue hypoxia or interference with antibiotic reaching the site. Moreover, blood loss did not appear to be affected. It seems that this practice should be discarded.] ◀

10–8 **Management of Postoperative Vaginal Hemorrhage.** D. M. Rosenthal, J. L. Harkins, G. Garzo, T. A. Doran, and R. Colapinto (Toronto Genl. Hosp.) reviewed experience over 6 years with management of postoperative vaginal bleeding in 17 patients. Mean age of the 17 was 39 years, and mean parity was 2.3. All initial procedures were done for benign disease. Many patients required several at-

(10–8) Obstet. Gynecol. 61(Suppl.):42S–46S, March 1983.

tempts at achieving hemostasis. One patient had two separate episodes of postoperative bleeding. Bleeding was eventually controlled in all 18 instances, and all patients survived. Mean estimated blood loss was 2 L. Vaginal packing was effective in 4 of 14 attempts, and repacking succeeded in 1 of 3 attempts. Suture ligation of the vaginal vault or a bleeding vessel succeeded in 6 of 7 attempts. Laparotomy was necessary in 4 instances; 1 of 2 resuturings of the vaginal vault and 1 of 2 ligations of the hypogastric artery succeeded. Four patients required hysterectomy, and 1 had bleeding after hysterectomy. Angiographic methods were used in 3 cases. Two patients were treated simply and effectively by selective angiographic embolization of the bleeding vessel with a Gianturco minicoil.

Vaginal packing with gauze and a topical hemostatic agent may be especially effective in patients with venous oozing after operation, but its role in cases of arterial bleeding is questioned. Suture ligation is effective if an arterial bleeder is clearly identified. Angiographic embolization is a rapid, safe, and effective procedure. The site of bleeding can be localized if flow exceeds 0.5 ml per minute. Surgery and its complications are avoided, and the procedure is safer than ligature in treating brittle atherosclerotic vessels. Risks are minimal in experienced hands. Laparotomy can be reserved for use when embolization fails. The efficacy of angiographic embolization in cases of postconization bleeding remains to be determined. Hysterectomy in this setting may itself be complicated by postoperative bleeding.

▶ [Several papers in recent years have described the use of selective arterial embolization for control of pelvic hemorrhage. The technique seems appealing and in experienced hands may turn out to be the preferable choice initially, to avoid major surgery in a hemodynamically unstable patient. Of course, in the patient whose bleeding persists or recurs after operation, it may well be the "only game in town."] ◀

10–9 **Forces Required For Surgical Dilatation of the Pregnant and Nonpregnant Human Cervix.** G. S. Anthony, J. Fisher, J. R. T. Coutts, and A. A. Calder (Glasgow, Scotland) measured the force required for surgical cervical dilatation in pregnant, nonpregnant, premenopausal, and postmenopausal women and in women using different types of hormonal contraceptives. The study comprised 240 women who had cervical dilatation with the use of general anesthesia; 200 were not pregnant and 40 were in the first trimester of pregnancy undergoing therapeutic abortion by suction curettage. The instrument used was designed specifically to measure the force required to pass a dilator through the cervix. Measurements were summated by a microprocessor, which resulted in an index of cervical resistance (CRI).

A progressive lowering of the CRI was seen with increasing parity; the CRI was significantly lower in women with parity of greater than 3 compared with nulliparous women. Pregnant women showed a lower CRI than nonpregnant women. Although lowest resistance was seen in the menstrual phase in the cycling patients, no significant differences existed between any phases of the menstrual cycle. Pa-

---

(10–9) Br. J. Obstet. Gynaecol. 89:913–916, November 1982.

tients on the combined pill showed slightly lower resistance than those using an intrauterine contraceptive device and slightly higher resistance than the menstrual cycling group. These differences were not significant, but those patients receiving Depo-Provera showed a significantly lower level of cervical resistance than did the cycling group. Postmenopausal women showed a significantly higher mean CRI than the premenopausal cycling group.

The purpose of developing the instrument used in this study was to obtain information on forces necessary to achieve surgical dilatation of the human cervix. This will allow long-term assessment of therapy designed to lower cervical resistance to reduce the risk of permanent damage to the cervix. The results from this study are used to establish baseline values for women who are cycling, using contraceptives, pregnant, and postmenopausal.

▶ [These findings are probably exactly what most gynecologists would predict: cervical dilatation is easier in parous than in nulliparous women, in pregnant than in nonpregnant women, in premenopausal than in postmenopausal women, and maybe during the menstrual phase than during other phases of the menstrual cycle.] ◀

10–10 **Peroperative Electrocoagulation of Endocervical Mucosa and Later Carcinoma of Cervical Stump.** The incidence of carcinoma of the cervical stump after subtotal hysterectomy is, according to the literature, 0.39% to 1.9%. Pentti Kilkku and Matti Grönroos (Turku Univ., Turku, Finland) studied the possibility that peroperative electrocoagulation of the endocervical mucosa has a protective effect against cervical carcinoma.

In 1952 to 1978, 2,712 subtotal hysterectomies for benign conditions included electrocoagulation of the endocervical mucosa before the stump was closed. Carcinoma of the cervical stump developed in 3 patients 4 to 11 years later, an incidence of 0.11%.

These 3 patients underwent hysterectomy in the 1950s, before the techniques of vaginal smear examination and colposcopy became widespread. Since 1963, subtotal hysterectomy has been performed only in patients with normal findings in these respects. Thus, it is impossible to prove that electrocoagulation of the endocervical mucosa was the only reason for the low cancer risk shown in the present study. Nevertheless, the authors feel that this technique should be used when subtotal hysterectomy is performed. However, they emphasize the importance of the preoperative vaginal smear and colposcopy.

▶ [The authors of this report suggest that if colposcopy and cytology are negative, electrocoagulation of the endocervical mucosa at the time of subtotal hysterectomy will be associated with a low incidence of cancer developing in the cervical stump. This may be so, but the incidence of stump cancer will be zero if total hysterectomy is performed.] ◀

10–11 **Ectopic Pregnancy in the United States: 1970 Through 1978.** Most reports on ectopic pregnancy (EP) in the United States have been based on individual hospital or state data. George L. Rubin, Herbert B. Peterson, Sally Faith Dorfman, Peter M. Layde, Joyce M. Maze, Howard W. Ory, and Willard Cates, Jr. (Centers for Disease

(10–10) Acta Obstet. Gynecol. Scand. 61:265–267, 1982.
(10–11) JAMA 249:1725–1729, Apr. 1, 1983.

Control) reviewed two data sets from the National Center for Health Statistics: the National Hospital Discharge Survey and national vital statistics on mortality by cause. Nearly 225,000 medical records, or about 1% of all patients discharged from short-stay hospitals, are reviewed annually in the Discharge Survey. Each record represents about 160 hospital discharges.

About 262,000 women aged 15–44 years were discharged from US hospitals between 1970 and 1978 with a diagnosis of EP. The rate per 1,000 reported pregnancies more than doubled in this interval. The final rate was 9.4 EP per 1,000 reported pregnancies.The risk of EP was higher for older women and for nonwhites. More than 2.5% of all reported pregnancies in nonwhite women aged 35–44 years were ectopic. The death-to-case rate for EP decreased by nearly 75% over the study period, but it remained higher for nonwhite women than for whites. The overall death-to-case rate for nonwhite women was 3.4 times that for white women.

The rate of EP more than doubled in the United States from 1970 through 1978. The risk increases with age and is greater for nonwhite women. An increase in pelvic inflammatory disease is a probable cause of the increase in incidence of EP documented in this survey. Clinicians must be especially aware of the possibility of EP in nonwhite women aged 35 and older who report menstrual irregularity and abdominal pain. Mortality from EP has declined, but it remains substantially greater in nonwhite than in white women.

▶ [This national survey documents a substantial increase in the incidence of ectopic pregnancy over the period 1970–1978. Among the possible reasons, an increased incidence of pelvic inflammatory disease (perhaps compounded by partially effective antibiotic therapy) seems most likely as a cause. Other factors, such as increased use of intrauterine contraceptive devices, and induced abortion may also play roles. It is of some encouragement that, while the rate doubled, the death-to-case rate fell by 75%.

In a related study, Glebatis and Javoerich (*JAMA* 249:1730, 1983) examined an upstate New York data base and found almost precisely the same trends as those noted in the national study.] ◀

10–12 **β-Subunit of Human Chorionic Gonadotropin, Ultrasound, and Ectopic Pregnancy: Prospective Study.** An accurate, nonoperative means of diagnosing ectopic pregnancy would be helpful. S. C. Peter Bryson (Toronto) undertook a prospective study of the usefulness of screening for the β-subunit of human chorionic gondadotropin (β-hCG) and of the selective use of ultrasound in diagnosing ectopic gestation in symptomatic, clinically stable women. The study included 81 consecutive patients seen in a 14-month period with signs and symptoms suggestive of ectopic pregnancy. Patients with acute severe symptoms requiring emergency operations and those with pelvic symptoms suggesting other pathology were not included. A qualitative β-hCG screen was carried out, and pelvic ultrasonography was done in patients with unsatisfactory results on pelvic examination. A qualitative radioimmunoassay for β-hCG was used.

Sixteen women had an ectopic pregnancy. All 16 had abnormal uterine bleeding, and 7 also had pelvic pain, amenorrhea, and an ad-

---

(10–12) Am. J. Obstet. Gynecol. 146:163–165, May 15, 1983.

nexal mass. These 16 patients were among the 27 having positive results on β-hCG screening. Ten of the others had confirmed intrauterine pregnancies, and 1 had a spontaneous abortion just before evaluation. The most common diagnosis in patients with negative results on β-hCG screening was rupture or torsion of an ovarian cyst. There were no false results of β-hCG screening. All 13 patients with positive screening results and no intrauterine pregnancy detected on ultrasound study had ectopic pregnancies. Only 6 of these ultrasonograms showed adnexal pathology.

The β-hCG screen and the selective use of pelvic ultrasonography can diagnose ectopic pregnancy before operation with nearly 100% accuracy in hemodynamically stable women in whom the condition is suspected. Unnecessary delay in treatment is avoided with this approach, and morbidity and mortality are reduced. Also, unnecessary surgery is avoided in a large number of patients with benign conditions. Surgery with preservation of the tubes may be possible in patients with small unruptured ectopic pregnancies.

▶ [This is another enthusiastic report on the combination of a β-hCG subunit assay and ultrasound examination in the diagnosis of ectopic pregnancy. If the former is positive, it means there's a pregnancy somewhere. If it is negative, pregnancy is very unlikely, although, as with any other laboratory test, it is not *absolutely* ruled out. The latter is helpful if an intrauterine location of the pregnancy is demonstrated. If not, laparoscopy is indicated. Operation is, of course, also indicated in the absence of this sort of diagnostic evaluation in unstable patients and in those with severe acute symptoms.] ◀

10–13 **α-Fetoprotein and Ectopic Pregnancy.** Measurement of maternal serum α-fetoprotein concentrations is a well-established screening test for fetal neural tube defects. These defects and other birth defects, including omphalocele and congenital nephrosis, result in increased concentrations of α-fetoprotein in the amniotic fluid due to migration of the protein from the fetal serum through the congenital defects. It then crosses the fetal membranes into the maternal circulation. Elevated serum α-fetoprotein concentrations also may be found after amniocentesis as a result of fetal serum leaking into the maternal circulation after breakdown of the fetomaternal barrier. Lars L. Cederqvist, Maureen A. Killackey, Nagwa Abdel-Latif, Rakesh Gupta, and Brij B. Saxena (Cornell Univ., New York) studied α-fetoprotein concentrations in 5 women with a 7- to 9-week pregnancy clinically suspected of being ectopic.

Ultrasonography demonstrated adnexal masses in all 5 patients, and α-fetoprotein was detected in maternal serum in all 5. In 2 patients, the concentration of α-fetoprotein was above the 95th percentile of the normal distribution of values in maternal serum. Human chorionic gonadotropin was detected by radioreceptor assay in 4 of the 5 patients. Tubal pregnancy was confirmed at operation in all 5 cases.

The elevated maternal serum α-fetoprotein concentrations in 2 of the patients can be explained by a breakdown in the fetomaternal barrier. Although normal placental implantation does not occur in tubal pregnancy, the villi grow freely and deep into the tubal tissue,

---

(10–13) Br. Med. J. 286:1247–1248, Apr. 16, 1983.

causing a breakdown in the fetomaternal barrier and allowing fetal α-fetoprotein to reach the maternal circulation more easily. Absorption of fetal blood after tubal abortion is another possibility. The results support the use of Rh_0 (D) immune globulin in Rh-negative women with ectopic pregnancy. Measurement of α-fetoprotein concentration may also prove to be useful as an adjunctive procedure in the diagnosis of ectopic pregnancy.

▶ [We agree with the authors that the elevated α-fetoprotein concentrations noted in 2 of their 5 patients with tubal pregnancies probably reflect breakdown in the fetomaternal barrier. We doubt, however, that α-fetoprotein determinations will prove useful in the diagnosis of ectopic pregnancy.] ◀

10–14 **Conservative Surgery for Tubal Pregnancy.** Rami Langer, Ian Bukovsky, Arie Herman, Dan Sherman, Gad Sadovsky, and Eliahu Caspi (Assaf Harofeh Hosp., Zerifin, Israel) report on 57 conservative surgical procedures for unruptured tubal pregnancy performed in 54 patients. Salpingotomy was performed in 44 cases and fimbrial expression of the ectopic gestation in 13.

Five patients in this study did not desire to conceive postoperatively and were using contraception. The other 49 patients had a total of 71 pregnancies, 65 of which were intrauterine (91.5%). Intrauterine pregnancies occurred in 39 patients. Of these intrauterine pregnancies, 48 culminated in viable births to 35 patients. Of the other intrauterine pregnancies, 4 terminated in induced abortions and 13 miscarried (20%). Repeat tubal pregnancy occurred in 6 patients (12%). In 4 cases, 3 salpingectomies and 1 salpingotomy were performed in the contralateral tube. The table compares fertility outcome and contralateral tubal status as found during surgery for ectopic pregnancy. Ninety percent of patients with a normal contralateral tube conceived normal intrauterine pregnancies, as compared with 64% of patients who underwent additional surgical correction of the contralateral tube due to either adhesions or distal end occlusion. Where the contralateral tube was absent or severely damaged, the intrauterine pregnancy rate was 62.5%.

The authors conclude that the increasing frequency of ectopic gestations offers the physician an opportunity to evaluate less radical operative procedures than previously performed. In particular, conservative salpingotomy and expression of tubal pregnancy continue to be procedures of proved safety and value for future fertility performance. They also should be considered in those cases where there is a normal contralateral tube.

▶ [Because there isn't a control group treated by salpingectomy, this study doesn't establish that a conservative operation for an unruptured tubal pregnancy in a patient with an apparently normal contralateral tube is better than the more traditional salpingectomy. The reported results, however, are excellent, and the ectopic pregnancy recurrence rate is very low. A conservative procedure, rather than salpingectomy, is indicated in the patient with an unruptured tubal pregnancy. The following article describes a technique for this type of management.] ◀

10–15 **"Milking": Conservative Surgical Technique for a Tubal Gestation.** The expression of tubal gestations by milking has been con-

---

(10–14) Fertil. Steril. 38:427–430, October 1982.
(10–15) Int. J. Fertil. 28:49–51, 1983.

CONTRALATERAL TUBE STATUS DURING SURGERY FOR TUBAL PREGNANCY AND FERTILITY OUTCOME IN 49 PATIENTS

Status of contralateral tube	No. of patients	Intrauterine pregnancies (no. of patients)	Live birth (no. of patients)	Extrauterine pregnancies (no. of patients)
Normal	30	27 (90%)	24 (80%)	2 (6.6%)
Periadnexal adhesions or sactosalpinx surgically corrected	11	7 (63.6%)	6 (54.5%)	2 (18.2%)
Previous salpingectomy or severely damaged tube*	8	5 (62.5%)	5 (62.5%)	2 (25%)
Total	49	39	35	6†

*Six patients had salpingectomy, and 2 had severely damaged oviducts incompatible with normal function.
†Two patients had a live birth followed by recurrent tubal pregnancy.
(Courtesy of Langer, R., et al.: Fertil. Steril. 38:427–430, October 1982.)

troversial. R. Langer, I. Bukovsky, A. Herman, Y. Lifshits, and E. Caspi managed 54 cases of unruptured tubal pregnancy by conservative surgical methods between 1972 and 1979. Thirteen patients underwent expression of a tubal pregnancy. The ova were adherent in the outer part of the ampulla in 7 and attached to the fimbria in 6. The ova were removed manually by exerting direct pressure on the tube just beneath the implantation site. Hemostasis was necesary in 5 instances; electrocoagulation was used in 3 cases. A solution of hydrocortisone and antibiotics then was instilled into the abdominal cavity. Hydrotubations and corticosteroid therapy were used postoperatively.

Mean patient age was 25 years. Six of the 13 patients were nulligravidas. A fimbrioplasty was done on the contralateral tube in 2 patients. Twelve intrauterine pregnancies occurred in 9 of the 13 study patients on follow-up. There were no subsequent ectopic pregnancies. Eight patients delivered 10 live infants. There was 1 elective abortion, and 1 spontaneous abortion occurred. Two pregnancies occurred in patients lacking the contralateral tube. There were no operative complications, and no patient required transfusions.

Tubal milking may be a valuable conservative treatment of ectopic pregnancy. A 75% rate of intrauterine pregnancy and a 67% rate of live births without ectopic recurrences were obtained in this series. The results compare favorably with those of conservative salpingectomy for ectopic gestation.

▶ [In this report of "milking" (i.e., digital expression of the conceptus), 9 of 12 patients conceived and there were no repeat ectopic pregnancies. The numbers are small but there does seem to be some reason for encouragement. Adjunctive measures that may be important included intraperitoneal instillation of hydrocortisone and antibiotics intraoperatively and hydrotubation and steroid therapy postoperatively.

In another report, Valle and Lifchez (*Fertil. Steril.* 39:316, 1983) described a 6-year experience with conservative surgery (usually salginostomy) for tubal pregnancy in patients who had only one tube. Of 11 patients, 1 was lost to follow-up, 1 intentionally avoided pregnancy, and 9 subsequently had at least one term gestation.] ◀

10–16 **Comparison of Different Laparoscopic Sterilization Occlusion Techniques in 24,439 Procedures.** Pouru P. Bhiwandiwala, Stephen D. Mumford, and Paul J. Feldblum (Res. Triangle Park, N.C.) reviewed data from the International Fertility Research Program covering 24,439 laparoscopic sterilizations performed by 5 methods since 1971 at 64 facilities in 27 countries.

The rates of surgical difficulties due to a patient characteristic (e.g., obesity or a pathologic condition) or to a problem with equipment or anesthesia ranged from 2.4% with open laparoscopy and tubal ring to 12.5% with the prototype spring-loaded Hulka-Clemens clip (overall, 5.1%). No important differences were noted in the rate of surgical complications among the five groups; they ranged from 0.7% with the prototype clip to 2.7% with the Rocket clip (overall, 1.7%). The rates of technical failure were uniformly low, ranging from 0.6% to 1.0% (overall, 0.8%). Twelve-month life-table pregnancy rates were less

---

(10–16) Am. J. Obstet. Gynecol. 144:319–331, Oct. 1, 1982.

TABLE 1.—PELVIC OPERATIONS AFTER LAPAROSCOPIC STERILIZATION

Follow-up rate* according to type of operation and indication	Follow-up: 6 month (N = 11,662) (49.8%)		12 month (N = 8,134) (34.7%)		18 month (N = 2,157) (9.2%)		24 month (N = 3,291) (14.0%)		Total
	No.	%	No.	%	No.	%	No.	%	No.
Hysterectomy:									
Carcinoma in situ (cervix)	3	0.03	3	0.04	1	0.05	3	0.09	10
Fibroids	0	—	3	0.04	0	—	3	0.09	6
Irregular bleeding	0	—	4	0.05	0	—	1	0.03	5
Adenomatous hyperplasia	1	0.01	0	—	0	—	0	—	1
Endometriosis	0	—	1	0.01	0	—	0	—	1
Prolapse	0	—	0	—	0	—	1	0.03	1
Unspecified	4	0.03	2	0.02	1	0.05	4	0.12	11
Subtotal	8	0.07	13	0.16	2	0.09	12	0.36	35
Curettage:									
Irregular bleeding	4	0.03	4	0.05	1	0.05	1	0.03	10
Retained products	3	0.03	0	—	0	—	0	—	3
Abortion	1	0.01	0	—	0	—	0	—	1
Unspecified	6	0.05	0	—	1	0.05	0	—	7
Subtotal	14	0.12	4	0.05	2	0.09	1	0.03	21
Repeat sterilization after failure	6	0.05	11	0.14	0	—	6	0.18	23
Cervical biopsy	4	0.03	7	0.09	0	—	0	—	11
Salpingo-oophorectomy (tubo-ovarian cysts)	4	0.03	2	0.02	2	0.09	1	0.03	9
Cervical cautery	1	0.01	2	0.02	1	0.05	3	0.09	7
Exploratory laparoscopy/laparotomy	1	0.01	2	0.02	0	—	1	0.03	4
Removal of cervical polyps	1	0.01	1	0.01	0	—	0	—	2
Repair of vaginal/uterine prolapse	0	—	1	0.01	0	—	1	0.03	2
Reversal of sterilization	1	0.01	0	—	0	—	0	—	1
Unspecified	19	0.16	21	0.26	1	0.05	1	0.03	42
Total	59	0.51	64	0.79	8	0.37	26	0.79	157

*Follow-up rates exclude open laparoscopy cases from denominator.
(Courtesy of Bhiwandiwala, P. P., et al.: Am. J. Obstet. Gynecol. 144:319–331, Oct. 1, 1982.)

TABLE 2.—STANDARDIZATION OF FINDINGS

Parameter	No.	Rate per 100 women: Unstandardized	Standardized*
Surgical difficulties (N = 24,439):			
Laparoscopy/electrocoagulation	12,643	3.89	3.94
Laparoscopy/tubal ring	7,766	5.02	4.94
Laparoscopy/prototype clip†	2,324	12.52	12.30
Laparoscopy/Rocket clip	702	6.70	6.91
Open laparoscopy	1,004	2.39	2.44
Surgical complications/injuries (N = 24,439):			
Laparoscopy/electrocoagulation	12,643	1.61	1.58
Laparoscopy/tubal ring	7,766	2.15	2.14
Laparoscopy/prototype clip†	2,324	0.65	0.65
Laparoscopy/Rocket clip	702	2.71	2.61
Open laparoscopy	1,004	1.20	1.17
Technical failures (N = 24,439):			
Laparoscopy/electrocoagulation	12,643	0.62	0.64
Laparoscopy/tubal ring	7,766	0.93	0.93
Laparoscopy/prototype clip†	2,324	0.99	0.99
Laparoscopy/Rocket clip	702	0.71	0.74
Open laparoscopy	1,004	0.07	0.07
Method failure‡ (N = 12,218)§:			
Laparoscopy/electrocoagulation	6,542	0.26	—
Laparoscopy/tubal ring	5,046	0.47	—
Laparoscopy/Rocket clip	630	0.18	—

*Standardized for patient category (interval, postabortion, postpartum) by indirect method.
†The Hulka-Clemens spring-loaded clip.
‡These rates are 12-month life-table failure rates. These rates were not standardized for timing of sterilization, since events among various categories were too rare to make this standardization analysis useful.
§Only patients with long-term follow-up were included. Patients with a Hulka clip were excluded in view of a manufacturing error which led to a high rate of failure.
(Courtesy of Bhiwandiwala, P. P., et al.: Am. J. Obstet. Gynecol. 144:319–331, Oct. 1, 1982.)

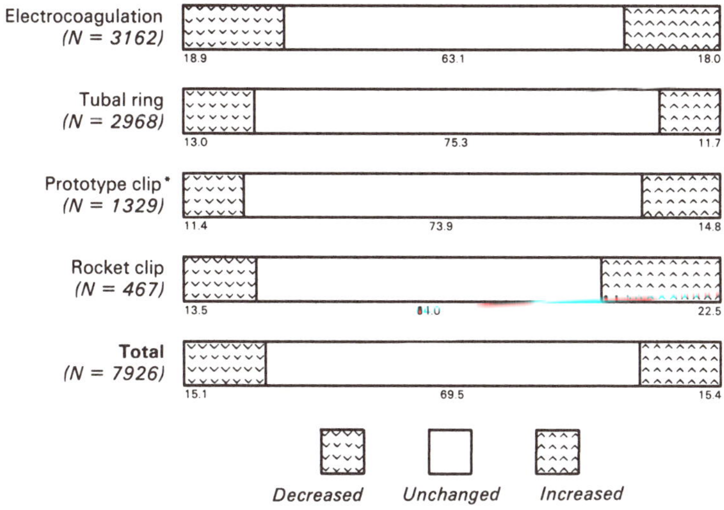

**The Hulka-Clemens spring-loaded clip.*

Fig 10–4.—Percentage of women with change in amount of menstrual flow from admission to 12-month follow-up. (Courtesy of Bhiwandiwala, P. P., et al.: Am. J. Obstet. Gynecol. 144:319–331, Oct. 1, 1982.)

than 1 per 100 woman-years with all methods. These results are summarized in Table 1.

Prospective data on six menstrual parameters showed that the menstrual cycles of most women were unchanged after sterilization. Of women who reported a change, about half reported an increase in the amount of menstrual flow (Fig 10–4) or severity of dysmenorrhea

Fig 10–5.—Percentage of women with change in severity of dysmenorrhea from admission to 12-month follow-up. (Courtesy of Bhiwandiwala, P. P., et al.: Am. J. Obstet. Gynecol. 144:319–331, Oct. 1, 1982.)

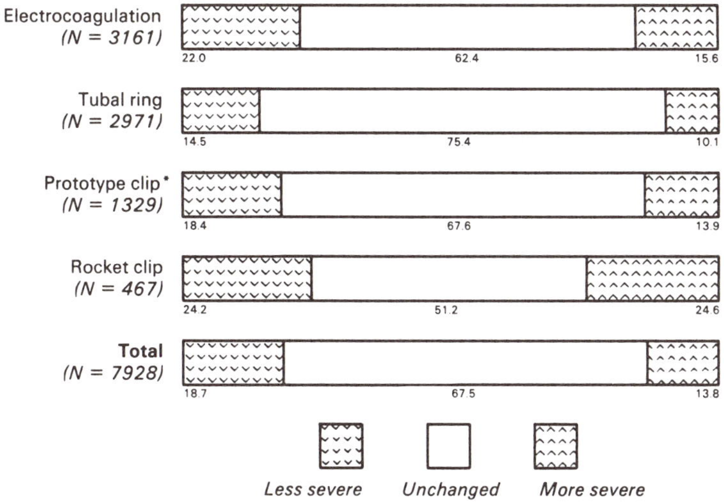

**The Hulka-Clemens spring-loaded clip.*

(Fig 10–5) and about half reported decreases. These changes were generally those to be expected when the method of contraception previously used by the patient was considered. The reported incidence of subsequent pelvic operations was less than 1% at each long-term follow-up, and most subsequent operations were not related to the sterilization procedure (Table 2).

Although several statistically significant differences were found in this study, the clinical implications are minimal because the differences in absolute rates are very small and may be overridden by clinical and other considerations. Laparoscopic sterilization is safe and effective. None of the studied techniques has a distinct advantage; open laparoscopy appears promising and needs further study. The physician should continue to use the method with which he is most familiar and comfortable; differences in techniques usually can be overridden by experience. The fact that the number of luteal phase pregnancies in the series almost equaled the number of pregnancies reported at follow-up due to method failure indicates the desirability of proper scheduling of sterilization procedures with regard to the menstrual cycle of the patient.

► [This large multinational study demonstrates the excellent results of laparoscopic sterilization. There is apparently not much difference between the various techniques (reversibility was not considered). The data concerning menstrual function after sterilization and the need for subsequent pelvic surgery are reassuring. There were nearly as many luteal-phase pregnancies (i.e., the sterilization was performed after fertilization, but before the "missed menses") as there were method failures. Some workers advocate routine dilation and curettage or suction curettage in conjunction with laparoscopic tubal sterilization, but, as the authors of this report point out, 840 such procedures would be performed to prevent 1 luteal-phase pregnancy, hardly a cost-effective measure.

Our usual practice is to perform closed laparoscopy with the use of general anesthesia and bipolar electrocoagulation. Clips are used in certain younger women. The concluding sentence of this article is very likely to be true, is applicable to many surgical procedures, and yet is rarely written. It reads: "At the present time, each physician should continue to use the method with which he is most familiar and comfortable; differences in techniques can usually be overridden by experience."] ◄

10–17 **Complications of Interval Laparoscopic Tubal Sterilization.** Tubal sterilization is one of the most common elective intra-abdominal operations performed on women of reproductive age in the United States. Frank Destefano, Joel R. Greenspan, Richard C. Dicker, Herbert B. Peterson, Lilo T. Strauss, and George L. Rubin (Centers for Disease Control, Atlanta) reviewed the findings in a prospective, multicenter study begun by the CDC in 1978 to evaluate the safety of various female sterilizing operations. A total of 3,500 women who underwent interval laparoscopic tubal sterilization by electrocoagulation or Silastic banding were enrolled in the first 31 months. Most were white and aged 25 to 34 years.

The overall rate of intraoperative and postoperative complications was 1.7/100 women. The most common complication was unintended major surgery; most of the laparotomies were done because of technical difficulties in completing sterilization by laparoscopy. Febrile morbidity was infrequent. The median postoperative hospital stay

---

(10–17) Obstet. Gynecol. 61:153–158, February 1983.

was 2 nights for women with complications. Factors increasing the risk of complications by at least twofold included diabetes, previous abdominal or pelvic surgery, pulmonary disease, a history of pelvic inflammatory disease, and obesity. The relative risk of general anesthesia relative to local anesthesia exceeded 4. Complications were not closely related to the method of tubal occlusion, although electrocoagulation was associated with more complications than was Silastic banding. Age, gravidity, number of previous abortions, and reported reason for tubal sterilization were not significant factors in the risk of complications.

Interval laparoscopic tubal sterilization appears, in general, to be a safe procedure, with a risk of complications of less than 2/100 women. Because so many women have tubal sterilization, however, morbidity and health care costs could be substantially reduced by making the procedure even safer. The safest procedures are those done with local anesthesia.

▶ [Laparoscopic tubal sterilization has become the most common of gynecologic operations. It is also one of the safest, although, as evidenced by this large survey, almost any complication will be encountered if the numbers are large enough. The overall incidence of significant complications was 1.7/100. One of the surprising findings is that complications were 4–5 times more frequent with general than with local anesthesia. We suspect this reflects a tendency to reserve local anesthesia for simple uncomplicated cases, perhaps done by experienced surgeons, with general anesthesia more likely to be used in difficult cases or by those surgeons with less experience.] ◀

10–18 **Deaths Attributable to Tubal Sterilization in the United States, 1977 to 1981.** Tubal sterilization was the most common method of contraception for women in the 1970s. Despite its overall safety, tubal sterilization does result in death in some instances. Herbert B. Peterson, Frank DeStefano, George L. Rubin, Joel R. Greenspan, Nancy C. Lee, and Howard W. Ory (Centers for Disease Control) reviewed data concerning 29 such deaths that occurred in the United States between 1977 and 1981. Complications of general anesthesia, usually hypoventilation and intraoperative cardiorespiratory arrest, accounted for 11 deaths; 3 of 4 women dying of intraoperative arrest had conditions that may have been contributory. Sepsis was responsible for 7 deaths, including 3 in women with apparent bowel injury after unipolar coagulation. Four deaths were attributed to hemorrhage, 3 after major vessel lacerations occurring during laparoscopic sterilization. Three women died after myocardial infarction. One death may have been associated with oral contraceptive use, and 1 followed pulmonary embolism. One patient died after intraoperative complete heart block developed, and 1 after complications of Eisenmenger's syndrome occurred.

Thus, complications of general anesthesia are the leading cause of recent deaths attributable to tubal sterilization in the United States, with sepsis and hemorrhage also being important. The frequency of these deaths may be reduced by using endotracheal intubation with general anesthesia, especially for laparoscopic sterilization, and by

(10–18) Am. J. Obstet. Gynecol. 146:131–136, May 15, 1983.

the safer application of unipolar coagulation or the use of alternative methods. In addition, careful insertion of the needle and trocar for laparoscopy is necessary. Oral contraception should be discontinued before sterilization. Continued surveillance for sterilization-related deaths will help make tubal sterilization an even safer option for fertility control.

▶ [There are no real surprises here. That intubation should be a requisite for laparoscopic sterilization with general anesthesia is easier for us to buy than the suggestion that patients should discontinue oral contraceptives for 1 month prior to operation. For certain patients (intelligent, motivated, compliant), this would be ideal. For others, confusion, concern, and pregnancy are likely to result.] ◀

10–19 **Hysteroscopic Tubal Occlusion With Formed-in-Place Silicone Plugs.** Richard M. Houck and Jay M. Cooper (Phoenix Baptist Hosp., Phoenix, Ariz.) discuss their experience with formed-in-place silicone rubber plugs in 161 patients who requested permanent sterilization from December 1980 through July 1981. This nonsurgical method involves allowing catalyzed silicone to flow into the oviduct through a silicone rubber obturator tip positioned at the tubal ostium. Average patient age was 30.08 years; gravida, 2.37; and para, 1.8.

In each case, an initial procedure was attempted in the office with the patient under paracervical block consisting of 150 mg of 1% lidocaine, with or without 1:100,000 epinephrine. Additional sedation or anesthesia was rarely required. Immediately after the tubal occlusion, all patients walked to the outpatient radiology department, where a film of the pelvis was taken to evaluate placement of the formed-in-place silicone plugs (Fig 10–6). All patients agreed to continued use of contraceptives and reevaluation with a repeat film of the pelvis 3 months after the procedure, in accordance with the protocol approved by the FDA.

Thirty-two patients required more than one attempt to place normal plugs. Bilateral normal plugs were noted on films of the pelvis of 135 patients immediately after the procedure. A unilateral normal

Fig 10–6.—Radiograph of bilateral normal-appearing silicone rubber plugs in place. (Courtesy of Houck, R. M., and Cooper, J. M.: Obstet. Gynecol. 60:641–644, November 1982. Reprinted with permission from The American College of Obstetricians and Gynecologists.)

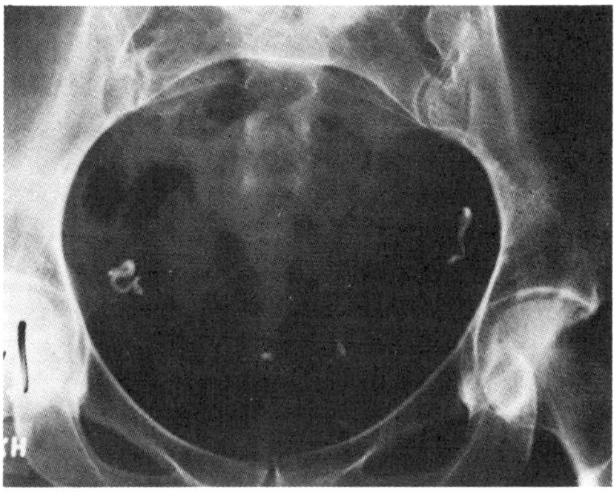

(10–19) Obstet. Gynecol. 60:641–644, November 1982.

plug was placed in 4 patients with confirmed contralateral tubal occlusion. Therefore, 139 patients (86%) underwent a successful procedure (based on radiographic appearance of the plugs).

Seventy-three of the 139 returned after 3 months for radiographic examination. Migration of a seemingly normal plug into the peritoneal cavity was detected in 1 patient, but the 72 others have been advised to discontinue contraceptive methods and are relying on the plugs for sterilization. The procedure was not successful in 22 patients. There were no complications requiring hospitalization, but 3 patients sustained a midline uterine perforation. Three patients were successfully treated with oral antibiotics for suspected endometritis. Patient discomfort was rated from none (0 patients) to severe discomfort (3); average was 1.08. Average duration of the procedure was 38 minutes.

This new technique offers an easily performed office procedure that is quickly accomplished with the patient under paracervical block and minimal discomfort. Careful patient selection has allowed only women wishing permanent sterilization to undergo the procedure. As a result, the authors have no experience with purposeful removal of the plugs to restore tubal patency and function. However, they anticipate that further evaluation will demonstrate easy reversibility.

▶ [Hysteroscopic means of tubal sterilization are appealing—outpatient setting, minimal anesthesia, low cost, etc. Caustic chemicals, electrocautery techniques, and cryotherapy haven't caught on. Perhaps silicone plugs will, but much more experience is needed.] ◀

10–20 **Hysteroscopic Resection of Intrauterine Scars Using a New Technique.** Robert S. Neuwirth, Amtul R. Hussein, Bruce M. Schiffman, and Hussein K. Amin (St. Luke's-Roosevelt Hosp. Center, New York) describe a new technique for resection of intrauterine adhesions in which Jako microlaryngeal scissors and the hysteroscope are advanced together into the uterus.

METHOD.—High molecular weight 32% dextran 70 is used to distend the uterus because its high viscosity reduces the rate of backflow through the cervix. When adhesions are densely blended into the myometrium, laparoscopy is used to prevent inadvertent perforation and to keep the uterus away from other structures by mechanical means. The Jako scissors and hysteroscope are advanced simultaneously into the uterine cavity with the scissors slightly ahead of the hysteroscope to permit constant visualization of the scissors during free range of dissection in the endometrial cavity. The scissors allow easier cutting of adhesions than do flexible instruments designed for the operative channel of the standard hysteroscope. To keep transected scar surfaces apart, an intrauterine device, or a Silastic balloon if bleeding is excessive, is left in the uterine cavity at the end of the procedure. Broad-spectrum antibiotics are administered for 5 days. Two 21-day courses of conjugated estrogens, 5 mg/day, separated by a 7-day rest period are given to stimulate the endometrium to resurface the area of transected scar before bands reform. The intrauterine device is removed within 2 months.

In 1974 to 1979, this method was used to treat 27 women with hysterographically and hysteroscopically confirmed intrauterine adhesions. One patient had primary infertility and 26 had a history of induced abortion, spontaneous abortion with curettage, or postpartum curettage.

(10–20) Obstet. Gynecol. 60:111–113, July 1982.

Of the 27 women, 14 became pregnant. Four of the 14 became pregnant twice. The pregnancies ended in 15 living children (1 was premature), 2 spontaneous abortions, and 1 ectopic pregnancy. Six women gave birth to living children by normal vaginal delivery and 8 by cesarean section (1 patient twice) for various obstetric indications. Two women required repeat hysteroscopic dissection before resuming normal menses and achieving pregnancy. Only one third-stage complication, postpartum hemorrhage, occurred; there was no histologic evidence of abnormal placentation.

Of the 13 women who did not conceive, all resumed regular menses but regular flow subsequently became cyclic spotting in 7, suggesting scar recurrence. These 13 women had more extensive adhesions than the 14 who conceived, and several may have had additional pathology.

10–21 **Hysteroscopic Metroplasty: Surgical Technique and Obstetric Outcome.** Congenital müllerian abnormalities such as septate uterus can result in recurrent abortion and premature labor. Douglas C. Daly, Clifford A. Walters, Carlos E. Soto-Albors, and Daniel H. Riddick (Univ. of Connecticut, Farmington) reviewed the results of hysteroscopic metroplasty in 25 patients with hysterosalpingographic findings consistent with either septate or bicornuate uterus. Seventeen patients had had 40 pregnancies, which resulted in 28 spontaneous deliveries, 6 second-trimester deliveries, and 5 premature third-trimester deliveries. Only 4 infants survived. Eight patients had a history of primary infertility. Two of them had otherwise normal infertility studies. Laparoscopy confirmed normal external uterine fusion in all cases. All the metroplasties were done by using the laparoscope as an external guide to the hysteroscope. Dextran 70 was used to expand the uterine cavity. A videotape camera facilitated the surgery. Patients received Premarin and medroxyprogesterone acetate after operation. Hysterosalpingography was repeated.

All patients had hysteroscopic metroplasty with general anesthesia; the operation lasted less than 1 hour. None had significant bleeding. Three patients with septal bleeding that obscured the field had repeat metroplasty after 2 months, with a successful outcome. All patients were discharged by the second postoperative day. Of 11 patients who had previously been pregnant and were followed for more than 6 months, 10 conceived, resulting in 6 term pregnancies and 1 preterm and 1 immature delivery; 2 pregnancies are in progress. One of 6 other patients with primary infertility conceived and had a spontaneous abortion of a 69 XXX fetus. Five of 7 patients have delivered vaginally. Cesarean sections were done for cases of postdatism with an unfavorable cervix and a history of previous sections.

Hysteroscopic metroplasty causes less morbidity than abdominal metroplasty, has a similar anatomical outcome, and precludes the need for cesarean section. If follow-up studies confirm a favorable pregnancy outcome, hysteroscopic metroplasty could become the preferred treatment for the septate uterus.

10–22 **Hysteroscopic Management of Intrauterine Lesions and Intractable Uterine Bleeding.** Hysteroscopy is used chiefly as a diagnostic technique, but the cystoscope-resectoscope provides a means of

(10–21) Fertil. Steril. 39:623–628, May 1983.
(10–22) Obstet. Gynecol. 61:392–397, March 1983.

transvaginal surgical management of many intrauterine lesions and intractable bleeding. Alan DeCherney and Mary Lake Polan (Yale Univ.) reviewed treatment with this instrument in 40 women during a 2-year period. The 15 who had a history of repeated or habitual abortion were shown by hysterography to have müllerian fusion defects, either an arcuate or a septate uterus. Fourteen patients had abnormal uterine bleeding not attributable to a hormonal or malignant cause. Eleven had intractable bleeding unresponsive to intravenous administration of conjugated estrogens. Six of the latter patients were extreme anesthesia risks, and 2 refused definitive surgical treatment. The patients with intractable uterine bleeding were treated with the use of diazepam or ketamine anesthesia, with occasional supplemental N_2O. The others were operated on with the use of general anesthesia. The patients with uterine defects had simultaneous laparoscopy.

None of the patients with uterine defects had serious complications from surgery. The septum was removed in 11 patients, 9 of whom had term pregnancies during follow-up; 8 of them delivered vaginally, and 1 delivered by cesarean section because of fetal distress. One patient had 2 subsequent first-trimester abortions, and another has been infertile. The patients with abnormal uterine bleeding had submucous myomas or polypoid endometria. All of the lesions were removed successfully, without notable sequelae. Cauterization of the entire endometrial cavity was carried out within 30 minutes in the patients with intractable bleeding. Three patients required temporary catheter tamponade; there were no long-term complications. No recurrent heavy bleeding occurred in the 9 patients followed up for 6–18 months postoperatively.

The resectoscope can be used to treat a variety of uterine abnormalities. The operating time is short, and complications are infrequent and not severe. The transcervical approach is a major advantage, obviating the need for abdominal surgery. Operator experience is a major consideration. Patients with large polyps or myomas or a thick uterine septum still require abdominal surgery, however.

▶ [Hysteroscopy is increasing in popularity, as indicated by this article and the two preceding it. The technique finds perhaps its most useful application in Asherman's syndrome, the subject of the report by Neuwirth and colleagues, where it permits direct resection of the intrauterine synechiae, rather than blindly (and hopefully) trying to break them down. The pregnancy rate reported by Neuwirth et al.—14 of 27 patients—is reasonably good for this condition.

Hysteroscopic resection of uterine septa, addressed in the papers by Daly, et al. and DeCherney and Polan, is appealing because, in comparison with the Jones and Tompkins procedures, neither laparotomy nor subsequent cesarean section is required. Laparoscopy should be done concomitantly with hysteroscopy to assess the external configuration of the uterus.] ◀

10–23 **Prevention of Postoperative Pelvic Adhesions: Animal Study Comparing Barrier Methods With Dextran 70.** Chemical and barrier methods have been used to prevent development of postoperative pelvic adhesions. Theoretically, chemical methods (e.g., dextran) prevent formation of adhesions by a surface-coating or hydroflotation ef-

---

(10–23) Am. J. Obstet. Gynecol. 143:829–834, Aug. 1, 1982.

fect, whereas barrier methods either prevent or mask adhesions by covering and isolating the injured area with an inert substance. Michael R. Soules, Larry Dennis, Alvin Bosarge, and Donald E. Moore compared the efficacy of dextran 70 (6% and 32%) and 7 barriers (3 natural and 4 synthetic) in preventing pelvic adhesions in female rabbits.

Symmetric cut and scrape lesions were made on both sides of the uterus. In barrier-treated animals, the lesions on one side of the uterus were covered with Gelfilm, Surgicel, Silastic, Gelfoam paste, amnion, peritoneum, or omentum, and the contralateral side served as control. The dextran-treated animals received 10 mg of 6% or 32% dextran 70 per kilogram intraperitoneally, and animals undergoing similar surgery without dextran treatment served as controls. About 4 weeks later, the severity of adhesions was graded.

The 7 barrier methods generally resulted in increased formation of adhesions when compared with control and dextran-treated animals. The degree of adhesion formation in dextran-treated rabbits did not differ significantly from that in controls, although animals treated with 32% dextran 70 had the lowest mean adhesion score of all groups tested.

Thus, barrier methods may actually promote adhesion formation, whereas use of dextran 70 gives inconclusive results.

▶ [Given the caveat that this is a rabbit study and that extrapolation of the reported findings may not be appropriate, the results suggest that a variety of barrier methods advocated for preventing adhesions actually promote them! The jury is still out on 32% dextran 70. In contrast to other reports involving animal models, although the adhesion scores were lower in the dextran group, they were not significantly different from those of the controls.] ◀

10–24 **Adnexal Adhesions: Prognostic Staging and Classification System Based on 5-Year Survey of Fertility Surgery Results at Chapel Hill, North Carolina.** A classification system for adnexal adhesive disease, based on findings at hysterosalpingography and laparoscopy, has been in use at the University of North Carolina since 1976. Jaroslav F. Hulka used this system to prospectively classify 108 patients who underwent microsurgical lysis of adnexal adhesions with (61) or without (47) salpingostomy in 1976 to 1980. Follow-up of 6 to 48 months in regard to pregnancy outcome was obtained in 90% of the patients.

Hulka has now proposed a simplified staging system based on four independent observations: extent of ovarian involvement in adhesive disease, nature of the adhesions, fimbrial patency, and isthmic patency (Fig 10–7). Each adnexa is staged separately, and patients are classified according to the operation performed on the more favorable side.

In an analysis of the results as defined by live births, use of this system showed a significant gradient from minimal adhesions (46.7% births) to extensive adhesions (no births). A similar strong gradient was demonstrated with salpingostomies, with a 30% birth rate with no adhesions ranging to no births with extensive adhesions.

(10–24) Am. J. Obstet. Gynecol. 144:141–148, Sept. 15, 1982.

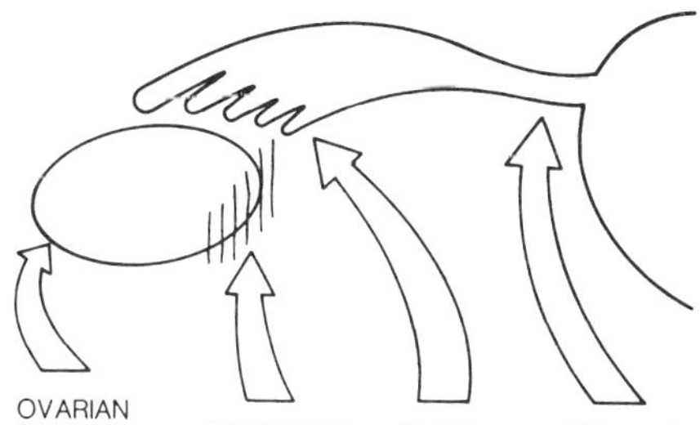

	OVARIAN SURFACE	ADHESIONS	FIMBRIA	ISTHMUS
NORMAL	( ) 100% seen	( ) None	( ) Open	( ) Open
30-50% PROGNOSIS	I over 50%	A Thin	F Closed	i Closed
POOR PROGNOSIS	II under 50%	B Thick		

Fig 10–7.—Staging of adnexal adhesive disease. Four independent observations are made on each adnexa. Poor prognoses are associated with extensive or thick adhesions or with combinations of adhesions and tubal obstruction. After laparotomy for correction of adhesive disease, the following patient classification conventions apply: 1. Revise staging after laparotomy; e.g., fimbrial occlusion due to adhesions around patent fimbria would be staged IAF at laparoscopy but would be revised to IA because no salpingostomy was required at laparotomy. 2. Classify patient according to most favorable adnexa; e.g., a patient staged as IIAF-IIA after laparotomy would be classified IIA for prognostic purposes. (Courtesy of Hulka, J. F.: Am. J. Obstet. Gynecol. 144:141–148, Sept. 15, 1982.)

This staging and classification system is particularly useful in offering realistic prognoses to patients contemplating adnexal operations. The criteria are simple in that they require only a yes/no clinical judgment concerning each of the four aspects.

▶ [This classification is somewhat complex, but it takes into account the factors involved in fertility and thus should prove useful in assessing patients preoperatively.] ◀

10–25 **Transplantation and Replantation of Fallopian Tubes and Ovaries: Technique for Patients Undergoing Pelvic Irradiation.** Fertility may be compromised in women who require irradiation in the pelvic region for neoplasia. Bernard Cantor (Univ. of Miami) describes a method of maintaining tubo-ovarian vascular and anatomical relationships in a patient requiring pelvic irradiation for an aneurysmal bone cyst.

Woman, 18, experienced paresthesias over the lateral digits of the left foot, followed by pain and muscle weakness in the left calf and a sense of fullness in the lower back. A mass 7–8 cm in size was noted on rectal examination, extending across the entire sacrum; sacral tomography showed a destructive lesion involving the midportion of the sacrum. Angiography and computed tomography showed extension to at least L5. Transsacral biopsy, causing loss of about 1,500 ml of blood, showed an aneurysmal bone cyst, and irradiation of a large pelvic field to 3,500 rad administered over a 4-week period was recommended. Bilateral transplantation of the fallopian tubes and ovaries was carried out as shown in Figures 10–8 and 10–9. The descending colon was moved medially as the infundibulopelvic vessels were skeletonized and mobilized.

(10–25) Fertil. Steril. 39:231–234, February 1983.

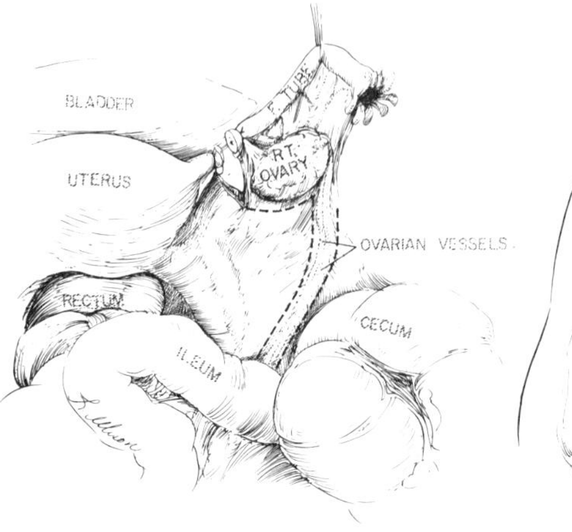

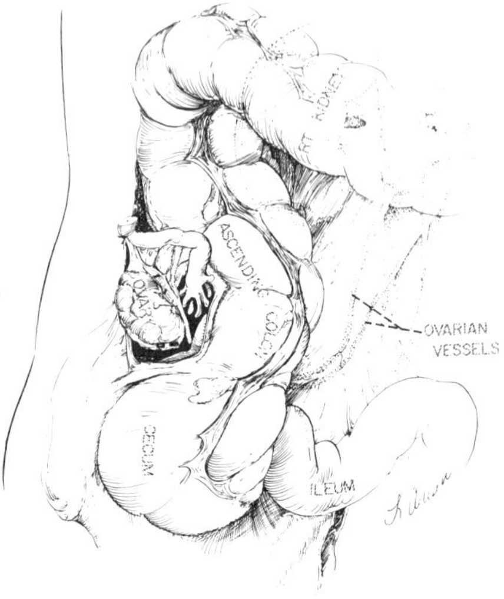

Fig 10–8 (left).—Mobilization of right tube and ovary.
Fig 10–9 (right).—Right tube and ovary after transplantation.
(Courtesy of Cantor, B.: Fertil. Steril. 39:231–234, February 1983.)

The menses resumed normally, with ovulation confirmed. Radiotherapy led to gradual ossification of the lesion and a return of muscle strength and sensation. Replantation subsequently was carried out in the proliferative phase of the cycle. A new defect was made in the bowel mesentery through which the right tube and ovary were drawn into a retroperitoneal position. The scarred ends of the tube were resected and standard microsurgical reanastomosis was carried out. Extensive fibrous adhesions were present on the left side, and the tube and ovary were excised. Normal menses continued, and the patient conceived 6 months after marrying. However, cervical incompetence complicated the pregnancy, and a stillbirth resulted.

This approach offers a significant chance of successful pregnancy after pelvic irradiation. Normal tubo-ovarian relationships are maintained while the adnexa are removed from the field of irradiation, reducing the risks of ovarian failure and oocyte exposure. The procedure may be useful for patients with Hodgkin's disease or other pelvic lymphomas, unilateral dysgerminomas, or sacral teratomas, and possibly for those with cervical and endometrial carcinomas.

▶ [This report illustrates an alternative to lateral ovarian transposition as a means of maintaining potential fertility in young women who require pelvic radiotherapy.] ◀

10–26 **Drug Monitoring of Surgical Patients.** David A. Danielson, Jane B. Porter, Barbara J. Dinan, Patrick C. O'Connor, David H. Lawson, Gavin S. M. Kellaway, and Hershel Jick (Boston Univ.) conducted intensive monitoring of drugs in surgical patients in selected wards in five hospitals in the United States, Scotland, and New Zealand from 1977 to 1981. Their report describes the methods and findings from the monitoring of drugs in 5,232 such patients.

Patients were interviewed shortly after admission to the surgical

(10–26) JAMA 248:1482–1485, Sept. 24, 1982.

ward. All drugs prescribed for each patient were recorded from the physicians' order books. When use of a drug was discontinued, reasons for discontinuation were obtained along with the physician's impression of the drug's efficacy. The monitor reviewed the operating and recovery room logs, anesthetist's records, and medical records to compile a list of surgical or endoscopic procedures and drugs administered during surgery and recovery. Final editing for quality of data was performed by a computer check of biologic data for plausibility as well as completeness.

Among the 5,232 monitored patients, 4,358 (83%) underwent a surgical procedure during their hospital stay. Sixty percent of the study patients were women; 78% were younger than 66 years. The average number of exposures to drugs for all patients was 9.0. On the average, more drugs per patient were prescribed in United States hospitals than in Scotland or New Zealand hospitals. Older patients in all countries received more drugs. Drugs for pain and preoperative medication each accounted for one sixth of all drugs prescribed. In operating rooms, an average of 6 drugs were used per patient. In recovery rooms, an average of about 1.1 drugs were prescribed.

Among 46,868 drugs received on surgical wards, 1,150 (2.5%) were associated with an adverse reaction. Most of these reactions were "minor" or "moderate" in severity (95%). Twenty patients were categorized as having "life-threatening" adverse reactions. Among 5,232 patients, only 76 (1.5%) died during the monitored hospitalization. In no case was a drug implicated as the primary cause of death.

▶ [The incidence of adverse drug reactions, 2.5%, in this large series of surgical patients was lower than we would have guessed. The most common "life-threatening" adverse reactions were respiratory depression, pseudomembranous colitis, and pulmonary edema.] ◀

10–27 **Estrogens and Surgery in Women With von Willebrand's Disease** are discussed by Jack B. Alperin (Univ. of Texas Med. Branch, Galveston). von Willebrand's disease, an autosomal dominant trait, involves spontaneous bleeding from mucocutaneous surfaces and excessive blood loss after operation. Some women have less spontaneous bleeding and improved coagulation when taking oral contraceptives or when pregnant, presumably because of estrogens. The author encountered three women who, while receiving estrogen therapy, had significantly less bleeding and improved hemostasis. All had classic type I von Willebrand's disease and had previously received infusions of fresh frozen plasma or cryoprecipitate for postoperative bleeding. Two patients used oral contraceptives, whereas one took estrogen to prevent menopausal symptoms. The patients underwent major operations, while receiving estrogen therapy, with no abnormal bleeding and no need for blood component administration. Two other women with type I von Willebrand's disease also exhibited improved hemostasis on coagulation testing while taking oral contraceptives. One of them used ethynodiol diacetate with ethinyl estradiol, and the other used norethindrone with mestranol.

These women had a lifelong bleeding diathesis associated with clas-

(10–27) Am. J. Med. 73:367–371, September 1982.

sic type I von Willebrand's disease that had necessitated blood transfusions for postoperative bleeding. Each had a prolonged bleeding time and reduced plasma factor III-related coagulant, factor VIII-related antigen, and factor VIII-related von Willebrand factor values. The patients were able to undergo major operations without excessive bleeding while receiving estrogen therapy. The bleeding time improved in all clinical cases, though not to normal. The other women studied during oral contraception had increased factor VIII values. Treatment with combination oral contraceptives or conjugated estrogens for 1 to 2 months may help prepare some women with von Willebrand's disease for elective operations. Estrogen therapy may preclude the need for cryoprecipitate or fresh frozen plasma to insure hemostasis, thereby eliminating the risk of transfusion-induced hepatitis and reducing surgical costs.

▶ [These three women with von Willebrand's disease each experienced substantially less than expected bleeding with surgical procedures when they had been taking estrogen. The mechanism of improved hemostasis is unknown but the message seems clear that in a patient with this congenital disorder who is facing an elective operation, estrogen therapy should be considered.] ◀

10–28 **Thromboembolism Complicating Surgery for Cervical and Uterine Malignancy: Incidence, Risk Factors, and Prophylaxis.** Daniel L. Clarke-Pearson, Frederick R. Jelovsek, and William T. Creasman (Duke Univ.) note that venous thromboembolism is a leading cause of death and morbidity after extended surgery for early malignant conditions of the cervix and uterus. They retrospectively reviewed the data on 281 patients who underwent such surgery, evaluating for associated risk factors, incidence of clinically significant thromboembolic complications, and prophylactic value of low-dose heparin and antiembolism stockings. Diagnostic tests were interpreted by physicians who were unaware of the prophylactic methods used.

Noteworthy venous thromboembolic complications developed postoperatively in 22 (7.8%) patients. There were 3 postoperative deaths directly attributed to pulmonary embolism, and 1 patient died of multiple complications, including acute pulmonary emboli. Of these 22 patients, 10 (45%) had symptoms of thromboembolism that developed after discharge from the hospital. Preoperative risk factors found to be associated with thromboembolism, in order of statistical significance, were weight in excess of 85.5 kg, advanced clinical stage of malignant change, and radiation therapy within 6 weeks of the operative procedure. Low-dose heparin therapy and use of antiembolism stockings as preventive measures did not appear to reduce the incidence of thromboembolic complications.

Identification of these high-risk factors should lead to clinical strategies to provide optimal prophylaxis. To determine whether absence of benefit from low-dose heparin therapy and use of antiembolism stockings was due to unrecognized bias or to failure of prophylactic methods in this group of patients, a randomized controlled prospective trial has been begun.

(10–28) Obstet. Gynecol. 61:87–94, January 1983.

10–29 **Venous Thromboembolism Prophylaxis in Gynecologic Oncology: Prospective, Controlled Trial of Low-Dose Heparin.** Deep vein thrombosis and pulmonary embolism are significant complications after surgery for gynecologic malignancy. Daniel L. Clarke-Pearson, R. Edward Coleman, Ingrid S. Synan, Wanda Hinshaw, and William T. Creasman (Duke Univ.) undertook a prospective trial of low-dose heparin prophylaxis in 185 patients undergoing major surgery for known or presumed gynecologic malignancy. In addition to having the foot of the bed elevated, 88 patients received 5,000 units of sodium heparin subcutaneously 2 hours preoperatively and every 12 hours postoperatively for 1 week. The other 97 patients had the foot of the bed elevated only and were ambulated soon after the surgery. Thromboembolism was sought by ^{125}I-fibrinogen counting and impedance plethysmography and confirmed by venography.

About half of the patients had advanced or recurrent malignancy at the time of surgery. Over 75% were aged 40 or older, and nearly 32% had venous varicosities. Venous thromboembolism was diagnosed within 42 days after operation in 12 controls and 13 patients given heparin (table). Seven heparin-treated patients and 2 controls had proximal deep vein thrombosis or pulmonary embolism. One patient had a fatal pulmonary embolism. The time course for development of venous thromboembolic complications is shown in Figure 10–10. Thromboemboli occurred later in heparin-treated patients. Sev-

INCIDENCE AND LOCATION OF VENOUS THROMBOEMBOLI

	Study group				
	Control		*Low-dose heparin*		
	No.	*%*	*No.*	*%*	*Significance*
No thromboembolism	85	87.6	75	85.2	$p > 0.05$
Any thromboembolism	12	12.4	13	14.8	
Site of thromboembolism:					
Calf vein thrombi only	10		6		
Proximal DVT only	1		3		
Proximal DVT and PE	0		2		
PE only	1*		2		
Total thromboemboli	12	12.4	13	14.8	

DVT = deep venous thrombosis; PE = pulmonary embolus.
*Fatal PE arising from internal iliac vein.
(Courtesy of Clarke-Pearson, D. L., et al.: Am. J. Obstet. Gynecol. 145:606–613, March 1983.)

(10–29) Am. J. Obstet. Gynecol. 145:606–613, Mar. 1, 1983.

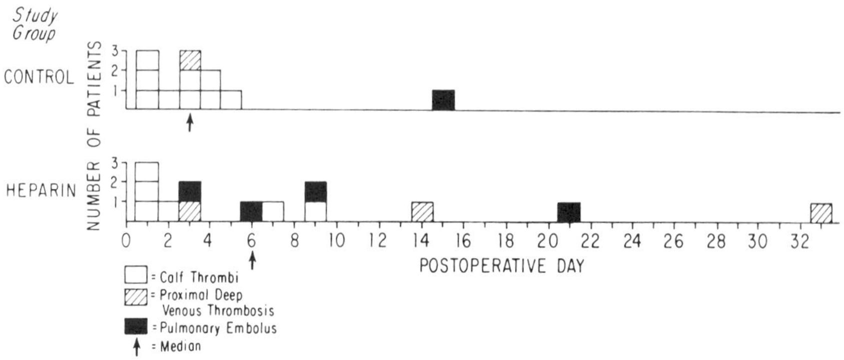

Fig 10–10.—Day postoperatively on which thromboembolism was diagnosed in control and low-dose heparin groups. (Courtesy of Clarke-Pearson, D. L., et al.: Am. J. Obstet. Gynecol. 145:606–613, Mar. 1, 1983.)

eral complications in the study group developed after heparin was discontinued.

Low-dose heparin therapy offered no significant protection against venous thromboembolism in this study of patients having major operations for gynecologic malignancy. Other studies report that low-dose heparin does not prevent thromboembolism after urologic and vascular operations. Prospective surveillance by ^{125}I-fibrinogen counting and impedance plethysmography remains the best means of detecting and treating thrombi before clinically significant thromboembolism develops.

▶ [Cancer patients have long been recognized to be predisposed to thromboembolic complications postoperatively, and obesity, an advanced stage of malignancy, and preoperative radiation are high-risk factors. This article and the one preceding it, one a retrospective study and the other prospective, come from the same authors and both seem to cast doubt on the efficacy of minidose heparin in preventing postoperative thromboembolism. In the case of the retrospective study, the lack of protection with low-dose heparin and stockings may not be surprising because it is entirely possible, perhaps even likely, that these measures were used in patients regarded as high risk and omitted in those at low risk. The lack of clear benefit in the prospective study is harder to explain and of more concern. In both reports, a large proportion of thromboembolic events in heparin-treated patients occurred after the drug was discontinued, raising the possibility of a "rebound" hypercoagulability and suggesting that heparin prophylaxis for longer than 7 days might give different results. Higher doses also should be tested.

For evaluation of a more mechanical approach to prophylaxis, read on. . . .] ◀

10–30 **Use of Graduated Compression Stockings in Prevention of Postoperative Deep Vein Thrombosis.** A. Allan, J. T. Williams, J. P. Bolton, and L. P. Le Quesne (London) examined the efficacy of thromboembolic deterrent (TED) stockings in controlling postoperative deep vein thrombosis (DVT) in 211 patients aged at least 40 years who underwent elective abdominal surgery lasting for at least 30 minutes. None had varicose veins, superficial vein thrombosis or a history of DVT or pulmonary embolism. None was receiving steroid or anticoagulant therapy. Deep vein thrombosis was diagnosed by the

(10–30) Br. J. Surg. 70:172–174, March 1983.

^{125}I-fibrinogen uptake test. Study patients were fitted the night before surgery and wore the stockings for at least a week afterward.

Stockings were worn by 97 of the 200 evaluable patients. The study and control groups were clinically comparable. Deep vein thrombosis developed in 36% of controls, bilaterally in 17, and in 15.5% of study patients, bilaterally in 2. The difference was significant. The difference in incidence of DVT was apparent both in patients younger than age 65 years and in older patients, but was more marked in the latter group. Deep vein thrombosis was less frequent in stockinged limbs both in patients operated on for benign disease and in those with malignancy.

Graduated compression stockings appear to provide an effective and safe means of preventing DVT in surgical patients. The simplicity of use of TED stockings, their relatively low cost, and the complete lack of complications associated with their use make them the most suitable means of preventing DVT in routine practice.

▶ [It is important to note that the end point here was not pulmonary embolism or clinical venous thrombosis, but a positive radioactive fibrinogen uptake test. Keeping this caveat in mind, the results reported here support the postoperative use of graduated compression stockings.] ◀

10–31 **Double-Blind Controlled Trial of Indomethacin as an Adjunct to Narcotic Analgesia After Major Abdominal Surgery.** Many of the analgesic methods used to replace or supplement opiate analgesia postoperatively provide only short-term relief or require expensive equipment or highly trained staff. Nonopiate anti-inflammatory agents can be effective in controlling postoperative pain. P. G. Reasbeck, M. L. Rice, and J. C. Reasbeck (Univ. of Otago, Dundein, New Zealand) evaluated indomethacin in a prospective, double-blind, placebo-controlled trial in patients older than age 16 who underwent laparotomy or thoracolaparotomy. They received either 100-mg indomethacin suppositories every 8 hours per rectum for 3 days, starting with the first dose of postoperative opiate analgesia, or placebo suppositories. Morphine and oral dextropropoxyphene administration were used as conventional analgesia, and antiemetics were used as required.

Forty-four of 90 patients received indomethacin suppositories. The groups were clinically comparable. Indomethacin-treated patients had significantly less pain on each of the first 4 postoperative days than did placebo patients, and they required fewer doses of morphine. Respiratory function was consistently better in the indomethacin group on the second and third postoperative days. Hospital mortality did not differ significantly in the two groups, and there were no important differences in chest infections or wound, thromboembolic, or urologic complications.

The use of indomethacin suppositories after major abdominal operations is effective in reducing the need for opiate analgesia. It is easy for staff, requires no special training, is acceptable to patients, and seems to be safe if used for short periods. Indomethacin may still be useful even where opiate can practicably be given intravenously or

---

(10–31) Lancet 2:115–117, July 17, 1982.

opiate analgesia is made more effective in controlling postoperative pain. Hemorrhagic complications have been more frequent in indomethacin-treated patients, but the significance of this finding is unclear.

▶ [Indomethacin given in large doses per rectum was a useful adjunct in providing pain relief in the postoperative period. Pain scores and morphine requirements were lower in those patients who received active drug. Does this mean we should be prescribing antiprostaglandins as postoperative analgesics? Not necessarily. These are potent drugs with effects apart from analgesia. More information is needed concerning the safety of this therapy in terms of postoperative infections, wound healing, and other factors. The indomethacin group did have an excess of hemorrhagic complications in the present study. Current means of providing pain relief to patients postoperatively are not ideal. Perhaps future studies will demonstrate that antiprostaglandin therapy is safe as well as effective.] ◀

11. Gynecologic Urology

11-1 **Unstable Female Urethra.** Ulf Ulmsten, Lars Henriksson, and Serafim Iosif (Sweden) attempted to determine the prevalence and significance of urethral instability in female patients referred for urodynamic investigation because of symptoms of urinary incontinence. Four hundred forty-seven patients with urinary incontinence were examined at the outpatient clinic and then referred and divided into two groups. Group 1 was composed of 239 women referred at the Malmö General Hospital; group 2 was composed of 208 women referred at University Hospital, Lund. Table 1 gives the diagnoses after urodynamic investigation. All patients were examined with simultaneous urethrocystometry.

Results showed urethral instability in 55 (12.3%) of the 447 patients investigated (Table 2). In group 1, 20 (8.3%) of the patients had signs of urethral instability. In group 2, urethral instability was found in 35 patients (16.8%). Urethral instability was found in 15 patients with stress incontinence, 23 with urge incontinence, and 13 with combined stress and urge incontinence (i.e., signs and symptoms of both stress and urge incontinence). In 4 patients, urethral instability was the only pathologic finding when the recordings were made. From the pressure recordings, three types of urethral instability could be recognized: type 1, relatively small fluctuations in urethral pressure at large bladder volumes; type 2, relatively large variations in urethral pressure with frequent decreases in the pressure, often combined with signs of unstable bladder; type 3, great variations in urethral pressure that had appeared already at the start of urethrocystometry, i.e., at low bladder volumes.

TABLE 1.—Diagnoses After Simultaneous Urethrocystometry in Patients With Symptoms of Urinary Incontinence

Diagnosis after simultaneous urethrocystometry	*Group 1* *No. of patients*	*Group 1* *%*	*Group 2* *No. of patients*	*Group 2* *%*
Stress incontinence	140	58.5	109	52.4
Urge incontinence	45	18.9	30	14.4
Combined stress and urge incontinence	22	9.2	31	14.9
Normal (continent)	32	13.4	38	18.3
Total	239	100.0	208	100.0

(Courtesy of Ulmsten, U., et al.: Am. J. Obstet. Gynecol. 144:93–97, Sept. 1, 1982.)

(11–1) Am. J. Obstet. Gynecol. 144:93–97, Sept. 1, 1982.

TABLE 2.—URETHRAL INSTABILITY RELATED TO SYMPTOMS OF URINARY INCONTINENCE

Diagnosis after simultaneous urethrocystometry	*No. of patients*	*Group 1*	*Group 2*
Unstable urethra only	4	3	1
Unstable urethra plus stress incontinence	15	3	12
Unstable urethra plus urge incontinence	23	10	13
Unstable urethra plus combined stress and urge incontinence	13	4	9
Total No.	55		

(Courtesy of Ulmsten, U., et al.: Am. J. Obstet. Gynecol. 144:93–97, Sept. 1, 1982.)

At present, no definitive explanation for urethral instability can be given, but it appears that urethral pressure is dependent on urethral striated muscles, urethral smooth muscles, and the vascular bed of the urethra. The disorder might then be ascribed to causes occurring within the striated and smooth muscles. Urethral instability might also be secondary to a bladder defect.

▶ [Bladder instability is recognized as a cause of female urinary incontinence, particularly nonstress type, and this large series suggests that the unstable urethra also may be responsible for urinary symptoms. Although an unstable urethra was found in all types of patients, it was more common with urge than with stress incontinence (23 of 75, or 31%, vs. 15 of 249, or 6%). Much more information about the pathophysiology of this condition is needed before anything about treatment can be suggested, but it does not seem likely that drugs used for the unstable bladder (i.e., agents to suppress the detrusor muscle) will prove effective if the urethra is at fault.] ◀

11-2 **Suburethral Diverticulum: Classification and Therapeutic Considerations.** Urethral diverticula are found in 2% to 5% of patients with genitourinary complaints. David Ginsburg and Rene Genadry (Johns Hopkins Hosp., Baltimore) reviewed the records of 70 patients (average age, 37.5 years) seen in 1955–1979 with a suburethral diverticulum. Ten patients were nulliparous. More than 90% of patients had symptoms of urinary tract infection, and 36 had a history of recurrent infections. A mass was palpated in 46 patients. All patients had a suburethral diverticulum documented by examination, urethrography, or urethroscopy.

Usually, the diverticulum was excised by dissecting the sac completely off the vaginal mucosa, excising the urethral mucosa lining the sac to the urethral communication, and closing over a transurethral catheter in a transverse plane. Acute urinary tract infection was treated before operation. Patients with chronic infection were operated on with the use of additional antibiotic coverage. Marsupialization was performed in 6 patients, and one diverticulum was managed by imbrication. Thirteen patients had recurrences. A fistula developed in 4 of 26 patients having excision of a diverticulum in the

(11–2) Obstet. Gynecol. 61:685–688, June 1983.

middle third of the urethra. One patient in this group had a postoperative stricture. In 2 patients stress incontinence developed within 2 years of the operation, and in 2 others within 1 month.

Suburethral diverticula have been ascribed to congenital, infectious, and traumatic causes. The symptoms are nonspecific and often mimic those of other urologic disorders. Excision is the most frequent form of management. Recurrences developed in 25% of patients after diverticulectomy. Some recurrences may be the result of missed or developing diverticula that are incompletely excised. Restoration of a positive closure pressure is the key factor in avoiding incontinence. Marsupialization is useful in treating distal urethral diverticula, but a tissue diagnosis must be obtained to exclude neoplasm, especially in patients with hematuria.

11-3 **Diverticulum of the Female Urethra: Postoperative Complications and Results.** Raymond A. Lee (Mayo Clinic) reports the results and complications of operations in 85 female patients with diverticulum of the urethra. The retrospective study comprised 91 patients who underwent surgical excision of the diverticulum by means of the anterior approach to the vaginal wall. The 85 patients included in this report have been followed up for 2–15 years.

Symptoms varied but most patients had urgency, frequency, dysuria, and dyspareunia. A history of urinary tract infection was common. The table shows the location of the ostium of the urethral diverticulum in the 85 patients. After surgical resection of the diverticulum, most patients (82%) had prompt and complete relief of all symptoms. A urethrovaginal fistula developed in only 1 patient after resection of 3 apparently separate diverticula. In 2 patients, urinary stress and urgency incontinence occurred during the immediate postoperative period; both patients underwent repair by the vaginal route. In 11 patients, stress incontinence developed 2 years or longer after diverticulectomy. Eight patients required 10 operations for a recurrence (or persistence) of a diverticulum.

TECHNIQUE.—A vertical incision is made in the vaginal wall; the underlying pubocervical fascia is exposed and lateral vaginal wall flaps are mobilized. The dissection of the diverticulum must be sharp, accurate, and metic-

LOCATION OF OSTIUM OF DIVERTICULUM OF FEMALE URETHRA

Site	No. of patients (N = 85)
Distal (external) third of urethra	10
Middle third of urethra	38
Proximal third of urethra (including vesical neck)	13
Multiple sites	18
Unknown	6

(Courtesy of Lee, R. A.: Obstet. Gynecol. 61:52–58, January 1983. Reprinted with permission from the American College of Obstetricians and Gynecologists.)

(11–3) Obstet. Gynecol. 61:52–58, January 1983.

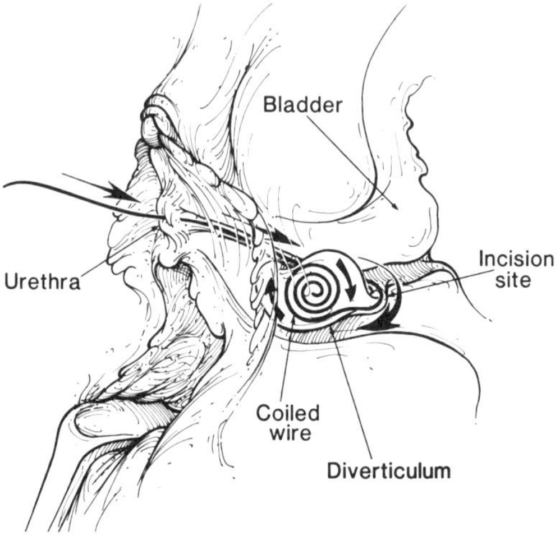

Fig 11–1.—Coiled ureteral catheter distends diverticulum and aids in identification and dissection. (Courtesy of Lee, R. A.: Obstet. Gynecol. 61:52–58, January 1983. Reprinted with permission from The American College of Obstetricians and Gynecologists.)

ulous. Preoperative placement (coiling) of a ureteral catheter within the diverticulum to distend its wall (when this can be accomplished) may enhance the identification and dissection of the diverticulum (Fig 11–1). The diverticulum is often in immediate apposition to or even perforating the pubocervical fascia. If the diverticulum is not readily apparent, a linear incision of the exposed urethral floor and passage of a probe through the ostium can aid identification. Occasionally, the sac of the diverticulum extends laterally and upward around the urethra. After closure of the urethra, and after two additional supporting layers are provided and superimposed suture lines are avoided, this method diminishes the possibility of fistular formation.

With properly selected urethral diverticula, marsupialization may provide excellent long-term results. At present, except for an occasional diverticulum located in the distal third of the urethra, transvaginal excision of the diverticulum is preferred. Resection has provided a relatively good long-term cure rate (82%) along with a low incidence of fistula (1.2%).

▶ [A suburethral diverticulum, the subject of this article and the preceding one, presents difficulties in both diagnosis and treatment. The article by Ginsburg and Genadry points out the importance of proximal or distal location of the diverticulum with respect to the choice of operative technique; marsupialization is generally simpler and better than excision for lesions arising from the distal third, but any more proximal origin requires excision.

Lee's article provides an excellent description of a technique of excision used in a large series. Figure 11–1 illustrates the neat trick of placing a coiled ureteral catheter in the diverticulum to aid in its identification in the meticulous and often tedious dissection required. The interested reader is referred to the original article for a series of very good illustrations of each step of the operative technique. The results reported are impressive indeed.] ◀

11–4 **Incompetent Urethral Closure Mechanism in Females: Experimental and Clinical Studies With Special Reference to Diagnosis and Classification.** Most operative failures after common sur-

(11–4) Urol. Int. 37:34–41, 1982.

gical techniques are found in grade III stress incontinence (incontinence in standing without strain, but continent when lying down). E. Fossberg and H. O. Beisland (Oslo) hypothesized that an endourethral weakness was causing the leakage in a great number of patients. An in vitro model system with a dual microtransducer catheter placed in a reservoir to simulate the abdominal cavity was used to test this hypothesis. Seventy-one female patients aged 12–93 years with symptoms of stress incontinence or sensory urge were observed. After the patient was asked to empty the bladder before the investigation, the proximal transducer was placed at the point of maximal urethral pressure. The bladder was filled with carbon dioxide at a rate of 50 ml per minute. Coughing vigorously provoked leakage and the pressure profile was measured. The procedure was repeated with the patient standing upright and with the bladder full.

Results show the use of water or carbon dioxide as a filling medium was indifferent because only the relation between the rise in urethral pressure and in bladder pressure was of practical importance. The increase in transmitted pressure was 25% lower when carbon dioxide was used. Incompetent urethral closure mechanism was found in three categories of female patients: (1) those with sensory urge who have an unstable urethra; (2) those with genuine stress incontinence; and (3) those who have a sphincteric insufficiency due to low maximal urethral closure pressure and atrophy of urethral mucosa. These categories were separated urodynamically with the use of simultaneous urethracystometry combined with transmission studies. Among 20 patients with sensory urge, 16 had an unstable urethra (table). Transmission studies in 51 women with symptoms of stress incontinence showed positive transmission. These patients were all elderly women with low maximal urethral closure pressure and leakage of urine due to endourethral weakness. The remaining 28 patients had negative transmission and, therefore, genuine stress incontinence. Figure 11–2 shows typical examples of sphincteric insufficiency.

Classification of the three different types of incompetent urethral closure mechanisms requires simultaneous urethracystometry, in

MAXIMAL URETHRAL CLOSURE PRESSURE IN PATIENTS WITH SENSORY URGENCY (n = 20), SPHINCTERIC INSUFFICIENCY (n = 23), AND GENUINE STRESS INCONTINENCE (n = 28)

Patient groups	Empty bladder		Full bladder		Upright position	
	mean	range	mean	range	mean	range
Sensory urgency (mean age 38 years, range 12–59)[1]						
MUCP	71	40–112	73	40–104	76	36–100
Sphincteric insufficiency (mean age 73 years, range 55–93)[2]						
MUCP	26	16–45	23	10–40	27	14–40
Genuine stress incontinence (mean age 50 years, range 33–72)[3]						
MUCP	50	24–80	41	10–72	46	16–72

[1]Negative transmission: 1 patient; unstable urethra: 16 patients.
[2]None of these patients had negative transmission in any position.
[3]Four patients had positive transmission in lithotomy position but negative trar mission when standing.
(Courtesy of Fosseberg, E., and Beisland, H. O.: Urol. Int. 37:34–41, 1982.)

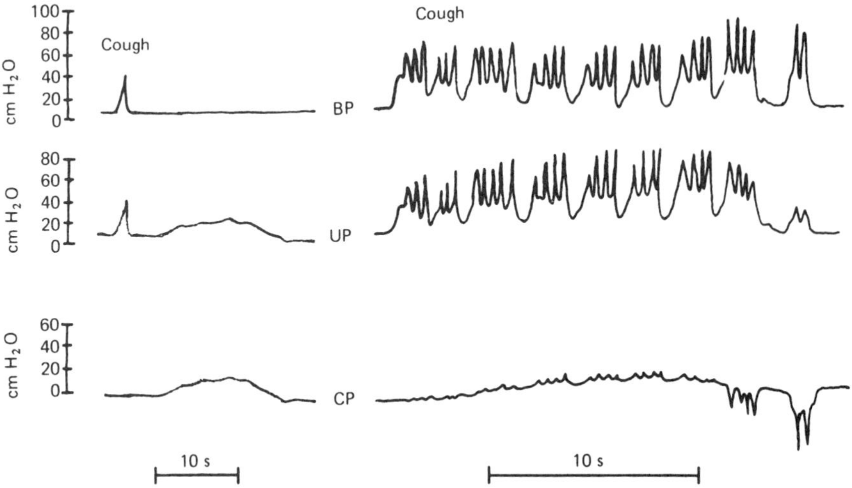

Fig 11–2.—Sphincteric insufficiency in woman, aged 65, with maximal urethral closure pressure of 16 cm H_2O and positive transmission. (Courtesy of Fossberg, E., and Beisland, H. O.: Urol. Int. 37:34–41, 1982.)

which transmission studies are mandatory; this is the most appropriate way to distinguish between patients who will benefit from an operation and patients who will not.

11–5 **Significance of Urethral Vascular Pulsations in Genuine Stress Urinary Incontinence.** Several factors help maintain a positive closure pressure in the female urethra at rest: smooth urethral sphincter, striated urethral sphincter, suburethral vascular plexus, and intrinsic elasticity of urethral mucosa. Figure 11–3 shows that urethral pressure recordings frequently contain low-amplitude pressure pulsations in the area of peak urethral pressure. David B. Hebert, Larry N. Francis, and Donald R. Ostergard (Univ. of California, Irvine) attempted to delineate the relationship between loss of vascular pulsations in the urethra and the presence of urethral sphincter weakness in genuine stress incontinence. One hundred women with this condition were selected for the study; 50 controls also were selected, 25 were asymptomatic and the other 25 had urinary tract symptoms but were stress continent. All patients underwent detailed urodynamic analysis by means of microtip catheter transducers and multichannel recording techniques.

Among the 100 study subjects, 85 lacked urethral vascular pulsations on the resting urethral closure pressure profile, which showed characteristic urodynamic findings of genuine stress incontinence. Seventy-six (89%) had a decrease in urethral closure pressure when the profile was performed with the patient in the sitting position with a full bladder. Fifteen patients with objective clinical evidence of genuine stress incontinence had urethral vascular pulsations on the resting pressure profile. The difference was statistically significant. Mean

(11–5) Am. J. Obstet. Gynecol. 144:828–835, Dec. 1, 1982.

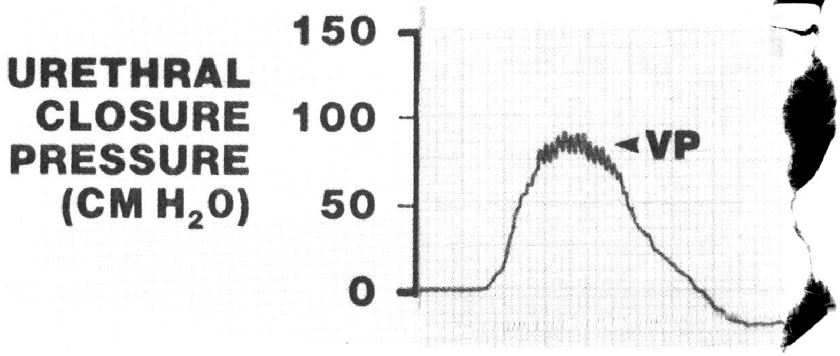

Fig 11–3.—Vascular pulsations *(VP)* in urethral closure pressure profile. Pulsations occur in synchrony with pulse rate of subject. (Courtesy of Herbert, D. B., et al.: Am. J. Obstet. Gynecol. 144:828–835, Dec. 1, 1982.)

functional urethral length in patients with vascular pulsations was 3.1 cm in the supine position. This measurement was significantly longer than that in those patients without vascular pulsations. The subgroup of genuine stress incontinence with vascular pulsations at rest was younger (42.3 years vs. 52 years) and more often premenopausal (93% vs. 36%) than those without vascular pulsations (table). Only 13% of patients with vascular pulsations had undergone a previous operation for incontinence.

Urethral sphincter weakness is a major cause of failure in operations for incontinence. Further studies are necessary to determine whether the woman with a normal sphincter and genuine stress incontinence responds differently to therapy than the woman with genuine stress incontinence and urethral sphincter weakness, although physiologic measurements suggest that the presence of urethral vascular pulsations is a good prognostic sign for successful surgical cure of genuine stress incontinence.

▶ [This report from California and the preceding one from Norway make similar points. Patients with apparent stress incontinence may have normal or low urethral closure pressures. In the first situation (associated with vascular pulsations in the California study), the problem is that there is descent of the urethrovesical junction

Age, Gravidity, Parity, and Menopausal Status of Patients With Genuine Stress Incontinence*

	GSI with vascular pulsations (n = 15)	*GSI without vascular pulsations (n = 85)*	*Significance*
Age	42.3 ± 7.0	52.0 ± 12.4	$p < 0.01$
Gravidity	4.8 ± 4.1	3.8 ± 3.3	NS
Parity	3.8 ± 2.3	2.9 ± 1.7	NS
Premenopausal (%)	93	36	$p < 0.001$
Postmenopausal (%)	7	64	$p < 0.001$

*GSI = genuine stress incontinence; NS = not statistically significant.

(Courtesy of Hebert, D. B., et al.: Am. J. Obstet. Gynecol. 144:828–835, Dec. 1, 1982.)

with poor transmission of intra-abdominal pressure to the upper urethra. An operation that restores the urethrovesical junction to its proper location will work. In the second situation, there is "sphincteric" weakness of the urethra and the closure pressures are low, even though in certain patients there is appropriate transmission of intra-abdominal pressure, as Figure 11–2 indicates. Most patients in the second report had low closure pressures, suggesting to the authors that most patients with stress incontinence have urethras disadvantaged by more than just their position. In both series, urethral closure pressures were lower in older women. Those patients with stress incontinence and low closure pressures apparently require more than just replacement of the bladder neck. Possible adjunctive measures are Kegel's exercises, estrogen therapy, and urethral plication. Studies of the effects of various therapies on the urethral pressure profile are needed.] ◀

11–6 **Diagnosis of Lower Urinary Tract Disorders in Postmenopausal Patients.** Gynecologists are seeing increasing numbers of postmenopausal patients with urinary tract symptoms. A. E. Bent, D. A. Richardson, and D. R. Osteegard (Irvine, Calif.) evaluated 100 consecutive patients older than age 60 who were referred to a gynecologic-urology unit with urinary tract symptoms. Hysterectomy had been performed in 50, anterior repair in 32, and a retropubic operation for incontinence in 16. The primary diagnoses are listed in Table 1 and all diagnoses in Table 2. Patients with the most common primary diagnoses had great overlap in symptoms. True stress incontinence was confirmed by urodynamic testing in two thirds of patients with this symptom. In 40% of patients who had both urgency and urge incontinence, an unstable bladder was demonstrated by water cystometry. The Q-tip test was not specific for true stress incontinence. Urethral syndrome was more frequent in patients younger than age 70 years and unstable bladder in older patients.

The urodynamic findings in women older than age 60 with lower urinary tract symptoms cannot be predicted from the history and physical findings. Over two thirds of the patients in this study had primary diagnosis of urethral syndrome, true stress incontinence, or unstable bladder. Extensive evaluation of these postmenopausal pa-

TABLE 1.—PRIMARY DIAGNOSES IN 100 POSTMENOPAUSAL PATIENTS

	<70 yr		*>70 yr*			
Primary diagnosis	*No.*	*%*	*No.*	*%*	*Total*	*Significance**
Urethral syndrome	23	40	6	14	29	$p < 0.01$
Genuine stress incontinence	14	25	7	16	21	N/S
Unstable bladder	6	10	13	30	19	$p < 0.05$
Hypoestrogenism	2	4	5	12	7	N/S
Pelvic relaxation	5	9	1	2	6	N/S
Other	7	12	11	26	18	
Total	57		43		100	

*Age < 70 years compared with age > 70 years.

(Courtesy of Bent, A. E., et al.: Am. J. Obstet. Gynecol. 145:218–222, Jan. 15, 1983.)

(11–6) Am. J. Obstet. Gynecol. 145:218–222, Jan. 15, 1983.

TABLE 2.—ALL DIAGNOSES IN 100 POSTMENOPAUSAL PATIENTS

Hypoestrogenism	41
Urethral syndrome	38
Genuine stress incontinence	33
Unstable bladder	24
Pelvic relaxation	11
Distal urethral stenosis	10
Radiation changes	5
Unstable urethra	4
Urinary tract infection	3
Rigid urethra	3
Other	27
Total	199

(Courtesy of Bent, A. E., et al.: Am. J. Obstet. Gynecol. 145:218–222, Jan. 15, 1983.)

tients is necessary to determine the cause of incontinence before operation is undertaken. Operation, where indicated, is individualized. Patients who are not candidates for operation may be significantly improved by treatment with an α-adrenergic stimulator such as phenylpropanolamine. Most patients with unstable bladder remain continent as long as the urethral sphincter mechanism is intact. These patients can be treated with an anticholinergic, dicyclomine, or imipramine. Those who fail to respond are managed by bladder drill, pelvic floor stimulation, or both.

▶ [This is a nice summary of urinary complaints in postmenopausal women. The most common primary diagnoses, in order of frequency, were urethral syndrome, genuine stress incontinence, and unstable bladder. However, among all diagnoses, hypoestrogenism was the most frequent. The value of urodynamic studies is illustrated by the fact that only two thirds of the patients with symptomatic stress incontinence had genuine stress incontinence by urodynamic criteria. Perhaps the most important clinical finding is that less than 30% of the patients were candidates for a surgical procedure.] ◀

11–7 **Clinical and Urodynamic Effects of Anterior Colporrhaphy and Vaginal Hysterectomy for Prolapse With and Without Incontinence** were assessed by Stuart L. Stanton, Paul Hilton, Christine Norton (St. George's Hosp., London) and Linda Cardozo (King's College Hosp., London) in a prospective study of 73 women (mean age, 53 years) who had anterior colporrhaphy with or without vaginal hysterectomy. Independent peak flow rate was measured and videocystourethrography (VCU) was performed before operation and at 3 to 4 months after operation. Follow-up continued for 2 years by using clinical methods and the Urilos test.

Before operation, 47 women complained of stress incontinence, but on clinical examination and VCU such a condition could be confirmed in only 29 patients. As shown in the table, symptoms of urge and stress incontinence and prolapse were significantly improved after operation, but VCU and Urilos testing showed stress incontinence was

(11–7) Br. J. Obstet. Gynaecol. 89:459–463, May 1982.

SYMPTOMATOLOGY AND SIGNS BEFORE OPERATION (PRE-OP.) AND AT 3 MONTHS AND 2 YEARS AFTER OPERATION

	Incontinent patients			Continent patients		
Details	Pre-op. ($n = 29$)	3 months	2 years ($n = 11$)	Pre-op. ($n = 44$)	3 months	2 years ($n = 24$)
Symptoms						
Urgency	6	8	3	9	6	3
Urge incontinence	16*	8*	5	12*	6*	1
Frequency	7	4	1	7	3	0
Stress incontinence	27*	8*	4	20*	8*	3
Voiding difficulty	5	3	4	8	3	2
Prolapse	16*	3*	1	39*	7*	0
Vaginal findings						
Cystocele	8	1	0	6	0	3
Cystourethrocele	12	2	0	28	0	2
Cervix or vault descent	4	0	0	15	1	0
Enterocele	3	0	0	1	2	2

*Significance of difference (X^2 test): $P < .01$.
(Courtesy of Stanton, S. L., et al.: Br. J. Obstet. Gynaecol. 89:459–463, May 1982.)

still present in 20 patients who were initially incontinent and in 5 who were initially continent. Prolapse recurred in some patients as early as 3 months after operation; later recurrences were also found, confirming the need to extend follow-up to at least 1 year to detect these later failures. Urodynamic data showed that for both initially incontinent and continent women, surgery had minimal effect on bladder function. For the incontinent group, milkback and elevation of the bladder neck were improved. For the continent group, first sensation was delayed and bladder neck elevation improved.

Overall, there was no evidence that bladder and urethral function was compromised by anterior colporrhaphy and vaginal hysterectomy. No increases were found in detrusor instability or voiding difficulties as measured by flow rate, maximum voiding pressure, or residual urine volume.

▶ [The proper operative approach for urinary stress incontinence has recently become a matter of considerable controversy. The traditional view that the woman with any significant degree of pelvic relaxation should be approached vaginally is being challenged by arguments that stress incontinence, regardless of whether or not a cystocele is present, should be dealt with by an abdominal approach. The results of this study seem to support traditional teaching, for incontinent women were clinically improved after colporrhaphy. The urodynamic studies did not seem to shed much light on the problem of why some patients fail to improve, or actually get worse, with vaginal repair.

In a related study, Walter and colleagues (*Br. J. Urol.* 54:377, 1982) described urodynamic evaluations before and after vaginal repair or retropubic suspension. Vaginal repair led to a decrease in urethral resistance, whereas the retropubic operation resulted in increased outflow resistance, indicating that the latter should be avoided in patients with poor detrusor function.] ◀

11–8 **Anatomical Explanation for Bladder Dysfunction Following Rectal and Uterine Surgery.** Previous reports indicate that bladder

(11–8) Br. J. Urol. 54:501–504, October 1982.

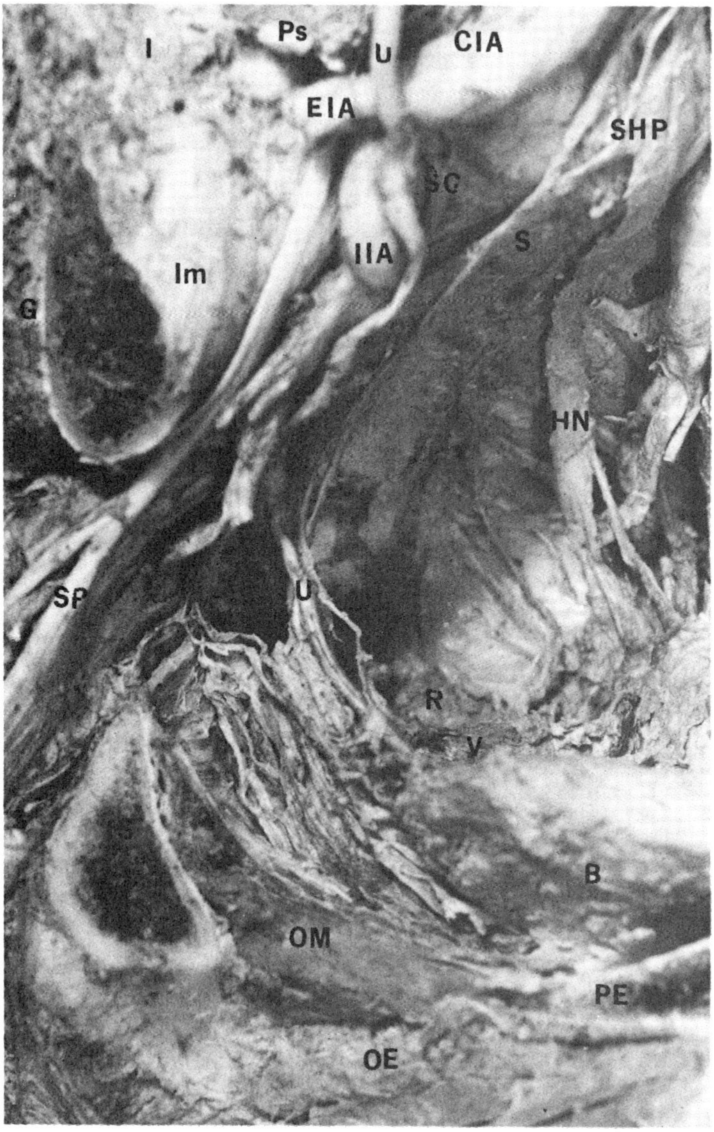

Fig 11–4.—Female pelvis, right anterior oblique view. To show the position of the pelvic plexus, the acetabulum and adjacent bone of the right lateral pelvic wall have been removed. The uterus, cervix, upper two thirds of the rectum, iliac venous system, and distal ramifications of the iliac arteries on the right also have been removed. (*Im,* ilium; *Is,* ischium; *Ps,* psoas; *OM,* obturator membrane and obturator internus; *OE,* obturator externus; *G,* gluteal muscles; *I,* iliacus; *IIA,* internal iliac artery, *CIA,* common iliac artery; *HN,* hypogastric nerves; *SHP,* superior hypogastric plexus (presacral nerve); *SC,* sacral sympathetic chain; *PE,* pubis; *SP,* sacral plexus. (Courtesy of Mundy, A. R.: Br. J. Urol. 54:501–504, October 1982.)

dysfunction can result from previous abdominoperineal resection of the rectum, but probably not from previous hysterectomy. A. R. Mundy (Guy's Hosp., London) assessed by pelvic dissections in 3 male and 9 female cadavers the vulnerability of the pelvic nerves and pelvic plexus to damage during these two procedures. In only one dissection did the S2 nerve root contribute to the pelvic parasympathetic nerves. The presacral fascia becomes the posterior layer of the hypogastric sheath shortly after the nerves enter it; the nerves then pass into the sheath to run below and medial to the visceral branches of the internal iliac vessels (Fig 11–4). In the female, the bulk of the pelvic plexus lies below the broad ligament on the lateral wall of the upper third of the vagina, although its upper fibers usually extend into the cardinal ligament that forms the base of the broad ligament. In males, the medial aspect of the pelvic plexus is more closely related to the lower rectum. In both sexes, the pelvic nerves are "tented" away from the posterolateral pelvic wall when the rectum is pulled anteriorly or to one side, but this does not occur if the capsule is first separated from the rectum.

The pelvic parasympathetic nerves and pelvic plexus appear to be much more vulnerable during rectal surgery than during uterine surgery. Only if the cardinal ligaments or an unusually long cuff of upper vagina is removed at hysterectomy is the field of excision likely to involve the pelvic plexus. The pelvic parasympathetic nerves and posterior pelvic plexus can be damaged directly during dissection on the anterolateral aspect of the lower rectum, especially in men. In addition, traction injury of the pelvic nerves can occur during mobilization of the lower rectum. This may cause only a temporary disorder of bladder function if the axons are not actually disrupted. Greater care during mobilization of the rectum and during dissection in this region could reduce the occurrence of complications from disruption of the pelvic nerves.

▶ [This article is proof that there is still something to be learned from gross anatomical studies. We were all taught that the pelvic plexus or ganglion of Frankenhäuser lies in the base of the broad ligament, but this careful dissection demonstrates that it is mostly somewhat lower than this, lateral to the upper vagina. Thus, it is usually not touched during ordinary hysterectomy. Radical hysterectomy, on the other hand, involves removal of both the cardinal ligament and upper vagina, and this is apparently the reason that bladder dysfunction is a fairly frequent postoperative occurrence.] ◀

11–9 **Pathologic Effect of Ureteral Ligation, With Clinical Implications.** Iatrogenic ureteral injury from radical pelvic surgery continues to occur. J. I. Gurin, Roger L. Garcia, Arnold Melman, and Elliot Leiter (Beth Israel Med. Center, New York) examined the effects of ureteral ligations of various durations on the ureter of the male rat. Placement of a chromic gut ligature around the ureter in its lower third was followed by deligation after periods ranging from 5 minutes to 72 hours. Simple deligation of a ureter tied for as long as 24 hours resulted in complete resolution of injury, with no gross or microscopic evidence of trauma. Hydroureter was seen after 48 and 72 hours of ligation, besides classic hydronephrosis. The dilatation improved only slightly in up to a month after deligation.

The findings suggest that if a crush injury of the ureter is appreciated at the time of a pelvic operation, removal of the crushing clamp,

---

(11–9) J. Urol. 128:1404–1406, December 1982.

and/or removal of the constricting ligature, should be adequate. If ureteral obstruction is unsuspected at operation and becomes apparent more than 24 hours after crash injury, deligation with ureteral stenting should yield a satisfactory outcome. Ureteral catheter drainage should not be necessary for much longer than 2 weeks. The advisability of deligation versus resection and reconstruction for injuries of more than 72 hours' duration remains unclear.

▶ [This study was done in rats, so the usual caveat concerning extrapolation to women must be made. The implication here is that ureteral ligation or clamping noted at operation, or within 24 hours, probably can be managed safely simply by removing the offending suture or clamp. Histologic evidence of repair is seen within 24 hours of injury. Initially, this involves proliferation of the lining epithelium in the adjacent uninjured ureteral segments.

Another approach to ureteral obstruction secondary to absorbable suture entrapment (nephrostomy and observation) was described in the 1983 YEAR BOOK (p. 266).] ◀

11–10 **Single Ectopic Ureter.** In contrast to reports in the English literature, most reports of ectopic ureters in Japan describe single collecting systems; also, the anomaly is more frequent in females in Japan, with drainage to the vagina. Toshiaki Gotoh, Hajime Morita, Sohei Tokunaka, Tomohiko Koyanagi, and Ichiro Tsuji (Hokkaido Univ., Sapporo, Japan) report data on single ureteric ectopia in 17 female and 4 male patients seen in Japan from 1962 to 1981. The condition was bilateral in 2 patients. Incomplete duplication was present in 2 ureters. One patient was a neonate, 3 others were younger than age 1 year, 8 were aged 1–7 years, and 9 were aged 26 or older. Wetting and fever were frequent findings. Nine ureters in females drained to the vagina. Usually, endoscopic or operative confirmation of ectopia is necessary. Endoscopy localized 9 ectopic ureteral orifices in the present series. Vaginography or administration of intravenous contrast medium showed reflux or staining in 5 instances. The kidney was not visualized on urography in 16 patients. Twenty patients had malformed kidneys, and 15 had dysplasia. Several ectopic ureters refluxed. Three patients had spina bifida occulta.

Treatment depends on the functional state of the kidney and the condition of the contralateral urinary tract. Most unilateral conditions require nephroureterectomy. If the ipsilateral kidney has useful function or the other side is abnormal, reimplantation of the ureter into the bladder is indicated. Nephrectomy was done on the ectopic side in 11 patients with unilateral ectopia, and all but 1 did well. Five patients had total nephroureterectomy. Six ureters underwent renal-conserving procedures, and 4 patients had ureteral reimplantation to the bladder.

Two thirds of ectopic ureters in Japan are associated with single collecting systems. Renal dysplasia in vaginal ectopia has not been as severe as in males with a comparable degree of genital ectopia. Total excision of the ureteral stump is necessary in patients with urethral ectopia in order to avoid postoperative problems.

▶ [This report describes 17 women with single ectopic ureter, of which 9 had a vaginal orifice, a large series because, according to the authors, the English language

---

(11–10) J. Urol. 129:271–274, February 1983.

literature contains only 16 reported cases. The presenting symptom was usually incontinence, making it likely that the gynecologist might see this problem initially. Diagnosis is difficult. Treatment depends on the functional status of the kidneys and the location of the orifice; if the ipsilateral kidney is impaired and the contralateral one is normal, nephroureterectomy is usually the best choice.] ◀

11–11 **Control of Recurrent Lower Urinary Tract Infection in the Postmenopausal Woman.** Management of recurrent infection of the lower urinary tract in postmenopausal women can be a difficult problem, especially among diabetics. Long-term suppressive antibacterial therapy may fail because of infection with various bacterial species other than *Escherichia coli.* C. Lowell Parsons and Joseph D. Schmidt (Univ. of California, San Diego) evaluated a treatment approach based on the work of Cox et al., indicating that bacteria migrate from the rectum to colonize the perineum and urethra as a prelude to cystitis. Augmentation of vaginal antibacterial defenses should interrupt this process. Low-dosage intravaginal estrogen treatment was evaluated in 5 postmenopausal women, aged 46–66 years, who had culture-proved recurrent cystitis that had resisted conventional treatment for 1½–4 years. All had had at least three infectious episodes in the past 3 months. Antibiotic therapy was given for 3 days if initial vaginal cultures were positive, followed by a nightly dose of suppressive therapy with an appropriate antibiotic until the pathogen disappeared. Conjugated estrogen was delivered intravaginally in a dosage of 0.3 mg daily for 7 days, followed by 0.3 mg every 2 days for a week, and then 0.3 mg every third day until a normal vaginal flora returned. The dose then was reduced to maintain a vaginal pH of 4.0–4.6.

Growth of enterobacteria in the vagina was reduced or eliminated in all 5 patients during estrogen therapy. The vaginal pH regularly declined to 4.0–4.6. Usually maintenance therapy was necessary at 4- to 7-day intervals. On follow-up for 10–15 months, 4 patients have had no urinary tract infections. One patient had a urinary tract infection during a flare of colitis, requiring antibiotics and an increased dosage of estrogen.

Growth of pathogens in the vagina in postmenopausal women with recurrent cystitis can be controlled by low-dosage intravaginal estrogen therapy. A rapid decrease in vaginal pH, disappearance of enterobacteria from the vagina, and a marked reduction in the frequency of urinary tract infections result from this treatment. The brief course of antibiotics used to clear cystitis is not thought to have had much if any sustained effect on the vaginal flora.

▶ [This is a small series, but the suggestion to treat postmenopausal women with recurrent urinary tract infections with intravaginal estrogen therapy in an attempt to alter the vaginal and perineal flora makes sense and is probably worth a try. If this therapy is utilized over the long-term and if the uterus is in situ, a supplemental 7- to 10-day course of a progestin should become part of the monthly regimen.] ◀

11–12 **Single-Dose Amoxicillin Therapy With Follow-up Urine Culture: Effective Initial Management for Acute Uncomplicated Urinary Tract Infections.** There is no single widely accepted protocol for the management of acute symptomatic urinary tract infections

(11–11) J. Urol. 128:1224–1226, December 1982.
(11–12) Am. J. Med. 73:808–813, December 1982.

in female patients. Marie Savard-Fenton, Bradley W. Fenton, L. Barth Reller, Brian A. Lauer, and Richard L. Byyny (Univ. of Colorado) undertook a prospective comparison of a single dose of amoxicillin with 2 weeks of amoxicillin therapy with follow-up culture for initial treatment of uncomplicated, acute urinary tract infections in female patients aged 16 and older. Patients randomly received either 3 gm of amoxicillin trihydrate orally or 250 mg three times daily for 2 weeks. The single dose was taken under observation. Significant bacteriuria was present in about half of the 388 patients in the study, and 162 bacteriuric women returned for follow-up urine cultures at 1 week.

The single dose of amoxicillin led to negative cultures at 1 week in 61% of patients. The cure rate for patients without antibody-coated bacteria in the urine was 77%. Treatment with amoxicillin for 2 weeks led to negative cultures in 74% of patients and in all patients without antibody-coated bacteria in the urine. Four of 12 patients with ampicillin-resistant organisms were cured by single-dose therapy and 6 of 15 by conventional treatment over 2 weeks. Adverse effects were half as frequent with single-dose therapy as with conventional treatment. Three conventionally treated patients were withdrawn because of side effects. No patient had to be hospitalized because of complications of urinary tract infection.

One 3-gm of amoxicillin with follow-up urine culture constitutes effective, safe management for nonpregnant female patients, with acute, uncomplicated urinary tract infections. The follow-up culture can be done by dipslide 3 to 7 days after treatment to identify women who require further specific antimicrobial therapy. Single-dose treatment could lead to substantial cost savings.

▶ [A single 3-gm dose of amoxicillin performed nearly as well as a 14-day regimen in this study of women with acute urinary tract infections. The authors recommend follow-up urine cultures 3–7 days after treatment to identify those patients with persistent infections who require additional therapy. A different view concerning follow-up urine cultures was presented in the 1982 YEAR BOOK (pp. 275–276). In the present series, only half of the patients treated had significant bacteriuria on initial culture. Many different management plans have been advocated for the treatment of acute urinary tract infections in women; we don't think there is a clear-cut "best" choice.] ◀

11–13 **Nonoperative Supravesical Urinary Diversion in Obstetrics and Gynecology.** Indwelling ureteral stent catheters have been used successfully to treat ureteral obstruction and fistula. Hugh A. G. Fisher, Alan H. Bennet, Donald J. Rivard, Thomas Caputo, and Martin Goldman (Albany Med. College, New York) evaluated various types of stent catheters in 25 obstetric-gynecologic patients who required relief of upper urinary tract obstruction. Twenty-one patients had advanced cervical cancer, 2 had hydronephrosis of pregnancy, and 1 each had endometrial cancer and a ureteral stricture due to node dissection for endometrial cancer. Fifteen patients had bilateral obstruction. Eleven patients were azotemic or uremic at the time of presentation. Eight had flank pain. Ureteral obstruction generally was diagnosed by means of intravenous pyelography. A Gibbons cath-

(11–13) Gynecol. Oncol. 14:365–372, 1982.

eter was used in 1 patient, the Cook double pigtail polyethylene catheter in three cases, and the Finney double J type in 19. In 2 patients the catheter was made from 7 F opaque, open-ended polyethylene tubing and fed to the renal pelvis over a wire stylet. Four patients underwent percutaneous nephrostomy after endoscopic placement failed.

Initial endoscopic placement was successful in 17 of the 22 patients with carcinoma. Renal function improved in 8 of 9 azotemic patients, and pain was relieved in all 9 patients affected. Most failures were attributable to difficulty in visualizing the ureteral orifices because of edema, tumor involvement of the trigonal region, or acute angulation of the intramural ureter. Only 1 patient with cancer eventually required placement of a surgical stent. The patients with benign conditions were successfully treated by placement of an endoscopic stent. Two patients had flank pain on the stented side without evidence of infection or obstruction. One patient had febrile urinary tract infection, and another, intermittent gross hematuria. Three patients had minor urinary frequency due to trigonal irrigation. Seven patients had stent obstruction after 4–12 weeks; all stents were readily replaced while the patient received local anesthesia.

An indwelling ureteral stent can be placed endoscopically using local anesthesia to palliate ureteral obstruction. External urine-collecting devices are not necessary. The procedure permits radiotherapy or chemotherapy to be administered. Complications are relatively minor. Several patients have been able to return to normal activities for significant periods after nonoperative treatment.

▶ [Semantically, it is arguable whether insertion of a ureteral catheter or percutaneous nephrostomy is "nonoperative," but—in any event—it is less "operative" than a more major procedure. This collection indicates that it usually works well enough in most cases to allow more definitive therapy to take place. The majority of applicable cases will involve malignant disease, and it is the patient whose initial presentation is uremia due to ureteral obstruction who is most likely to benefit. This article doesn't provide a breakdown between primary and recurrent cancer cases, but it does mention that four patients are in long-term remission following radiation therapy.] ◀

12. Tumors

12–1 **Expression of Herpes Simplex Virus Type 2 Antigens in Premalignant and Malignant Human Vulvar Cells.** Not only has the incidence of in situ and invasive carcinoma of the vulva increased, a higher frequency of vulvar carcinoma in association with other genital cancers also has been reported. This suggests that a common pathogenic factor may be involved in these malignancies. G. A. Cabral, F. Marciano-Cabral, D. Fry, C. K. Lumpkin, L. Mercer, and D. Goplerud (Med. College of Virginia, Richmond) examined vulvar biopsies and explants from patients with vulvitis, hyperkeratosis, condyloma acuminatum, severe dysplasia, and squamous cell carcinoma for the presence of herpes simplex virus type 2 (HSV2) antigens.

Indirect immunoperoxidase staining for VP143, an early nonstructural polypeptide of HSV2, was readily seen in 1 of 3 biopsy specimens showing severe dysplasia, 3 of 7 specimens exhibiting carcinoma in situ, and in 1 of 3 specimens with invasive squamous cell carcinoma (Fig 12–1). The staining was localized in areas showing dysplasia or carcinoma cells and was especially prominent in the basal layer of the dermis in biopsy specimens from patients with severe dysplasia or carcinoma in situ. Staining for VP119, the major envelope glycoprotein of HSV2, revealed a similar but less intense pattern of staining and was observed only in specimens that were positive for VP143. Both VP143 and VP119 were expressed in the absence of staining for virus capsid proteins, demonstration of virus structures by electron microscopy, and isolation of infectious virus by cocultivation. In addition, staining for VP157, the major capsid protein of HSV2, was negative, indicating that only a fraction of the virus genome was expressed. Explants from patients with invasive squamous cell carcinomas showed staining for VP143 and VP119. The staining for VP143 showed a prominent perinuclear pattern within the cytoplasm, but staining for VP119 was generally dispersed throughout the cytoplasm. Biopsy specimens from patients with vulvitis, hyperkeratosis, or condyloma acuminatum did not stain for VP143 or VP119.

The fact that 38% of the biopsy specimens derived from patients with premalignant and malignant vulvar disease stained positive for VP143 and VP119, despite the absence of productive viral infection, indicates that a close relationship may exist between HSV2 and squamous cell carcinoma of the vulva.

▶ [These findings of localization of HSV2 antigens in some specimens of dysplasia and invasive carcinoma of the vulva suggest that herpesvirus plays a role in the development of vulvar cancer, as previously has been proposed in the case of cervical cancer.] ◀

(12–1) Am. J. Obstet. Gynecol. 143:611–619, July 15, 1982.

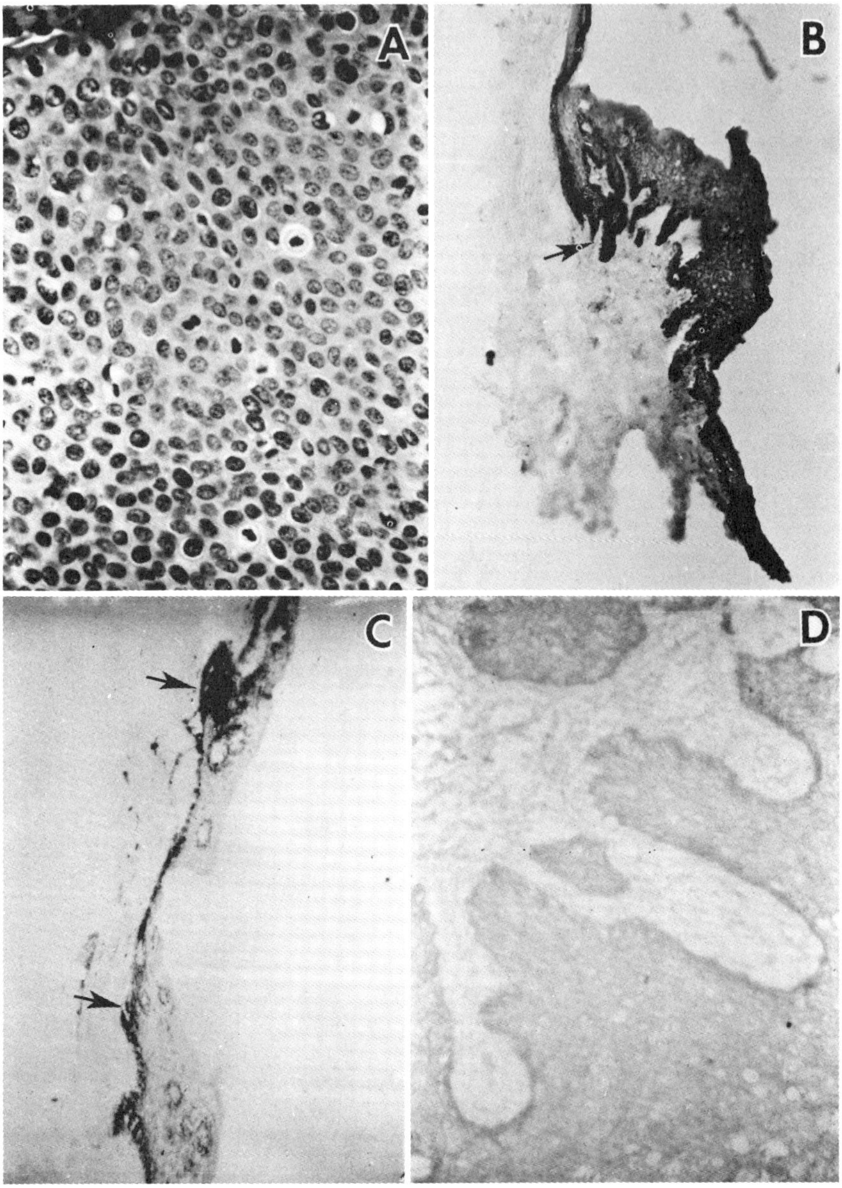

Fig 12–1.—**A,** in situ squamous cell carcinoma of vulva of patient aged 21 years. Hematoxylin-eosin; ×600. **B,** immunoperoxidase staining of same biopsy specimen for VP143. There is intense staining for this early nonstructural β-polypeptide of HSV2 *(arrow)*; ×200. **C,** immunoperoxidase staining of same specimen with VP119. Although staining is distributed throughout dermis, it is most preponderant in basal layer *(arrows)*; ×200. **D,** vulvar biopsy specimen from patient aged 19 years with condyloma acuminatum and stained for VP143 as control. There is absence of staining, especially in basal layer, in contrast to that seen in in situ squamous cell carcinoma. (Courtesy of Cabral, G. A., et al.: Am. J. Obstet. Gynecol. 143:611–619, July 15, 1982.)

12–2 **Verrucous Carcinoma of the Vulva: Study of 24 Cases.** Hugo Japaze, Tung van Dinh, and J. Donald Woodruff (Johns Hopkins Hosp., Baltimore) describe the important histopathologic features and clinical course of 24 cases of verrucous carcinoma of the vulva. Age range of the patients was 29 to 86 years (average, 54 years). Three patients (12.5%) had evidence of syphilitic infection manifested by positive serology.

The lesions were prominent gray-white fugating cauliflower-like masses resembling large condylomata acuminata. In 9 cases (37%) there were varying degrees of ulceration. Most lesions were localized to the labia majora. In 5 cases the lesions were so extensive that recognition of the site of origin was impossible. The tumors were composed of papillary fronds of mature stratified squamous epithelium that locally infiltrated the stroma with pushing bulbous rete pegs. Hyperkeratosis was often extensive.

Treatment included simple vulvectomy, radical vulvectomy, and bilateral lymph node dissection followed by irradiation. Lymph nodes were not involved in any of the 17 patients treated by radical vulvectomy and regional lymph node dissection. Recurrences developed in 9 patients, 5 of whom had undergone previous irradiation. The shortest interval between surgery and recurrence was 5 months, the longest was 10 years. Among the 17 patients who were treated by surgery alone, there were 5 deaths, only 1 of which was due to tumor. Thus, the corrected 5-year survival rate in the group which had surgery alone was 94%. In contrast, 4 of 7 patients treated by surgery and irradiation died of disease, a survival rate of only 42%.

The finding of massive condylomata acuminata that are resistant to treatment, particularly in patients older than age 40, should suggest the possibility of verrucous carcinoma of the vulva. Extensive biopsy specimens that include the underlying tissue should be taken. The tumor should be treated by wide local excision. Radiation therapy has not proved to be therapeutically useful.

▶ [Verrucous carcinoma of the vulva, recognized over the past 15 years, is a bulky, cauliflower-like tumor, biopsies of which are often too superficial to demonstrate invasion, leading to a misdiagnosis of condyloma or papilloma. This report of a large series from Johns Hopkins Hospital emphasizes the pertinent clinical and pathologic points. Most significant is the finding that lymph node metastases were absent in all patients in the series and in the literature in whom nodes were removed. Thus, lymphadenectomy is probably unnecessary.] ◀

12–3 **Primary Carcinoma of the Bartholin Gland: A Report of 14 Cases and Review of the Literature.** Ronald S. Leuchter, Neville F. Hacker, Richard L. Voet, Jonathan S. Berek, Duane E. Townsend, and Leo D. Lagasse reviewed data on all patients with a primary malignancy in the Bartholin gland who were seen between January 1955 and December 1980 at the University of California, Los Angeles, Medical Center.

Of the 14 patients, 12 were white and 2 black. The average parity was 1. The right Bartholin gland was involved in 8 cases and the left in 6. The most common presenting complaint was a vulvar mass (10

(12–2) Obstet. Gynecol. 60:462–466, October 1982.
(12–3) Ibid., pp. 361–368, September 1982.

TABLE 1.—PELVIC LYMPH NODE STATUS BY INGUINAL LYMPH NODE STATUS IN CANCER OF BARTHOLIN'S GLAND

	Inguinal femoral lymph nodes	Pelvic lymph nodes	
		Negative	Positive
Negative	14	14	0
Positive	11	9	2
Total	25	23	2
Percent		92	8

(Courtesy of Leuchter, R. S., et al.: Obstet. Gynecol. 60:361–368, September 1982. Reprinted with permission from The American College of Obstetricians and Gynecologists.)

cases). Nonspecific perineal pain was noted in 2 patients. Duration of symptoms before diagnosis was 1–12 months (mean, 4 months). There were 7 squamous carcinomas, 5 adenocarcinomas, 1 mixed adenosquamous carcinoma, and 1 transitional cell carcinoma. In 13 cases the primary lesion was limited to the vulva. Treatment was radical vulvectomy in 13 of 14 cases. Radiation therapy was used in 1 case because of extensive disease and the patient's poor medical condition. Twelve patients underwent removal of the inguinal-femoral lymph nodes. Of these 12, histologically positive lymph nodes were found in 4 (33%). Three recurrences occurred in 2 patients. Five patients remain disease-free at more than 5 years after therapy, and 5 others at more than 10 years.

The literature review showed 90 cases of primary carcinoma of the Bartholin gland available for analysis, including the 14 cases in the present series. Patients' median age was 57 years, and duration of symptoms ranged from 2 weeks to 180 months. The most common complaints were vulvar mass or perineal pain. Adenocarcinoma and squamous cell carcinoma were the most common histology, occurring in 85.6% of the cases. No patient had metastatic involvement of the

TABLE 2.—RELATIONSHIP OF HISTOLOGIC TYPE TO INGUINAL-FEMORAL NODE METASTASES

Histology	Total No.	No. positive	Percent	
Squamous	27	12	44.4	$P = .59$ (Squamous vs. Adenocarcinoma)
Adenocarcinoma	16	5	31.3	
Adenoid cystic	7	1	14.3	
Mixed	3	2	66.6	
Transitional	3	2	66.6	
Anaplastic	3	0	0	
Total	59	22		
Percent		37.3		

(Courtesy of Leuchter, R. S., et al.: Obstet. Gynecol. 60:361–368, September 1982. Reprinted with permission from the American College of Obstetricians and Gynecologists.)

pelvic lymph nodes when the groin nodes were negative, but when the inguinal-femoral nodes were positive for tumor, 18% demonstrated pelvic lymph node metastases (Table 1). Table 2 outlines the association of the histologic types of Bartholin gland cancer to inguinal-femoral node involvement. Most patients (64.5%) underwent radical vulvectomy and inguinal-femoral node dissection. Twenty-one of 33 patients are alive and well 6–36 months after treatment. The finding of positive inguinal-femoral nodes (37.3%) adversely affected survival. Optimal treatment of this cancer requires wide and radical removal of the primary lesion, best accomplished by radical vulvectomy. Regardless of histologic type, routine removal of the inguinal-femoral lymph nodes is indicated.

▶ [This is a nice review of a rare neoplasm. The prognosis of cancer of the Bartholin gland—when nodes are negative, 65% 3-year survival and 52% 5-year survival—seems somewhat better than that with other forms of vulvar malignancy. Standard surgical therapy consists of radical vulvectomy and inguinal-femoral lymphadectomy; removal of pelvic nodes is not necessary unless more than one or two inguinal nodes are involved.] ◀

12–4 **Topographic Relation of Cervical Ectropion and Vaginal Adenosis to Clear Cell Adenocarcinoma.** To study this relationship, Stanley J. Robboy, William R. Welch, Robert H. Young, Geri Y. Truslow, Arthur L. Herbst, and Robert E. Scully (Registry for Research on Hormonal Transplacental Carcinogenesis) serially blocked and sectioned 20 specimens of uterus and vagina removed because of clear cell adenocarcinoma of the cervix or vagina in women exposed prenatally to diethylstilbestrol (DES).

Three tumors, 0.5 to 2.0 cm in greatest diameter, were cervical; 17 were vaginal. Iodine staining on 2 cervical and 6 vaginal cancer specimens showed the inferior borders of the tumor to lay just above the junction of the stained and nonstained cervical and vaginal surfaces, corresponding to the boundary between the native squamous epithelium of the vagina or ectocervix and the metaplastic squamous epithelium. Each of the 20 specimens contained both microscopically documented cervical ectropion and vaginal adenosis.

In the 17 cases of vaginal carcinoma, the percentage of blocks that showed adenosis varied from 2% to 100%, and in 11 cases it was present in more than 66% of the blocks. The adenosis was either confined to the portion of the vagina that failed to stain with iodine or extended for a short distance into the part that stained normally. Ten of the vaginal cancers were situated where the concentration of glands was greatest.

Correlation of the distance between tumor and cervical external os with quantity of glandular epithelium and its cytologic type revealed that tumors that were progressively more caudal were associated with increasing numbers of tuboendometrial glands and higher proportions of such glands to those lined by mucinous epithelium. The frequency of tuboendometrial glands in any given location in the vagina and cervix was increased if tumor was present at that level. Thus, 7% of the blocks of the cervix had tuboendometrial glands in

---

(12–4) Obstet. Gynecol. 60:546–551, November 1982.

cases with cervical carcinoma, in contrast to none if tumor was absent. Similar differences were also observed in the upper, middle, and lower vaginas.

A clinically significant finding in this study is that clear cell adenocarcinomas in DES-exposed women develop consistently near the distal border of the vaginal or cervical mucosa that fails to stain with iodine. The appearance of this region usually reflects the presence of glandular epithelium undergoing squamous metaplasia. This finding indicates that the gynecologist should focus attention on this portion of abnormal mucosa in a search for early malignant transformation.

▶ [This article provides important information concerning the pathology of adenosis as related to clear cell carcinoma. The tuboendometrial, rather than mucinous, epithelium is apparently the culprit. The cancers tend to develop near the distal border of the mucosa that fails to stain with iodine, or the distal limit of colposcopic abnormality. Special attention should be focused on this area when one evaluates the diethylstilbestrol-exposed patient.] ◀

12–5 **Paired Cervical Smears: A Method of Reducing the False Negative Rate in Population Screening.** J. O. W. Beilby, R. Bourne, J. Guillebaud, and S. T. Steele (London) compared the use of the Ayre wooden spatula and the Armovical plastic spatula, which has a central boss, for obtaining material for the detection of dysplastic cervical epithelium and endocervical cells. The value of taking duplicate smears also was assessed. Paired cervical smears were obtained at a single visit from 21,352 women by using the two types of spatulas in four different sequences.

Individually, the Armovical spatula was superior to the Ayre spatula for the collection of endocervical epithelial material, but this advantage was not accompanied by any marked improvement in detection of cervical dysplasia. Paired smear sampling, however, was clearly more rewarding in this respect. A difference was found between the total number of smears found to be abnormal on the first sample alone and on the two smears combined. Paired smear sampling also allowed the introduction of laboratory quality control when each preparation of any given pair was examined by a different technician. The false negative rate in the first smear was 18.5%, composed of an 11.1% sampling error (patients with no dysplastic cells on the first smear) and a 7.4% screening error (dysplastic cells overlooked in the first preparation but found in the second).

Paired smear sampling would significantly reduce the false negative rate in population screening and offer convenience and economy for both the patient and the clinician.

▶ [This study confirms a report published several years ago (Cathy et al.: *Obstet. Gynecol.* 51:713, 1978) indicating that the false negative rate with Papanicolaou screening for cervical intraepithelial neoplasia can be reduced substantially by taking two smears. False negativity can result from either not collecting dysplastic cells in the sample or missing them in the laboratory screening. The average false negative rate with the various methods of taking the first smear was 18.5%, representing a sampling error of 11.1% and a laboratory screening error of 7.4%. The diagnosis of dysplasia seems to have been made on smears only—at least nothing is said about histologic studies—so it is not entirely certain that these represent "true" false negative rates.] ◀

(12–5) Obstet. Gynecol. 60:46–48, July 1982.

12-6 **False Negative Cytology Rates in Patients in Whom Invasive Cervical Cancer Subsequently Developed.** In 1980 the American Cancer Society proposed that cervical cytologic screening be performed every 3 years for low-risk patients. To evaluate the advisability of such screening every 3 years rather than every year, Nicholas D. Morell, James R. Taylor, Richard N. Snyder, Harry K. Ziel, Arthur Saltz, and Samona Willie (Kaiser-Permanente Med. Center, Los Angeles) analyzed retrospectively the clinical and pathologic data for 85 patients diagnosed in 1977 through 1979 as having invasive or microinvasive squamous or epidermoid cell cervical cancer. These patients were among those seen at seven hospitals in southern California and their outlying clinics. The data base included 909,357 Papanicolaou smears. All patients younger than age 20 years and older than age 65, those with previously abnormal cervical cytology or pathology, and those with invasive endocervical adenocarcinoma were excluded from the study.

Several patients had had no documented cytologic screening prior to the diagnosis of invasive cancer. Seventeen patients (20%) had had 2 or more negative Papanicolaou smears, the last within 3 years of the diagnosis; 9 of the 17 patients had had 3 or more negative smears, the last within 3 years of the diagnosis. An additional 9 patients (11%) had had 1 negative smear within 3 years of the diagnosis. Examination of 36 slides available for review for 17 patients who had had 2 or more negative smears showed 26 slides to be truly negative, 7 exhibited nondysplastic epithelial changes consistent with repair or inflammation, 2 had obviously malignant cells, and 1 had been mislabeled. A negative binomial probability model was found to provide a better fit to the observed sample data than a geometric probability model. When both models as well as the study data were used, the percentage of positive cases that would not be detected during an 8-year period was estimated for various sampling intervals. It was found that sampling once a year over an 8-year period would result in a 1.17% frequency of positive cases missed by Papanicolaou smear (table). With a sampling interval of 2 years, it would be expected that

ESTIMATED PERCENTAGE OF POSITIVE CASES MISSED BY PAPANICOLAOU SMEAR DURING EIGHT-YEAR PERIOD OF ASSUMED STABILITY*

Interval between Papanicolaou smears (yr)	Sample estimate (%)	Geometric estimate (%)	Negative binomial estimate (%)
1	1.17 (±1.92)	0.09	0.96
2	3.53 (±3.29)	3.16	5.74
3	10.59 (±5.49)–20.0 (±7.14)	7.50–17.79	9.45–16.32
4	20.0 (±7.14)	17.79	16.32

*As determined by sampling frequency.

(Courtesy of Morell, N. D., et al.: Obstet. Gynecol. 60:41–45, July 1982. Reprinted with permission from The American College of Obstetricians and Gynecologists.)

(12–6) Obstet. Gynecol. 60:41–45, July 1982.

3.53% of the positive cases would be missed. However, the difference between the number of cases expected to be missed at 1- and 2-year sampling intervals was not statistically significant. The difference became statistically significant only at and beyond the 3-year sampling interval.

A possible explanation for the high false negative rate in this series may be sampling error at the time of Papanicolaou smear and misinterpretation of the smear. The authors recommend that cervical cytologic screening be performed every year or at least every 2 years to decrease the chance of missing an early lesion.

▶ [The mathematical considerations involved in probability estimates are complex and, at least in this study, difficult for us to understand fully. Assuming the approach used here to be valid, the results constitute a potent argument against the American Cancer Society's recommendation for Papanicolaou screening every 3 years in low-risk patients under certain conditions. The risk status of the subjects in this study is not stated, probably because it was not known, as is often the case—and therein lies the rub in treating patients differently depending on such factors as age at first coitus and number of sexual partners. From the data presented, it appears that the risk of missing a case is about 1% with annual screening, 3%–5% with a 2-year interval, 7%–20% with a 3-year interval, and 16%–20% with a 4-year interval.] ◀

12–7 **Cervical Intraepithelial Neoplasia and "Warty" Atypia: A Study of Colposcopic, Histologic, and Cytologic Characteristics.** Recent evidence suggests that a significant proportion of intraepithelial lesions of the cervix may be related to the influence of human papillomavirus. These warty changes simply may be a self-limiting manifestation of viral infection with no long-term sequelae or they may be involved etiologically in cervical intraepithelial neoplasia (CIN). To assess the features that may be characteristic of these possibly distinct disease processes, W. Kirkup, A. S. Evans, A. K. Brough, J. A. Davis, T. O'Loughlin, G. Wilkinson, and J. M. Monaghan reviewed data on a consecutive series of 168 patients referred to the colposcopy clinic because of abnormal cervical cytology.

A relatively large number of positive associations were found between histologic features previously related to possible human papillomavirus infection of cervical epithelium, particularly koilocytosis, double nucleation, and dyskeratosis. Only koilocytosis was associated with a colposcopic finding, that being a recorded impression of a warty lesion. In addition, the overall histologic appearance of a warty lesion was associated with the colposcopic finding of an outline of a finger-like lesion and an appearance of open mosaic, but not with other colposcopic appearances such as an indefinite margin of the lesion or the presence of satellite lesions. The presence of looped capillaries seemed to be associated with the histologic findings of dyskaryosis and prominent mitoses. A colposcopic finding of nonopen mosaic was associated histologically with prominent rete pegs.

Pure CIN was seen in 28 patients; warty lesions histologically associated with koilocytosis, double nucleation, or dyskeratosis were present in 62 patients; and mixed lesions were found in 35. (However, more than 67% of patients with warty lesions did not exhibit the associated colposcopic features.) The remaining 43 patients had lesions

---

(12–7) Br. J. Obstet. Gynaecol. 89:571–577; July 1982.

that could not be construed as either CIN or warty lesions. Histologic features representative of CIN were rarely seen in women whose first intercourse had occurred less than 10 years previously, whereas lesions with warty characteristics appeared to be distributed evenly among patients presenting at more than or less than 10 years from first intercourse.

A self-consistent group of histologic changes, characterized by koilocytosis, double nucleation, and dyskeratosis, may be related to infection of the cervical epithelium by human papillomavirus. Cytologic detection of these lesions and their differentiation from CIN may be difficult and their true incidence may be underestimated. Colposcopy in itself is not a reliable technique for predicting the occurrence of these warty changes in the cervical epithelium. The true nature and significance of these changes are uncertain and warrant further investigation.

▶ [Cytologists and histopathologists are beginning to recognize an entity, variously referred to as warty atypia or atypical condylomata, thought to be due to infection with the human papillomavirus. This study indicates that warty atypia is probably different biologically from CIN but the differentiation is very difficult cytologically, colposcopically, or histologically. A finger-like outline of a lesion seen with the colposcope is suggestive, and the histologic signs of value include koilocytosis, double nuclei, and dyskeratosis.] ◀

12–8 **Morphometric Study of Intraepithelial Neoplasia of the Uterine Cervix.** The primary cause of treatment failure for intraepithelial neoplasia of the uterine cervix after electrocautery, cryosurgery, or carbon dioxide laser therapy is incomplete eradicaton of the lesion. This may be related to the depth of crypt involvement, the linear extent of the lesion, or the site of the abnormal epithelium. Fadi W. Abdul-Karim, Yao S. Fu, James W. Reagan, and W. Budd Wentz (Case Western Reserve Univ., Cleveland) analyzed 319 cervical conization specimens to determine the maximal depth, linear extent, and location of varying grades of intraepithelial abnormalities.

Mild dysplasias were classified as cervical intraepithelial neoplasia (CIN) I, moderate dysplasias as CIN II, and severe dysplasias and carcinomas in situ as CIN III. Mean age of the patients, mean depth of the lesions, and mean linear extent of the lesions are listed in the table. To eradicate 99.7% of the CIN I, CIN II, and CIN III lesions, it would have been necessary to destroy tissue up to 2.08, 3.06, and 4.80 mm in depth, respectively, and to a linear extent of 11.54, 18.23, and 20.56 mm, respectively. A positive correlation was observed between the depth and linear extent of the lesions. Fifty-nine percent of the lesions between 1 and 2 mm in depth had a linear extent greater than 6 mm, and 71.9% of the lesions greater than 2 mm in depth had a linear extent greater than 6 mm. A proportional increase in depth and linear extent of the lesions was observed with increasing age. There was no correlation between the location of the lesion and the severity of CIN. Regardless of the severity, most lesions involved the new transformation zone (zone 3, 46.7%), the original transformation zone (zone 2, 20.7%), or both (zone 4, 19.8%). Less common was in-

---

(12–8) Obstet. Gynecol. 60:210–214, August 1982.

CORRELATION OF SEVERITY AND EXTENT OF CERVICAL INTRAEPITHELIAL NEOPLASIAS

CIN	No. of patients	Age* (yr)	Depth* (mm) mean ± SD	Length* (mm) mean ± SD	Depth (mm) Mean + 1.96 SD	Depth (mm) Mean + 3 SD	Length (mm) Mean + 1.96 SD	Length (mm) Mean + 3 SD
I	84	32.7 ± 7.8	0.42 ± 0.28	4.10 ± 2.84	0.97	1.26	9.67	11.54
II	152	35.0 ± 9.8	0.93 ± 0.71	5.84 ± 4.13	2.32	3.06	13.93	18.23
III	83	35.3 ± 10.6	1.35 ± 1.15	7.60 ± 4.32	3.60	4.80	16.07	20.56
Total	319	34.5 ± 9.6	0.92 ± 0.88	5.84 ± 4.09	2.65	3.56	13.86	18.11

*Mean ± SD.

(Courtesy of Abdul-Karim, F. W., et al.: Obstet. Gynecol. 60:210–214, August 1982. Reprinted with permission from The American College of Obstetricians and Gynecologists.)

volvement of the ectocervix alone (zone 1, 3.1%) or a proximal site in the cervical canal (zone 5, 9.7%). Lesions in zone 4, which involved the ectocervix and endocervix, were more extensive and were largely composed of CIN II and CIN III changes. The lesion was located high in the cervical canal in 28.6% of women older than age 51 years and in less than 10% of younger women.

The magnitude of intraepithelial neoplasia of the uterine cervix is related closely to the severity of the lesion. It is recommended that appropriate cytologic samples, endocervical curettage, and colposcopic examination be used in evaluating CIN and that strict criteria should be applied in selecting patients for conservative management.

▶ [This study nicely demonstrates positive correlation between the severity of CIN and the linear extent and depth of the lesion. The authors point out that autoradiographic studies indicate increasing proliferative activity of CIN with advancing severity. Does the large size and greater depth of CIN III lesions explain the higher failure rate of cryotherapy in this situation compared with that observed in patients with CIN I and CIN II?] ◀

12–9 **Behavior of Moderate Cervical Dysplasia During Long-Term Follow-up.** It is well known that dysplastic changes of the squamous epithelium of the uterine cervix are potentially precancerous and that cellular morphology does not give an accurate prognosis in individual cases. To further study the biologic behavior of cervical dysplasia, Karen Nasiell, Magnus Nasiell, and Vlasta Václavinková (Sabbatsberg Hosp., Stockholm) followed by cytology without major treatment 894 consecutive women with cytologically established moderate cervical dysplasia.

At the end of follow-up (February 1980), 54% of the lesions had regressed, 16% had persisted, and 30% had progressed (table). The average follow-up time was 78 months for patients with regression of dysplasia and 53 months for patients with continuous normal cytology after disappearance of dysplasia. Patients with moderate or mild persisting dysplasia were followed for an average of 50 months, during which 37 of 140 patients exhibited periods of normal smears for more than 12 months. Dysplasia progressing to more severe lesions did so after an average follow-up of 51 months. Fewer lesions showed

Follow-up of Patients With Untreated Moderate Cervical Dysplasia

Status	No.	Percent	Follow-up time (mo)
Regression to normal	483	54	78*
Persistence of dysplasia	140	16	50
Progression	271	30	51
Total	894	100	

*Continuous cytologic normalcy after disappearance of dysplasia: 53 months.

(Courtesy of Nasiell, K., et al.: Obstet. Gynecol. 61:609–614, May 1983. Reprinted with permission from The American College of Obstetricians and Gynecologists.)

(12–9) Obstet. Gynecol. 61:609–614, May 1983.

progression in patients older than age 51 years than in younger age groups; the time of progression was also significantly longer in older patients. Biopsy specimens were obtained in 54% of all patients. Significantly more biopsied (57%) than nonbiopsied (50%) lesions regressed during follow-up and fewer biopsied (27%) than nonbiopsied (35%) lesions progressed to more severe lesions ($P < .05$). Based on life-table techniques, the probability of progression of moderate dysplasia to a more severe lesion for all patients increased from 8% after 2 years of follow-up to 33% after 12 or more years of follow-up. For patients who did not undergo biopsy, the probability of progression after more than 12 years of follow-up was 38%. The annual risk for a woman with moderate dysplasia to progress to a more severe lesion was 5/100 to 9/100 women/year, which is about 2,000 times greater than for a woman with normal cervical epithelium.

It is concluded that the follow-up period in patients with continuously normal cytology should be at least 2 to 3 years long before the disappearance of dysplasia should be considered established. The rate of progression is lower in postmenopausal women aged 51 and older, as well as in women aged 20 and younger. Punch biopsy, cervical curettage, or both appear to decrease the frequency of progressing lesions and to increase the frequency of regression. For the patient with moderate persisting dysplasia, the risk of developing a more severe lesion increases if she has had three or more initial abnormal smears.

▶ [Reliable data regarding the biologic behavior of cervical intraepithelial neoplasia (CIN) are hard to come by. Repeated follow-up visits and long periods of time are necessary. Moreover, histologic sampling done for diagnosis inevitably has therapeutic potential. This study by Nasiell et al. used cytology, complimented by colposcopy, as primary methodology, avoiding the problem of inadvertent therapy but adding one of relative imprecision in diagnosis. The figures reported for moderate dysplasia (i.e., CIN 2)—regression to normal in 50%, progression to CIN 3 in 35%, and persistence in 15%—are somewhat more optimistic than previous studies would suggest.] ◀

12–10 **Cryotherapy and Carbon Dioxide Laser Management of Cervical Intraepithelial Neoplasia: A Controlled Comparison.** Duane E. Townsend (Los Angeles) and Ralph M. Richart (New York) treated 200 patients with cervical intraepithelial neoplasia alternately by cryotherapy and carbon dioxide laser therapy on an outpatient basis after appropriate triage with colposcopy, cervical biopsy, and endocervical curettage. The study was designed to compare objectively results of management with cryotherapy and carbon dioxide laser therapy.

Results show that every patient treated with cryotherapy had abnormal sensations during the course of treatment; 5% had severe cramps and 20% had vasomotor effects, particularly light-headedness. Patients treated with carbon dioxide laser all experienced some pain; 6% had severe menstrual-like cramps or a needle-like sensation, 4% had barely noticeable discomfort, and 90% had tolerable discomfort. None of the laser-treated patients had vasomotor symptoms. Patients treated with cryotherapy had discharge of water; 80% described the

(12–10) Obstet. Gynecol. 61:75–78, January 1983.

RESULTS OF TREATMENT ACCORDING TO HISTOLOGIC DIAGNOSIS

	Cryotherapy			CO_2 Laser Therapy		
		Failure			Failure	
Diagnosis	No. treated	No.	Percent	No. treated	No.	Percent
CIN I	10	0	0	10	1	10
CIN II	37	2	5	37	3	9
CIN III	53	5	10	53	7	13
Total	100	7	7	100	11	11

(Courtesy of Townsend, D. E., and Richart, R. M.: Obstet. Gynecol. 61:75–78, January 1983. Reprinted with permission from The American College of Obstetricians and Gynecologists.)

discharge as profuse and lasting as long as 14 days. No significant bleeding occurred in this group. Among laser-treated patients, 9% had a slight malodorous discharge; 31% had spotting or bleeding. Among cryotherapy patients, 47% showed healing at the 6-week follow-up; among laser-treated patients, 90% were healed after 6 weeks. The table shows the results of treatment according to histologic diagnosis. The failure rate was 7% for cryotherapy and 11% for laser treatment.

There appears to be no advantage in replacing cryotherapy with carbon dioxide laser therapy. If therapeutic results are equivalent, the modality that provides an equivalent grade of care for the least possible cost is the logical choice and, in the office setting, this would favor cryotherapy over laser treatment.

▶ [These results seem to indicate that it is pretty much "six of one, half dozen of the other," in terms of cure rate and side effects, with respect to cryotherapy and carbon dioxide laser in treating cervical intraepithelial neoplasia. For another therapeutic possibility, see the following article.] ◀

12–11 **Electrocoagulation Diathermy for Cervical Dysplasia and Carcinoma in Situ: A 15-Year Survey.** William Chanen and Robert M. Rome (Melbourne) reviewed experience with electrocoagulation diathermy for cervical dysplastic lesions over a 15-year period (1966–1981). Abnormal results of cervical smear examination were assessed in 5,250 patients, and either cervical intraepithelial neoplasia (CIN) or preclinical invasive carcinoma was confirmed histologically in 2,934. More than 50% of the patients were younger than age 30 years, and nearly 25% were nulliparous. Treatment methods for 2,504 patients are listed in the table. The number of patients managed by cone biopsy declined markedly during the study period. Electrocoagulation diathermy was possible in more than 90% of patients younger than age 30 with confirmed CIN. All 6 patients in this age group who required hysterectomy had invasive carcinoma. Severe dysplasia or carcinoma in situ was present in 62.5% of the diathermy group. A modified endocervical speculum was useful in viewing the

(12–11) Obstet. Gynecol. 61:673–679, June 1983.

METHOD OF TREATMENT IN 2,504 PATIENTS WITH HISTOLOGICALLY PROVED CERVICAL INTRAEPITHELIAL NEOPLASIA OR PRECLINICAL INVASIVE CANCER

Method of treatment	No. patients (%)
Electrocoagulation diathermy	1864 (74.4)
Cone biopsy	425 (17.0)
Other (laser, cryosurgery, cervical amputation, etc.)	26 (1.0)
Hysterectomy (primary or interval)	93 (3.7)
Treated for invasive carcinoma	96 (3.8)
Total	2504 (100)

(Courtesy of Chanen, I., and Rome, R. M.: Obstet. Gynecol. 61:673–679, June 1983. Reprinted with permission of The American College of Obstetricians and Gynecologists.)

upper boundary of the abnormal transformation zone in some instances.

Of 1,734 patients seen within a year after electrocoagulation diathermy, 2.7% had confirmed residual CIN. The lesion was visible with the colposcope in all but 2 of these 47 patients. Cytology findings were falsely negative in 5 instances, but results were positive in both patients with residual disease in the endocervical canal. Treatment failures were not related to the histologic severity of the original lesion. Fifteen patients (0.8%) had recurrent CIN confirmed by target biopsy after at least a year of follow-up. Recurrences also were unrelated to the severity of the original CIN. Twenty-two patients with residual or recurrent disease were cured by biopsy alone and 22 others by a second diathermy. Complications followed diathermy in 2.5% of patients. Twelve patients (0.6%) had acute pelvic infection; all responded rapidly to antibiotic therapy. No long-term adverse effects on subsequent fertility or pregnancy were apparent.

A single application of electrocoagulation diathermy is a safe and effective means of treating most patients with premalignant disease of the cervix, regardless of its extent or severity. The risk of subsequent invasive cancer in these patients has been virtually eliminated.

▶ [Of the various "conservative" treatments of CIN, cryotherapy is probably the most widely used in the United States, with laser a recent challenger. By contrast, in this series the most common method was electrocoagulation diathermy. The results seem quite good. It should be noted that this technique is more extensive than the old-fashioned electrocautery of the cervix; anesthesia is required.] ◀

12–12 **Microinvasive Carcinoma of the Cervix.** J. R. van Nagell, Jr., N. Greenwell, D. F. Powell, E. S. Donaldson, M. B. Hanson, and E. C. Gay (Univ. of Kentucky, Lexington) related several histomorphological variables to nodal metastasis and tumor recurrence in 177 patients seen from 1966 to 1980 with squamous cell cancer invading the

(12–12) Am. J. Obstet. Gynecol. 145:981–991, Apr. 15, 1983.

TABLE 1.—HISTOMORPHOLOGICAL VARIABLES RELATED TO TUMOR RECURRENCE

Variable	*No. of patients*	*No. of recur-rences*	*Significance*
Depth of invasion (mm):			
≤3.0	145	2	$p < 0.001$
3.1-5.0	32	6	
Pattern of invasion:			
Confluent	42	2	NS
Infiltrative	135	6	
Cell type:			
Large cell nonkeratinizing	155	5	
Keratinizing	16	1	NS
Small cell	6	2	
Lymphoplasmacytic infiltrate:			
Mild	145	7	NS
Marked	32	1	
Lymph–vascular space invasion:			
Positive	33	4	$p < 0.04$
Negative	144	4	

(Courtesy of van Nagell, J. R., et al.: Am. J. Obstet. Gynecol. 145:981–991, Apr. 15, 1983.)

cervical stroma to 5 mm or less. Treatment was by vaginal or abdominal hysterectomy or by radical hysterectomy with pelvic lymphadenectomy. Patients with positive nodes received 5,000–6,000 rad of pelvic radiation.

Mean patient age was 38 years and mean gravidity was 4.5. All patients having hysterectomy initially had tumors with less than 3 mm of stromal invasion. Tumor was found in lymph nodes in 9.3% of 32 patients with stromal invasion of 3–5 mm, but in none of 52 patients with less than 3 mm of stromal invasion. The most important histologic factor related to risk of tumor recurrence was the depth of stromal invasion (Table 1). All 3 patients with carcinoma in situ were treated successfully, but 2 of the 3 with recurrent invasive cancer failed to respond to radiotherapy or chemotherapy and died of their disease.

The depth of stromal invasion is the most critical factor in defining microinvasive cancer and also in predicting whether nodal metastases will be present (Tables 2 and 3). Microinvasive carcinoma should be defined as a lesion invading the cervical stroma to a depth of 3 mm or less without lymph-vascular space invasion. Conization is necessary to make the diagnosis. True microinvasive cancer can be treated adequately by vaginal or abdominal hysterectomy. Colposcopy should be done before hysterectomy to identify any areas of vaginal extension. If there is any doubt as to the depth of stromal invasion, or whether lymph-vascular space invasion is present, radical surgery or radiotherapy is indicated.

▶ [This study demonstrates convincingly that the overwhelmingly important prog-

TABLE 2.—FREQUENCY OF LYMPH NODE METASTASES IN PATIENTS WITH STROMAL INVASION OF 3.0 MM OR LESS

Study	*No. of patients*	*No. of patients with positive nodes*
Smith Foushee et al. (1969)	16	0
Roche and Norris (1975)	9	0
Leman et al. (1976)	32	0
Seski et al. (1977)	37	0
Taki et al. (1979)	55	0
Yajima and Noda (1979)	90	0
Hasumi et al. (1980)	106	1
Van Nagell et al. (1982)	52	0
Total	397	1

(Courtesy of van Nagell, J. R., et al.: Am. J. Obstet. Gynecol. 145:981–991, Apr. 15, 1983.)

TABLE 3.—FREQUENCY OF LYMPH NODE METASTASES IN PATIENTS WITH STROMAL INVASION OF 3.1 TO 5.0 MM

Study	*No. of patients*	*No. of patients with positive nodes*
Smith Foushee et al. (1969)	13	1
Roche and Norris (1975)	21	0
Leman et al. (1976)	3	0
Hasumi et al. (1980)	29	4
Van Nagell et al. (1982)	32	3
Total	98	8

(Courtesy of van Nagell, J. R., et al.: Am. J. Obstet Gynecol. 145:981–991, Apr. 15, 1983.)

nostic feature in microinvasive carcinoma of the cervix is depth of stromal invasion. With 3 mm or less invasion from the basement membrane, the risks of lymph node metastases and later recurrence of invasive disease are negligible; therefore, simple hysterectomy is adequate treatment. When invasion extends more than 3 mm, however, a small but definite risk of nodal spread and later recurrence exists and more radical therapy is needed. Histopathologic features other than depth of invasion—cell type, pattern of invasion, a round cell infiltrate—bore no relation to prognosis. Invasion of lymph-vascular spaces did relate to outcome, but here again it was mediated by invasion depth; lymph-vascular involvement with less than 3 mm of invasion was seemingly benign, whereas that with 3.1–5.0 mm of invasion was not.] ◀

12–13 **Cytoplasmic Estrogen and Progesterone Receptors in Primary Cervical Carcinoma: Clinical and Histopathologic Correlates.** Cytoplasmic estrogen receptors (ERc) and progesterone receptors (PRc) have been demonstrated in cervical carcinoma, but they have not been quantitated and correlated with possible prognostic pa-

(12–13) Am. J. Obstet. Gynecol. 146:299–306, June 1, 1983.

rameters. Yong Liang Gao, Leo B. Twiggs, Benjamin S. Leung, Winston C. Y. Yu, Roger A. Potish, Takashi Okagaki, Leon L. Adcock, and Konald A. Prem (Univ. of Minnesota) studied 39 cases of primary cervical carcinoma seen in 1977–1981 to determine the presence or absence of ERc and PRc. A saturation point dextran-coated charcoal assay was used. Criteria for positive tests were 5 fmol/mg of cytosol protein for ERc and 10 fmol/mg for PRc. Survival was computed by the product-limit analysis method.

Mean receptor levels were relatively consistent between histologic types of cancer. The PRc level tended to increase with increasing histologic grade. Levels of PRc were higher in premenopausal cases, whereas ERc levels were slightly higher in postmenopausal women. About 80% of all tumors were PRc positive; 55% were ERc positive. A significant difference in survival in the PRc-positive and PRc-negative groups was evident in premenopausal patients only. Survival rate was significantly better in PRc-positive cases.

Putative prognostic parameters such as stage, grade, and histologic type could not be related to PRc status in the present series, but survival appeared to be compromised in premenopausal patients who were PRc negative. Identification of such patients permits distinction of a group at high risk of treatment failure. Carcinomas negative for PRc may behave more aggressively than others.

▶ [Interest in steroid hormone receptor status as an index of prognosis has been high in the case of endometrial cancer, but the matter has received little attention with respect to cervical malignancy. These findings are suggestive of some value in that, among premenopausal patients, those with higher levels of cytoplasmic progesterone receptors had better survival than those with lower levels.] ◀

12–14 **Influence of Patients' Age and Tumor Grade on Prognosis of Carcinoma of the Cervix.** Thongbliew Prempree, Vinita Patanaphan, Wilfred Sewchand, and Ralph M. Scott (Univ. of Maryland) examined the effects of age and tumor grade on disease-free survival in 561 patients treated by irradiation for histologically proved invasive squamous cell cervical cancer seen from 1969 to 1974. Ninety-four patients aged 23–29 years at diagnosis staged by the International Federation of Gynecology and Obstetrics (FIGO) system were followed up for 5 or more years. Whole pelvis external irradiation was delivered, with parametrial boosts when appropriate. The usual pelvic dose was 4,000 rad in 4 weeks. A dose of 5,000 rad often was delivered in patients with stage II or stage III disease. The dose of intracavitary radium therapy was about 4,500–5,000 mg/hour.

The absolute disease-free survival at 5 or more years was 70.2% for those with stage I disease, 54% for those with stage II disease, and 17% for those with stage III disease. None of 3 patients with stage IV disease survived for 5 years. The overall disease-free survival was 53.2%. Patients aged 23–29 years had a lower survival rate than those aged 30–39 years for all stages of disease. Local treatment failure was more frequent in younger patients. Tumor grade also was a factor in survival. Local failures often occurred concomitantly with

---

(12–14) Cancer 51:1764–1771, May 1, 1983.

distant disease. Distant failure occurred in 26%, 42%, and 33% of patients with disease in stages I, II, and III, respectively. Most distant failures occurred within 2 years of diagnosis. Visceral failure predominated in patients with stage I cancer, but in those with stage II lesions, para-aortic and inguinal node involvement was frequent.

Tumor grade is a significant factor in younger patients with cervical carcinoma. Laparotomy with node sampling should be done to determine the true extent of disease in patients younger than age 40 with poorly differentiated squamous cancer or anaplastic or small cell cancer of the cervix. In inoperable patients, computed tomography is a useful study. Isotope scanning can identify visceral distant disease. Patients younger than age 30 with stage I or IIA disease are best managed by radical operation, with an attempt to identify para-aortic node involvement. When residual disease may be present, radiotherapy can be given postoperatively. Patients aged 30–40 years can be treated by either radical surgery or irradiation.

▶ [The findings reported here are consistent with those of other recent studies of cervical cancer (1982 YEAR BOOK, pp. 304–305; and 1983 YEAR BOOK, pp. 278–279). The prognosis is poorer in younger women; this may be due to a higher prevalence of undifferentiated tumors.] ◀

12–15 **Stage IB Carcinoma of the Cervix, The Norwegian Radium Hospital: II. Results When Pelvic Nodes Are Involved.** The incidence of pelvic lymph node metastases in stage I carcinoma of the cervix reportedly varies from 10% to more than 30%. Pierre W. Martimbeau, Kjell E. Kjorstad, and Torbjorn Iversen (Norwegian Radium Hosp., Oslo) reviewed retrospectively the results of radical hysterectomy with pelvic lymphadenopathy in 562 patients with stage IB squamous cell carcinoma of the cervix according to ratings of the International Federation of Gynecology and Obstetrics treated from 1967 through 1972. Primary surgery was performed in 20 patients with relatively small tumors. Beginning with 1970, lymphography was performed before treatment, and 271 patients had an average of 31 lymph nodes excised. If pelvic metastases were detected at operation, external beam supervoltage irradiation was applied. Generally, patients with metastases in the common iliac nodes were given 5,000 rad; those with metastases below this level received 4,000 rad.

Metastases were found in the pelvic lymph nodes in 120 (21.3%) of the 562 patients. Periaortic node involvement was present in 6 patients (1.1%); all but 1 of the 6 had pelvic node metastases. Overall, patients with pelvic lymph node metastases had a 5-year survival of 53%, whereas those with no demonstrable metastatic disease had a 5-year survival of 92%. Five of 6 patients with periaortic disease died within 4 to 20 months after treatment. Of 6 other patients who had an incomplete operation, 5 died and 1 is alive at 6 years without evidence of disease.

Metastases were found in the common iliac nodes in 32 patients (5.7%), only 2 of whom were alive without evidence of disease at 5 years (table). In contrast, 52 (59%) of 88 patients with metastases in the external iliac and obturator nodes were alive at 5 years without

(12–15) Obstet. Gynecol. 60:215–218, August 1982.

SURVIVAL AND SITE OF RECURRENCE FOR PATIENTS WITH PELVIC LYMPH NODE METASTASES FOUND AT OPERATION

Highest level of metastases	No. of patients	Recurrence			5-year survival (%)	NED‡ (%)
		Pelvis	Other*	Distant†		
Obturator, unilateral	21	4	1	4	71	57
Obturator, bilateral	9	2	0	1	67	67
External iliac, unilateral	46	7	4	5	65	61
External iliac, bilateral	12	4	0	2	58	50
Common iliac, unilateral	26	9	7	6	23	8
Common iliac, bilateral	6	6	0	0	—	—
Total	120	32	12	18		

*Unspecified site or suspected pelvic recurrence without histologic proof.
†No evidence of concomitant pelvic recurrence.
‡Alive at 5 years, no evidence of disease.
(Courtesy of Martimbeau, P. W., et al.: Obstet. Gynecol. 60:215–218, August 1982. Reprinted with permission from The American College of Obstetricians and Gynecologists.)

evidence of disease. In patients with metastases in only the external iliac or the common iliac nodes, without other metastatic involvement, the respective 5-year survival was 65% and 14%. When there was no involvement of the common iliac nodes, there was little difference in survival among patients with different sites of metastases. In addition, the presence of unilateral or bilateral involvement did not seem to significantly affect survival. Failure of regional tumor control in the pelvis occurred in 47% of patients with metastases in the common iliac nodes and in 19% of those with metastases below the common iliac levels. Distant metastases, without pelvic recurrence, occurred with approximately the same frequency, regardless of the level of metastases in the pelvic nodes.

Patients with pelvic node metastases below the common iliac nodes have a considerably better prognosis than patients with metastatic disease in the common iliac nodes. Patients with disease limited to one node or one group of nodes below the common iliac level do not have a better prognosis than patients with multiple metastatic nodes at this level.

▶ [In this large series of patients with stage IB cervical cancer, survival rates were similar with external iliac, obturator, or external iliac and obturator nodal metastases. The prognosis was much worse if the common iliac nodes were positive.] ◀

12–16 **Stage IB Cervical Carcinoma and Pregnancy: Report of 49 Cases.** Jeffrey A. Nisker and Michael Shubat (London, Ont.) reviewed 49 cases of stage IB cervical carcinoma associated with pregnancy seen between 1955 and 1980. Twenty-five patients were managed by radiotherapy alone, 11 had radical hysterectomy and node dissection, 5 had operation and adjuvant radiotherapy for involved nodes, and 2 had simple hysterectomy with radiotherapy. The diagnosis was made in the first trimester of pregnancy in 13 patients, including 6 in whom therapeutic abortion was performed. Mean age was 34 years. Forty-seven squamous cell cancers and 2 adenocarcinomas were diagnosed.

Overall 5-year survival was 69.8%. Pelvic node dissection yielded tumor-positive nodes in 5 of 20 cases. Three of 4 node-positive patients given postoperative radiotherapy lived 5 years, whereas both patients given no further treatment died. Serious complications occurred in 22.5% of patients, and 1 patient died during radiotherapy. The method of delivery did not influence 5-year disease-free survival. Ten of 11 women with a diagnosis in the second or third trimester had cesarean section, and 1 underwent termination with hypertonic glucose. Five of 6 patients who had radical operations at the time of cesarean section survived. When cesarean section was followed by radiotherapy, only 1 of 4 patients survived. With 1 exception, all deaths of patients with a diagnosis in the second or third trimester were of women given post-cesarean section radiotherapy as the only treatment.

Pregnancy may have an adverse effect on the course of stage IB cervical carcinoma. The best approach seems to be radical hysterec-

(12–16) Am. J. Obstet. Gynecol. 145:203–206, Jan. 15, 1983.

tomy and pelvic adenectomy, with radiotherapy if tumor-positive nodes are found. This plan is especially appropriate when the diagnosis is made in the second or third trimester of pregnancy.

▶ [Traditional teaching has been that the results of treatment of carcinoma of the cervix, stage by stage, are not affected by the coexistence of pregnancy. This study, however, suggests otherwise. The incidence of positive nodes was higher and the 5 year survival rate lower than those customarily reported with stage IB disease. Caveats to be acknowledged are that the number of subjects is relatively small and the comparison group is not a concomitant one from the same time period.] ◀

12–17 **Survival Among Women With Endometrial Cancer: Comparison of Estrogen Users and Nonusers.** Joseph Chu, Abraham I. Schweid, and Noel S. Weiss (Seattle) studied the role of postmenopausal estrogen use in survival of patients with endometrial cancer. A population-based tumor registry identified 363 white women, aged 50 to 74 years, in whom endometrial cancer developed between January 1975 and April 1976. Of these women, 285 (79%) had used menopausal estrogens for 1 or more years and 78 (21%) had not used them or had used them for less than 1 year.

The 4-year relative survival ratio was 1.05 in estrogen users and 0.898 in nonusers. Overall, after adjustment for age, survival in estrogen users was significantly better than in nonusers. The tumors in estrogen users were lower in stage, histologic grade, and depth of myometrial invasion, suggesting that the improved survival in users relative to nonusers was due to the fact that users had tumors with relatively favorable characteristics at the time of diagnosis.

Although estrogen use may predispose to an increased incidence of endometrial cancer, it appears that such use does not lead to an increased mortality from this condition. This could be due to the fact that endometrial cancer is diagnosed earlier in estrogen users than in nonusers, perhaps because the women are already under medical surveillance or there is greater awareness by physicians of women who are using estrogens. Another factor may be that estrogen-associated tumors are biologically less aggressive than those that arise without estrogen. The fact that estrogen users had a better 4-year survival than expected is probably due to selection of "healthier" women for exogenous estrogen therapy rather than to the fact that estrogen-related endometrial cancer leads to a lower mortality.

▶ [Several reports have shown, as does this one, that while exogenous estrogen may predispose to development of endometrial cancer, the prognosis is considerably better than with estrogen-unrelated tumors. Is this a reflection of earlier diagnosis (due to the patient already receiving regular medical care or to the physician being aware of the increased risk) or is the estrogen-related neoplasm of inherently lower biologic risk? The association of estrogen use with tumors of earlier stage and less myometrial invasion is compatible with either hypothesis, but the characteristically better differentiation suggests a lesser degree of virulence as the factor responsible.] ◀

12–18 **Stage I Endometrial Adenocarcinoma: Treatment Results in 835 Patients.** The optimal management of endometrial adenocarcinoma remains uncertain. R. J. Lotocki, L. J. Copeland, A. D. DePetrillo, and W. Muirhead (Hamilton, Ont.) reviewed the results of treatment of endometrial cancer in 835 patients seen from 1960 to

---

(12–17) Am. J. Obstet. Gynecol. 143:569–573, July 1, 1982.
(12–18) Ibid., 146:141–145, May 15, 1983.

TABLE 1.—MENSTRUAL STATUS RELATED TO GRADE

Menstrual status	*No. of patients*	*Grade 1 (%)*	*Grade 2 (%)*	*Grade 3 (%)*
Premenopausal or menopausal	41	68.3	14.6	17.1
Postmenopausal	771	49	26.5	22.1

(Courtesy of Lotocki, R. J., et al.: Am. J. Obstet. Gynecol. 146:141–145, May 15, 1983.)

1975 with stage I disease. Five-year follow-up was available in 820 patients. Abdominal hysterectomy and bilateral salpingo-oophorectomy were carried out as part of initial treatment in 86.4%, sometimes after radium therapy. External irradiation was used selectively for deep myometrial invasion or disease outside the uterus. The 113 patients considered to be inoperable had a single radium insertion.

The actuarial 5-year survival of patients having initial operation was 87.7%. Addition of radium therapy to surgery was associated with improved survival compared with surgery alone. The actuarial 5-year survival of "inoperable" patients was 64%, and absolute survival was 45%. Older patients tended to have less-differentiated tumors. Well-differentiated lesions were more frequent in premenopausal and menopausal patients (Table 1). The 118 patients with recurrent disease had a generally poor outcome. Survival is related to grade and depth of tumor invasion in "operable" patients in Table 2. These factors were additive in affecting the prognosis adversely. Preoperative radium therapy may obscure the depth of myometrial invasion. Ten of 18 patients with vault recurrences died of disease despite treatment of recurrences. Radium therapy reduced the rate of vault recurrences.

Surgery is the mainstay of treatment of stage I endometrial adenocarcinoma. Internal radium insertion reduces vault recurrences. The value of external radiation remains uncertain, because in this series it was used selectively in patients with a high risk of recurrence and in those with persistent disease.

TABLE 2.—FIVE-YEAR ACTUARIAL SURVIVAL RELATED TO GRADE AND DEPTH OF TUMOR INVASION IN 718 "OPERABLE" PATIENTS

	Actuarial survival		
Depth of invasion	*Grade 1 (%)*	*Grade 2 (%)*	*Grade 3 (%)*
No residual	97.6	98	79.9
Endometrial	97.1	97.5	79.8
Myometrial (<⅓)	92.6	87	61.1
Myometrial (>50%)	90.9	71	26.3

(Courtesy of Lotocki, R. J., et al.: Am. J. Obstet. Gynecol. 146:141–145, May 15, 1983.)

▶ [This retrospective study of patients with endometrial cancer confirms several generally accepted opinions. Tumor grade and depth of myometrial invasion independently relate to prognosis. Older and postmenopausal women tend to have less well-differentiated tumors than do younger and premenopausal women. "Estrogen use cancers" tend to be well differentiated and to be associated with a good prognosis. Endometrial cavity depth (stage IA vs. stage IB) doesn't affect survival. Finally, patients with recurrences fared poorly. Because of the lack of random assignment, the effects of adjunctive radiotherapy cannot be ascertained.] ◀

12–19 **Selective Use of Vaginal Hysterectomy in Management of Adenocarcinoma of the Endometrium.** Abdominal hysterectomy remains the standard management of endometrial adenocarcinoma, but vaginal hysterectomy has been recommended in selected patients with medical conditions placing them at high risk from abdominal surgery. William A. Peters III, Willie A. Andersen, W. Norman Thornton, Jr., and George W. Morley reviewed experience with vaginal hysterectomy in 56 patients with stage I endometrial adenocarcinoma, 20 at the University of Michigan Medical Center and 35 at the University of Virgina Medical Center. The chief medical complication in most of these patients was obesity. A colporrhaphy was performed in 12 patients. The adnexa were removed in about 20% of cases. Thirty-two patients received adjuvant radiation therapy. Median postoperative hospital stay was 1 week. One patient died of pulmonary embolism 15 days after operation. Overall 5-year survival rate was 94%; survival probability was 98% for patients with grade 1 tumors. Five patients without recurrent cancer have died of intercurrent disease.

Vaginal hysterectomy has a definite role in the management of endometrial carcinoma. It carries a low morbidity and mortality in high-risk patients, such as those with morbid obesity. It should not, however, be used routinely or indiscriminately. Addition of adjuvant radiation therapy to hysterectomy remains controversial. The authors plan to continue using preoperative irradiation in grade 2 and grade 3 cases, but there appears to be no benefit from radiation therapy in patients with grade 1 tumors.

▶ [The major disadvantages of vaginal hysterectomy for endometrial cancer are the inability to remove the adnexa, at least routinely, and the lack of surgical staging for possible additional therapy. In some cases, however, it is a reasonable consideration. Most often this will arise in massively obese women, in whom the high risk of abdominal wound infection can be avoided by a vaginal approach. Surely the outcome reported here—94% survival probability—is good.] ◀

12–20 **Risk Factors and Prognosis in Stage II Endometrial Cancer.** The classification of stage II endometrial cancer includes those cases in which the carcinoma has involved the corpus and the cervix but has not extended outside the uterus. In this stage, prognosis is poorer and there is greater likelihood of occult lymph node metastases than in stage I. Michael L. Berman, Muhammed Ali Afridi, Anisa I. Kanbour, and Harrison G. Ball (Pittsburgh) used life-table analysis to assess survival as a function of patient age, cell type, grade of tumor, depth of invasion, treatment, surgical stage, and extent of cervical involvement in 97 patients with stage II endometrial cancer identi-

(12–19) Am. J. Obstet. Gynecol. 146:285–291, June 1, 1983.
(12–20) Gynecol. Oncol. 14:49–61, August 1982.

fied in a retrospective review of data on 1,249 patients who received primary treatment for endometrial carcinoma at Magee-Womens Hospital between 1953 and 1977. All patients but 1 were followed up for at least 30 months; 85% were followed up for at least 5 years or until death.

For all 97 patients the actuarial 5- and 10-year survival rates were 65.9% and 57.9%, respectively. Cumulative 5-year survival fell progressively with age from 62.9% in patients aged 51 to 70 years to 54% in those older than age 70. Cumulative 5-year survival was 77% for the 31 patients treated with irradiation only, 66.1% for the 25 patients treated surgically, and 58.5% for the 41 patients who received combined therapy; these differences were not statistically significant. Patients with histologic grade 1 tumors had a 5-year survival of 79.3%, compared with a survival of 58% for patients with grade 2 and grade 3 tumors. Treatment regimens did not differ significantly among these patients. The grade of tumor was usually identical in specimens from both uterine curettage and hysterectomy, although in 2 of 19 patients with preoperative radiation, the curettage specimens were 1 grade higher than the hysterectomy specimens.

Five-year survival was 60.3% in 63 patients with adenocarcinoma, 88.4% in 21 patients with adenoacanthoma, and 71.1% in 9 patients with adenosquamous carcinoma. Two of 4 patients with clear cell carcinoma died. The difference in survival between patients with adenocarcinoma and those with adenoacanthoma could be explained only in part by differences in tumor grade.

Of 36 patients who did not receive preoperative radiation therapy, all with superficial tumors survived at least 5 years, compared with a 5-year survival of 57.9% for those with deeply invasive tumors. All 5 patients with deep myometrial invasion and penetration to the uterine serosa died of recurrent disease within 4 years after initial therapy. The depth of uterine invasion was independent of tumor grade in the 36 evaluable patients. Of 32 patients who were clinically stage II, only 50% were stage II at operation; 28% had no cervical involvement; and 22% had more advanced disease. In the 36 patients whose surgical stage was evaluable, 5-year survival was 88.9% in those with surgical stage I disease, 70% in those with stage II, and 0% in those with stage III and stage IV disease (Fig 12–2). All 12 patients who had recurrence by 12 months died of tumor at 0 to 20 months after recurrence; 24 patients who had recurrence after 12 months had a mean survival of 8 months after recurrence. Tumor grade had no effect on time to recurrence, distant metastases, and regional and local spread.

The wide range of frequencies for stage II disease and the frequent staging errors evident in this study support the contention that criteria for determining cervical extension of endometrial carcinoma are not well standardized. The results suggest that aggressive radiation therapy will cure many patients with stage II endometrial carcinoma.

▶ [The prognosis for patients with stage II endometrial cancer is significantly worse than that for patients with stage I disease. Tumor grade and extent of myometrial invasion are important predictors here just as they are in patients with stage I disease.

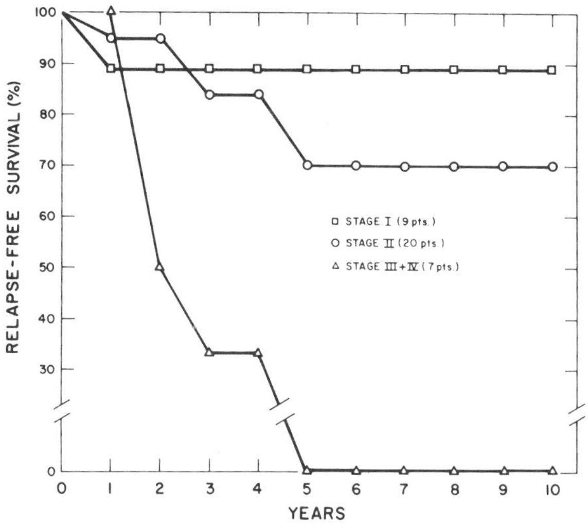

Fig 12–2.—Corrected actuarial survival by surgical stage in patients without preoperative radiation. (Courtesy of Berman, M. L., et al.: Gynecol. Oncol. 14:49–61, August 1982. Reprinted with permission from The American College of Obstetricians and Gynecologists.)

A discouraging finding reported in this article is the inaccuracy of the clinical staging. Of 32 clinical stage II patients, only half were stage II at operation, one-fourth had disease outside the uterus and one-fourth had no endocervical involvement. Of the 32 patients, 9 had gross cervical involvement, 1 had a positive cone, and 22 were diagnosed on the basis of endocervical curettage. Twelve in the last group had tumor confined to the corpus at hysterectomy. Thus, the endocervical curettage (which we emphasize to our residents and students) was frequently misleading. A better means of diagnosing endocervical involvement is required. Perhaps hysteroscopy is the answer. One might suggest primary hysterectomy in patients with positive endocervical curettage results in the absence of gross involvement of the cervix, but many think that patients with true stage II disease should have intracavitary radiotherapy prior to operation. We don't see a clear-cut solution to this problem.] ◀

12–21 **Importance of Gestagen, Tamoxifen, and Steroid Receptors in the Therapy of Endometrial Cancer: Report of an Experiment.** Breast cancer is currently managed by receptor-specific therapy using antiestrogenic and ablative hormonal methods, but data on receptors in endometrial cancer remain contradictory. W. Kleine, A. Fuchs, and A. Pfleiderer xenotransplanted 6 human endometrial cancers of differing clinical stage and histologic differentiation into thymus-aplastic nude mice, and treated them with medrogestone, gestonorone, tamoxifen, and estradiol. Tissue fragments were transplanted into the ventral chest wall subcutaneously, and hormonal therapy was begun when definite growth was documented. Female mice received medrogestone, 3 mg/kg, or tamoxifen, 2 mg/kg, daily for 4 weeks. Male animals were treated with estradiol, 3 mg/kg, or gestonorone, 20 mg/kg, every 3 days. All treatments were given intramuscularly.

Both estrogen and progesterone receptors were present in 2 of the endometrial cancers, whereas 4 lacked both receptors. The receptor-

---

(12–21) Acta Obstet. Gynecol. Scand. 61:449–453, 1982.

negative tumors grew faster in nude mice than in receptor-positive mice. Receptor-positive tumors tended toward greater differentiation. Tamoxifen therapy significantly retarded the growth of a receptor-positive tumor, but medrogestone led to only minimal retardation of growth of this lesion. The cancers without steroid receptors had no significant retardation of growth with medrogestone or tamoxifen. Estradiol accelerated the growth of a cancer with estrogen receptors. Typical hormonal effects were observed in the treated mice.

These findings show the importance of hormone receptor determination as a prognostic measure. Tamoxifen can be used to treat endometrial carcinoma when estrogen-receptor-positive tumor tissue is present. Experiments in the nude mouse are of limited value in predicting the response of various types of endometrial cancer to different hormonal manipulations.

▶ [These results in nude mice add support to the suggestion that the estrogen receptor status of endometrial cancers may be predictive of the response of these tumors to hormonal therapy.] ◀

12–22 **Leiomyosarcoma of the Uterus.** Conflicting opinions exist as to the precise histopathologic features for diagnosis of leiomyosarcoma. Tung Van Dinh and J. Donald Woodruff (Johns Hopkins Hosp., Baltimore) report a study of 43 uterine leiomyosarcomas in an attempt to clarify some of the controversial features. Forty-one of the 43 patients in this study were observed for 2 or more years; 17 patients (40%) were postmenopausal and 26 (60%) were premenopausal.

Abnormal uterine bleeding and pelvic discomfort were the most common presenting symptoms. The largest tumor measured 19 × 15 × 7.5 cm and weighed 695 gm. Lesions were described as whitish gray or pale pink with cystic, hemorrhagic, or necrotic soft areas. A solitary tumor was found in 45% of the cases, and multiple myomas in 42%. In this series, at least 2 mitotic figures per any high-power field were necessary to validate diagnosis of leiomyosarcoma. Total hysterectomy with or without salpingo-oophorectomy was performed in 37 (86%) cases. Myomectomy only was performed in the remaining 6 cases (14%).

The overall 5-year survival for the 41 patients followed up for 2 or more years was 73%. When survival was related to number of mitoses per 1 or 10 high-power fields (Tables 1 and 2), no tumor-related deaths occurred in patients with 2 or 3 mitoses in any high-power field or 1 to 4 mitoses in 10 high-power fields; however, 1 patient is alive with recurrence in the latter category. Pleomorphism did not influence prognosis. The 5-year survival rate was equal for patients with tumors with and without high degrees of pleomorphism (77%). Borders of tumor (infiltrating or pushing) and vascular invasion by malignant cells did not affect survival. Localization of tumor was possibly the most prognostic feature. Whereas the 5-year survival rate was similar for patients with submucous (80%), intramural (88%), and subserous tumor (100%), it was dismal for patients with tumors occurring de novo in the myometrium (25%) and in those patients

(12–22) Am. J. Obstet. Gynecol. 144:817–823, Dec. 1, 1982.

TABLE 1.—SURVIVAL RELATED TO MOST MITOSES IN ANY HIGH-POWER FIELD

	2 Years after diagnosis			5 Years after diagnosis		
*No. of mitoses per high-power field**	*No. of patients*	*No. of deaths*	*Survival (%)*	*No. of patients*	*No. of deaths*	*Survival (%)*
2-3	14	0	100	11	0	100
4-5	19†	1	95	13†	4	69
6-7	3	0	100	3	2	33
8-9	5	2	60	3	2	33
Total	41			30		

*Number of mitotic figures in most anaplastic high-power fields.
†One patient living with recurrence.
(Courtesy of Dinh, T. V., and Woodruff, J. D.: Am. J. Obstet. Gynecol. 144:817–823, Dec. 1, 1982.)

with tumors that extended beyond the uterus (33%) at initial operation. Premenopausal patients had a 5-year survival rate of 93%; postmenopausal patients had a 50% 5-year survival rate. Myometry alone was performed in 6 cases, with one recurrence. The role of adjunctive chemotherapy with use of Adriamycin and dacarbazine is still unclear.

TABLE 2.—SURVIVAL RELATED TO NUMBER OF MITOSES PER 10 HIGH-POWER FIELDS

	2 Years after diagnosis			*5 Years after diagnosis*		
No. of mitoses per 10 high-power fields	*No. of patients*	*No. of deaths*	*Survival (%)*	*No. of patients*	*No. of deaths*	*Survival (%)*
1-4	12	0	100	9*	0	100
5-9	22*	2	91	16	4	75
≥10	7	1	86	5	4	20
Total	41			30		

*One patient living with recurrence.
(Courtesy of Dinh, T. V., and Woodruff, J. D.: Am. J. Obstet. Gynecol. 144:817–823, Dec. 1, 1982.)

Uterine leiomyosarcoma is rare and the basic therapy is surgery. No evidence exists that adnexectomy alters survival. Factors indicating a good prognosis are premenopausal status, localization of tumor in a myoma, low mitotic count, presence of hyalinization around the tumor, and absence of necrosis. Tumors arising de novo in the myometrium have a poorer prognosis than lesions developing in a leiomyoma.

▶ [This large series of cases of uterine leiomyosarcoma generally confirms what is known from earlier studies, particularly the prognostic importance of the number of mitotic figures. Other clinical or pathologic features that correlated with outcome were age (premenopausal was better than postmenopausal) and location of the tumor (one situated in a myoma was better than one arising de novo in myometrium). Histologic differentiation, by contrast, had no prognostic import. Figure 1 in the original article illustrates a highly pleomorphic tumor with a moderate mitotic count; the patient survived with only myomectomy.] ◀

12-23 **Metastases to Uterine Corpus From Extragenital Cancers: Clinicopathologic Study of 63 Cases.** Neelam B. Kumar and William R. Hart (Univ. of Michigan) reviewed data on 63 patients with cancer metastatic from extragenital sites to the uterine corpus. There were 43 autopsy cases and 20 surgical cases in the series. The mean patient age was 60 years. Primary sites are listed in Table 1, and the

TABLE 1.—Sites of 63 Primary Extragenital Cancers Causing Metastases to the Uterine Corpus

Site of primary neoplasm	Autopsy Cases No. (%)	Surgical Cases No. (%)	All Cases No. (%)
Breast	20 (46.5)	7 (35.0)	27 (42.9)
Colon	3 (7.0)	8 (40.0)	11 (17.5)
Stomach	6 (13.9)	1 (5.0)	7 (11.1)
Pancreas	6 (13.9)	1 (5.0)	7 (11.1)
Gallbladder	3 (7.0)	0 (0)	3 (4.8)
Lung	2 (4.7)	1 (5.0)	3 (4.8)
Melanoma of skin	2 (4.7)	0 (0)	2 (3.2)
Urinary bladder	1 (2.3)	1 (5.0)	2 (3.2)
Thyroid	0 (0)	1 (5.0)	1 (1.6)
Total	43 (100)	20 (100)	63 (100)

(Courtesy of Kumar, N. B., and Hart, W. R.: Cancer 50:2163–2169, Nov. 15, 1982.)

TABLE 2.—Anatomical Distribution of metastases Within Uterine Corpus in 52 Patients*

Location in uterine corpus	Autopsy cases No. (%)	Hysterectomy cases No. (%)	All cases No. (%)
Myometrium only†	25 (58.1)	8 (88.9)	33 (63.5)
Endometrium and myometrium	16 (37.2)	1 (11.1)	17 (32.7)
Endometrium only	2 (4.7)	0 (0)	2 (3.8)
Total	43 (100)	9 (100)	52 (100)

*In 11 other patients, disease was diagnosed by endometrial curettage without subsequent hysterectomy or autopsy.

†Included are 6 patients with metastases restriced to myometrial leiomyomas.

(Courtesy of Kumar, N. B., and Hart, W. R.: Cancer 50:2163–2169, Nov. 15, 1982.)

(12–23) Cancer 50:2163–2169, Nov. 15, 1982.

distribution of metastases in the uterus is shown in Table 2. All patients also had node metastases, and most had metastases in the lungs, liver, bone, or adrenals. The urinary bladder was involved in about 25% of the patients. Metastases were present in an ovary in 65%, in the uterine cervix in 41%, and in the vagina in 35%. In 5 patients who underwent surgery, uterine metastases were the first indication of an extragenital primary cancer. The microscopic features of the metastases closely resembled those of the respective primary tumors. In the endometrium, metastases were typically in the stroma adjacent to normal endometrial glands.

Uterine bleeding may be caused by metastases from an extragenital primary neoplasm to the uterine corpus. The breast was the most common primary site in the present series. Rarely, uterine metastasis may be the first indication of an extragenital primary cancer. The myometrium is involved more frequently than the endometrium is. Metastases to leiomyomas were present in several patients.

▶ [This is a nice summary of a rare condition that the gynecologist may encounter sometime. The primary tumors seem to be represented in about their frequency distribution; lung cancer may seem to occur more commonly than the frequency here, but it was actually an unusual malignancy in women through most of the 60-year period covered by this report.] ◀

12–24 **Ovarian Cystadenofibromas in Three Women With Antenatal Exposure to Diethylstilbestrol.** Grant Schmidt and Wesley C. Fowler, Jr. (Univ. of North Carolina, Chapel Hill) report that, of 350 women with in utero exposure to synthetic estrogen diethylstilbestrol (DES) followed up at the University of North Carolina, 3 had removal of ovarian cystadenofibromas, of which 1 showed severe epithelial atypia (borderline malignancy—World Health Organization classification).

CASE 1.—Woman, 28, nulligravid, DES-exposed, had primary infertility and underwent laparoscopy for an asymptomatic pelvic mass. An ovarian tumor was identified. Microscopic examination of the tumor and nodules showed a papillary cystadenofibroma, but with intraglandular tufting, papillation, and some cell detachment, after unilateral oophorectomy. After subsequent conception and delivery by cesarean section, histologic study of multiple ovarian cysts were again consistent with borderline malignancy. Eight weeks post partum, the patient underwent hysterectomy, left salpingo-oophorectomy, and staging biopsies, with findings limited to tumor foci in the left ovary.

CASE 2.—Woman, 26, nulligravid, DES-exposed, had primary infertility and an asymptomatic pelvic mass. During laparotomy, bilateral ovarian cystic tumors with extensive intra-abdominal papillomatosis were identified. A panhysterectomy and omentectomy were performed, which showed bilateral ovarian and multicentric omental cystadenofibromas. Two-year follow-up has been without complications.

CASE 3.—Woman, 21, nulligravid, DES-exposed, underwent laparotomy for an asymptomatic enlarging pelvic mass that had been unresponsive to hormonal suppression. An ovarian cyst was excised, which showed microscopic cystadenofibroma without atypical epithelium. Five-year follow-up has been uneventful.

(12–24) Gynecol. Oncol. 14:175–184, October 1982.

The cystadenofibroma is believed to arise from the germinal epithelium of the ovary and comprises about 4% of all ovarian tumors. The appearance of 3 ovarian cystadenofibromas among 350 unselected women exposed to DES in utero is most unusual, especially in a group of women whose average age is 24 years. A self-selection bias seems remote considering the rarity of the tumor, and all 3 patients were asymptomatic. Two had primary infertility and all had classic DES-related cervicovaginal changes. The pathogenesis of cystadenofibroma remains unresolved, but the apparent increased incidence in a group of young DES-exposed women may be contributory. Conservative surgical therapy remains the method of management for this condition.

► [This may be only coincidence, but finding 3 young women with this relatively unusual ovarian tumor (cystadenofibromas were considered in the 1981 YEAR BOOK, pp. 304–305) among 350 cases of intrauterine DES exposure suggests that there may be an association. One of the patients described here had a borderline malignancy. Other investigators interested in the consequences of in utero DES exposure are certain to report their experience concerning this ovarian lesion.] ◄

12–25 **Primary Cytoreductive Surgery for Epithelial Ovarian Cancer.** Ovarian cancer spreads chiefly by exfoliation of tumor cells and their implantation throughout the peritoneal cavity, presenting a unique surgical challenge. Many remain skeptical regarding the value of cytoreductive surgery. Neville F. Hacker, Jonathan S. Berek, Leo D. Lagasse, Roberta K. Nieberg, and Robert M. Elashoff (Univ. of California at Los Angeles) reviewed experience with primary cytoreductive surgery in 47 patients with stage III or stage IV epithelial carcinoma of the ovary operated on in 1974 to 1979. The mean age was 58 years and the mean parity was 1.5. Three patients had stage IV disease. Serous carcinomas predominated. Ascites was present in 30 patients. The mean diameter of the primary tumor was 11 cm. Fourteen patients had been considered inoperable.

Thirty-one patients (66%) had optimal cytoreduction, with no residual tumor mass more than 1.5 cm in diameter. Ten of the 14 patients previously operated on had optimal cytoreduction. Fifteen patients required only abdominal hysterectomy, bilateral salpingo-oophorectomy, and omentectomy. Bowel resection was necessary in 5 patients. Resectability was not significantly influenced by tumor grade. Major complications occurred in 8 patients having optimal cytoreduction, but there was no operative mortality in this group. Most of the patients having optimal cytoreduction received a single alkylating agent. Five patients were alive without disease and 4 with disease after optimal cytoreduction. After optimal cytoreduction, median survival was 40 months when residual nodules were less than 0.5 cm in size and 18 months when they were larger, compared with 6 months in the other patients. All of the latter patients died of disease within 18 months. Survival without disease ranged up to 7½ years postoperatively. The chief determinants of outcome in the optimal cytoreduction group were size of the largest metastatic nodule before operation and the presence of clinical ascites.

Optimal cytoreduction can be achieved in at least two thirds of pa-

(12–25) Obstet. Gynecol. 61:413–420, April 1983.

tients with invasive epithelial ovarian cancer, with acceptable morbidity. Survival is significantly prolonged in patients with small residual tumor, and some of them are cured. A primary attempt at aggressive cytoreductive surgery is warranted in these patients. The value of preoperative or postoperative chemotherapy remains unclear; the authors favor cytoreductive surgery before intensive chemotherapy is tried.

▶ [Cytoreductive surgery or "debulking" in advanced ovarian cancer is controversial, but several recent studies seem to indicate that it improves the subsequent response to chemotherapy. In this report, patients who could have enough tumor removal so that remaining masses were less than 1.5 cm in diameter clearly did better in terms of survival than those in whom this was not possible. The degree of resection needed may be extensive (e.g., 25% of all cases involved bowel and/or bladder resection) but the operative and postoperative morbidity was not alarming. At present, it appears that an aggressive approach to removing as much tumor as possible is indicated.] ◀

12–26 **Prognostic Importance of Psammoma Bodies in Adenocarcinomas of the Ovaries.** Areas of microscopic calcification called "psammoma bodies" are commonly found in serous papillary adenocarcinomas of the ovary. Some investigators think that tumors with such bodies have a markedly better prognosis than those without. Bengt Sorbe and Bo Frankendal (Örebro, Sweden) assessed retrospectively the prognostic importance of psammoma bodies in serous papillary adenocarcinomas in a review of data on 501 patients treated for epithelial ovarian carcinoma from 1964 through 1979. Treatment consisted of hysterectomy and bilateral salpingo-oophorectomy, followed by abdominal radiation or chemotherapy, or both. Microscopic specimens were reexamined for tumor histology, grade, and presence of psammoma bodies. Prognosis was measured as the probability of survival according to actuarial life-table analysis.

Mean age of the patients was 59 years and the overall 5-year survival rate was 38%. Histologically, serous papillary adenocarcinoma (type 1c) accounted for 48.9% of the cases, endometrioid adenocarcinoma (type 3c) for 14.2%, and mucinous adenocarcinoma (type 2c) for 12.8%. Psammoma bodies were present in 68 (13.6%) of the 501 cases. Of the 68, 61 (24.9%) cases occurred among 245 patients with histologic type 1c. These calcifications were more than twice as common in clinical stages III and IV than in stage I; stage II was intermediate. There was no clear-cut association between tumor grade and the presence of psammoma bodies.

Life-table analysis showed that the presence of psammoma bodies did significantly influence the prognosis for serous papillary adenocarcinomas. When analyzed by tumor stage, the presence of psammoma bodies again was not of statistical significance for cumulative life-table survival.

The results do not confirm the finding of a significantly better prognosis for adenocarcinomas with these calcifications. Supportive evidence suggests that psammoma body formation is a result of dystrophic calcification associated with ischemia rather than tumor host hypersensitivity-related cell death.

(12–26) Gynecol. Oncol. 14:6–14, August 1982.

▶ [Some have suggested that the presence of psammoma bodies in papillary serous cystadenocarcinomas of the ovary is associated with an improved prognosis. This large series doesn't support that view.] ◀

12–27 **Cyclophosphamide Plus *cis*-Platinum in Combination: Treatment Program for Stage III or IV Ovarian Carcinoma.** David G. Decker, Thomas R. Fleming, George D. Malkasian, Jr., Maurice J. Webb, John A. Jefferies, and John H. Edmonson (Mayo Clinic and Found.) compared treatment of 42 patients with stage III or stage IV ovarian carcinoma with cyclophosphamide only (21 patients) or with cyclophosphamide plus *cis*-platinum (21 patients). Cytoreductive surgery was performed in most patients in the study before the chemotherapy regimen was initiated. Second-look surgery was performed after a year of chemotherapy, which was given on an outpatient basis.

The time to progression of tumor and the duration of survival were markedly improved in patients receiving combination chemotherapy. Toxicity to the bone marrow was obviously increased with combination chemotherapy, but in no patient was it life threatening, and recovery was rapid after the nadir. Severity of vomiting differed little between the two groups. Cystitis was mild and cleared spontaneously. Diarrhea was increased with combination chemotherapy but was manageable. At 2 years, 52.4% of patients receiving combination therapy had no progression of tumor, whereas only 9.5% of those receiving cyclophosphamide alone had no progression. Survival at 2 years was 61.9% for the combination chemotherapy group and 19.0% for those treated with cyclophosphamide alone. Figure 12–3 shows that patients treated with cyclophosphamide and *cis*-platinum have an apparent advantage in long-term survival compared with those treated with cyclophosphamide alone. The 17 patients with residual tumor smaller than 2 cm at initiation of chemotherapy tended to have longer survival than those with residual tumor larger than 2 cm, but this was not significant.

Fig 12–3.—Survival of patients with stage III or stage IV ovarian cancer treated with cyclophosphamide only *(C)* or with a combination of cyclophosphamide and *cis*-platinum *(CP)*. (Courtesy of Decker, D. G., et al.: Obstet. Gynecol. 60:481–487, October 1982. Reprinted with permission from The American College of Obstetricians and Gynecologists.)

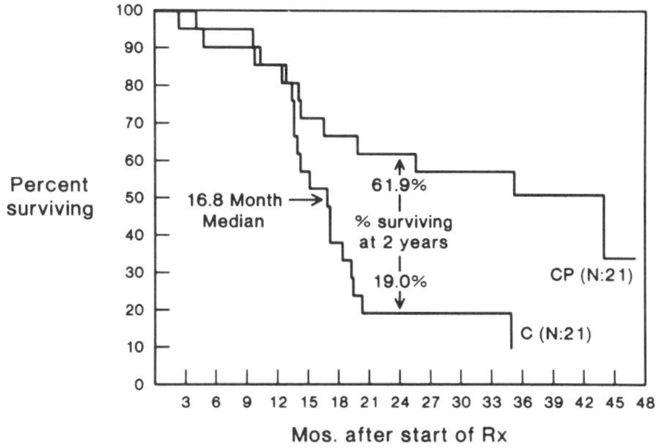

(12–27) Obstet. Gynecol. 60:481–487, October 1982.

Combination chemotherapy with cyclophosphamide and *cis*-platinum appears to be a treatment program that involves reasonable toxicity, that can be administered in an outpatient setting, and that produces an increased response rate over single-agent treatment in patients with proved stage III or stage IV epithelial ovarian cancer.

12–28 **Improved Therapy With Cisplatin Regimens for Patients With Ovarian Carcinoma (FIGO Stages III and IV) as Measured by Surgical End-Staging (Second-Look Operation).** Carmel J. Cohen, Judith D. Goldberg, James F. Holland, Howard W. Bruckner, Gunter Deppe, Saul B. Gusberg, Robert C. Wallach, Bernard Kabakow, and John Rodin (City Univ. of New York) reviewed the outcome in 273 patients with epithelial cancer of the ovary, International Federation of Gynecology and Obstetrics (FIGO) stages III and IV, seen from 1974 to 1982. The patients were randomized to four therapeutic trials, all including cisplatin and other drugs such as cyclophosphamide, Adriamycin, hexamethylmelamine, and thiotepa. Of this series, 74% had FIGO stage III tumors and 14% had FIGO stage IV tumors.

Overall, 73 second-look operations were done on randomized patients after achieving complete clinical remission and the completion of at least 10 cycles of chemotherapy. Another 43 nonrandomized patients also had second-look procedures. Fifteen percent of patients had microscopic residual disease, none of which was diagnosed by laparoscopy. From 40% to 46% of patients treated with cisplatin regimens had no disease at second look. The outcome was not related to cell differentiation or to volume of disease present postoperatively. Two treatment-related deaths occurred, but no deaths resulted from surgical end-staging. Comparison of survival in randomized and nonrandomized patients having second-look operations suggested that, once at least 10 courses of cisplatin-containing chemotherapy are given and complete clinical remission is obtained, survival after second-look operations remains constant.

An optimistic attitude toward the treatment of advanced ovarian cancer does not seem unreasonable today. Although the authors previously have not been very aggressive in recommending surgical end-staging, there is still reason to reduce chemotherapy as soon as cure has been achieved, because the impact of new second-line chemotherapy has not yet been assessed and the late adverse effects of prolonged chemotherapy may not be manifest for years.

▶ [This article and the preceding one both confirm the value of *cis*-platinum, probably the most efficacious agent presently available for disseminated ovarian cancer. The study by Decker and colleagues from the Mayo Clinic and Foundation demonstrates clearly that the addition of *cis*-platinum to cyclophosphamide improves outcome. Toxicity, evident mainly in leukopenia and thrombocytopenia, was not especially serious.

The study by Cohen and associates from New York found, among patients receiving cisplatin combined with Adriamycin or thiotepa after cytoreductive surgery, an objective response rate at 3 months of 80% or better. Moreover, nearly half of patients undergoing "second-look" laparotomy after a cisplatin regimen had negative findings. It is somewhat disconcerting, however, that the median length of survival did not reflect a clear superiority for cisplatin over other chemotherapy regimens.

For a suggestion of how *cis*-platinum may work, read on. . . .] ◀

(12–28) Am. J. Obstet. Gynecol. 145:955–967, Apr. 15, 1983.

12–29 **Histologic Correlates of Virulence in Ovarian Adenocarcinoma: I: Effect of Differentiation.** Patients with ovarian tumors that are better differentiated histologically are thought to survive longer and respond better to chemotherapy. The degree of maturation of a tumor (grading) and the topographic extent of the tumor (staging) are considered to be important determinants of its prognosis. The dramatic change in the natural history of ovarian adenocarcinoma produced by more effective chemotherapeutic agents, such as cisplatin, has created the need to review the morphological parameters traditionally believed to be related to survival.

Allan J. Jacobs, Liane Deligdisch, Gunter Deppe, and Carmel J. Cohen (Mount Sinai School of Medicine, New York) reviewed the data on 87 patients with stage III or stage IV ovarian adenocarcinoma whose treatment, which began in 1974 to 1978, included cisplatin, either alone or in combination with other agents.

Cumulative survival rates for the 87 patients were 86% at 1 year, 49% at 2 years, and 38% at 3 years. Histologic differentiation of the tumor made no difference with regard to response to treatment or to survival. The cytologic factors of mitotic activity, cellular pleomorphism, and giant cells appeared to be parameters of tumor grade and were related to histologic differentiation. The presence of psammoma bodies may also be an indicator of tumor differentiation.

Elimination of differentiation as an element affecting survival of patients with adenocarcinoma may be a consequence of a change produced by cisplatin in the biologic performance of this disease.

▶ [In cancer generally, the degree of histologic differentiation is an important prognostic characteristic. The relationship has been found to hold in a number of studies of ovarian cancer, but in this report of data on patients with stage III or stage IV adenocarcinoma of the ovary treated with cisplatin alone and with other chemotherapeutic agents, there did not seem to be a correlation between histology (differentiation, mitotic activity, and pleomorphism) and survival or response. The authors postulate that cisplatin may eliminate histologic differentiation as a determinant of response by altering the biology of the neoplasm.] ◀

12–30 **Cyclic GMP in Urine to Monitor the Response of Ovarian Cancer to Therapy.** G. A. Turner, R. D. Ellis, D. Guthrie, A. L. Latner, W. M. Ross, and A. W. Skillen (Newcastle Genl. Hosp., Newcastle upon Tyne, England) report on their retrospective study in which they measured guanosine 3′:5′-phosphate (cyclic GMP) repeatedly in a group of patients with ovarian cancer receiving chemotherapy. Single urine specimens were collected from 33 women with ovarian cancer at random times between 9 A.M. and 5 P.M. Only patients showing either complete clinical remission (21 women) or no signs of remission (12 women) were selected for study.

In each case, urine cyclic GMP levels appeared to follow a definite pattern of two phases. In the first phase, after an initial fall, the level remained around the upper limit of the normal reference range. In the second phase, the level gradually rose and was generally maintained at an elevated value. At the end of this phase, cancer recurrence was detected and the patient's death followed soon afterward.

(12–29) Am. J. Obstet. Gynecol. 143:574–580, July 1, 1982.
(12–30) Br. J. Obstet. Gynaecol. 89:760–764, September 1982.

Clinical disappearance of the tumor was associated with a decrease in urine cyclic GMP in 19 of 21 patients. Conversely, in 15 of 16 patients who had a recurrence, the urine cyclic GMP level was increased on the day the recurrence was detected as compared with the value obtained for the day the remission was detected ($P < .01$). In those patients who did not respond to chemotherapy, urine cyclic GMP levels remained above the upper limit of the reference range in most specimens assayed.

The authors conclude that measurement of cyclic GMP levels in urine could have considerable value in monitoring ovarian cancer during chemotherapy. A changing cyclic GMP level could predate any clinical detection of the cancer by as much as 10 months. Early detection of a recurrence of ovarian cancer would allow the clinician to change the mode of therapy before the tumor burden becomes large. Cyclic GMP is stable at room temperature for long periods of time, provided a preservative is present, and it is excreted in quantities far exceeding the detection limits for radioimmunoassay.

▶ [More experience is required to establish the value of cyclic GMP concentrations in urine in monitoring the course of patients with ovarian cancer who are receiving chemotherapy. The track record of other biochemical markers of tumor activity hasn't been too hot, with the exception, of course, of human chorionic gonadotropin and trophoblastic neoplasms.] ◀

12–31 **Surgical Management of Bowel Obstruction in Advanced Ovarian Carcinoma.** Bowel obstruction is a frequent complication of advanced ovarian cancer. Some suggest aggressive surgical treatment for delayed obstruction, whereas others advise individualized management because of the high operative mortality and morbidity in these patients. Hans-B. Krebs and Dean R. Goplerud (Med. College of Virginia, Richmond) reviewed experience with 118 surgical procedures in the treatment of bowel obstruction associated with advanced ovarian cancer in 98 patients seen from 1960 to 1980. All received three or more courses of chemotherapy before bowel obstruction developed, and 42 received radiotherapy. Twenty patients had a second operation for recurrent bowel obstruction. Most operations were done to relieve small bowel obstruction. Eleven enteroenterostomy bypasses were done. Large bowel obstruction was managed by various bypass procedures.

The median postoperative survival in surgically treated patients was 12½ weeks. Fatal complications occurred within a month postoperatively in 12 of 104 episodes managed by bowel surgery. The most common complication was dehiscence of the bowel anastomosis. Median survival in 92 patients in whom surgery was feasible without postoperative mortality was 18 weeks. Patients benefited from surgery in two thirds of instances. Benefit was less likely to occur with increasing age, nutritional deprivation, more extensive tumor spread, and presence of ascites and in patients receiving previous chemotherapy or radiotherapy (table).

Operations for bowel obstruction caused by advanced ovarian cancer result in high mortality and morbidity rates; in some cases cor-

---

(12–31) Obstet. Gynecol. 61:327–330, March 1983.

PROGNOSTIC PARAMETERS IN OVARIAN CARCINOMA COMPLICATED BY BOWEL OBSTRUCTION

Parameters	No benefit from surgery	*P* value*	Assigned risk score
Age (yr)			
<45	11/48 (23%)		0
45–65	21/58 (36%)	<.025	1
>65	9/12 (75%)		2
Nutritional status† (deprivation)			
None or minimal	5/42 (12%)		0
Moderate	13/39 (33%)	<.001	1
Severe	23/37 (62%)		2
Tumor status			
No palpable intraabdominal masses	4/38 (11%)		0
Palpable intraabdominal masses	23/56 (41%)	<.005	1
Liver involvement or distant metastases	14/24 (58%)		2
Ascites			
None or mild (asymptomatic, abdomen not distended)	10/59 (17%)		0
Moderate (abdomen distended)	18/43 (42%)	<.001	1
Severe (symptomatic, requires frequent paracenteses)	13/16 (81%)		2
Previous chemotherapy			
None, or no adequate trial	2/18 (11%)		0
Failed single drug therapy	7/35 (20%)	<.025	1
Failed combination drug therapy	32/65 (49%)		2
Previous radiation therapy			
None	18/76 (24%)		0
Radiation therapy to pelvis	6/15 (40%)	<.025	1
Radiation therapy to whole abdomen	17/27 (63%)		2

*Test for homogeneity.
†Based upon criteria according to Dudrick et al.
(Courtesy of Krebs, H.-B., and Goplerud, D. R.: Obstet. Gynecol. 61:327–330, March 1983. Reprinted with permission from The American College of Obstetricians and Gynecologists.)

rective surgery is not possible because of extensive tumor involvement. Surgery is not likely to be helpful if the patient is expected to live for less than 2 months or contrast studies show evidence of impaired bowel motility because of diffuse intraperitoneal carcinomatosis. Irradiated patients and those with rapidly reaccumulating ascites requiring repeated paracentesis also have done poorly. Nutritional deprivation is another important factor. A comprehensive assessment of all prognostic parameters is necessary in each patient to determine the possible benefit from surgical intervention.

▶ [Bowel obstruction is a common occurrence with ovarian cancer, and the outcome in patients with this complication is not very good. This article identified six risk factors and developed a scoring system based on them. Outcome was pretty good (75%–100% survival for at least 8 weeks) when the score was 4 or less, but not so good (0%–25%) when it was 7 or more.] ◀

12–32 **Natural History of Dysgerminoma.** Giuseppe De Palo, Silvana Pilotti, Rado Kenda, Elisabetta Ratti, Renato Musumeci, Constantino

(12–32) Am. J. Obstet. Gynecol. 143:799–807, Aug. 1, 1982.

Mangioni, Francesco Di Re, Angelo Lattuada, Umberta Conti, Francesco Cefis, Liliana Recanatini, Silvestro Carinelli, and Gianfranco Rossi (Milan) reviewed the records of 56 patients with pure dysgerminoma seen from January 1958 to June 1980. Nineteen patients were new, 30 were seen for reassessment after undergoing unilateral ovariosalpingectomy elsewhere 45 to 60 days previously, and 7 were seen for restaging after being treated elsewhere more than 60 days previously.

The patients were aged 8 to 45 years (mean, 21 years) at the time of histologic diagnosis; 48 were younger than age 30, and 14 were younger than age 16. Seven patients were premenarchal, 49 were postmenarchal, and only 10 were parous. The tumor was often asymptomatic. Nonspecific pelvic discomfort or swelling of the lower abdomen or both were the most frequent symptom and sign. Duration of symptoms exceeded 6 months in only 2 patients. The disease was bilateral in 8 cases. Tumor diameter was unknown in 27 patients, greater than 10 cm in 25, and less than 10 cm in 4. The tumor capsule was ruptured in 2 patients.

Results of lymphography, performed in 47 patients, were positive in 14 (31.8%) of 44 new and reassessment cases and in 12 (31.6%) of 38 patients with clinical stage I or stage II disease. Results of peritoneoscopy, performed in 18 patients, showed the peritoneum, diaphragm, and liver capsule of all 18 to be free from metastases. Peritoneal cytologic testing, performed in 32 patients, gave positive results in 4. Seventeen patients had reassessment or restaging laparotomy. Radiologic and histologic correlation of retroperitoneal node examination was possible in 20 patients.

Treatment protocols varied. Of the 31 patients with stage 1A, 1B, or 1C disease (mean follow-up, 45 months), total survival was 100% and 5-year recurrence-free survival was 91%. Of the 18 patients with stage III disease (mean follow-up, 29 months), total survival was 81% and 4-year recurrence-free survival was 56%. Four-year survival was 74% in patients with stage III retroperitoneal disease and only 24% in those with stage III peritoneal disease with or without retroperitoneal involvement. Disease recurred in 1 of 31 patients with stage 1A, 1B, or 1C disease, and in 2 of 12 with stage III retroperitoneal disease.

Dysgerminoma usually spreads by the lymphatic route to the nodes near the left kidney, to the para-aortic region at the level of the right third lumbar vertebra. Only chest roentgenography and lymphography are mandatory for determining local, regional, and distant extent of disease. A chest film can show adenopathy in the mediastinum and pulmonary metastases. The authors consider lymphography the most important staging procedure although the International Federation of Gynecology and Obstetrics does not presently accept it for staging ovarian tumors. Laparoscopy with diaphragmatic inspection is theoretically useful for staging. Peritoneal cytologic testing sometimes shows malignant disease. Surgical inspection of the contralateral ovary with wedge biopsy is as important as surgical lymph node assessment. Abdominal exploration must be performed through a vertical rather than Pfannenstiel incision to permit removal of the tumor without rupture and to adequately explore the entire abdominal cavity.

The prognosis for pure dysgerminoma is good. If staging is accurate, stage I disease has a favorable prognosis whether or not adjuvant radiation therapy is used. The prognosis for stage III retroperitoneal disease is good if adequate radiation therapy is given to involved sites and to other sites as a precaution. The prognosis for stage III peritoneal disease is poor, and it may be necessary to use, besides surgery, radiation therapy and chemotherapy, with *cis*-diamminedichloroplatinum alone or in combination with Adriamycin or with vinblastine and bleomycin for the best chemotherapy. The prognosis for patients with recurrence is good if therapy is adequate.

▶ [This report of a large series of patients with dysgerminomas reaffirms certain points. The patients are often young and the tumors unilateral. Para-aortic lymph node metastases were common (32% in stages I and II). In contrast to a recent report involving patients with cervical cancer (1981 YEAR BOOK, pp. 284–285), lymphography accurately identified nodal involvement. Survival was good even in the presence of nodal metastases, reflecting the radiosensitive nature of this lesion. Two patients with recurrences in the contralateral ovary are free of disease after its removal.] ◀

12–33 **Krukenberg Tumors of the Ovary: Clinicopathologic Analysis of 27 Cases** was made by Fred Holtz and William R. Hart (Ann Arbor, Mich.). The typical Krukenberg tumor of the ovary is characterized by mucinous, signet ring carcinoma cells in a cellular, nonneoplastic stroma. Mean age at diagnosis was 46 years. Clinical signs and symptoms usually were related to an abdominal or pelvic mass or to peritoneal, osseous, or pulmonary metastases. Three patients were asymptomatic. Two patients had a history of breast cancer, and 1 had had an ovarian "fibroma" removed 4 months before. Eight patients had proved osseous metastases. Two had lymphangitic pulmonary metastases, and at least 1 patient had leukoerythroblastosis associated with bone marrow metastases. A primary cancer responsible for the ovarian tumor was identified in 20 of the 22 adequately followed patients. Most of the extraovarian primaries that were verified arose in the stomach; the rest were in the colon. In only 5 patients was the primary carcinoma diagnosed first.

In over half the patients at least one involved ovary was 10 cm or more in size. Both ovaries were involved in all 18 evaluable patients. The typical microscopic appearance is of signet ring carcinoma cells arranged in linear streaks and small aggregates, with abundant mucin. Small glands or tubules were seen in about a third of cases. Small acinar structures with poorly formed or abortive lumina were not infrequent. The stroma often appeared to be reactive or hyperplastic in at least some areas. In the cortex the proliferating stromal cells often assumed a storiform pattern with dense collagenization. Intracytoplasmic mucosubstances were identified histochemically in the tumor cells in all cases studied. Intravascular tumor cell emboli were identified in half the cases.

All women with a typical Krukenberg tumor of the ovary should be

---

(12–33) Cancer 50:2438–2447, Dec. 1, 1982.

considered to have metastatic carcinoma, usually from the stomach, until proved otherwise. The tubular Krukenberg tumor appears to be an unusual histologic variant with prominent tubular or glandular formations.

▶ [This series serves as a nice review of Krukenberg tumors. It is noteworthy that half of the patients were aged 40 years or younger. Of the 20 extraovarian primary cancers, only 5 had been diagnosed before the ovarian tumors were found.] ◀

12–34 **Natural History of Hydatidiform Mole After Primary Evacuation.** John R. Lurain, John I. Brewer, Elizabeth E. Torok, and Bernard Halpern (Northwestern Univ.) followed up 738 patients after hydatidiform mole evacuation performed between 1962 and 1978. Serial human chorionic gonadotropin (hCG) tests were carried out at intervals of 10–15 days after termination of the molar gestation for 2 months, and then every 2 weeks until no hCG was detectable. Follow-up ranged from 4 to 18 years. A mouse uterine weight bioassay for urinary hCG determination was superseded by a serum radioimmunoassay and a specific radioimmunoassay for the β-subunit of hCG. Patients with a diagnosis of invasive mole or choriocarcinoma were treated mainly with intravenous administration of methotrexate or actinomycin D.

About 80% of patients experienced spontaneous remission after evacuation of the hydatidiform mole (table). Chemotherapy was given to 125 patients with a diagnosis of invasive mole and 17 with choriocarcinoma. Metastatic disease was present in 18 of the former patients and in 4 of the latter. All patients in whom hCG titers fell spontaneously to normal levels remained free of disease. All of those given chemotherapy entered permanent remission. In all patients with progressive disease, a rise in the hCG concentration identified disease more rapidly and accurately than did physical or roentgenographic findings.

About 20% of patients with hydatidiform mole can be expected to require further treatment after evacuation. Serial hCG testing with a sensitive assay can identify patients with progressive disease more

FOLLOW-UP IN 738 PATIENTS AFTER EVACUATION OF HYDATIDIFORM MOLE

	Patients			
	Normal hCG level		*Treated*	
Days after evacuation	*No.*	*%*	*No.*	*%*
0-30	135	18.3	3	0.4
31-60	255	34.6	23	3.1
61-170	206	27.9	116	15.7
Total	596	80.8	142	19.2

(Courtesy of Lurain, J. R., et al.: Am. J. Obstet. Gynecol. 145:591–595, Mar. 1, 1983.)

(12–34) Am. J. Obstet. Gynecol. 145:591–595, Mar. 1, 1983.

specifically than can physical findings. All patients in whom hCG titers declined spontaneously to normal levels remained well without treatment, and all of those with progressive disease were cured by chemotherapy.

▶ [This large experience with hydatidiform mole indicates that there is nothing magic about the 60-day mark after evacuation, so long as the hCG titer is falling. Nearly two thirds of the patients with detectable hCG levels at 60 days did not require chemotherapy.] ◀

12–35 **Treatment of Nonmetastatic Gestational Trophoblastic Disease: Results of Methotrexate Alone Versus Methotrexate and Folinic Acid.** Ellen Blair Smith, John C. Wood, Jr., Lee Tyrey, and Charles B. Hammond (Duke Univ.) compared the effects of two treatments for nonmetastatic gestational trophoblastic disease in a retrospective study. The course of nonmetastatic gestational trophoblastic disease in 39 patients treated with methotrexate alone is compared with the course in 29 patients who were treated with methotrexate alternated with folinic acid.

Among those patients initially treated with methotrexate alone, 7.7% had methotrexate-resistant disease and required a change in chemotherapy for induction of remission. In contrast, 27.5% of patients initially treated with methotrexate and folinic acid had methotrexate-resistant disease and required a change in chemotherapy to achieve remission. Remission was ultimately achieved in all patients. Those patients treated initially with methotrexate alone were later treated with actinomycin D. No patient in this series required hysterectomy because of resistance to chemotherapy. Those patients requiring actinomycin D subsequent to methotrexate received an average total of 7 treatments. The group of 29 patients treated with methotrexate and folinic acid averaged 3.5 treatments. Four of 39 patients (10.3%) required a change in therapy from methotrexate to actinomycin D solely because of toxic reactions. All 4 patients had distinct myelosuppression with methotrexate. Two of these 4 also had severe dermatitis. The difference in need to change therapy because of toxicity is not statistically significant between the two chemotherapeutic regimens.

The differences among peak serum glutamic oxaloacetic transaminase levels in patients receiving methotrexate, methotrexate and folinic acid, and actinomycin D subsequent to methotrexate or methotrexate and folinic acid are statistically significant. Among those 32 patients treated with methotrexate alone, who did not require further therapy with actinomycin D, 30 have been in remission for longer than 1 year. All patients who required actinomycin D in addition to methotrexate have achieved remission for longer than 1 year. Among 21 patients in remission after treatment with only methotrexate and folinic acid, 14 have been in remission for longer than 1 year. No statistically significant difference exists in the incidence of recurrence between those patients treated with methotrexate alone and those requiring actinomycin D in addition to methotrexate to produce remission.

(12–35) Am. J. Obstet. Gynecol. 144:88–92, Sept. 1, 1982.

Methotrexate and folinic acid is not as effective as methotrexate alone in inducing remission in nonmetastatic gestational trophoblastic disease. However, the markedly decreased toxicity of the combination regimen promotes continued use of the two drugs, although a change in therapy may be required to achieve remission.

▶ [This study suggests that methotrexate with folinic acid "rescue," while substantially less toxic than methotrexate alone, is also less effective. However, a couple of aspects are of concern. In the first place, the two groups came from different time periods and it is conceivable that something other than drug treatment (e.g., type of disease, sensitivity of assay, etc.) might be involved. Second, and probably more importantly, 4 patients in the group having methotrexate and folinic therapy subsequently proved to have lung metastases, and 3 of these patients were among the 8 failures. In any event, however, the question has been raised and a firm answer is needed.] ◀

12–36 **Fatal Gestational Trophoblastic Disease: Analysis of Treatment Failures.** John R. Lurain, John I. Brewer, Michael T. Mazur, and Elizabeth E. Torok (Chicago) reviewed the records of the 399 patients admitted to the trophoblastic disease center at Northwestern University during 1962 to 1978 for treatment of invasive mole or choriocarcinoma and found that 48 (12%) died. These 48 were aged 14 to 59 years (mean, 29 years). All had histologically documented choriocarcinoma and elevated levels of human chorionic gonadotropin (hCG).

Presenting symptoms included abnormal uterine bleeding in 22 patients, pulmonary symptoms in 6, uterine and pulmonary symptoms in 9, neurologic symptoms in 4, and abdominal pain in 5; 2 patients were asymptomatic. Term pregnancy, abortion, or ectopic pregnancy, rather than hydatidiform mole, preceded development of choriocarcinoma in 71% of the 48 fatal cases as compared to 51% of patients who were cured. The interval from the pregnancy event to initial treatment of trophoblastic disease was greater than 4 months in 62% of patients who died, compared to 23% of patients who were cured. Levels of hCG at initiation of treatment were in excess of 100,000 IU/L in 54% of patients who died, compared to 22% of those who were cured. Metastases were demonstrable prior to treatment in 44 patients and within 43 months after the start of treatment in 4. Pulmonary metastases were present in 77% of the patients. In 50% of the patients there was metastatic spread to the brain, liver, or peritoneal cavity upon presentation for treatment.

Treatment included 1 or more courses of chemotherapy in 43 patients, radiation therapy in addition to chemotherapy in 18, and 1 or more surgical procedures in 29. The most common cause of death was hemorrhage from one or more sites of metastasis (table).

Failure to cure patients with gestational trophoblastic disease is mainly due to the presence of extensive disease at the time of initial treatment; lack of initial, appropriately aggressive treatment in high-risk patients; and failure of presently used chemotherapy protocols to control advanced disease. Less than optimal treatment had been given to 10 of 15 patients who were referred after undergoing therapy

(12–36) Am. J. Obstet. Gynecol. 144:391–395, Oct. 15, 1982.

CAUSES OF DEATH IN 48 PATIENTS WITH METASTATIC GESTATIONAL CHORIOCARCINOMA

Cause of death	*Patients* *No.*	*%*
Hemorrhage	20	42
Pulmonary insufficiency	15	31
Drug toxicity	5	10
Sepsis	1	2
Uremia	1	2
Acute tubular necrosis (postoperative)	1	2
Pulmonary embolism (postoperative)	1	2
Unknown	4	8

(Courtesy of Lurain, J. R., et al.: Am. J. Obstet. Gynecol. 144:391–395, Oct. 15, 1982.)

elsewhere (wrong choice of chemotherapeutic agents or wrong drug dosages and treatment time schedules, or both). This shows the value of a center for study and treatment of gestational trophoblastic disease.

Some of the patients who died early in the series might have been cured with more modern and aggressive combination chemotherapy. Secondary chemotherapy in patients with gestational trophoblastic disease has been found to yield poor results. Whole brain irradiation (3,000 to 3,600 rad in 10 to 12 fractions) in combination with chemotherapy plays an important role in the treatment of patients with brain metastases but irradiation to other sites is not beneficial. The role of adjuvant surgery in the treatment of high-risk metastatic trophoblastic disease is uncertain, but such treatment did not appear to prolong survival or markedly decrease hCG levels, and 2 patients died from postoperative complications.

▶ [Deaths from gestational trophoblastic disease are unusual nowadays. This report from the Brewer Center at Northwestern University indicates that prognosis was influenced by type of antecedent pregnancy (term gestation, spontaneous abortion, and ectopic pregnancy are worse than hydatidiform mole), length of time until diagnosis, and pretreatment hCG titer. The most frequent causes of death, in order, were hemorrhage, pulmonary insufficiency, and drug toxicity. It seems clear that the key to lowering death rates further rests with earlier diagnosis and treatment.] ◀

12–37 **The Efficacy of Radionuclide Liver and Bone Scans in the Evaluation of Gynecologic Cancers.** John C. Harbert, Luis Rocha, Fred P. Smith, and Gregorio Delgado (Georgetown Univ. Hosp., Washington, D.C.) studied the frequency of positive liver and bone scans at the time of initial staging of patients with cervical, ovarian, and uterine malignancy. Between 1978 and 1980, 28 patients with uterine cancer, 33 with cervical cancer, and 40 with ovarian cancer underwent clinical diagnostic staging. Fifty-four patients had bone scans; 101 had liver scans.

Results showed no positive bone scans were found. Among the 101 patients who had liver scans, only patients with stage III or stage IV

(12–37) Cancer 49:1040–1042, Mar. 1, 1982.

disease determined by staging laparotomy had positive results of the scan, including 3 patients with uterine, 2 with cervical, and 4 with ovarian cancer. Eight of 33 patients with stage IV disease had positive results of liver scans consistent with hepatic metastases. Only 1 of 69 patients with stage I–III disease had a positive test for metastases.

The value of liver scanning in patients with abnormal liver function tests, hepatomegaly, jaundice, or ascites and the use of bone scanning in patients with bone pain or elevated alkaline phosphatase levels are recognized. The value of these diagnostic tests in the clinical staging protocol, however, must be questioned. Results of other studies have shown that bone scanning does not appear warranted as a screening test in asymptomatic patients with stage 0–II cervical cancer. Although the numbers of bone scans in ovarian and uterine cancer are too small for statistical certainty, one could infer that bone scanning has a limited use in staging of these cancers, at least in patients without evidence of bone disease. This same conclusion could also be applied to liver scanning.

▶ [The message here seems clear: Radionuclide scans for bone and liver metastases are not sufficiently productive in other than advanced gynecologic cancer to include them in the usual "tumor workup."] ◀

12–38 **Acute Nonlymphocytic Leukemia After Therapy With Alklating Agents For Ovarian Cancer: A Study of Five Randomized Clinical Trials.** Mark H. Greene, John L. Boice, Jr., Benjamin E. Greer, John A. Blessing, and Alon J. Dembo evaluated the rate of occurrence of acute nonlymphocytic leukemia (ANL) among 1,399 women with ovarian cancer.

Among 998 women treated with alkylating agents, 12 cases of ANL were observed; the expected number was 0.18. The mean latent period between diagnosis of ovarian cancer and diagnosis of ANL was 47 months (range, 2 to 7 years). Most patients had a preleukemic phase, and survival after diagnosis of ANL was a median of 4 months. Only 84 patients were followed up for more than 7 years, precluding a meaningful estimate of cumulative risk at longer intervals.

All 12 patients with ANL had been exposed to alkylating agents; 10 patients had received melphalan and 2, chlorambucil. Acute nonlymphocytic leukemia was not observed in 401 women treated with surgery or radiation, or both, without alkylating agents. The excess risk of ANL associated with alkylating-agent therapy was 5.8 cases per 1,000 women per year, and the cumulative 7-year risk of ANL was 9.6 ± 3.3% (± SE). The risk of ANL among patients treated with chemotherapy alone was not significantly different from that observed in patients receiving both radiation and chemotherapy.

A positive correlation between initial drug dose and risk of ANL was suggested. Nine of the 10 patients treated with melphalan received more than 700 mg. The lowest melphalan dose associated with ANL was 420 mg. Both chlorambucil-treated patients received more than 2,000 mg. All melphalan-related cases occurred in patients re-

---

(12–38) N. Engl. J. Med. 307:1416–1421, Dec. 2, 1982.

ceiving 12 or more cycles of therapy; the 2 chlorambucil-related cases developed in patients who received daily therapy for more than 18 months. Dose and duration of treatment were so highly correlated that separate effects of each could not be distinguished.

The data underscore the need to assess other cytotoxic agents and regimens of drug administration to identify those that do not have harmful late effects.

▶ [That alkylating agent (specifically, melphalan and chlorambucil) therapy is associated with a small risk of the subsequent development of acute nonlymphocytic leukemia seems clear. As the authors of this article point out in their discussion, this shouldn't dotor one from using these drugs in patients with advanced ovarian cancer, but should be given weight in the risk-benefit analysis when these agents are considered for an adjunctive role in patients whose risk of cancer recurrence is low or in patients who suffer from nonneoplastic conditions. There is an apparent association between the dose and duration of drug therapy and the subsequent development of leukemia.] ◀

12–39 **No Increase in Second Tumors After Cytotoxic Chemotherapy for Gestational Trophoblastic Tumors.** Many anticancer agents are known carcinogens, and the chemotherapy or radiotherapy used to treat one cancer may induce a second cancer. Gordon J. S. Rustin, Frances Rustin, Joan Dent, Margaret Booth, Sandra Salt, and Kenneth D. Bagshawe (London) studied the incidence of second tumors after cytotoxic chemotherapy in 457 long-term survivors treated for choriocarcinoma or invasive mole between 1958 and 1978. At the start of therapy the women were aged 14–55 years (mean, 27.8 years).

The drug regimens changed considerably over the 21-year period, but all regimens were intermittent (cytotoxic agents usually were given in courses of 2–10 days, followed by drug-free intervals of 5–15 days), there was no long-term daily drug administration or maintenance therapy, and all but 2 women received methotrexate (mean dose, 1,562 mg), with 261 of them (57%) also receiving other cytotoxic drugs, usually dactinomycin, vincristine, cyclophosphamide, mercaptopurine, and 6-azauridine. Mean duration of chemotherapy was 4 months.

After a mean of 7.8 years since the beginning of treatment (total of 3,522 patient-years of risk), second neoplasms developed in only 2 women (acute leukemia in 1 and carcinoma of the breast in 1). The fact that 3.5 cancers would have been expected in this group suggests that use of methotrexate as chemotherapy for choriocarcinoma is not carcinogenic or cocarcinogenic in the medium term. Trophoblastic tumors do not appear to be associated with development of second primary neoplasms.

▶ [Previous reports, including the preceding article by Greene et al., have noted an increased incidence of second tumors, typically lymphoma or leukemia, after successful cancer chemotherapy. This large series demonstrates no such sequelae with cytotoxic therapy of trophoblastic disease. The difference may be that the positive studies generally have involved alkylating agents used in ovarian cancer, whereas methotrexate is an antimetabolite.] ◀

(12–39) N. Engl. J. Med. 308:473–476, Mar. 3, 1983.

12–40 **Natural History of Radiation-Induced Proctosigmoiditis: Analysis of 88 Patients.** Radiation injury of the gastrointestinal tract is a recognized complication of treatment delivered to the abdomen and pelvis. N. H. Gilinsky, D. G. Burns, G. O. Barbezat, W. Levin, H. S. Myers, and I. N. Marks (Univ. of Cape Town) reviewed 88 cases of radiation-induced proctosigmoiditis seen between 1974 and 1981. All but 4 patients had been treated for gynecologic malignancies. All patients had had rectal bleeding for over a month and had radiation injury confirmed sigmoidoscopically. Mean age was 52 years. Thirty-nine patients had low-grade rectal bleeding; 32 required transfusions but had minimal bowel dysfunction; and 17 had significant changes in bowel habits, especially constipation, and pain refractory to oral medication. Most patients had received combined external cobalt teletherapy and radium brachytherapy.

The peak incidence of onset of rectal bleeding was 9 months after radiotherapy. Mean follow-up was 34 months. Over 80% of patients received topical corticosteroid and oral salazopyrine therapy, and a number also used antifibrinolysins. Barium enema studies showed abnormalities attributable to radiation injury in the rectum, sigmoid or both in all but 2 of 72 patients examined. Radium doses and total rectal doses were comparable in the different clinical groups. Urinary tract involvement was apparent in 28% of patients. Only 2 patients with low-grade bleeding required operation for radiation-induced bowel damage. All patients with bowel dysfunction who survived required operation. About one third of surviving patients who needed transfusions but had minimal bowel dysfunction required operation. About 80% of operations were complicated. Mortality ranged from 15% in the least affected patients to 41% in those with bowel dysfunction.

Operation appears to predispose to radiation-induced bowel injury in patients with gynecologic malignancy. Radiation dose could not be related to severity of disease in this series. Associated urinary tract damage is frequent. Conservative management is preferred where possible.

▶ [This large series of patients with radiation-induced proctosigmoiditis underscores how significant a problem this treatment complication is. Rectal bleeding was the common presenting symptom and most frequently occurred 9 months from the start of therapy. Operation was required in nearly one third of the patients; operative and postoperative complications were frequent and severe.] ◀

(12–40) Q. J. Med. 52:40–53, Winter 1983.

13. Infections

13–1 **Condyloma Acuminata: An Unusual Presentation of Child Abuse.** Sexual abuse is found in 12% of all reported cases of child abuse and is generally underreported, and condyloma acuminata is not well recognized as a sign of child abuse. Christopher R. McCoy, Harry Applebaum, and Arthur S. Besser (Detroit) report data on 2 girls and 2 boys, aged 14 months to 11 years, with condyloma acuminata that required surgical treatment. Two of them required multiple procedures for control of the lesions. Both girls had perineal and perivaginal lesions, and one had a history of dysuria and recurrent urinary tract infections. Both boys had perianal and intrarectal vegetations; 1 had rectal pain, and the other had rectal bleeding. The indications for operation included the need for histologic identification and tissue for immunotherapy and the presence of large, recurrent, or refractory lesions.

Young infants of both sexes may have condyloma acuminata resulting from sexual abuse. Lesions develop within 2–3 months in most inoculated cases. The cutaneous vegetations are found in the moist anogenital regions and may be painful or secondarily infected. Small external lesions readily are treated with 4 to 6 weekly applications of 20% podophyllin. Newer surgical methods include cryosurgery with liquid nitrogen and use of the carbon dioxide laser. Immunotherapy is another option. Cessation of sexual abuse is necessary to prevent a continued threat to the patient's physical and emotional well-being. Involved families often are hostile and tend to resist care for the child.

▶ [The point of this article is that vulvar condyloma accuminata in a prepubertal girl—which we do not recall ever seeing—should raise the suspicion of sexual abuse.] ◀

13–2 **Vulvovaginitis in Premenarcheal Girls: Clinical Features and Diagnostic Evaluation.** Jan E. Paradise, Joseph M. Campos, Harvey M. Friedman, and Gertrude Frishmuth (Univ. of Pennsylvania, Philadelphia) describe unselected outpatients with symptoms or signs of vulvovaginitis who were systematically interviewed and examined with the use of a standardized format, underwent microbiologic studies, and were followed up prospectively.

A total of 54 premenarcheal patients (median age, 5.8 years) with symptoms or signs of vulvovaginitis were studied. Results of the cultures of vaginal secretions were compared with those from an age-matched control group. Vaginal discharge was found during examination in 24 of 42 patients who complained of discharge and in 2 of 12 patients who had no such complaint. Convincing evidence of bac-

---

(13–1) J. Pediatr. Surg. 17:505–507, October 1982.
(13–2) Pediatrics 70:193–198, August 1982.

terial or monilial infection was found in 14 of the 26 patients with discharge during examination, but in none of the 28 patients without discharge ($P < .001$). In the latter group, pinworm infestation was present in 1 patient. Moniliasis occurred exclusively in girls who were pubertal. Four patients were found to have gonorrhea. No patient appeared to have symptoms or signs caused by *Bacteroides* sp., *Chlamydia trachomatis,* viruses, or *Trichomonas vaginalis*. Noninfectious causes were identified in 4 patients with and 13 without discharge; the most common cause was poor hygiene, which was implicated in 6 patients. Use of bubble bath was implicated in only 1 patient. In 22 patients, no specific cause could be identified. All patients with poor hygiene as the only cause, as well as most with no demonstrable cause, recovered after being advised to improve perineal hygiene.

Patients with vaginal discharge are likely to have specific infections, and, therefore, cultures should be taken, particularly for *Neisseria gonorrhoeae*. Genital pruritus in prepubertal girls has little or no etiologic specificity, but in pubertal girls with vaginal discharge, it suggests the presence of monilial vaginitis. At all ages, culture of vaginal discharges is indispensable for accurate etiologic diagnosis.

▶ [This article provides an excellent review of what can cause vaginal discharge (and similar symptoms) in premenarcheal girls. Monilial infection was encountered only in pubertal girls, and typically in those whose predominant symptom was pruritis. Viruses and *Chlamydia* and *Trichomonas* organisms were not isolated in any case, making it seem unlikely that they are frequent causes of vulvovaginitis prior to menarche. Moreover, *Bacteroides* organisms were isolated with similar frequency from both subjects and controls, so their pathogenic role in this age group is also suspect.] ◀

13–3 **Sexual Contact in Children With Gonorrhea.** David L. Ingram, Susanne T. White, Michael F. Durfee, and Anna W. Pearson (Univ. of North Carolina) conducted a study to test the hypothesis that gonorrhea in children aged 1–12 years often is associated with sexual contact. From July 1976 through June 1981, data were reviewed on all children aged 1–12 years who had gonorrheal infections and who lived in Wake County, North Carolina. As many "extended family" members as could be located were interviewed, and cultures for gonorrhea were taken. The term "extended family" includes relatives, caretakers, friends, baby-sitters, and neighbors who had frequent contact with the children.

Two boys and 29 girls with gonorrhea were examined. There were 26 black and 5 white children. The boys, aged 3 years and 12 years, respectively, had symptomatic gonorrheal urethritis. All 29 girls had symptomatic gonorrheal vaginitis, with positive vaginal cultures. Six girls had a history of attempted or definite vaginal intercourse, and 8 others had histories that were too vague to allow differentiation among vaginal intercourse, rectal intercourse, and genital or digital manipulation in the perineal area. Five girls had histories of being isolated with older male persons under suspicious circumstances. Seventeen girls had rectal cultures taken, of which 7 (41%) were positive for gonorrhea, and 16 had oropharyngeal cultures taken, of which 3

(13–3) Am. J. Dis. Child. 136:994–996, November 1982.

(19%) were positive. None of the children had signs or symptoms of pharyngitis. One hundred extended family members were interviewed; 35 had gonorrhea or had been treated for gonorrhea in the previous 3 weeks. Identifying extended family members with gonorrhea, together with further interviews, proved to be a useful procedure for ascertaining the names of sexual contacts of the children. Of the 29 girls with gonorrhea, only 5 had a sexual contact named during the initial interview; after further interviews and identification of those extended family members with gonorrhea, sexual contacts were revealed in 14 more cases. All children older than age 4 years had a named sexual contact. Only 6 of 17 children aged 1–4 years had a named sexual contact.

Hospitalization of the children and identification of extended family members with gonorrhea, followed by additional interviews, were useful procedures in determining who had had sexual contact with the children. Nonsexual child-to-child contamination was not found in this study.

▶ [The "bottom line" of this study is that gonorrhea in children older than age 4 years is virtually always acquired sexually, usually as a result of contact with an older male person in the extended family. Before the age of 4, however, evidence indicating sexual transmission was found in only about one third of the cases; others may represent nonsexual transmission or perhaps simply the difficulty of history-taking under such circumstances.] ◀

13–4 **Vaginal Spermicides and Gonorrhea.** Hershel Jick, Marian T. Hannan, Andy Stergachis, Fred Heidrich, David R. Perera, and Kenneth J. Rothman compared the incidence of gonorrhea among recent spermicide users with the incidence among presumably sexually active nonusers. All those evaluated were born between 1940 and 1960 and were members of the Group Health Cooperative of Puget Sound, Seattle, from December 20, 1978, through December 31, 1980. At this consumer-owned health facility about 80% of prescriptions filled for vaginal spermicide contain octoxynol and about 20% contain nonoxynol 9. Observations for women using spermicides or oral contraceptives were limited to the 90-day period after the filling of each prescription. Cases of gonorrhea were identified by reviewing all laboratory slips reporting a culture for *Neisseria gonorrhoeae.*

The incidence rate of gonorrhea among spermicide users was 5.7 cases per 10^6 woman-days at risk; among oral contraceptive users, it was 29 cases per 10^6 woman-days at risk; among surgically sterilized women, it was 16 cases per 10^6 woman-days at risk. The risk ratio estimate for spermicide users compared with others, taking year of birth and marital status into account, was 0.23 (90% confidence interval). Among 77 women with a positive culture, 4 (5%) had had a prescription for spermicides filled within 90 days, 56 (73%) had had a prescription for oral contraceptives filled within 90 days, and 17 (22%) were surgically sterilized.

The rate of metronidazole prescriptions among spermicide users was 169 per 981,804 woman-days at risk. Among the remainder, it was 961 per 4,260,706 woman-days at risk. The risk ratio estimate,

---

(13–4) JAMA 248:1619–1621, Oct. 1, 1982.

taking into account year of birth and marital status, was 0.81 (90% confidence limit).

The data show that recent spermicide users at the Group Health Cooperative of Puget Sound have positive cultures for *N. gonorrhoeae* at about one-fourth to one-eighth the rate of recent users of oral contraceptives and women with surgical sterilization. The results are consistent with a substantial protective effect of these drugs of the order of 75% or higher against gonorrhea.

▶ [This epidemiologic study indicates an inverse relationship between the use of vaginal spermicides and the incidence of gonorrhea. In vitro studies indicate that these preparations inhibit the growth of *Neisseria gonorrhoeae*. Alternative explanations for the reported results include the protection afforded by barrier methods (condom or diaphragm) often used in conjunction with spermicides and a possible difference in sexual behavior, including the number of partners, among subjects in the three contraceptive groups.] ◀

13–5 **Treatment of First Episodes of Genital Herpes Simplex Virus Infection With Oral Acyclovir: Randomized Double-Blind Controlled Trial in Normal Subjects.** An effective outpatient treatment for genital herpes would be most practical, because most patients with first episodes of infection do not require hospitalization. Administration of topical acyclovir has exhibited activity in such cases. Yvonne J. Bryson, Maryanne Dillon, Michael Lovett, Guillermo Acuna, Stephen Taylor, James D. Cherry, B. Lamar Johnson, Edward Wiesmeier, William Growdon, Terri Creagh-Kirk, and Ronald Keeney conducted a double-blind, placebo-controlled trial of orally administered acyclovir in the treatment of first-episode genital herpes in young adults. The trial included 48 patients, about half of whom had first-episode primary herpes simplex infections. Study patients received 200 mg of acyclovir 5 times daily for 10 days. Herpes simplex virus type 2 was isolated from genital lesions in 43 cases, and type 1 virus in 5.

The duration of virus shedding was significantly shorter in acyclovir-treated patients than in placebo patients. New lesion formation was reduced significantly in acyclovir-treated men and women. Both the duration and severity of symptoms were reduced in the study group. No adverse reactions were observed. Recurrence was noted on follow-up for 4–9 months in 68% of acyclovir-treated patients and in 72% of placebo patients.

Oral treatment with acyclovir significantly reduced virus shedding, symptoms, and new lesion formation compared with placebo in this study of young adults with genital herpes. The clinical course was shortened by about a week with acyclovir therapy, and this is of practical clinical importance. Further studies are planned to evaluate oral treatment in pregnant women near term. Orally administered acyclovir did not reduce the frequency of recurrence in the present study; its effect on the natural history of genital herpes simplex infection remains to be determined.

13–6 **Efficacy of Oral Acyclovir in Treatment of Initial and Recurrent Genital Herpes.** Genital herpes is becoming increasingly prev-

---

(13–5) N. Engl. J. Med. 308:916–921, Apr. 21, 1983.
(13–6) Lancet 2:571–573, Sept. 11, 1982.

TABLE 1.—EFFECTS OF ORAL ACYCLOVIR TREATMENT ON INITIAL GENITAL HERPES

—	All patients			Culture positives			Females			Males		
	ACV† n = 17	PCB‡ n = 14	p value	ACV n = 16	PCB n = 11	p value	ACV n = 10	PCB n = 7	p value	ACV n = 7	PCB n = 7	p value
Viral shedding*	1	13	<0·001	1	13	<0·001	1	10	<0·01	1	15	<0·01
Crusting time*	4	6	NS	4	6	<0·05	4	6·5	<0·01	7	5	NS
Assessed healing time*	6	11	<0·01	6	11	<0·01	4·5	6	<0·05	7	11	0·06
Averaged healing time*	7	11·5	0·08	7·5	14	<0·05	6	7	NS	7·5	14	<0·05
Itching duration*	1·5	5	<0·01	1·5	6	<0·01	1	5	<0·05	2	7·5	NA
Pain duration*	4	8	<0·001	3	7	<0·01	3·5	7	<0·05	4	9	<0·05
Combined sympton duration*	4	9	<0·05	4	9	NS	5	8	NS	3	9	<0·05
New lesion formation (%)	0	43	<0·01	0	55	<0·01	0	29	NS	0	57	<0·05

NS: not significant; NA, not analyzable (too few patients).
*Median time in days.
†ACV: acyclovir.
‡PCB: placebo.
(Courtesy of Nilsen, A. E., et al.: Lancet 2:571–574, Sept. 11, 1982.)

alent, and current treatments are far from satisfactory. Acyclovir is an antiviral agent with considerable specific activity against herpes simplex viruses types 1 and 2. Arvid E. Nilsen, Tor Aasen, Arne M. Halsos, B. Rugh Kinge, Enok A. L. Tjøtta, Kjell Wikström, and A. Paul Fiddian undertook a double-blind trial of acyclovir versus placebo in 31 patients with initial and 85 with recurrent genital herpes. Seventeen patients with initial disease and 42 with recurrent herpes

TABLE 2.—EFFECTS OF ORAL ACYCLOVIR TREATMENT ON RECURRENT GENITAL HERPES

	All patients			Males		
—	ACV n=41	PCB n=42	p value	ACV n=32	PCB n=34	p value
Viral shedding*	1	2	<0·001	1	2	<0·001
Crusting time*	4	4	NS	4	4	NS
Assessed healing time*	5	6	<0·001	5	6	<0·001
Averaged healing time*	5	6	<0·01	5	6	<0·05
Itching duration*	1	2	NS	1	2	NS
Pain duration*	3	2·5	NS	3	2	NS
Combined symptom duration*	3	3	NS	3	2·5	NS
New lesion formation (%)	2	19	<0·05	3	18	0·07

ACV: acyclovir; PCB: placebo.
*Median time in days.
(Courtesy of Nilsen, A. E., et al.: Lancet 2:571–574, Sept. 11, 1982.)

were treated with 200 mg of acyclovir orally five times daily for 5 days. All patients were aged 16 or older. Those with initial herpes were seen within 5 days of the onset of symptoms and those with recurrent herpes within 48 hours. Treatment groups were stratified for sex and for a past history of genital herpes. The treatment and control groups were clinically quite comparable.

Viral shedding lasted a much shorter time in patients with first attacks who were treated with acyclovir (Table 1). New lesion formation was completely prevented by acyclovir in all cases. Lesion progression was clearly curtailed by acyclovir therapy. The duration of all symptoms was significantly shorter in the acyclovir-treated patients. In the group with recurrent genital herpes, viral shedding again was curtailed by acyclovir therapy and new lesion formation was prevented, except in 1 case (Table 2). The effects of treatment on lesion progression were less marked than in the group with initial attacks. Healing times were significantly shorter in actively treated patients. One acyclovir-treated patient with a history of renal stones developed renal colic during treatment.

Acyclovir given orally is the best specific outpatient treatment for initial genital herpes. Less dramatic results have been obtained in cases of recurrent infection, but initiation of therapy in the prodromal phase of an attack would likely give better results. Prophylaxis might be indicated for patients with frequent or easily predictable recurrences of genital herpes.

▶ [This article and the preceding one demonstrate that orally administered acyclovir is effective in the treatment of genital herpes, especially initial episodes.] ◀

13–7 **Intravenous Acyclovir for the Treatment of Primary Genital Herpes.** Topical acyclovir therapy has shortened the time of viral shedding and accelerated the healing of genital lesions of herpes, but it has not influenced the duration of systemic symptoms or reduced

(13–7) Ann. Intern. Med. 98:914–921, June 1983.

the rate of new lesion formation. Lawrence Corey, Kenneth H. Fife, Jacqueline K. Benedetti, Carol A. Winter, Anita Fahnlander, James D. Connor, Marie A. Hintz, and King K. Holmes evaluated intravenous acyclovir in a double-blind, placebo-controlled study in which 31 patients with first episodes of genital herpes received acyclovir, 5 mg/kg every 8 hours for 5 days, or a saline placebo. Twenty-seven patients had primary genital herpes, and 4 had nonprimary first-episode genital herpes. All were treated at University Hospital, Seattle. Mean time from onset of lesions to the start of treatment was 3.7 days.

Median duration of viral shedding from genital lesions was significantly shorter in acyclovir-treated patients than in the placebo group (2 versus 13 days). Viral shedding from the pharynx, cervix, and urethra also lasted a shorter time in acyclovir-treated patients. Median times to complete crusting and healing of genital lesions were 6 and 9 days, respectively, in the acyclovir group, and 13 and 21 days, respectively, in placebo patients. Formation of new lesions was less frequent in treated patients. Local and systemic symptoms lasted a mean of 5 days less in the acyclovir-treated group. Complications of herpes occurred in 4 patients, all in the placebo group. One acyclovir-treated patient had mild phlebitis. Nine of 15 acyclovir-treated patients and 14 of 16 placebo patients had clinical recurrences during follow-up.

Intravenous acyclovir therapy substantially reduces the symptoms of primary genital herpes, the duration of lesions, and the complications. The ultimate role of intravenous acyclovir in the treatment of primary genital herpes remains to be defined by further clinical experience and evaluation of toxicity. Studies are needed to estimate the risk of emergence of acyclovir-resistant mutants.

▶ [Corey and his associates at the University of Washington have been at the forefront of herpes research and have demonstrated previously that topical administration of acyclovir is efficacious in treating primary genital infections. In this study, they tested the intravenous route of administration and found a marked effect on duration of viral shedding and local and svstemic symptoms.] ◀

13–8 **Nonspecific Vaginitis: Diagnostic Criteria and Microbial and Epidemiologic Associations.** Previous studies of nonspecific vaginitis report conflicting results regarding its cause and clinical manifestations. Richard Amsel, Patricia A. Totten, Carol A. Spiegel, Kirk C. S. Chen, David Eschenbach, and King K. Holmes (Univ. of Washington) studied 397 consecutive unselected female university students, excluding only those who were menstruating and those who had received antibiotics or any treatment for vaginitis in the preceding month. The most common presenting features were symptoms of vaginitis, including discharge, vaginal odor, and vulvovaginal irritation or itching. The criteria for diagnosing nonspecific vaginitis included a thin, homogeneous discharge; a vaginal pH above 4.5; release of a fishy odor from the discharge after treatment with 10% potassium hydroxide (KOH); abnormal amines in the vaginal fluid; and vaginal epithelial cells heavily coated with bacilli, or clue cells.

The findings are summarized in the table. Asymptomatic disease

(13–8) Am. J. Med. 74:14–22, January 1983.

Diagnostic Classification of 311 Consecutive* Patients According to Various Criteria for Nonspecific Vaginitis

	Patients with Nonspecific Vaginitis			Normal Patients		
Criteria†	No. (%)	Clue Cells Present	G. vaginalis Isolated‡	No. (%)	Clue Cells Present	G. vaginalis Isolated‡
A	36 (12)	35	21/21	275 (88)	37	80/183
B	69 (22)	61	41/44	242 (78)	11	64/160
C	64 (21)	—§	39/40	247 (79)	—§	62/164
D	77 (25)	—§	45/48	234 (75)	—§	56/156

*Excludes 72 patients with other genital infections and 14 with incomplete data.

†Criteria sets used for diagnosis of nonspecific vaginitis: **A** = pH above 4.5, nonspecific vaginitis discharge, and positive potassium hydroxide (KOH) odor; **B** = any 3 of the following: pH above 4.5, nonspecific vaginitis discharge, positive KOH odor, abnormal amines; **C** = any 3 of the following: pH above 4.5, nonspecific vaginitis discharge, positive KOH odor, clue cells; **D** = any 3 of the following: pH above 4.5, nonspecific vaginitis discharge, positive KOH odor, abnormal amines, clue cells.

‡Isolation on selective medium (HB agar).

§Not given; clue cells included in diagnostic criteria.

(Courtesy of Amsel, R., et al.: Am. J. Med. 74:14–22, January 1983.)

was recognized in more than 50% of the women with nonspecific vaginitis. The diagnosis correlated with the presence and concentration of *Gardnerella vaginalis* in the vaginal discharge and with characteristic biochemical findings on gas-liquid chromatography. The presence of nonspecific vaginitis also correlated with a history of sexual activity, previous trichomoniasis, and the current use of nonbarrier contraceptive methods, especially an intrauterine device (IUD). An IUD was used by 19% of patients with nonspecific vaginitis and 5% of normal women. Half of all IUD users had nonspecific vaginitis.

The criteria proposed for clinical use in diagnosing nonspecific vaginitis include a vaginal pH above 4.5, a characteristic discharge, a positive KOH odor test, and the presence of clue cells on a saline wet mount. At least three of these criteria should be present. Although a clinical entity, nonspecific vaginitis may be multifactorial in cause and may have a clinical spectrum merging with normal.

▶ [It has been 30 years since the initial description by Gardner and Dukes of *Hemophilus* (now *Gardnerella*) *vaginalis* vaginitis, yet the clinical and microbiologic place of this condition is still unsettled. However, there is reason to hope that the picture will be clarified by work such as that being done by Holmes and his associates in Seattle. This carefully done study contains a wealth of information about "nonspecific vaginitis" and, more importantly, it suggests as diagnostic criteria any three of four findings: vaginal pH above 4.5, characteristic vaginal discharge, release of a fishy amine odor on addition of KOH, and clue cells on wet mount.] ◀

13–9 **Single Oral Dose Metronidazole Therapy for *Gardnerella Vaginalis* Vaginitis in Adolescent Female Patients.** William L. Minkowski, Charles J. Baker, Delores Alleyne, Mohammad Baghai, Louis Friedlander, and Biruta Schultz (Los Angeles) examined the efficacy of a single 2-gm oral dose of metronidazole in 882 symptomatic adolescent girls seen in a 20-month period with positive cultures for *Gardnerella vaginalis.* The subjects, all postmenarcheal, were in the juvenile detention system of Los Angeles County. Mean age was 16 years. Caucasians comprised about half the sample, with the rest being mostly blacks and Hispanics. No other vaginal pathogens were isolated in 609 subjects, or 48% of a total of 1,273 subjects with nonspecific vaginal infection.

(13–9) J. Adolesc. Health Care 4:113–116, June 1983.

Of the 531 girls followed up after metronidazole therapy, 95% had negative posttreatment cultures coincident with resolution of vaginal symptoms. Twenty-two of 26 girls whose vaginal cultures remained positive for *G. vaginalis* were retreated with metronidazole, in the same-sized dose, and all but 2 had negative cultures subsequently. These 2 patients were later cured with a standard 7-day course of metronidazole. The only side effects were transient nausea in 5 patients and a single episode of vomiting in 2. No neurologic or dermatologic sequelae were observed.

A single 2-gm oral dose of metronidazole appears to be highly effective in the treatment of *G. vaginalis* vaginitis in adolescent girls, with infrequent and minor side effects. The cost per patient is lower than with the 1-week treatment. The single-dose approach offers assurance of compliance by patients who are unable or unwilling to complete a 1-week course of treatment.

▶ [This report confirms the efficacy of single-dose metronidazole treatment of *Gardnerella vaginalis* vaginitis. The reported incidence of side effects was negligible. The single-dose approach has obvious advantages in ease and cost over a 7- or 10-day regimen.] ◀

13–10 **Treatment of Vaginal Candidosis With Natamycin and Effect of Treating the Partner at the Same Time.** Annette Buch and Else Skytte Christensen (Copenhagen) undertook a prospective double-blind study in which the partners of women with vaginal candidosis were treated with either 2.5% natamycin cream or a placebo cream, and all the patients with 25 mg natamycin vaginal tablets. Forty-two patients aged 20–45 years were included in the study. Nearly all had clinical signs of vaginitis, and none had other infectious conditions. All patients had ordinary sexual lives with 1 partner who agreed to be treated for 10 days. Thirty-three of the patients completed the study; 16 had partners treated with natamycin. The two groups were comparable.

All but 1 of the 16 patients with actively treated partners and 15 of the 17 with placebo-treated partners had negative cultures at the initial follow-up evaluation, for respective cure rates of 94% and 88%. Five patients with treated partners and 4 in the placebo group had a recurrence or reinfection. Four of 20 patients followed up a second time had positive cultures but no symptoms. Eight of 13 patients with recently acquired symptoms had positive cultures. Use of oral contraception did not influence the outcome of treatment.

Treatment of the sexual partners of patients with vaginal candidosis appears not to influence the primary cure rate or the rate of recurrence-reinfection significantly. Early recurrence-reinfection was considerably more frequent in patients in the present study than in patients in previously reported studies. Apart from direct infection, intercourse may predispose to recurrence-reinfection through mechanical injury to the vaginal mucosa.

▶ [The results reported here are consistent with the view that autoinfection, presumably from a colonized colon or rectum, rather than genital transmission from a partner, explains most recurrences of monilial vulvovaginitis.] ◀

(13–10) Acta Obstet. Gynecol. Scand. 61:393–396, 1982.

13–11 **Comparative Study of Piperacillin Versus Cefoxitin in Treatment of Obstetric and Gynecologic Infections.** The polymicrobial nature of obstetric and gynecologic infections suggests the use of broad-spectrum antibiotics such as the new semisynthetic penicillin, piperacillin sodium. Richard L. Sweet, Marilyn O. Robbie, Marilyn Ohm-Smith, and W. Keith Hadley (Univ. of California, San Francisco) compared the effects of piperacillin with those of cefoxitin in 48 women with acute genital tract infections. Twenty-three received 4.5 gm of piperacillin intravenously every 6 hours, and 25 received 2 gm of cefoxitin on the same schedule. Both drugs were infused in 5% dextrose solution over a 30-minute period. Acute salpingitis and endomyometritis were the most common diagnoses.

Both aerobes and anaerobes were isolated from more than 80% of

TABLE 1.—AEROBIC MICROORGANISMS ISOLATED FROM PRETREATMENT CULTURES IN 41 WOMEN WITH PELVIC INFECTIONS TREATED WITH PIPERACILLIN OR CEFOXITIN

	No. of isolates		
Aerobic bacteria	*Piperacillin group*	*Cefoxitin group*	*Total*
Gram-positive cocci:			
Group A streptococci	0	1	1
Group B streptococci	2	5	7
Group D streptococci, not enterococci	2	4	6
Enterococci	3	2	5
Other nonhemolytic streptococci	5	4	9
α-Hemolytic streptococci	3	2	5
β-Hemolytic streptococci, not groups A, B, or D	0	1	1
Staphylococcus aureus	2	2	4
Coagulase-negative staphylococci	7	5	12
Micrococci	1	0	1
Gram-negative cocci:			
Neisseria gonorrhoeae	9	8	17
Gram-negative rods:			
Escherichia coli	1	4	5
Proteus mirabilis	0	1	1
Unidentified nonfermenting gram-negative rods	0	2	2
Gardnerella vaginalis	3	4	7
Gram-positive rods:			
Lactobacilli	11	10	21
Diphtheroids	3	5	8
Yeast:			
Candida albicans	0	1	1
Total aerobes	51	62	113

(Courtesy of Sweet, R. L., et al.: Am. J. Obstet. Gynecol. 145:342–349, Feb. 1, 1983.)

(13–11) Am. J. Obstet. Gynecol. 145:342–349, Feb. 1, 1983.

TABLE 2.—ANAEROBIC MICROORGANISMS ISOLATED FROM PRETREATMENT CULTURES IN 41 WOMEN WITH PELVIC INFECTIONS TREATED WITH PIPERACILLIN OR CEFOXITIN

Anaerobic bacteria	*No. of isolates* *Piperacillin group*	*Cefoxitin group*	*Total*
Gram-positive cocci.			
Peptococcus prevotii	7	9	16
Peptococcus asaccharolyticus	7	8	15
Peptococcus magnus	1	3	4
Peptostreptococcus anaerobius	5	10	15
Peptostreptococcus productus	0	1	1
Streptococcus morbillorum	3	1	4
Unidentified anaerobic gram-positive cocci	5	2	7
Gram-negative cocci:			
Veillonella parvula	2	2	4
Unidentified anaerobic gram-negative cocci	2	2	4
Gram-negative rods:			
Bacteroides bivius	6	6	12
Bacteroides disiens	1	1	2
Bacteroides fragilis group	0	4	4
Bacteroides melaninogenicus	2	5	7
Bacteroides corrodens	0	2	2
Bacteroides sp.	10	5	15
Fusobacterium sp.	0	2	2
Unidentified anaerobic gram-negative rods	0	4	4
Gram-positive rods:			
Clostridium perfringens	0	1	1
Lactobacillus sp.	1	3	4
Bifidobacterium sp.	4	2	6
Eubacterium sp.	0	5	5
Unidentified anaerobic gram-positive non-sporing rods	4	3	7
Total anaerobes	61	80	141

(Courtesy of Sweet, R. L., et al.: Am. J. Obstet. Gynecol. 145:342–349, Feb. 1, 1983.)

genital tract cultures. The organisms isolated are detailed in Tables 1 and 2. A clinical response to initial therapy occurred in 91% of the piperacillin-treated patients and in 92% of the cefoxitin group. About 60% of the organisms were eradicated by piperacillin in evaluable patients, whereas cefoxitin eliminated 90%. No hematologic toxicity or nephrotoxicity occurred in either group, and patient tolerance of both drugs was excellent.

Piperacillin appears to be an effective, safe single drug for use in treating female genital tract infections associated with a variety of aerobic and anaerobic organisms. A clinical cure was obtained in more than 90% of the present patients without additional treatment being necessary. The results were similar to those obtained using cefoxitin. It seems appropriate to replace standard first-line regimens with the newer cephalosporins and penicillins in treating most genital tract infections. Colonization by piperacillin-resistant *Escherichia coli* is a possible problem, but may not be of clinical importance.

▶ [The tables nicely document the organisms present in the mixed infections we all see. Both cefoxitin (a second-generation cephalosporin) and piperacillin (a new semisynthetic penicillin) performed well except when abscesses were present. Using a single antibiotic has theoretical and practical advantages over combination therapy. One concern is that these new agents are expensive. The "triple therapy" most often ordered on our service consists of ampicillin, gentamicin, and clindamycin. The first two are inexpensive, but clindamycin is not. A course of cefoxitin would cost about what our usual regimen does. Cefoxitin doesn't cover enterococci. The authors of this report imply that this may not matter. We remember patients with enterococci on culture who did not respond to a cephalosporin, and who subsequently responded to ampicillin. This issue isn't resolved.

As new antibiotics continue to come onto the market at a rapid pace (it's easier to remember the names of United States Football League players or return obstetric patients!), some price competition is inevitable. A final question: How do the various single agents or combination regimens stack up concerning their antichlamydial activity?] ◀

13–12 **Necrotizing Fasciitis: Preventable Disaster.** Necrotizing fasciitis (NF) is a serious soft tissue infection characterized by widespread necrosis of the fascia and subcutaneous tissue and, ultimately, of muscle and skin. Thomas M. Rouse, Mark A. Malangoni, and William J. Schulte (Med. College of Wisconsin, Milwaukee) reviewed findings in 27 patients with 28 episodes of NF occurring between 1969 and 1981. The 20 men and 7 women had a mean age of 61 years. All patients initially had cellulitis and skin edema (Table 1). The diagnosis was based on surgical findings of aggressively spreading liquefactive necrosis of the fascia and subcutaneous tissues. Twenty-one patients had associated chronic conditions such as diabetes, obesity, and atherosclerotic cardiovascular disease. Perineal disease and postoperative infection also were frequent. Nine patients had postoperative NF, usually limted to the abdomen.

Twenty patients (73%) died, most from either persistent wound sepsis or systemic septic complications despite apparent local control of infection. All patients with uncontrolled wound sepsis died within 10

TABLE 1.—CLINICAL FINDINGS IN 28 PATIENTS

Physical examination	*n*	*Laboratory data*	*n*
Cellulitis	28	Leukopenia or leukocytosis	18
Edema	28	Anemia (hematocrit < 30%)	12
Cutaneous gangrene	15	Hyperglycemia	12
Crepitus	12		
Temperature > 38.3°C	8		
Altered sensorium	7		
Blood pressure < 80 mm Hg	3		

(Courtesy of Rouse, T. M., et al.: Surgery 29:765–770, October 1982.)

(13–12) Surgery 92:765–770, October 1982.

TABLE 2.—ORGANISMS

Aerobes (n = 68)		*Anaerobes (n = 42)*	
E. coli	14	*Bacteroides*	17
Enterococci	12	*Clostridia*	10
Pseudomonas	6	*Peptostreptococcus*	8
Klebsiella	6	*Peptococcus*	4
S. epidermidis	6	Other	3
α-Streptococcus	5		
Proteus	4		
Other	15		

(Courtesy of Rouse, T. M., et al.: Surgery 29:765–770, October 1982.)

days of admission. In 8 patients nosocomial infections developed. The organisms isolated are listed in Table 2. Five of 12 patients whose disease was controlled by a single debridement survived, as did only 2 of 15 who required more than 1 debridement. Only 1 of 12 patients in whom surgery was delayed for more than 12 hours survived. No single antibiotic or drug combination was associated with a reduction in mortality or in the incidence of septic complications.

Antimicrobial therapy directed against anaerobes and aerobes is appropriate in NF. Early diagnosis of NF is essential, because chronic debilitating disease may contribute to uncontrollable local and systemic infection in these patients. Strict adherence to principles for the management of contaminated procedures may prevent the development of NF.

▶ [We have seen a few cases of necrotizing fasciitis after gynecologic operations and we agree that the condition is a potential disaster. We're not so sure, however, whether or not it's always a "preventable disaster." Surely the key is early and extensive debridement, and too often the problem is the familar one of too little, too late. Antibiotic therapy should be based on the polymicrobial nature, and the possible need for *Clostridia* antitoxin should be kept in mind.] ◀

13–13 **Role of Mycoplasmas in Reproduction.** Some studies have implicated mycoplasmas in human reproductive failure. Meena Upadhyaya, Bryan M. Hibbard, and Sheila M. Walker (Welsh Natl. School of Medicine, Cardiff) examined the incidence of genital *Mycoplasma* infection in 167 pregnant women before 20 weeks' gestation at admission to an antenatal clinic (group I) and in 334 women attending an infertility clinic (group II) and 174 of their partners. *Mycoplasma* cultures were carried out on cervical swab specimens. Women in group II with positive cultures received 200 mg of doxycycline on the first day of the menstrual cycle, followed by 100 mg daily for 2 weeks.

Mycoplasmas were found in 38% of group I women and in 60% of group II, a highly significant difference (Table 1). Ureaplasmas were isolated most frequently in both groups. When *M. hominis* was present, it often was associated with *Ureaplasma*. Infection developed

(13–13) Fertil. Steril. 39:814–818, June 1983.

TABLE 1.—FREQUENCY OF ISOLATION OF MYCOPLASMAS

Group	Total no.	*Ureaplasma* only	*M. hominis* only	*Ureaplasma* and *M. hominis*	Total positive *Mycoplasma*
I. Pregnant	167	56 (33%)	2 (1%)	6 (4%)	64 (38%)
II. Infertile women	334	162 (48.5%)	10 (3.5%)	28 (8%)	200 (60%)
Infertile men	174	65 (37%)	10 (6%)	8 (5%)	83 (48%)

(Courtesy of Upadhyaya, M., et al.: Fertil. Steril. 39:814–818, June 1983.

TABLE 2.—RELATIONSHIPS OF *Ureaplasma* WITH BIRTH WEIGHT AND GESTATIONAL AGE

Group	No.	Mean birth weight	Birth weight percentile		Birth weight < 2500 gm	Mean duration of gestation	Gestation < 37 completed
			< 5	< 10			
		gm				*wks*	*wks*
Ureaplasma-negative	75	3358	3	7	3	40.02	3
Ureaplasma-positive	60	3327	3	5	2	40.01	1

(Courtesy of Upadhyaya, M., et al.: Fertil. Steril. 39:814–818, June 1983.)

during pregnancy in 5% of group I women. Mycoplasmas did not appear to influence mean duration of gestation or birth weight (Table 2). Cultures from 48% of partners of infertile women were positive. Mycoplasmas were isolated from both partners in 44% of cases. In cases that had complete fertility studies, pregnancy rates did not differ significantly in treated *Mycoplasma* positive cases and untreated positive cases.

These findings strongly suggest that mycoplasmas, in general, are not associated with either poor pregnancy outcome or infertility. Isolation of mycoplasmas was not associated with prematurity or infants small for gestational age in the present study. Doxycycline therapy eradicated mycoplasmas in more than 90% of infertile couples treated, but the subsequent pregnancy rate was not improved, compared with untreated cases.

► [Genital *Mycoplasma* infection has been associated with a variety of reproductive problems–infertility, habitual abortion, preterm labor—in previous studies. These results seem to indicate no correlation with infertility, prematurity, or fetal growth retardation. Thus, the role of mycoplasmas remains uncertain. A different view is presented in the following article.] ◄

13–14 **Efficacy of Antibiotic Therapy in Preventing Spontaneous Pregnancy Loss Among Couples Colonized With Genital Mycoplasmas.** An increased incidence of asymptomatic genital tract *Mycoplasma* colonization has been found in women who have had spontaneous abortions and stillbirths. Because mycoplasmas are sensitive to antibiotics, fetal loss due to the organism might be preventable. P. A. Quinn, A. B. Shewchuk, J. Shuber, K. I. Lie, E. Ryan, M. L. Chipman, and D. M. Nocilla (Univ. of Toronto) evaluated doxycycline therapy before conception and erythromycin stearate therapy during pregnancy for preventing spontaneous abortion in 71 couples with a history of pregnancy wastage. A total of 95 pregnancies in 62 women with *Mycoplasma*-positive cultures were assessed. The women had

(13–14) Am. J. Obstet. Gynecol. 145:239–244, Jan. 15, 1983.

lost a total of 237 pregnancies previously. Doxycycline was given in a dosage of 100 or 200 mg daily until cultures became negative, and the couples used condoms for intercourse to prevent cross-infection. Erythromycin was given starting at 2 to 3 months' gestation in a dosage of 250 mg four times daily until term.

Doxycycline therapy was associated with a significant reduction in the risk of pregnancy loss. Combined treatment and erythromycin therapy only reduced the risk of loss to a greater degree. There was no evidence of significant interaction between the two drugs. The efficacy of treatment appeared to be independent of maternal age and of past obstetric history. Pregnancy losses were reduced by about half with doxycycline therapy before conception and to less than 20% with erythromycin or combined treatment.

Appropriate treatment of *Mycoplasma* infection may prevent recurrent spontaneous abortions in couples with positive cultures. Because the fetal risk of long-term erythromycin therapy is unknown, it is best to treat the couple before a conception and to use the drug during pregnancy only for those women confirmed as being *Mycoplasma* positive at that time.

▶ [These findings suggest a role of asymptomatic *Mycoplasma* colonization in pregnancy wastage. However, it should be noted that the study is not randomized and the "control" group is the subjects in their previous pregnancies. A prospective investigation with random assignment to treatment and no treatment is needed. Until this is done, culture of habitual aborters with a preconceptional course of antibiotics for colonized patients seems worthy of consideration.

In a comparison study, these same authors (Quinn et al.: *Am. J. Obstet. Gynecol.* 145:245, 1983) found that both mothers and fetuses responded to mycoplasmal infections serologically and that *Ureaplasma* serotypes 6 and 8 seemed more likely to be associated with pregnancy wastage.] ◀

13–15 **Subsequent Pregnancies Among 161 Couples Treated For T-Mycoplasma Genital Tract Infection.** The role of T-mycoplasma infection in reproductive failure remains unclear despite several claims that eradication of the organism by doxycycline improves fertility. Attila Toth, Martin L. Lesser, Constance Brooks, and Dominic Labriola (New York) for 3 years systematically cultured semen specimens from husbands of women attending a fertility clinic and have recommended treatment of both partners when T-mycoplasma infection was discovered. A total of 161 men with T-mycoplasma infection in the seminal fluid were treated, along with their wives, for 4 weeks with 100 mg of doxycycline twice daily. The indications for culture included request by the referring physician, a history of miscarriages, a history of genital tract infection in either partner, and generally poor semen quality, particularly decreased motility.

Eighty percent of the men had negative semen cultures at the end of treatment, and this correlated significantly with the pregnancy status. Nearly all men in couples who eventually conceived were free of mycoplasmas after treatment, compared with 66% of men in couples without successful pregnancies. A fairly strong trend toward a history of multiple fertility procedures was observed in women in the study. *Mycoplasma* status after therapy was the variable most closely asso-

---

(13–15) N. Engl. J. Med. 308:505–507, Mar. 3, 1983.

ciated with the time to successful pregnancy, followed by hysterosalpingography and tuboplasty.

The 129 couples in this series in which the men were treated successfully for *Mycoplasma* infection had a 3-year rate of successful pregnancy of 60%, compared with a rate of 5% for those who were not successfully treated. The median time to conception after successful treatment was less than a year. Most patients conceived without additional fertility tests or drugs. Apart from *Mycoplasma* status, a history of hysterosalpingography or tuboplasty was negatively associated with the time to conception.

▶ [The focus of this study of *Mycoplasma* in relation to reproductive failure is on the male partner, in contrast to most other reports in the literature. Of course, because the female partners were not cultured, the infection may well have been—indeed, probably was—mutual. In any event, the achievement of successful pregnancy was much more likely to be associated with bacteriologic cure than with persistence of infection. Unfortunately, the lack of "successful pregnancy" is not otherwise specified, so it is unclear whether any therapeutic benefit is directed against infertility or abortion or both.] ◀

14. Endocrinology

14–1 **Evidence for Involvement of β-Endorphin in the Human Menstrual Cycle.** Opiate receptors appear to be present in neuronal pathways that modulate activity in the hypothalamic-pituitary-LH axis, and β-endorphin immunoreactivity is present in normal human plasma. Keith W. Vrbicky, John S. Baumstark, Ibert C. Wells, Thomas W. Hilgers, Warren T. Kable, and Christopher J. Elias (Creighton Univ.) examined the possible role of β-endorphin in regulation of the human menstrual cycle. Serum β-endorphin concentrations were monitored daily over 26 hormonally normal menstrual cycles. The results are shown in Figure 14–1. A preovulatory peak and a postovulatory trough of β-endorphin concentrations were seen in 21 cycles. Two cycles had a postovulatory peak, and 3 had a postovulatory peak and sustained elevation. A composite plot of all cycles indicated a significant preovulatory peak of β-endorphin concentration occurring 2 days before the LH surge and a postovulatory trough occurring 5 days later.

β-Endorphin may have a significant role in neurochemical mechanisms of gonadotropin release. The rise and fall in serum β-endorphin concentration in the periovulatory period are statistically significant. β-Endorphin may have an initial stimulatory effect that results in LH secretion.

▶ [This study demonstrates a menstrual cyclicity of plasma β-endorphin levels, with higher values during the follicular phase and lower values during the luteal phase. Experiments in animals have suggested that β-endorphin plays a role (presumably inhibitory) in regulating LH production or release, or both, and the findings noted here of a slight decline just prior to the LH surge are consistent with that hypothesis. On the other hand, if β-endorphin were a major inhibitor of LH, one would not expect both to decline after ovulation.] ◀

14–2 **Effects of Obesity on Estradiol Metabolism: Decreased Formation of Nonuterotropic Metabolites.** Obesity has been associated with an increased incidence of reproductive dysfunction and an enhanced susceptibility to estrogen-related diseases. A recent study showed urinary excretion of 2-hydroxylated metabolites of estrogen to be diminished in obese women, though this does not necessarily reflect diminished 2-hydroxylative activity in the obese and may represent preferential excretion of the 2-hydroxyestrogens via the biliary route or an enhanced additional metabolism of these substances to unidentified compounds. To elucidate the role of body weight on estrogen metabolism, Jill Schneider, H. Leon Bradlow, Gladys Strain, Joseph Levin, Karl Anderson, and Jack Fishman (New York) studied the principal oxidative biotransformations of estradiol in 13 obese

(14–1) Fertil. Steril. 38:701–704, December 1982.
(14–2) J. Clin. Endocrinol. Metab. 56:973–978, May 1983.

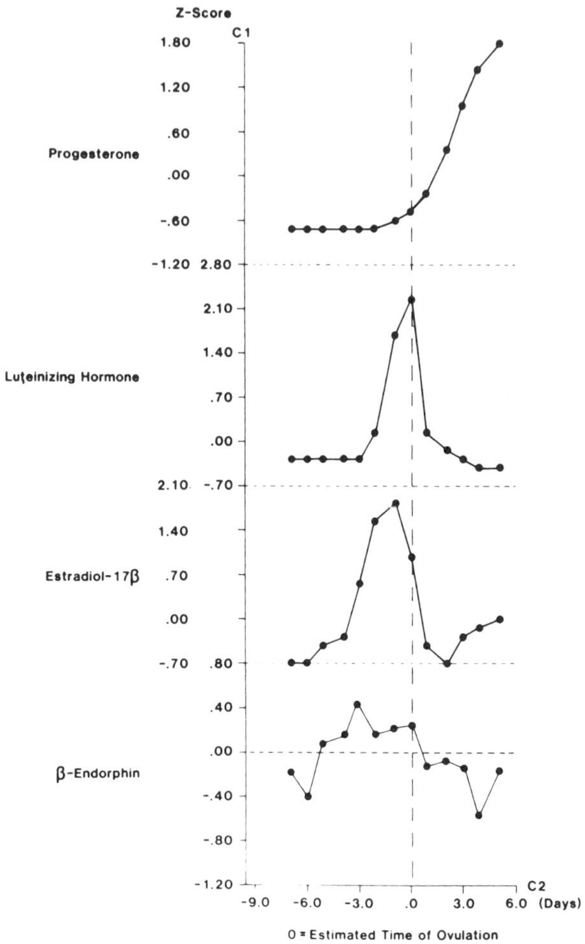

Fig 14–1.—Composite graph of 26 cycles, showing relationship of β-endorphin to LH, estradiol, and progesterone in periovulatory period with preovulatory β-endorphin peak. (Courtesy of Vrbicky, K. W., et al.: Fertil. Steril. 38:701–704, December 1982.)

premenopausal women (aged 25–43) and 10 obese men (aged 22–52) and compared the findings with those in 9 normal premenopausal women (aged 27–43) and 15 male (aged 23–56) control subjects. The studies were performed using a recently devised, sensitive radiometric method that allows assessment of the total in vivo oxidative metabolism of estradiol at specific sites (17α, 16α, and C-2) on the steroid molecule.

Compared with age-matched, normal weight, control subjects, both female and male subjects who weighed more than 160% of ideal body weight had significant decreases in hydroxylation at C-2 (women, $P < .001$; men, $P < .02$). The obese premenopausal women also showed a significant reduction in 17β-ol oxidation ($P < .05$) (table). These reductions in the oxidative metabolism of extradiol at C-2 and 17α did

METABOLISM OF ESTRADIOL AT POSITIONS 16α, 17α, AND C-2 IN NORMAL AND OBESE INDIVIDUALS

Subjects	% Oxidative metabolism		
	2-Hydroxylation	16α-Hydroxylation	17β-ol oxidation
1) Obese females	17.9 ± 3.1 (11)	11.3 ± 1.3 (12)	62.0 ± 5.9 (6)
2) Normal females	36.1 ± 3.2 (9)	11.6 ± 1.2 (9)	78.4 ± 3.7 (9)
3) Obese males	16.7 ± 2.6 (10)	8.9 ± 1.2 (7)	55.3 ± 2.9 (6)
4) Normal males	25.8 ± 2.2 (15)	7.6 ± 0.5 (15)	59.7 ± 2.6 (15)
P values			
1 *vs.* 2	<0.001	NS	<0.05
3 *vs.* 4	<0.02	NS	NS
1 *vs.* 3	NS	NS	NS
2 *vs.* 4	<0.02	<0.005	<0.002

Values are expressed as mean ± SE. Numbers of subjects are in parentheses.
(Courtesy of Schneider, J., et al.: J. Clin. Endocrinol. Metab. 56:973–978, May 1983.)

not correlate with either percent ideal body weight or daily caloric intake. Obesity did not affect the extent of hydroxylation at 16α significantly.

These metabolic alterations in obese subjects could result in a relatively hyperestrogenic state, because, unlike the other estrogen metabolites, the 2-hydroxyestrogen compounds possess relatively little peripheral estrogenic activity. On a prolonged basis, this metabolic alteration might contribute to the prevalence of certain hormonally related diseases in the obese.

▶ [Previous studies of estrogen metabolism and obesity have focused on peripheral aromatization of adrenal androgens to estrone, but these observations indicate that obesity affects estradiol metabolism as well. Obese women demonstrated a decreased tendency to hydroxylation at the C-2 position (which could lead to a hyperestrogenic state because 2-hydroxyestrogen compounds exhibit little estrogenic action) and oxidation at the 17α position.] ◀

14–3 **Effect of Body Weight Reduction on Plasma Androgens in Obese, Infertile Women.** Although various disorders are associated with polycystic ovarian disease, obesity, hirsutism, and menstrual dysfunction are the most frequent manifestations. G. William Bates and Neil S. Whitworth (Univ. of Mississippi, Jackson) investigated the possibility that obesity per se may give rise to androgen excess through alterations in estrogen metabolism and, consequently, through alterations in gonadotropin secretion. Eighteen obese, infertile women with polycystic ovarian disease were compared with 20 control women for levels of androstenedione, testosterone, follicle-stimulating hormone (FSH), and luteinizing hormone (LH). Sex-hormone-binding globulin was not measured.

Results of basal plasma androgen measurement showed that the level of plasma androstenedione in obese women was 252 ± 18 ng/dl compared with 173 ± 9 ng/dl in controls ($P < .001$). Plasma testosterone in obese women was 66 ± 5.7 ng/dl compared with 41 ± 3.0

(14–3) Fertil. Steril. 38:406–409, October 1982.

ng/dl in controls ($P < .001$). Plasma FSH and LH levels in obese women were 14.3 ± 1.2 mIU/ml and 43.2 ± 6 mIU/ml, respectively. Thirteen of the obese women (72%) lost more than 15% of their body weight by dietary restriction. Ten of these women (77%) became pregnant without additional therapy; 1 established regular ovulatory menses. Three of those who became pregnant conceived before measurement of androgens was repeated. The remaining 5 women would not participate in the weight reduction program and did not return for follow-up. Androgen levels were measured before and after weight loss in 7 women. Before weight loss, androstenedione and testosterone were 295 ± 19.1 ng/dl and 75 ± 8.3 ng/dl, respectively. After weight reduction, they were 179 ± 5.4 ng/dl and 39 ± 4.7 ng/dl, respectively ($P < 0.001$). After weight loss, random determinations of plasma androgen concentrations were similar to control values.

Simple weight loss to within 125% of ideal body weight is recommended for women with polycystic ovarian disease as the primary method of treatment, especially in those who wish to become pregnant. Current methods of treatment may be used as adjunctive therapy in women who do not respond to simple weight loss alone.

► ["Simple" weight loss may be hard to achieve. The lowered androgen levels and the return of ovulatory cycles in those who dieted successfully are not surprising.] ◄

14–4 **Polycystic Ovarian Syndrome: A Retrospective Study of the Therapeutic Effect of Ovarian Wedge Resection After Unsuccessful Treatment With Clomiphene Citrate.** O. Lunde (Univ. of Oslo) examined the value of ovarian wedge resection in a series of 92 women operated on in 1970–1980 for polycystic ovarian syndrome, which had been confirmed by ovarian biopsy. All had had problems in infertility for 1 to 15 years. Seven patients had previously been pregnant. All patients were treated with clomiphene citrate preoperatively; many responded with ovulations, but none established regular menstrual periods or conceived. Wedge resections were performed to the extent necessary to reduce the ovaries to apparently normal volume.

Ovulation was confirmed postoperatively in 94% of 62 evaluable women, compared with a frequency of 19% before wedge resection. Thirty-seven women conceived spontaneously, and 21 conceived after further treatment with clomiphene, gonadotropins, or bromocriptine. Seven of these 58 patients conceived both spontaneously and when induced. Eighty percent of the 92 pregnancies resulted in normal children. Fifty-three women had regular periods for more than a year after wedge resection. Nineteen others had more regular periods, but 18 failed to improve after the operation, although most of these patients ovulated and conceived or had vaginal bleeding after treatment with gonadotropin or bromocriptine.

Ovarian wedge resection should be considered after an unsuccessful trial of clomiphene citrate in women with polycystic ovary syndrome. Wedge resection is performed longitudinally, with attention to meticulous hemostasis and atraumatic handling of the tissues. The risk of

(14–4) Ann. Chir. Gynaecol. 71:330–333, 1982.

pelvic adhesions developing after wedge resection is currently under study. Wedge resection proved to benefit significantly both menstrual irregularities and infertility in patients in this series.

▶ [When clomiphene became available, the treatment of polycystic ovarian syndrome shifted dramatically from surgical to medical, and many endocrinologists said that the wedge resection was gone, completely and forever. Not quite, says this report. We also believe that there is a small but definite place for wedge resection, but we're not sure that this retrospective study proves it. Although a pregnancy rate of 63% among clomiphene failures seems impressive at first glance, in the absence of any control or comparison group, it's difficult to interpret. Moreover, we would ask whether failure to conceive with a clomiphene regimen of 50–100 mg per day for 5 days and for an average of four cycles really constitutes "clomiphene failure."] ◀

14–5 **Failure of Bromocriptine to Restore the Menstrual Cycle in Normoprolactinemic Postpill Amenorrhea.** Bromocriptine has been reported to restore menstruation in women with normoprolactinemic amenorrhea, but these reports did not issue from double-blind placebo-controlled studies. Herjan J. T. Coelingh Bennink and Henk J. van der Steeg (Utrecht, The Netherlands) examined the efficacy of bromocriptine in a double-blind, placebo-controlled, randomized study in 29 patients who had amenorrhea for 6 months or longer after discontinuance of oral contraception and plasma prolactin levels below 0.6 mU/ml. No cause of anovulation was found after extensive endocrinologic screening. The patients received either 3 mg of bromocriptine daily or placebo tablets for 12 weeks, or until the second vaginal bleeding occurred. Thirteen women received bromocriptine and 16, placebo.

Menstruation occurred in 4 of the 13 bromocriptine-treated patients. Ovulation was likely in 1 of these women. Vaginal bleeding was reported by 9 of the 16 placebo-treated women, and ovulation seemed likely in 8 of these cases. One woman conceived at the first ovulation.

Results of this controlled study clearly show that bromocriptine has no effect on restoration of the menstrual cycle in women with normoprolactinemic postpill amenorrhea. The results reported in previous studies are attributable to placebo effects. There is increasing evidence that a small but significant proportion of cases of postpill amenorrhea can be attributed to the previous use of oral contraceptives.

▶ [In this double-blind, placebo-controlled trial of bromocriptine in normoprolactinemic patients with postpill amenorrhea, 8 of 16 women in one group ovulated versus only 1 of 13 in the other. The kicker is that the placebo was the "effective" treatment. The efficacy of bromocriptine in normoprolactinemic patients with amenorrhea has been a matter of dispute (cf. 1980 YEAR BOOK, p. 351; and 1982 YEAR BOOK, pp. 377–379). The present report underscores the value of controlled trials. If the serum prolactin level is normal, bromocriptine apparently is without value.] ◀

14–6 **Secretion of Prolactin After Acute and Chronic Stimulation of the Breast: Effect of Timing During the Menstrual Cycle.** Robert E. Ratner, Stephen H. Sherry, and André T. Guay (Burlington, Mass.) observed that, because prolactin (PRL) assays have become a common screening test for the presence of pituitary disease, they at-

---

(14–5) Fertil. Steril. 39:238–240, February 1983.
(14–6) Ibid., 38:410–414, October 1982.

tempted to clarify the relationship between stimulation and secretion of PRL in a normal nonpostpartum population. The effect of acute and chronic stimulation of the breast in 11 nonpostpartum women was studied in both follicular and luteal phases of menstruation. All the women entered the study on days 3–5 of their monthly cycles. Subjects ranged in age from 23–40 years and all had normal menstrual cycles. All subjects in the study had normal baseline PRL and normal thyroid-stimulating hormone values.

The mean of all values drawn at equivalent times in the menstrual cycle showed no overall change in PRL level as a result of single or multiple episodes of stimulation during a 24-hour period. Examination of individual responses showed that in 1 patient a rise in PRL level occurred after a single stimulation and in another patient, after 24 hours of stimulation. After 2 weeks of daily breast stimulation, mean PRL value rose from a baseline mean of 10.2 ng/dl to 13.0 ng/dl and remained within normal limits of the assay. From these data, it was unclear whether the rise was secondary to chronic stimulation or to altered hormonal milieu associated with a change from follicular to luteal phase. Effects in 3 patients were restudied. Despite elevation in the lutel phase baseline PRL value, compared with the follicular phase baseline value, a further rise during acute stimulation occurred in only 1 patient.

The data suggest that the elevation of PRL in these patients is more of a function of the hormonal milieu of the luteal phase than of the duration of stimulation. With the increasing use of PRL determinations as a guide to diagnosis of pituitary disease, the importance of evaluating elevated PRL values in light of the menstrual phase, with less regard to a history of previous breast stimulation, is emphasized.

▶ [The suggestion has been made in the past that an assay of the serum prolactin level might be spuriously elevated if the blood specimen is drawn shortly after examination of the breasts. Not so, according to this study.] ◀

14–7 **Possible Prognostic Value of Serum Prolactin Increment During Pregnancy in Hyperprolactinemic Patients.** The progressive rise in serum prolactin that occurs during pregnancy is believed to be due to increased estrogen secretion. Nonpregnant hyperprolactinemic patients have a heterogeneous prolactin response to exogenous estradiol, and pregnant patients could be expected to have a heterogeneous increase in prolactin levels during pregnancy. A. Nyboe Andersen, J. Starup, AnnTabor, H. Kålund Jensen, and J. G. Westergaard attempted to correlate the prolactin response in pregnancy with the hyperprolactinemic state after pregnancy in 15 hyperprolactinemic, infertile patients in Denmark who achieved 17 pregnancies while receiving bromocriptine therapy. The mean duration of treatment before pregnancy was 3½ months. Bromocriptine was withdrawn after 4–10 weeks' gestation. All patients delivered healthy infants after 36–42 weeks' gestation. Sixteen normal women with uncomplicated pregnancies also were examined.

Five patients had a prolactin increment during pregnancy that was

(14–7) Acta Endocrinol. (Copenh.) 102:1–5, January 1983.

similar to or augmented compared with that seen in normal women. All had higher prolactin levels after pregnancy than before treatment. The other 10 patients had no rise in serum prolactin levels in the third trimester like that seen in normal women, and their postpartum prolactin levels were significantly lower than levels before treatment. Two patients with long-standing amenorrhea before treatment had distinct reductions in serum prolactin levels, and began menstrual bleeding after pregnancy; 1 was oligomenorrheic, whereas the other patient had a regular cycle.

Some hyperprolactinemic patients may benefit from pregnancy. These patients probably can be identified by their lack of significant changes in serum prolactin levels during pregnancy. The cause of decreasing prolactin levels during gestation is unclear, although both adenoma apoplexy and infarction have been suggested. The correction of a minor "functional" defect during bromocriptine therapy has also been considered.

▶ [This interesting report points to a possible prognostic relationship of the effect of pregnancy on serum prolactin levels in hyperprolactinemic patients. In 10 of 15 patients, levels did not increase during the third trimester and postpartum levels in these women were lower than those before treatment, suggesting that pregnancy had exerted some beneficial effect in these hyperprolactinemic patients. On the other hand, gestation is known to be associated occasionally with marked growth of a prolactinoma, sometimes with disastrous consequences, so pregnancy should not be regarded in any way as therapeutic.] ◀

14–8 **Outcome in Patients With Postpill Amenorrhea.** M. H. Soltan (Cork, Ireland) and K. W. Hancock (Univ. of Leeds) report their results of the resumption of menstruation and pregnancy in women with postpill amenorrhea. Ninety-six patients with postpill amenorrhea lasting 12 months or more after discontinuation of oral contraceptives were included. Before oral contraceptive use, 45 patients had a reasonably regular cycle of between 28 and 40 days (group 1), whereas 51 patients had some form of menstrual irregularity (group 2).

Twenty-six of the 45 patients in group 1 resumed spontaneous ovulation and 6 achieved a pregnancy, whereas in group 2, 19 of 51 patients ovulated spontaneously and 7 conceived. Thirty-one of the 96 patients did not wish to conceive. Of the remaining 65 patients, 7 were lost to follow-up, 7 proved to have primary gonadal failure, and 4 had additional barriers to conception. If these 18 patients are excluded, the overall pregnancy rate was 82% (39 of 47 patients). These results show the prognosis in postpill amenorrhea to be favorable.

The authors conclude that the outcome in patients with postpill amenorrhea is good, and treatment does improve the prognosis for pregnancy, particularly in patients with preexisting menstrual dysfunction. They no longer counsel patients with a previous history of fully investigated postpill amenorrhea against resuming oral contraception when they desire both effective contraception and the reassurance provided by regular withdrawal bleeds.

▶ [Readers of past YEAR BOOKS will recall that the existence of postpill amenorrhea as

(14–8) Br. J. Obstet. Gynaecol. 89:745–748, September 1982.

a distinct entity is a matter of dispute. The prognosis for achieving pregnancy in the current series of patients so classified was good. Half of the patients, however, required gonadotropin therapy.] ◀

14–9 **Growth and Maturation of Patients With Turner's Syndrome.** Elizabeth Park, John D. Bailey, and Carol A. Cowell (Hosp. for Sick Children, Toronto) retrospectively examined the effects of sex chromosome constitution and estrogen treatment on increases in height and on skeletal and sexual maturation in 116 patients with female phenotype and at least one major feature of Turner's syndrome associated with an abnormality of an X chromosome.

Seventy-one patients had a pure 45 X karyotype (XO group), 33 had X chromosome mosaicism, and 12 had a structurally abnormal X chromosome (non-XO group). Birth weights in all gestations were similar for XO and non-XO patients, but were significantly lower than normal. Unexpectedly high correlations were observed between birth weight and adult height and weight (r = .96 and 0.92, respectively). Patients were significantly shorter than normal at all ages tested between 2 and 17 years ($P < .05$), though the difference was more pronounced after age 10 years. Mean adult height was 142.0 ± 7.6 cm. No consistent pattern of significant differences in height could be discerned between XO and non-XO or between Xp monosomic and Xp disomic patients. Thirteen patients, 2 XO and 11 non-XO, who had undergone spontaneous menarche had evidence of a slight premenarcheal growth spurt. In 11 of these 13 patients, the average annual growth rate increased from 3.00 to 4.83 cm in the year preceding menarche, although this was considerably below the mean pubertal growth rate of 9 ± 1.03 cm/year. This difference indicates that endocrine mechanisms associated with more normal pubertal sexual development also produce a more normal growth pattern. Patients treated with estrogen grew at a slower, fairly constant rate in the 2 years preceding and 1 year after treatment, with the total increase in height after estrogen treatment averaging only 3.6 cm. The rate of skeletal maturation was lower than normal (0.53 bone-age year/chronological year) in the 2 years preceding estrogen treatment and higher than normal (1.47 bone-age year/chronologic year) in the 2 years after treatment, which suggests that these patients may be hypersensitive to the skeletal maturing effects of estrogen. Prior to estrogen treatment, breast development was absent or more delayed than pubic hair development, though the delay in the development of both secondary sex characteristics was greater than the delay in skeletal maturation. Whereas the average normal girl at age 12 has moderate breast development, only 5.4% of the patients had moderate breast development and only 10.8% had moderate pubic hair growth at bone-age 12. Spontaneous menarche occurred in significantly more non-XO than XO patients, which suggests that even non-XO patients who require estrogen treatment may have a more normal level of ovarian function than XO patients, who have significantly less pretreatment breast development and later epiphyseal fusion.

The results indicate that the short stature characteristic of Turn-

---

(14–9) Pediatr. Res. 17:1–7, January 1983.

er's syndrome appears to be a consequence of intrauterine events. Because patients treated with estrogens showed fairly constant growth until an average age of 16.4 years, whereas patients in whom menarche occurred spontaneously had experienced a slight growth spurt but had stopped growing at an average age of 16.0 years, sex steroids may merely hasten the attainment of the predetermined growth potential.

▶ [It is well known that individuals with Turner's syndrome are short in adolescence and adulthood. This study indicates that they are small from birth onward. The correlation between birth weight and adult weight and height is astonishingly high (0.96 and 0.92, respectively), indicating that whatever the growth-limiting mechanism is, it apparently begins its effect in utero. It is interesting that growth did not seem to differ between patients with XO Turner's syndrome and those with some other chromosomal pattern.] ◀

14–10 **Relation of Menstrual Cycle Phase to Symptoms of Rheumatoid Arthritis.** Both progesterone and estrogen exhibit anti-inflammatory and antiarthritic activity, and women with rheumatoid arthritis may have fewer symptoms of arthritis in the postovulatory phase of the cycle when plasma levels of the hormones increase. Neal S. Latman (Weatherford, Okla.) evaluated daily symptoms during 69 menstrual cycles in 14 women, aged 18 to 45 years, with rheumatoid arthritis. An average of about 5 cycles per subject were evaluated. None of these women was using hormonal contraception.

Less morning stiffness occurred in the postovulatory phase in 57% of the cycles studied and in the preovulatory phase in 19%. Less pain occurred in 60% and 20% of the postovulatory phase and preovulatory phases, respectively. By within-patient analysis, 7 of the 14 patients had less morning stiffness in the postovulatory phase of the cycle, but no patient had less stiffness in the preovulatory phase. Significantly less pain occurred in the postovulatory phase in 7 patients, and less in the preovulatory phase in none. These differences were significant. Duration of morning stiffness was significantly less in the postovulatory phase than in the preovulatory phase of the cycle.

The morning stiffness and pain of rheumatoid arthritis often are less marked in the postovulatory phase of the menstrual cycle. In trials of anti-inflammatory and antiarthritic drugs the phase of the menstrual cycle should be taken into account. Awareness that symptoms may fluctuate during the menstrual cycle may keep the physician and patient from too rapidly discarding a new treatment modality. Any effect of plasma estrogen and progesterone levels is subtle and often is hidden by the many factors that determine the severity of symptoms in rheumatoid arthritis.

▶ [Patients with rheumatoid arthritis typically experience improvement in symptoms during pregnancy, a situation attributed to increased plasma levels of free cortisol. However, it could also be due to estrogen or progesterone, or both, and, if so, amelioration also should occur during the luteal phase of the menstrual cycle. It does, according to this study.] ◀

14–11 **Estrogen Excretion Patterns and Plasma Levels in Vegetarian and Omnivorous Women.** There is increasing evidence that nu-

---

(14–10) Am. J. Med. 74:957–960, June 1983.
(14–11) N. Engl. J. Med. 307:1542–1547, Dec. 16, 1982.

tritional status and diet can influence estrogen production and excretion in women. A positive correlation has been found between body weight and plasma estrone and estradiol concentrations, and there is experimental evidence that diet alters estrogen metabolism. Barry R. Goldin, Herman Adlercreutz, Sherwood L. Gorbach, James H. Warram, Johanna T. Dwyer, Linda Swenson, and Margo N. Woods examined estrogen metabolism in 20 premenopausal women, 10 of them vegetarians. All were nulliparas aged 20 to 30 years. The two groups were similar in age, height, weight, and mean caloric and protein intakes. The omnivores took 43% of their protein from animal sources and the vegetarians, 7% from fish. The vegetarians took more than twice as much fiber. The omnivores consumed significantly more total fat and saturated fat per unit food intake.

Fecal excretion of estrogens was twofold to threefold higher in the vegetarian women than in the omnivores. Urinary estriol excretion was significantly lower in vegetarians. Plasma estrone and estradiol concentrations were lower in the vegetarians. Fecal weight and fecal estrogen excretion correlated positively in both groups. β-Glucuronidase activity of fecal bacteria was significantly reduced in the vegetarians.

Vegetarian women have an increased fecal excretion of estrogen, due to increased fecal output, and decreased plasma estrogen concentrations. The reduced enterohepatic circulation of estrogen in vegetarians could be due to a higher intake of dietary fiber, producing a shielding effect, or to a decreased ability of the intestinal flora to deconjugate biliary estrogen conjugates.

▶ [A number of epidemiologic observations have suggested an association between diet and breast cancer incidence. This interesting and well-done study of estrogen metabolism in vegetarians points to a possible mechanism. Vegetarians, in comparison with omnivores, were found to excrete much more estrogen in feces (due to increased fecal bulk), leading to decreased levels of plasma concentrations.] ◀

14–12 **Amenorrhea Associated With Carotenemia.** Carotenemia can result from either excessive ingestion of carotene-rich vegetables or an impaired ability to metabolize carotenes. Ekkehard Kemmann, Samuel A. Pasquale, and Robert Skaf (Rutgers Med. School, New Brunswick, N. J.) diagnosed carotenemia in 10 amenorrheic hypogonadotropic women of normal weight, all of whom ate foods rich in carotene. Strenuous exercise was not an apparent factor in their amenorrhea, but all patients took a diet rich in raw vegetables and devoid of red meats. Nine women were ammenorrheic and were considered hypoestrogenic. None had elevated serum prolactin levels. One patient had mild hirsutism and normal androgen levels. Serum carotene levels ranged from 221 to 1,007 μg/dl. Only 1 patient reported significant weight loss. The dietary habits were attributed to both health concerns and a liking for vegetables, salads, and carrots.

The patients were encouraged to reduce their intake of carotene-rich foods and increase their protein intake. These suggestions were difficult to follow, but 8 patients made some changes; 2 continued to have high carotene levels and failed to menstruate. The other pa-

---

(14–12) JAMA 249:926–929, Feb. 18, 1983.

tients menstruated within 4 months of modifing their diets, and 1 conceived after having established regular cycles. In 2 women seen specifically for infertility, anovulation was the only cause. Both of these patients conceived, 1 after clomiphene therapy and 1 with exogenous gonadotropin therapy.

Carotenemia due to ingestion of a high-carotene diet may be associated with the development of amenorrhea. Further studies are needed concerning the possible relationship between carotene metabolism and reproductive function. The nature of this form of menstrual dysfunction is not clear, but carotene may exert a peripheral antiestrogenic effect. Low gonadotropin and prolactin levels are, however, compatible with a central, possibly hypothalamic, effect. Fertility readily has been restored to these patients.

▶ [The authors of this report think that the hypothalamic amenorrhea in these 10 patients with carotenemia did not occur on the basis of weight loss or exercise, but rather was diet induced, related either to an excess of carotene or a deficiency of some other nutrient. Vegetarian diets were the rule; one half of the women ate at least a pound of raw carrots daily. Menstrual function returned in those patients who modified their diets. Apparently, when taking a history from a nonpregnant patient with secondary amenorrhea, in addition to questioning her about weight gain or weight loss, we should determine just what she's been eating. Yellow palms were noted in 9 of the 10 women described here.] ◀

14–13 **An Epidemiologic Study of Young Women With Dysmenorrhea.** Björn Andersch and Ian Milsom (Univ. of Göteborg) studied the incidence of dysmenorrhea in a random sample of 19-year-old women from an urban Swedish population. A total of 656 women out of a population of 2,621 were included in the study. It was possible to compare 60 nonrespondents with the 596 respondents; no significant difference was found.

The incidence of dysmenorrhea in this population was 72.4%, 90 respondents (15.4%) suffered from dysmenorrhea that limited daily activity and was unrelieved by the use of analgesics. However, 162 women (27.6%) experienced no dysmenorrhea. Incidence and severity of dysmenorrhea were significantly reduced among users of oral contraceptives compared with users of intrauterine devices (IUDs) or women who did not use oral contraceptives or IUDs. A significant correlation was found between severity of dysmenorrhea and both menarcheal age and duration of menstrual flow. Severity and incidence of dysmenorrhea were unaffected by height, weight, or length of menstrual cycle. Incidence and severity of dysmenorrhea were significantly reduced in parous women compared with those who had never been pregnant or whose pregnancies had been terminated by abortion or miscarriage. The amount of menstrual bleeding was correlated significantly with severity of dysmenorrhea, which was also significantly correlated with maternal and sibling dysmenorrhea. Analgesics were regularly taken by 38.2% of the respondents, and oral contraceptives were used by 21.5%; 23.9% reported that they desired medical attention for dysmenorrhea. A total of 50.9% had been absent from work or school due to dysmenorrhea. Compared with nonsmokers, smokers had significantly less dysmenorrhea.

(14–13) Am. J. Obstet. Gynecol. 144:655–660, Nov. 15, 1982.

This cross-sectional study does not take into account time-related factors. The same population will be assessed in a longitudinal study to analyze the effect of time-related factors, such as increasing age and changes in parity, on dysmenorrhea.

▶ [This study of urban Swedish 19-year-old women may be limited in its applicability by cultural factors, but has the important advantages of being based on a random sample of the entire population and of a very high response rate. The findings are not surprising, except for the curious negative correlation between the severity of dysmenorrhea and cigarette smoking.] ◀

14–14 **Zomepirac Sodium in Treatment of Primary Dysmenorrhea Syndrome.** Zomepirac sodium, a potent inhibitor of prostaglandin synthesis, is a nonnarcotic, oral analgesic previously shown to relieve oral surgical pain, postoperative pain, pain of osteoarthritis, and acute orthopedic pain. Penny Wise Budoff (Woodbury, N.Y.) conducted a 6-month, double-blind, placebo-controlled, multiple crossover trial of its effectiveness in relieving abdominal cramping and 25 other symptoms of primary dysmenorrhea assessed daily.

The 47 study participants were aged 15 to 42 years (mean, 27 years) and had recurrent monthly abdominal cramping painful enough to require a prescription analgesic. Patients were randomly assigned to one of eight possible medication sequences (Fig 14–2). They took 1 capsule (100 mg) of zomepirac sodium or placebo at the first sign of menstrual pain and could repeat the dose every 4 hours as needed, to a maximum of 6 capsules per day for up to 5 days during each menstrual period. If adequate relief of symptoms was not obtained after 2 doses (8 hours), a supplemental analgesic was permitted.

Zomepirac was significantly more effective than placebo in relieving 12 of 13 primary symptoms and 6 of 13 associated symptoms. The severity of 9 primary symptoms was reduced by more than 50% (Fig 14–3). While taking zomepirac, patients were able to continue normal

Fig 14–2.—Medication sequences. Each patient took medications in one of these eight sequences. Every 2-month segment was a crossover, and no patient took the same medication 3 months in succession. (Courtesy of Budoff, P. W.: N. Engl. J. Med. 307:714–719, Sept. 16, 1982.)

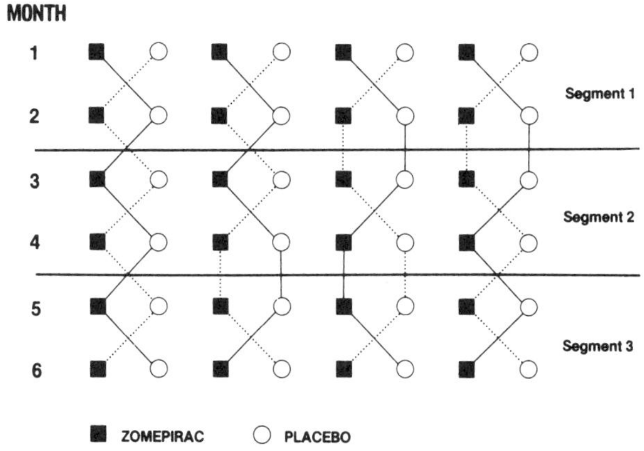

(14–14) N. Engl. J. Med. 307:714–719, Sept. 16, 1982.

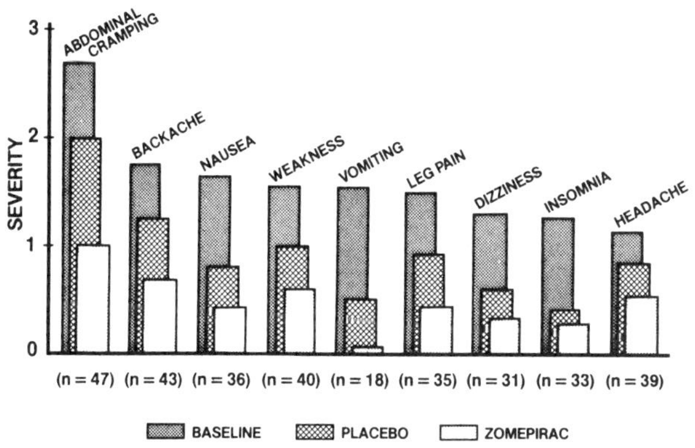

Fig 14–3.—Reduction in mean severity of nine primary symptoms. These symptoms were evaluated for severity at baseline and daily during treatment. Zomepirac provided significantly more relief of all nine symptoms than did placebo. (Scale: 3 = severe, 2 = moderate, 1 = mild, and 0 = none.) (Courtesy of Budoff, P. W.: N. Engl. J. Med. 307:714–719, Sept. 16, 1982.)

activities on a higher proportion of treatment days (86% vs. 59%) and required supplemental analgesics less often (on 7% vs. 50% of treatment days). Global evaluations significantly favored zomepirac over placebo. There were no unusual or unexpected side effects. As is generally the case with prostaglandin-synthesis inhibitors, the largest proportion of side effects were gastrointestinal disturbances that were generally mild and transient. No clinically significant changes in any laboratory value occurred. Although patients were permitted up to 600 mg of zomepirac per day, symptoms were relieved by a mean dose of 260 mg for an average of 2.1 days per month.

▶ [Again, a prostaglandin-synthesis inhibitor has scored better than the placebo in the treatment of primary dysmenorrhea. A new wrinkle here is the variety of medication sequences indicated in Figure 14–1. This should help minimize bias associated with a study subject guessing whether or not she is receiving active drug during a particular menstrual period.

This drug subsequently was withdrawn because of idiosyncratic reactions.] ◀

14–15 **Dose-Response Evaluation of Cyclic Estrogen/Gestagen in Postmenopausal Women: Placebo-Controlled Trial of Its Gynecologic and Metabolic Actions.** Merete Sanvig Christensen, Claus Hagen, Claus Christiansen, and Ib Transbøl (Univ. of Copenhagen) randomly administered a 12-month treatment with placebo or one of three different doses (high, medium, low) or natural estrogens (17 β-estradiol and estriol), sequentially combined with norethisterone acetate for 10 of the 28 cycle days (Fig 14–4), to 100 volunteers to study dose-response relationships of estrogen in normal postmenopausal women. A total of 87 women completed the trial with examinations every 3 months, between the 16th and 22d days of the tablet cycle.

The table shows the comparability of the four groups. Postmenopausal symptoms, estimated by the Kupperman index, were reduced in a dose-related pattern; the highest dose showed a 70% drop in symptoms and the lowest, a 33% drop. The reduction in FSH level was also

---

(14–15) Am. J. Obstet. Gynecol. 144:873–879, Dec. 15, 1982.

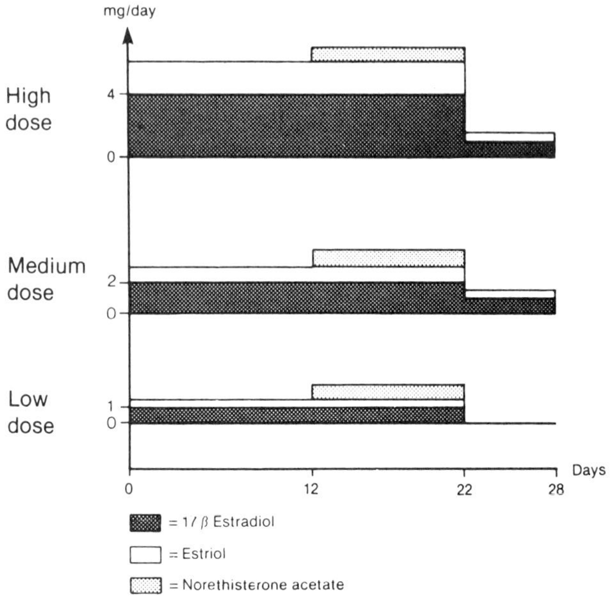

Fig 14–4.—Content (mg/day) of micronized 17 β-estradiol, estriol and norethisterone acetate in high-dose, medium-dose, and low-dose tablets. (Courtesy of Christensen, M. S., et al.: Am. J. Obstet. Gynecol. 144:873–879, Dec. 15, 1982.)

dose dependent, varying between 60% and 32% reductions. The percentage of women with regular cyclic bleeding was dose related. Changes in bone mass were small but also dose related. Cholesterol levels in serum were reduced in a dose-related manner; the highest drop was 10% for the highest hormone dose, with intermediate changes for the medium- and low-hormone groups. Blood pressure, body weight, and serum triglyceride concentration did not change significantly in any of the groups.

Results of this study clearly demonstrate that the beneficial effects of combined estrogen and gestagen treatment were related to the estrogen dose, although a somewhat smaller compliance was observed in the high-dose group. In most women the medium dose would be

CLINICAL DATA AND PRETREATMENT VALUES IN 87 POSTMENOPAUSAL WOMEN CLASSIFIED ACCORDING TO TREATMENT

	Age (yr)		*Menopausal age (mo)*		*Kupperman index (score)*		*Height (cm)*	*Serum FSH (U/L)*	*Serum Cholesterol (mmol/L)*	*Bone mass (units)*
Treatment	*Mean*	*Range*	*Mean*	*Range*	*Mean*	*Range*	*(mean ± 1 SD)*	*(mean ± 1 SD)*	*(mean ± 1 SD)*	*(mean ± 1 SD)*
High dose (n = 19)	50.6	45-53	40.1	29-59	5.6	0-18	162.2 ± 4.4	84.2 ± 23.4	5.9 ± 1.0	38.2 ± 5.3
Medium dose (n = 22)	52.7	49-55	44.6	30-61	8.4	0-25	161.2 ± 4.8	82.0 ± 31.4	6.2 ± 1.3	39.0 ± 7.8
Low dose (n = 23)	52.3	47-55	42.3	28-58	8.2	0-30	160.7 ± 6.7	84.3 ± 32.8	5.8 ± 1.2	36.4 ± 6.2
Placebo (n = 23)	50.4	46-55	44.1	29-62	7.2	0-25	162.9 ± 6.9	85.6 ± 34.2	5.6 ± 1.0	36.1 ± 6.0

(Courtesy of Christensen, M. S., et al.: Am. J. Obstet. Gynecol. 144:873–879, Dec. 15, 1982.)

sufficient to treat climacteric symptoms to insure regular vaginal bleeding, prevent postmenopausal bone loss, and maintain a low "premenopausal range" of serum cholesterol.

▶ [This study demonstrates a nice (in fact, almost too nice) dose-response relationship for postmenopausal estrogen therapy. The data do not permit firm conclusions about the important clinical issue of the best dosage, but it does seem that the low dose used here (1 mg of micronized estradiol and 0.5 mg of estriol) is too little. Whether the medium dose (2 and 1 mg, respectively) or the high dose (4 and 2 mg, respectively) is better cannot be stated.] ◀

14–16 **Randomized Double-Blind Crossover Trial Into the Effect of Norethisterone on Climacteric Symptoms and Biochemical Profiles.** Although cyclical estrogens are effective in the treatment of menopausal symptoms, they have been associated with an increased risk of endometrial cancer. This risk can be reduced and perhaps eliminated by the addition of a progestogen. M. E. L. Paterson (Birmingham and Midland Hosp. for Women, Birmingham, England) assessed the effectiveness of norethisterone (5 mg/day) in a randomized double-blind crossover study of 23 postmenopausal women with climacteric symptoms, including hot flushes and sweating.

Eighteen women completed the study. Ten initially received active treatment and 8 received placebo first. Active therapy significantly reduced the number of hot flushes experienced each week from more than 50 to less than 10, and this difference between active and placebo treatment was evident after 1 month of treatment. Blood pressure and body weight were not significantly affected by active treatment. The severity of hot flushes was also significantly reduced with active therapy and there was a slight improvement in memory, insomnia, and lack of energy. Other climacteric symptoms were not consistently altered. Side effects were usually minor, although 4 of 14 women who still had a uterus had vaginal bleeding during active therapy. Levels of serum calcium, alkaline phosphatase, cholesterol, triglycerides, FSH, and LH were significantly reduced during active therapy. The effect of active therapy on serum creatinine and urea levels was variable, but there were no significant changes in other biochemical parameters and liver function tests.

The results indicate that norethisterone (5 mg/day) is effective in alleviating the hot flushes and sweating associated with the climacteric. It is suggested that norethisterone exerts this beneficial effect directly, without being converted into ethinylestradiol.

▶ [Progestogens represent a viable alternative to estrogens in treating the menopausal syndrome. Medroxyprogesterone (Provera) has been used with good effect (see 1982 YEAR BOOK, pp. 416–419), and this study indicates that norethisterone is also effective in alleviating the symptomatology and reversing the biochemical consequences of the climacteric.] ◀

14–17 **Effect of Clonidine on Hot Flashes in Postmenopausal Women.** Larry R. Laufer, Yohanan Erlik, David R. Meldrum, and Howard L. Judd (Univ. of California, Los Angeles) examined the effectiveness of clonidine in suppressing postmenopausal hot flashes by using a dose-response study design and objective recordings of the

(14–16) Br. J. Obstet. Gynaecol. 89:464–472, June 1982.
(14–17) Obstet. Gynecol. 60:583–586, November 1982.

flashes. Patients with frequent flashes were studied before and after oral administration of placebo and 0.1, 0.2, and 0.4 mg of clonidine daily for 2 weeks at each dose level. Finger temperature and skin resistance were recorded as indices of hot flash episodes. Ten women with frequent severe hot flashes were included; 5 had entered menopause spontaneously; 5 had undergone surgical castration.

During administration of clonidine, 4 patients experienced side effects severe enough to withdraw from the study. One noted severe fatigue, nausea, headaches, and irritability; the others withdrew because of dizziness. An apparent dose-response relationship to clonidine was observed. Analysis of variance showed a significant reduction in the number of objectively recorded hot flashes in relation to baseline and placebo when clonidine was given. With the largest dosage (0.4 mg/day), mean reduction from baseline was 46%.

Of the 6 patients who completed the study, 5 complained of mouth dryness on the 0.2- and 0.4-mg dosages. Two patients reported insomnia on the same dosages and 1 experienced a syncopal episode on the 0.4-mg dosage.

In this study, the administration of clonidine reduced significantly the number of objectively measured hot flashes in symptomatic postmenopausal women. However, the reduction was of lesser magnitude than has been reported with estrogenic or progestational agents. Administration of clonidine was associated with several side effects, thus limiting the clinical acceptibility of this drug for treatment of hot flashes.

▶ [Clonidine had a modest effect in decreasing the number of objectively determined hot flashes in the study subjects. At the largest dose there was a 46% reduction. This compares with the complete elimination of hot flashes with estrogen and their nearly complete elimination with a progestin, as previously reported by these authors. Side effects were frequent. It is of interest that this centrally acting α-adrenergic agonist affects vasomotor symptoms, but it appears that there is little if any reason to choose this drug in the treatment of hot flashes.] ◀

14–18 **Estrogen Use and All-Cause Mortality: Preliminary Results From the Lipid Research Clinics Program Follow-up Study.** The well-established advantage women hold in total mortality is not well understood and is not explained by sex differences in behavior or known risk factors. Some investigators have suggested a protective effect of endogenous estrogens, and there is some evidence of a reduced mortality risk in postmenopausal women taking exogenous estrogens. Trudy L. Bush, Linda D. Cowan, Elizabeth Barrett-Connor, Michael H. Criqui, John M. Karon, Robert B. Wallace, H. Al Tyroler, and Basil M. Rifkind (Natl. Inst. of Health) report a study of prospectively collected data examining the association of both estrogen use and hysterectomy status with total mortality in a free-living population. Follow-up was made of 2,269 white women aged 40–69 years enrolled in the Lipid Research Clinics Program Follow-up Study; average follow-up was 5.6 years. Seventy-two deaths occurred during the study period.

The relative risk of death in estrogen users compared with nonus-

(14–18) JAMA 249:903–906, Feb. 18, 1983.

ers was 0.54 in gynecologically intact women, 0.34 in hysterectomized women, and 0.12 in bilaterally oophorectomized women. This risk of death in estrogen users regardless of hysterectomy status was 0.37. A significant negative association of estrogen use with mortality persisted after adjusting for possibly confounding factors. Hysterectomy status alone was not a significant predictor of mortality. When the high-density lipoprotein cholesterol level was considered, the effect of estrogen use was reduced but not eliminated. The reported use of various other medications was comparable in estrogen users and nonusers.

Exogenous estrogen use was associated with a lower risk of all-cause mortality in this study, as in others. The findings support a protective effect of exogenous estrogen use. Such an effect is consistent with the increase in the high-density lipoprotein cholesterol level associated with estrogen use and the corresponding reduction in risk of coronary heart disease, the chief cause of death in postmenopausal women. However, current estrogen-prescribing practices should not be altered before further controlled experimental studies are completed.

▶ [Noncontraceptive estrogen use was associated with decreased all-cause mortality regardless of hysterectomy status in this study population. Increased levels of high-density lipoprotein cholesterol in estrogen users accounted for some, but not all, of the lower risk of death. The results reported here suggest that the effects of estrogen on high-density lipoprotein cholesterol levels do have clinical significance. Today it is customary, when using estrogen to treat a woman who has not had a hysterectomy, to add a progestin on a cyclic basis in order to protect her endometrium against the development of hyperplasia and carcinoma. What we need to know is what dosage of what progestin at what frequency is sufficient to provide this protection with the least interference with the beneficial effect of estrogen on the serum lipoprotein pattern.] ◀

15. Infertility

ENDOMETRIOSIS—1984

ROBERT W. KISTNER, M.D.
ROBERT L. BARBIERI, M.D.
STEPHEN EVANS, M.D.

Department of Obstetrics and Gynecology, Brigham and Women's Hospital, Harvard Medical School, Boston, Massachusetts

Endometriosis is a rather ubiquitous, potentially disabling disease that seems to be increasing in incidence. It is a frequent cause of infertility and has been reported to account for 25% to 30% of fertility problems in the human female. If male factors were excluded, endometriosis would probably be the most common cause of infertility in women older than age 25.

Overview of Endometriosis

Although this disease may have always existed, the term "endometriosis" was first coined by John Sampson in 1922. Since then, it has been described, defined, and classified in over 2,000 reports. Yet it is still an enigmatic disease. At least a dozen theories attempt to explain the histogenesis of endometriosis, but the most logical, I believe, is still that of Sampson—namely, retrograde menstruation via the oviduct with recurrent peritoneal insult month after month, year after year, in women who unfortunately do not have periods of menstrual cessation. The disease is, therefore, common in the nullipara and uncommon in the multipara.

The most frequently involved areas are the ovaries and the cul-de-sac. This is consistent with the menstrual tubal reflux theory. Predisposing factors are undoubtedly of importance in the development of endometriosis. Recent studies indicate that race per se is not relevant. A familial tendency has been reported, particularly in sisters, but also in mothers and daughters.

Because all women menstruate into the peritoneal cavity simultaneously with vaginal efflux, the important question to be answered is, "Why does the menstrual effluvium attach and grow in some women, but not in others?" Undoubtedly, the former are not protected, immunologically speaking, whereas the latter are. Future research should be directed toward delineating the cause of this protection, rather than newer treatment methods.

Specific physical and psychologic characteristics have been attributed to patients with endometriosis. These women are tense perfectionists with an insatiable desire to excel. They express demanding and specific goals for their lives, usually are well dressed, and usually have trim figures. In one study, most of the patients were employed in responsible administrative positions or in professions such as law, medicine, and teaching. It should be noted, however, that these personality traits occur in career women who have elected a prolonged delay in initiating a family; perhaps it is the prolongation of peritoneal insult rather than the somatotype that is etiologic. However, when a planned delay has been accomplished with the use of oral contraceptives, the incidence of endometriosis seems to be diminished. Oral contraceptives effectively reduce the quantity and quality of tubal efflux.

What are the signs and symptoms of endometriosis? The classic symptom complex includes dysmenorrhea, deep dyspareunia, and infertility (Table 1). Progressive, acquired dysmenorrhea probably is due to "miniature menstruation" in areas of endometriosis with distention of overlying peritoneum. Patients with extensive endometriosis, especially ovarian, may have minimal pain; 30% of patients with endometriosis have no pain. Dyspareunia is related to active disease in the cul-de-sac with third-degree uterine retroversion. Premenstrual staining and hypermenorrhea may be associated with abnormal ovarian function, endometrial polyps, or adenomyosis. Urinary frequency, dysuria, and hematuria are due to extension of disease into the bladder, and painful defecation is due to involvement of the rectosigmoid. Only 30% of patients are completely asymptomatic. Because reliable and simple endoscopic procedures are now available, the diagnosis easily can be made visually or histologically. Laparoscopy provides an ideal method to demonstrate the extent and severity of the disease, thus permitting accurate classification prior to therapy (Table 2). The diagnosis should be suspected by the history, corroborated by pelvic examination, and verified by endoscopy or biopsy. Treatment should not be instituted until precise diagnosis and classification have been established.

TABLE 1.—SYMPTOMS OF ENDOMETRIOSIS

Pelvic pain	Progressive, acquired dysmenorrhea
Dyspareunia	Related to active disease in cul-de-sac with third-degree uterine retroversion
Premenstral staining and hypermenorrhea	May be associated with abnormal ovarian function, endometrial polyps, or adenomyosis
Painful defecation	Due to involvement of retrosigmoid
Urinary frequency, dysuria, hematuria	Due to disease extension into bladder

TABLE 2.—DIAGNOSIS OF ENDOMETRIOSIS

Diagnosis is suspected by history, corroborated by pelvic examination, and verified by endoscopy or biopsy

Pelvic exam	Tender, nodular uterosacral ligaments, with fixed third-degree uterine retroversion
Biopsy	Perineum, cervix, vagina, abdominal scars, umbilicus
Endoscopy	Laparoscopy or culdoscopy
Laparotomy	Not all "chocolate" cysts necessarily caused by endrometriosis; biopsy all "blue spots" and "powder burns"

Endometriosis must be differentiated from various other disorders (Table 3). Adenomyosis causes similar symptoms but usually occurs in an older age group: a multiparous uterus is enlarged, nodular, and tender. In pelvic inflammatory disease symptoms similar to those with endometriosis include infertility; examination reveals bilateral, tender, broad ligament masses, characteristically doughy or fluctuant; leukocytosis and an elevated sedimentation rate suggest infection. Ovarian carcinoma may present as solid nodules in the cul-de-sac; carcinoma may arise in endometriosis. Oxyuris vermicularis, splenosis (following ruptured spleen) and mesotheliomas may be calcified and present as nodules in the cul-de-sac. Classification in terms of severity, or stage, of the development of the disease, has proved to be useful, not only in selection of appropriate therapy, but also in evaluation and reporting of results of treatment. We introduced a classification in 1977, which has been augmented and approved by the American Fertility Society (Table 4).[1]

Endometriosis and Infertility

What is the mechanism of infertility in patients who have endometriosis? When endometriosis is extensive, the alteration of tubal and ovarian physiology is ominous, and the relationship to infertility easily is explained. However, in early stages, it is difficult to rationalize a cause. Prostaglandins may play a role in such patients. It has been suggested that degeneration of ectopic endometrial tissues releases prostaglandin $F_2\alpha$, resulting in local vasospasm, hypoxia, tissue destruction, and uterine contractions. Physiologic levels of prostaglandins have been shown to be necessary for ovum release, normal tubal motility, uterine relaxation and contractility, and steroidogenesis. An increased concentration of prostaglandins in peritoneal fluid may result in alterations in tubal motility, ovum release, and steroidogenesis.[2]

The objectives of treatment are to secure pain relief, permit adequate coitus, prevent abnormal bleeding, and, of course, to preserve or increase the possibility of pregnancy. Conservative surgery accomplishes all of this in many patients, but pregnancy itself has been

TABLE 3.—DIFFERENTIAL DIAGNOSIS OF ENDOMETRIOSIS

Adenomyosis	Similar symptoms but age group usually older; multiparous uterus is enlarged, nodular tender
Pelvic inflammatory disease	Similar symptoms, including infertility Bilateral, tender, broad ligament masses, usually doughy or fluctuant Leukocytosis and elevated sedimentation rate suggesting infection
Ovarian carcinoma	May present as solid nodules in cul-de-sac
Oxyuris vermicularis infection	May be calcified and present as nodules in cul-de-sac
Splenosis	
Mesotheliomas	

suggested as the optimum in prophylaxis and therapy. We suggested in 1958 that this improvement may be due in part to a transformation of the functioning endometriotic tissue into decidua by increased levels of chorionic estrogen and progesterone. This concept led to the combined use of synthetic estrogens and progestins to create a so-called pseudopregnancy. Subsequently, in 1971, danazol (Danocrine) was introduced; it creates a so-called pseudomenopause.

The introduction of "progestin-only" and pseudopregnancy regimens resulted in a marked improvement in the medical management of endometriosis.[3] The pseudopregnancy regimen provides symptomatic relief in 50% to 80% of patients with endometriosis and is associated with a smaller percentage of disturbing side effects than diethylstilbestrol or methyltestosterone therapy. The pseudopregnancy regimen remains the standard against which all new regimens are judged. The introduction of the synthetic steroid danazol creates another option in the medical management of endometriosis.[4]

Danazol Therapy

The medical management of endometriosis has been significantly advanced by the introduction of the synthetic steroid danazol. Danazol has at least four pharmacologic properties that could account for its therapeutic efficacy in the treatment of endometriosis: (1) suppression of gonadotropin-releasing hormone or gonadotropin secretion, or both; (2) direct interaction with endometrial androgen and progesterone receptors; (3) direct inhibition of ovarian steroidogenesis; and (4) increased metabolic clearance of estradiol and progesterone. These properties of danazol produce an endocrine environment that inhibits the growth of endometrial tissue. By a direct androgenic and antiprogestational action on the endometrial implants of endometriosis, danazol produces atrophy of this tissue. In addition, danazol blocks ovarian follicular growth by direct actions on the hypothalamic-pituitary axis and the ovary. The lack of ovarian follicular activity results in a hypoestrogenic-hypoprogestational environment that also inhibits endometrial growth. Finally, by producing amenorrhea, danazol pre-

TABLE 4.—STAGES I, II, III, AND IV IN DEVELOPMENT OF ENDOMETRIOSIS

STAGE I	STAGE II, A	STAGE II, B	STAGE III	STAGE IV
Broad Ligaments No implants >5 mm Tubes Avascular adhesions, fimbria free Ovaries Avascular adhesions, no fixation Cul-de-sac No implants >5 mm Bowel Normal Appendix Normal	Broad Ligaments No implants >5 mm Tubes Avascular adhesions, fimbria free Ovaries Endometrial cyst ≤ 5 cm (A1 stage); >5 cm (A2 stage); ruptured (A3 stage) Cul-de-sac No implants >5 mm Bowel Normal Appendix Normal	Broad Ligaments Covered by adherent ovary Tubes Adhesions not removed by endoscopy, fimbria free Ovaries Fixed to the broad ligament, implants >5 mm Cul-de-sac Multiple implants, no adherent bowel or fixed uterus Bowel Normal Appendix Normal	Broad Ligaments May be covered by adherent tube or ovary Bladder Normal Tubes Fimbria are covered by adhesions Ovaries Adherent with or without implants or endometriomas Cul-de-sac Multiple implants, no adherent bowel or fixed uterus Bowel Normal Appendix Normal	(Usually combined with stages I, II, III) Bladder Implants Uterus May be fixed and adherent posteriorly Cul-de-sac Covered by adherent bowel or fixed retrodisplaced uterus Bowel Adherent to the cul-de-sac, uterosacral ligaments or corpus Appendix May be involved

vents the peritoneal "reseeding" of endometrial tissue that could occur during the menses. Given these pharmacologic properties of danazol, it is not surprising that danazol therapy results in a significant degree of symptomatic and objective improvement in patients with endometriosis.

Barbieri, Evans, and Kistner analyzed data on 100 patients with endometriosis treated with danazol.[5] They presented a 4-year follow-up and noted symptomatic improvement in 89% and objective improvement in 94% as demonstrated by repeat laparoscopy or laparotomy. In those patients desiring pregnancy, the fertility rate was 46%. The overall recurrence rate was 46%.

Many of the results reported in this study confirm the original findings of Dmowski and Cohen.[4] Before these two studies are compared, one important difference in methodology needs to be emphasized: danazol therapy was combined with follow-up conservative laparotomy in a greater number of patients in our study than in the Dmowski and Cohen report. In this respect, the studies are not directly comparable. However, the findings of both studies are similar in the following respects: (1) danazol alone produced symptomatic and objective improvement in more than 85% of patients with endometriosis; (2) the overall recurrence rate of endometriosis after completion of a course of danazol (with or without conservative surgery) was 15% to 20% in the first year and 5% each year thereafter; (3) in those women who carried a full-term pregnancy after completing a course of danazol (with or without conservative sugery) the recurrence rate was approximately 15% over a 3-year follow-up period; (4) after danazol therapy was discontinued (with or without conservative surgery), approximately one-half the pregnancies occurred within 6 months of stopping the drug; and (5) the overall fertility rate was 46% in both studies.

Our findings differ from those of Dmowski and Cohen in the following respects: (1) in our study most patients (85%) complained of side effects while on drug therapy; and (2) in our experience, no increased incidence of spontaneous abortions, ectopic pregnancies, or stillbirths were noted in pregnancies occurring after the completion of danazol therapy. The reason for these discrepancies is unclear. The observation by Dmowski and Cohen that there was an increased incidence of second- and third-trimester intrauterine fetal deaths in those conceptions occurring within three cycles of discontinuing danazol therapy has yet to be confirmed. Dmowski and Cohen have postulated that their observed relationship between early conceptions after completion of danazol therapy and an increased stillbirth rate is due to abnormal placentation in an atrophic endometrium. In the late 1950s, Kistner observed that "progestin-only" and pseudopregnancy therapy for endometriosis resulted in a pseudodecidualization of the endometrium. Aware of the possibility of abnormal implantation in the decidualized endometrium, he cautioned that patients desiring a conception after completing a course of pseudopregnancy therapy should wait one menstrual period of normal flow and duration before attempting to conceive. Consequently, all patients in this study who were attempting to become pregnant after a course of danazol therapy were cautioned to avoid conception until one menses of normal length and flow had occurred. It is possible that this advice led to the low incidence of spontaneous abortions and stillbirths in our study. However, data recently reported by Daniell and Christianson[6] are in marked disagreement with the findings of Dmowski and Cohen.[4] Daniell and Christianson reported 36 pregnancies occurring in women after the completion of a course of danazol therapy. They advised their infertility patients to begin to attempt conception immediately after discontinuing danazol therapy. Overall, there were only 2 spontaneous abortions, 1 ectopic pregnancy, and no stillbirths. Five patients stopped danazol and became pregnant without an intervening menstrual period and all 5 had a normal full-term delivery. Daniell and Christianson conclude that because most conceptions after a course of danazol therapy occur within the first 6 months of completion of therapy, there is no advantage to waiting for one normal menstrual cycle before conceiving. In their opinion, the delay does not decrease the risk of spontaneous abortion or stillbirth but does prevent the patient from attempting conception during a very fertile time period. The observation that endometriosis itself is associated with an increased spontaneous abortion rate[7] further complicates the interpretation of the relationship between danazol and spontaneous abortions. It is of interest that all 5 spontaneous abortions that occurred in our study occurred more than 15 months after completing a course of danazol (with or without conservative surgery). It is possible that recurrent endometriosis was partly responsible for these spontaneous abortions. Further investigations will be needed to resolve this area of controversy.

Guidelines concering the use of danazol continue to evolve. Controversies remain concerning many aspects of the application of danazol in the treatment of endometriosis. However, one area of almost universal agreement is that a patient should have the diagnosis of endometriosis documented by laparoscopy prior to starting danazol therapy. Another point of consensus is that the patient should not be pregnant while taking danazol. Danazol and related isoxazole compounds cross the placenta and can induce significant urogenital abnormalities in human and laboratory animal offspring exposed in utero.[8, 9] The safest way to initiate danazol is to start therapy immediately after 5 days of normal menstrual flow. Alternatively, in the oligomenorrheic patient, pregnancy testing of blood with sensitive human β-chorionic gonadotropin measurements in conjunction with an appropriate period of abstinence from sexual exposure can be used to exclude an early pregnancy. Interestingly, we have observed 1 patient who initiated a "low-dose" danazol regimen (400 mg/day) after a normal menstrual period and became pregnant some time within the first 2 weeks of therapy. We are not aware of a similar occurrence in patients taking 800 mg of danazol per day. This has prompted us to caution all patients on low-dose danazol to use an alternative method of contraception or to practice abstinence during the first 2 weeks of therapy. In patients on low doses of danazol who have a history of poor medication compliance, vigilance should be maintained to exclude an unsuspected interval pregnancy.

Of the many areas of controversy that still remain regarding the therapeutic application of danazol, a major one concerns the appropriate dosage. The major early studies investigating the efficacy of danazol in the therapy of endometriosis used a dose of 800 mg/day.[4, 10–12] More recently, experienced clinicians have suggested that a dose of 400 mg/day results in symptomatic improvement, amenorrhea, and objective regression of disease in most patients.[13, 14] They have suggested that all patients given danazol be started on 400 mg/day and that the dosage be modified on the basis of symptom response and physical examination. If necessary, the dose can be increased to 600 to 800 mg/day. In the study reported here, all patients were treated with 800 mg/day. Since 1978 we have treated most patients with 400 mg of danazol daily. Experience with this dose of danazol in approximately 200 patients has been uniformly excellent. A major benefit of this reduction of dose is the important reduction in total cost of a course of danazol therapy. Another benefit is that the severity of side effects appears to be somewhat dose related. Recently, some clinicians have suggested starting all patients on 200 mg of danazol daily. Although this dose uniformly produces a decrease in symptoms, we have been reluctant to use it for two reasons: (1) most women on this dose continue to have uterine bleeding, and (2) a small percentage of women will ovulate on this dose of danazol.

As noted above, significant side effects were reported by 85% of the patients. The major side effects (in decreasing order of frequency) were weight gain, edema, decrease in breast size, acne, hirsutism, oily skin, and deepening of the voice. The acne, oily skin, hirsutism, and deepening of the voice are clearly due to the androgenic properties of danazol. The decrease in breast size probably reflects both a hypoestrogenic environment and the androgenic properties of danazol. The mechanisms by which danazol produces weight gain and edema are unclear. Although some of the weight gain might be due to "anabolic" properties of danazol, mineralocorticoid and glucocorticoid effects of the drug might be responsible for both the observed weight gain and the edema.[15] Although most patients taking danazol experience significant drug-related side effects, these side effects generally are not severe enough to require discontinuation of the drug. In our study, only one patient discontinued danazol therapy due to side effects (acne, oily skin), and this occurred after 12 weeks of therapy. Because most women taking danazol will experience side effects, it is reasonable to review these effects with the patient prior to instituting therapy.

In the nonpregnant, nonlactating woman, very few absolute contraindications to danazol therapy exist. Because danazol is metabolized by the liver and can produce modest elevations in serum glutamic oxaloacetic transaminase and serum glutamic pyruvic transaminase, its use in patients with liver disease is relatively contraindicated. In addition, the dramatic gain in weight and the fluid retention seen in some patients taking danazol make this drug relatively contraindicated in patients with cardiac or renal disease.

Many aspects of the application of danazol to the treatment of endometriosis should be tailored to the needs of the individual patient. In this regard, the length of treatment with danazol is an important variable. Courses of therapy as short as 3 months to as long as 24 months can be justified in certain clinical situations. For example, in the patient with advanced endometriosis and infertility who is scheduled for conservative laparotomy, a 12- to 14-week preoperative course of danazol might be appropriate. For the patient with painful endometriosis not desiring fertility who is adamantly opposed to surgery, an 18- to 24-month course of danazol is not unreasonable if side effects are monitored carefully.

An important finding of this study is that in the infertile patient with stage I and stage II endometriosis, a course of danazol alone resulted in a 50% uncorrected fertility rate. This observation confirms the findings of Van Zyl et al.,[16] who studied 20 infertile patients with mild to moderate endometriosis (staging system of Acosta et al.[17]); eight conceptions were obtained after a course of danazol without surgical intervention.

Although the mechanisms by which danazol enhances fertility in patients with mild to moderate endometriosis are unclear, it is possible that danazol decreases the production of prostaglandins by endometriostic tissue. Prostaglandins and related metabolites have been implicated as hormonal mediators of the infertility accompanying endometriosis.[18]

In patients with infertility and advanced stages of endometriosis, operation is usually necessary to remove implants of endometriosis and to repair anatomical abnormalities. Few experimental data are available concerning the value of danazol in the preoperative or postoperative management of endometriosis. In our experience, danazol is of significant value in the preoperative management of endometriosis because it decreases the number and size of endometriotic areas and thus reduces the extent of surgery needed. A reduction in the extent of surgery probably results in fewer postoperative adhesions and complications. In addition, the preoperative use of danazol eliminates the chance of traumatizing a corpus luteum. In general, we have limited the use of danazol in the postoperative management of the infertile patient. Most conceptions after surgical therapy occur within the first 6 months postoperatively.[19] Therefore, by treating the patient with danazol for a prolonged period postoperatively, part of the time interval with the greatest fertility potential is lost. For the patient not interested in conception, postoperative danazol therapy can prove helpful in reducing endometriosis in areas that could not be surgically resected and in delaying recurrent disease.

A controversial subject is the effect of danazol on endometriomas. No systematic study assessing this has been reported. Observations in this and other[5, 19] studies suggest that danazol can often reduce the size of endometriomas, but that it is unusual for danazol to cause their complete regression. Therefore, in most infertility patients with endometriomas surgical intervention will be required. Nevertheless, the use of danazol preoperatively will decrease the overall extent of the endometriosis and thereby probably reduce the extent of the operation. One cautionary observation must be made concerning the use of danazol in the preoperative management of the patient with an endometrioma: it is possible for the endometrioma to rupture preoperatively. If this should occur, chances for fertility probably are reduced.

A major problem in the treatment of endometriosis is that the disease tends to recur unless surgical therapy is definitive. In our study, there was a 16% recurrence in the first year. Thereafter, the rate of recurrence was 3% to 8% per year, for an overall recurrence rate of 33% during the 4-year follow-up. For those patients who carried a term pregnancy after completing danazol (with or without conservative laparotomy), the overall recurrence rate was only 15%. These observations are similar to the findings of Dmowski and Cohen.[4] Nine patients who had recurrent endometriosis after completing danazol therapy were treated with a second course of danazol (400 mg/day). All 9 patients responded with improvement in symptoms and physical findings. None of these patients experienced any unusual side effects from the second course of therapy. These observations suggest that recurrent endometriosis can be treated effectively with a second course of danazol therapy. Theoretically, the endometriotic implants could become "resistant" to multiple courses of danazol therapy. We have yet to observe this phenomenon.

One major controversy concerning the use of danazol in the treatment of endometriosis is the efficacy of danazol versus a pseudopregnancy regimen. Very little experimental data are available that directly address this issue.

The results of one small prospective randomized trial of danazol versus mestranol and norethynodrel has been reported by Noble and Letchworth.[20] They studied 42 patients with endometriosis documented by laparoscopy or laparotomy. Patients were randomly assigned to groups receiving danazol or mestranol and norethynodrel. Patients were started on low doses of danazol (200 mg/day), and the dose was increased until amenorrhea occurred. Patients in the pseudopregnancy group were started on mestranol, 150 μg/day, and norethynodrel, 10 mg/day.

The validity of the results of the study by Noble and Letchworth is difficult to evaluate because of numerous methodologic problems: (1) questionable comparability of the treatment groups; (2) unbalanced treatment groups—danazol, n = 25, and pseudopregnancy, n = 17; and (3) unclear length of follow-up. However, because this is the only randomized prospective study that examines this important question, the results are of interest. Eighty-six percent of the patients treated with danazol, but only 30% of the pseudopregnancy group, reported symptomatic improvement. Eighty-four percent of the patients treated with danazol had improvement in their objective findings, compared with only 18% of patients treated with the pseudopregnancy regimen. Eighteen percent of the pseudopregnancy group required hysterectomy, compared with only 4% of the danazol-treated group. Side effects were a major problem for patients receiving either therapeutic regimen. Four percent of the danazol-treated group and 41% of the pseudopregnancy group discontinued therapy due to side effects. The findings of Noble and Letchworth[20] suggest that danazol is more effective than pseudopregnancy in reducing the symptoms and objective findings of endometriosis. These findings are consistent with our clinical impression; for example, it has been our experience that patients with stage IIB endometriosis often have significant residual disease after a course of pseudopregnancy therapy. In contrast, most patients with stage IIB endometriosis have little or no endometriosis after a course of danazol. Danazol provides a further advantage for the infertile patient because ovulation resumes promptly after therapy is completed. Resumption of ovulation is often delayed in patients completing a course of pseudopregnancy. A major disadvantage of danazol therapy, however, is its cost.

Surgical Treatment

In contemplating surgical treatment of endometriosis, one should remember that functioning ovarian tissue is necessary for the continued activity of the disease. Therefore, successful treatment of endometriosis depends on a knowledge of when it is reasonably safe or desirable to maintain ovarian function and when it is necessary to destroy it. It is obvious that ovarian function should be preserved in treating very early, and perhaps symptomless, lesions, and hysterectomy should be performed only when the ovaries are destroyed by endometriosis. Unfortunately, most cases fall between these two extremes and may present problems in surgical judgment seldom encountered in any other pelvic disease. As our knowledge of the life history of endometriosis has increased, there has been a definite tendency to become more conservative, particularly in the treatment of the infertile patient. In general, it is believed that one should err on the side of conservatism; this belief is based on the facts that endometriosis (1) usually progresses slowly over a period of years, (2) is not, and rarely becomes, malignant, and (3) regresses at the menopause.

Early implantations on the surface of the peritoneum should be excised or fulgurated. Small endometrial cysts on the ovary may be excised or a portion of one or both ovaries may be resected. Small endometrial implants on the intestines should be excised. To aid in the prevention of recurrence, conservative operations should be accompanied by correction of uterine displacements, relief of cervical obstruction, and removal of any other concomitant pelvic pathologic changes. Endometriosis coexisting with uterine myomas, ovarian cysts, or other pelvic abnormalities may be insignificant; on the other hand, the extent or location of these may make conservative operations hazardous. Decisions cannot always be made prior to laparotomy, and the patient should be so informed.

Conservative Surgery (Ovarian Resection)

If childbearing function is to be preserved, operative procedures should be as conservative as possible. All surgical procedures should be preceded by a thorough curettage, and every patient should have had a cytologic examination to exclude possible malignancy of the cervix.

The approach usually should be through a transverse suprapubic incision. However, if the ovarian masses are large, a midline incision may be necessary. Thorough exploration of the pelvic and abdominal organs should be performed routinely, and the decision should be reached as to whether conservative or radical surgery is preferable.

Because of recurrent bleeding and fibrosis associated with the process of endometriosis, the ovaries are frequently adherent to the posterior leaf of the broad ligament and must be carefully displaced from this site before resection is possible.

When the disease is extensive, the uterus is usually fixed in third-degree retroversion, with both ovaries adherent to the uterus at the posterior leaf of the broad ligament and to the rectosigmoid. When this situation exists, it frequently is safer to displace the ovaries by gentle finger dissection rather than by sharp dissection with a knife or scissors. In extensive endometriosis, the ureter often is displaced medially and may be immediately adjacent or adherent to the fixed ovary. Knife or scissors dissection might inadvertently injure or divide the ureter.

If the ovarian masses are large, as with bilateral endometriomas, it is advisable to finger dissect both ovarian masses first and then elevate the uterus from its fixed position. In order to free the uterus, it often is necessary to place upward traction on the rectosigmoid so that its attachment to the back of the uterus and cervix may be identified.

Occasionally the ovary is attached intimately to the lateral peritoneum immediately over the course of the ureter. In this case, the posterior peritoneum is opened at the level of the promontory of the sacrum in the same way as for presacral neurectomy. We usually perform the presacral neurectomy first, so that the posterior peritoneum may be left open until all steps of the operation have been concluded. This prevents ureteral damage during mobilization of the fixed ovaries. Allis clamps then are placed on the edge of the peritoneum, and the right ureter is identified on the lateral flap. The left ureter lies below the superior hemorrhoidal vessels and is somewhat more difficult to locate. A right-angle clamp then is used to tease the ureter free from the peritoneum in the area where the ovary is attached. After this has been accomplished, the ovary may be mobilized by sharp dissection. Because the contents of endometriomas are irritating to the peritoneum and bowel serosa, several packs are placed above the pelvis to protect these structures.

Small areas of endometriosis often are found deep in the substance of the ovary and these are excised. Occasionally the major portion of the ovarian substance has been completely destroyed or replaced by endometriosis, and at the conclusion of the resection only a small fragment of ovarian cortex at the hilus remains. This should not be an absolute indication for oophorectomy, because we have observed pregnancies in women who have had a unilateral salpingo-oophorectomy and three fourths of the remaining ovary removed. In the ovarian reconstruction, the operator should attempt to reapproximate the cortical surface as closely as possible in order to prevent adhesions of omentum or small intestine to the ovary.

Areas of endometriosis on the posterior surface of the uterus and cervix or on the anterior surface of the rectosigmoid should be excised as completely as possible. This frequently results in large areas of denudation of the peritoneum and raw, oozing surfaces in the cul-de-sac. Although it is possible to cover these areas by reflecting the redundant sigmoid inferiorly and suturing it to the posterior aspect of the uterus, this results in obliteration of the cul-de-sac. In order to preserve the anatomical configuration of the cul-de-sac, we believe that it is advantageous to cover the raw surface with omental or peritoneal grafts. We have had the opportunity to observe these grafts at second operations and have found them to be intact and free of adhesions to the adnexal structures or intestines.

At the conclusion of the ovarian resection, the entire oviduct should be inspected carefully, and adhesions of the fimbriated portion of the distal oviduct to the ovary should be freed. Ligation of small blood vessels on the oviduct is accomplished with 6-0 vicryl. If the bowel lumen is entered, closure of the submucosal and seromuscular layers is done in the usual two-layer manner. After all areas of endometriosis have been excised, the edges of available peritoneum are closed with fine catgut. All denuded areas should be covered with peritoneal or omental grafts.

In conservative operations for endometriosis, a uterine suspension and presacral neurectomy usually are performed. We believe that it is important, from the viewpoint of subsequent fertility, to insure the anatomical normality of the cul-de-sac, and this is best accomplished by anterior uterine suspension.

Plication of the uterosacral ligaments is an adjunctive procedure to uterine suspension and improves the posterior deflection of the cervix, thus aiding anterior positioning of the uterus. In many cases the denuded area of the rectosigmoid is adequately peritonealized by plication of the uterosacral ligaments. This is accomplished with three interrupted sutures of 0 vicryl, the first suture being placed just at the insertion of the uterosacral ligaments and two sutures just below the first. After this has been completed, the sigmoid colon fits nicely into the arc of the uterosacral ligaments. When the uterosacral ligaments are being plicated, care must be taken not to place the sutures too far laterally, because of the possibility of kinking or obstructing the ureter. Because we advise doing the presacral neurectomy before the ovarian and cul-de-sac resections, it often is advantageous to leave the posterior peritoneum open until this has been concluded. The ureters then will be visualized easily during these dissections and reconstructions.

If subsequent pregnancy is not a prime factor or if there is evidence of extensive involvement of other pelvic structures, such as the bowel or ureter, a hysterectomy and bilateral salpingo-oophorectomy may be indicated.

Because leiomyomas of the uterus are found in approximately 15% of patients with endometriosis, single or multiple myomectomy should be carried out as part of the conservative approach. It has been our practice to perform a presacral neurectomy whenever the uterus is not removed. Even if the patient has not had dysmenorrhea or pelvic pain preceding surgery, these symptoms may develop subsequently, due to recurrent disease. The presacral procedure should be extensive, with excision of all nerve tissue between the right ureter and the superior hemorrhoidal vessels. In addition, we often remove a part of the uteroacral ligaments at their insertion into the uterus, thus accomplishing more complete pelvic denervation.

Appendectomy is performed at the time of surgical treatment because functioning endometriosis of the appendiceal serosa has been noted in many patients. Endometriosis of the terminal ileum is seen only rarely and may be treated by superficial excision. If the muscularis and mucosa are involved, resection and end-to-end anastomosis should be performed.

Danazol is given for a minimum of 3 months after operation if all areas of endometriosis cannot be excised, and then concerted efforts toward conception are made. Approximately 50% of women so treated will become pregnant if no other cause for infertility exists.

It has been our policy to perform a careful peritoneal toilet and irrigate the pelvis with Ringer's lactate solution with dexamethasone constantly during the operation. Because it is almost impossible to remove an endometrioma intact, without spillage, removal of the cellular debris and thick fluid contents is advised. In an effort to reduce the incidence of postoperative adhesions, we have, since 1966, used dexamethasone and promethazine preoperatively, intraperitoneally before closure, and postoperatively (20 mg of dexamethasone and 25 mg of promethazine 2 hours before the operation and then every 4 hours for 12 doses postoperatively; the same amount is placed in the cul-de-sac through a small catheter).

The incidence of pregnancy after conservative surgery varies widely and is dependent on such factors as extent of the disease, age of the patient and her husband, frequency of coitus, previous parity, and the presence of other pelvic pathology (leiomyomas, tubal disease, or adhesions) at the time of the operation.

Analysis of our results during the past 20 years indicates that a pregnancy rate of approximately 50% may be expected after pseudopregnancy or danazol therapy in patients whose only abnormality, as determined by endoscopy, is surface ovarian endometriosis without endometriomas or tubo-ovarian adhesions (50.8% in 186 patients.)[21] The pregnancy rate subsequent to surgical treatment of ovarian endometriomas, with or without peritoneal endometriosis involving the bladder, uterus, cul-de-sac, or lateral pelvic wall, was 76% in 232 patients.[22] It should be noted, however, that postoperative pseudopregnancy therapy was used in these patients only if all areas of endometriosis could not be excised during the operation. Furthermore, 96% of these patients were younger than age 32 and no other factors contributing to infertility were present. The incidence of pregnancy after surgical therapy in 106 patients who were found to have ovarian and peritoneal endometriosis complicated by tubo-ovarian, utero-ovarian, or sigmoido-ovarian adhesions was only 38%, however. Since 1966 we have administered dexamethasone and promethazine preoperatively, intraperitoneally, and postoperatively in all patients undergoing surgical treatment for infertility. Postoperative pseudopregnancy therapy also was used in this group of patients with adhesions only if all areas of endometriosis could not be excised. The pregnancy rate for those patients who received postoperative hormonal treatment was essentially the same as for those who did not. However, it is obvious that pseudopregnancy therapy was invariably used in patients with more extensive disease.

REFERENCES

1. Kistner R. W., Siegler A. M., Behrman S. J.: Suggested classification of endometriosis: Relationship to infertility. *Fertil. Steril.* 28:1008, 1977.
2. Drake T. S., O'Brien W. F., Ramwell P. W., Metz S. A.: Peritoneal fluid thromboxane B_2 and 6-keto-protaglandin F_1 in endometriosis. *Am. J. Obstet. Gynecol.* 140:401, 1981.
3. Kistner R. W.: The use of progestins in the treatment of endometriosis. *Am. J. Obstet. Gynecol.* 75:264, 1958.
4. Dmowski W. P., Cohen M. R.: Antigonadotropin (danazol) in the treatment of endometriosis. *Am. J. Obstet. Gynecol.* 130:41, 1971.
5. Barbieri R. L., Evans S., Kistner R. W.: Danazol in the treatment of endometriosis: Analysis of 100 cases with a 4-year follow-up. *Fertil. Steril.* 37:737, 1982.
6. Daniell J. F., Christianson C.: Combined laparoscopic surgery and danazol therapy for pelvic endometriosis. *Fertil. Steril.* 35:521, 1981.
7. Naples J. D., Bah R. E., Sadigh H.: Spontaneous abortion rate in patients with endometriosis. *Obstet. Gynecol.* 57:509, 1981.
8. Goldman A. S., Bongiovanni A. M., Yakorac W. E.: Production of adrenogenital syndrome in rats by initiation of 3β-HSD. *Proc. Soc. Exp. Biol. Med.* 121:757, 1966.
9. Duck S. C., Katayama K. P.: Danazol may cause female pseudohermaphroditism. *Fertil. Steril.* 35:230, 1981.
10. Friedlander R. L.: The treatment of endometriosis with danazol. *J. Reprod. Med.* 10:197, 1973.
11. Greenblatt R. B., Tzingounis V.: Danazol treatment of endometriosis: Long-term follow-up. *Fertil. Steril.* 32:518, 1979.
12. Lauersen N. H., Wilson K. H., Birnbaum S.: Danazol: An antigonadotropin agent treatment of pelvic endometriosis. *Am. J. Obstet. Gynecol.* 123:742, 1975.
13. Ward G. D.: Dosage aspects of danazol therapy in the treatment of endometriosis. *Postgrad. Med. J.* 55(S5):7, 1979.
14. Biberoglu K. O., Behrman S. J.: Dosage aspects of danazol therapy in endometriosis: Short-term and long-term effectiveness. *Am. J. Obstet. Gynecol.* 139:645, 1981.
15. Barbieri R. L., Lee H., Ryan K. J.: Danazol binding to rat androgen, glucocorticoid, progesterone, and estrogen receptors: Correlation with biological activity. *Fertil. Steril.* 31:185, 1979.

16. Van Zyl J. A., Muller M. S., Van Niekerk W. A.: Danazol in the treatment of endometriosis externa. *S. Afr. Med. J.* 58:591, 1980.
17. Acosta A. A., Buttram V. C., Besch P. K., et al.: A proposed classification of pelvic endometriosis. *Obstet. Gynecol.* 42:19, 1973.
18. Drake T. S., O'Brien W. F., Ramwell P. W., et al.: Peritoneal fluid thromboxane B_2 and 6-keto-prostanglandin F_1 in endometriosis. *Am. J. Obstet. Gynecol.* 140:401, 1981.
19. Buttram V. C., Jr.: Conservative surgery for endometriosis in the infertile female: A study of 206 patients with implications for both medical and surgical therapy. *Fertil Steril.* 31:117, 1979.
20. Noble A. D., Letchworth A. T.: Medical treatment of endometriosis: A comparative trial. *Postgrad. Med. J.* 55:37, 1979.
21. Kistner, R. W.: Management of endometriosis in the infertile patient. *Fertil. Steril.* 26:1151, 1975.
22. Kistner, R. W., Patton G. W.: *Atlas of Infertility Surgery.* Boston: Little, Brown & Co., 1975.

15–1 **Program for In Vitro Fertilization at Norfolk** is described by Howard W. Jones, Jr., Georgeanna Seegar Jones, Mason C. Andrews, Anibal Acosta, Clark Bundren, Jairo Garcia, Bruce Sandow, Lucinda Veeck, Charles Wilkes, Jeannine Witmyer, J. Edward Wortham, and George Wright (Norfolk, Va.). In phase I (1981) they used the following protocol: (1) The natural cycle was abandoned in favor of stimulated controlled ovulation. (2) For stimulated controlled ovulations, human menopausal gonadotropin (hMG) was used in preference to clomiphene. (3) Exogenous human chorionic gonadotropin (hCG) was used to substitute for the midcycle LH surge. (4) Use of real-time sector ultrasonography to monitor follicular growth became routine. (5) Quality control in the laboratory was tightened. (6) Early in 1981, supplementary maturation in vitro of oocytes prior to insemination was initiated. The 1981, phase I, pregnancies occurred in two patients.

CASE 1.—Woman, 27, had a ruptured right ectopic pregnancy in 1977, and the right tube was removed. In 1978, she had a left tubal pregnancy and in 1980 she had a left ruptured tubal pregnancy removal of the left tube. Hysterosalpingogram had shown normal uterine cavity. The couple was treated with Vibramycin in February 1981 for *ureaplasma urealyticum* and the woman received 10,000 IU of hCG on April 13. On April 15 (day 10 of menstrual cycle) laparoscopic aspiration of two right follicles was carried out. Cleavage occurred in only one follicle, which was transferred to the uterus. Ultrasonography was carried out 9 times during pregnancy. Because of small fetal size and cessation of weight gain, cesarean section was performed 9 days prior to term. A normal female infant weighing 5 lb 12 oz was delivered with Apgar scores of 9 and 10 at 1 and 5 minutes, respectively.

CASE 2.—Woman, 21, had had a right salpingectomy and a cuff salpingostomy on the left tube, but a hysterosalpingogram later showed tubal occlusion. Laparoscopy produced three follicles and three eggs. One egg progressed to the four-cell stage and was implanted. The pregnancy progressed normally and a normal male infant was born.

In 1981, changes were made in protocol (phase II), including: (1) Stimulated controlled ovulation was continued with the use of hMG

(15–1) Fertil. Steril. 38:14–21, July 1982.

RESULTS OF IN VITRO FERTILIZATION PROGRAM

		1980					Phase I—1981					Phase II—1981				
		No.	%A	%B	%C	%D	No.	%A	%B	%C	%D	No.	%A	%B	%C	%D
A	Laparoscopies	41					31					24				
B	Fertilizable eggs	19	46				26	84				22	92			
C	Eggs fertilized	ND*	ND	ND			ND	ND	ND			21	88	95		
D	Transfers	13	32	68	ND		12	39	46	ND		19	79	86	90	
E	Pregnancies	0	0	0	ND	0	2	6	8	ND	17	5	21	23	24	26

**ND,* not determined.
(Courtesy of Jones, H. W., et al.: Fertil. Steril. 38:14–21, July 1982.)

and hCG. (2) Serum estradiol values quickly determined became available on a daily basis. (3) Further improvement occurred in laboratory quality control. (4) The concept of supplementary oocyte maturation in vitro was continued and extended. With these changes, results were better. In 24 laparoscopic cycles, fertilizable eggs were obtained in 22, or 92%. There were 5 pregnancies (table), the outcomes of which are not yet determinable.

The authors note that supplementary incubation prior to fertilization is extremely beneficial in further maturing the immature oocyte. Also, ultrasound examination during pregnancy appeared to cause no detectable or recognizable damage.

▶ [The Norfolk, Virginia, group has had the largest U.S. experience with in vitro fertilization and embryo transfer, and this description of the evolution of their program is therefore of particular value. Noteworthy are the most recent statistics that 92% of cycles yielded fertilizable ova and 26% of transfers resulted in pregnancy. The chance of a "take" seems to be increased if two or three concepti are transferred. The ultimate plan of in vitro fertilization is, of course, not clear at this time, but figures such as those presented here suggest that it may turn out to be more than the gimmick it first appeared.

Mettler and associates from Germany reported on their experience with ovum recovery and in vitro fertilization (*Fertil. Steril.* 38:30, 1982). Success rates similar to those of the Norfolk group (with respect to successful embryo culture) were obtained.] ◀

15–2 **Clinical Features of Eight Pregnancies Resulting From In Vitro Fertilization and Embryo Transfer.** Carl Wood, Alan Trounson, John F. Leeton, Peter M. Renou, William A. W. Walters, Beresford W. Buttery, James C. Grimwade, John C. Spensley, and Victor Y. H. Yu (Melbourne) report the prenatal, intranatal, and postnatal progress of 8 pregnancies from in vitro fertilization (IVF) and embryo transfer, which resulted in the birth of 9 babies, including a set of twins.

Ultrasonic examination was carried out at 7½–8 weeks' gestation to check fetal viability, number of pregnancies, and presence of any associated pathology; at 12–13 weeks' gestation to check fetal viability, growth, and normality; at 16–17 weeks' gestation specifically to evaluate normality and the site of the placenta if amniocentesis was to be performed; and at 30 weeks' gestation to assess fetal growth.

Results show the clinical features of these pregnancies were not significantly different from those of a normal obstetric population, ex-

(15–2) Fertil. Steril. 38:22–29, July 1982.

cept that delivery occurred prior to 40 weeks in all but 1 case, and in 6 of the 8 pregnancies, delivery was by cesarean section.

CASE 2.—Infant, preterm, weighing 2,780 gm, had difficulty in breast-feeding and temperature control for several days. Sixteen days after birth, arm twitching occurred on the right side and the infant had a temperature of 37.4 C. Penicillin and kanamycin were given and no further clinical abnormality was observed.

CASE 4.—Woman, 31, had a corpus luteum cyst at 8 weeks of pregnancy which resolved in 4 weeks. Twins were born: a boy first and a girl second. The boy had an Apgar score of 7 at 5 minutes after birth despite oxygen administration and active ventilation. Cyanosis persisted despite 100% oxygen. Chest films showed a heart typical of transposition of the great vessels and this was confirmed by echocardiogram and cardiac catherization. The infant later developed peritonitis and underwent subtotal colectomy and ileostomy, after which cardiac failured occurred. He recovered and gained weight. The cardiac defect was corrected later.

CASE 5.—Woman, 27, had an uneventful pregnancy until 25 weeks, when threatened preterm labor occurred, with evidence of chorioamnionitis. Fever and a yellow vaginal discharge were present. At 28 weeks and at 3 days before term, labor recurred. Cesarean section was performed when the cervix was dilated 3 cm. Respiratory distress occurred in the infant soon after birth and pneumothorax occurred on both sides; intraventricular hemorrhage was diagnosed and a cardiac murmur later was found. The infant was normal when discharged to a country base hospital 45 days after birth.

CASE 8.—Woman, 27 had a twin pregnancy diagnosed. At 8 weeks, she was admitted because of vaginal bleeding. A repeat ultrasound study showed twin fetuses, but fetal movement was no longer detected in the second twin. At 12 weeks, the fetal sac of the second twin had shrunk, and it was reabsorbed.

One congenital malformation, transposition of the great vessels, occurred among 9 babies. It presently is not known whether or not this malformation is related to the technique of IVF. The method of sperm preparation in vitro does eliminate some of the abnormal spermatozoa. The possibility of an increased incidence of errors in second meiotic division or nondisjunction-induced trisomic embryos after fertilization is of concern in IVF. The cause of the more frequent birth of female infants (7 girls, 2 boys) cannot be determined. Long-term follow-up of the newborns is planned to study their physical, psychologic, and intellectual well-being.

▶ [This article summarizes the obstetric course and outcome of 8 pregnancies resulting from in vitro fertilization and embryo transfer, the largest series reported to date. Among the notable features are a female sex preponderance (7 of 9 infants) and premature labor in 2 of 8 cases, but the numbers are much too small to determine if these frequencies are unusual.] ◀

15–3 **Oocyte Recovery, In Vitro Insemination, and Transfer Into the Oviduct After Its Microsurgical Repair at a Single Laparotomy.** Jan Tesařík, Ladislav Pilka, Milan Dvořák, and Pavel Trávník (J. E. Purkyně Univ., Brno, Czechoslovakia) describe a method that combines recovery of a preovulatory oocyte, its in vitro insemination, and transfer into the oviduct with tubal microsurgery at a single laparotomy and report the results of its application in 6 women with a

---

(15–3) Fertil. Steril. 39:472–475, April 1983.

history of infertility persisting for several years, regular menstruation, and bilateral fimbrial occlusion.

TECHNIQUE.—Clomiphene citrate and human chorionic gonadotropin (hCG) were administered to stimulate follicle growth and oocyte maturation. Laparotomy was performed on day 14 of the menstrual cycle, 34 to 36 hours after injection of hCG. The type of microsurgery performed was either fimbrioplasty or salpingoneostomy. On the day before the operation, the insemination medium, consisting of Ham's F-10 tissue culture medium supplemented with lactate, pyruvate, bicarbonate, and penicillin, was freshly prepared. The insemination medium contained 0.15 volume units of the patient's heat-inactivated serum per 1 volume unit of the final medium. Spermatozoa from the husband, obtained 2 to 3 hours before planned surgery, were added to the insemination droplets at a final concentration of 1×10^6/ml. During laparotomy, large antral follicles were punctured and aspirated and the aspirated fluid immediately was transferred into Petri dishes. Oocytes were identified under a dissecting microscope, and preovulatory oocytes, surrounded by large mucified cumili oophori, were placed into the insemination droplets. The time from oocyte recovery to transfer into the insemination droplets did not exceed 3 minutes. After completion of tubal repair, the inseminated oocyte was aspirated into the oocyte-transfer set. The tip of the catheter was then inserted about 2 cm into the lumen of the recanalized fallopian tube and the inseminated oocyte was gently expelled from the catheter into the tubal ampulla.

No preovulatory oocyte was found in the follicular aspirate of 2 women, 2 preovulatory oocytes were obtained and transferred in each of 2 other women, and 1 preovulatory oocyte was obtained and transferred in each of the 2 remaining women. Two of the 4 women who underwent oocyte in vitro insemination and tubal transfer combined with tubal microsurgery became pregnant. It is not known whether fertilization occurred in vitro or in vivo. One of these women miscarried in the fifth week postoperatively. The other pregnancy continued without complication to term and a normal male infant was delivered. The infant has progressed normally.

This method is a possible alternative to in vitro fertilization and embryo transfer in some infertile women and as a supplemental procedure in some patients in whom tubal microsurgery is indicated.

▶ [As in vitro fertilization programs become more common, we are certain to read of new wrinkles, such as that reported here. The fertilized egg (or egg-semen mixture, to be more precise) is injected into the now patent tube. Is the in vitro fertilization or the tuboplasty the adjunct? Possible theoretical advantages of this one-shot approach are that transcervical instrumentation with its inherent risk of bacterial contamination is avoided and that the fertilized egg is offered repose in the tube, its natural habitat. One might guess that the risk of tubal pregnancy would be appreciable in this situation. More experience with this technique is necessary before its value can be determined.] ◀

15–4 **Ectopic Pregnancy Following Treatment With Human Gonadotropins** is discussed by Carl Gemzell, Jaques Guillome, and Chun Fu Wang. From 1960 to 1979, 604 anovulatory women were treated a total of 1,665 times with human pituitary gonadotropin (hPG) for the purpose of conception. Of these, 289 women conceived 379 times, and 9 had 10 ectopic pregnancies (2.7% of all conceptions),

(15–4) Am. J. Obstet. Gynecol. 143:761–765, Aug. 1, 1982.

all located in the fallopian tubes. Four of the tubal pregnancies occurred in association with an intrauterine pregnancy.

The 9 women with ectopic pregnancies were aged 23 to 33 years. Five had polycystic ovarian disease, 1 had hypogonadotropic hypogonadism with primary amenorrhea, 1 had pituitary microadenoma with hyperprolactinemia unresponsive to bromocriptine treatment, 1 had anorexia nervosa with long-lasting secondary amenorrhea, and 1 had amenorrhea after use of an oral contraceptive. None had tubal disease.

Treatment with human gonadotropins was started after a spontaneous bleeding or a bleeding after withdrawal of progesterone. Patients received 150 IU of FSH (2 ampules of Pergonal or an equivalent dose of hPG). Levels of plasma 17β-estradiol or total urinary estrogens were measured daily. The dose was adjusted every 5 days according to estrogen levels. When a suitable level of estrogen was reached after at least 6 or 7 days of continuous rise, 10,000 IU of human chorionic gonadotropin (hCG) was administered to induce ovulation. Usually, a second injection of 5,000 IU of hCG was given 1 week later.

The diagnosis of tubal pregnancy was made at 6 to 12 weeks' gestation. No tubal ruptures with intra-abdominal bleeding occurred. The tubal pregnancies were strongly suspected because of unilateral pain and tenderness and a slow rise in the level of serum or urinary hCG. Sonographic evidence of an empty uterine cavity confirmed the diagnosis. In women with intrauterine and tubal pregnancies, the diagnosis was more difficult, but the unilateral pain and tenderness could not be explained by the intrauterine pregnancy. The 10 tubal pregnancies were treated by salpingectomy or salpingostomy. The 4 intrauterine pregnancies in association with a tubal pregnancy ended in 2 abortions and 2 normal term births.

Five patients showed ovarian overstimulation, suggesting that hormonal modifications at the time of ovulation may explain the high incidence of tubal gestations. Combined ectopic and intrauterine pregnancies are very rare, but seem to have increased in frequency since the introduction of treatment with human gonadotropins.

▶ [The relatively high rate of tubal pregnancy after ovulation induction with gonadotropins reported here is consistent with that reported by McBain and co-workers a few years ago (1981 YEAR BOOK, p. 70). Again, ovarian hyperstimulation was found to increase the risk.] ◀

15–5 **Premature Ovulation After Ovarian Ultrasonography** J. Testart, A. Thebault, and R. Frydman (Clamart, France) report their experience with premature follicle rupture when ultrasonography was used during the 3 days preceding ovulation. A total of 57 patients (64 cycles) were hospitalized to collect oocytes for in vitro fertilization. Laparoscopy was planned to take place 30–37 hours after the onset of the LH surge (59 cycles) or human chorionic gonadotropin (hCG) administration (5 cycles). Four additional cycles in 3 volunteer nurses were studied by frequent ovarian ultrasonography to establish time

(15–5) Br. J. Obstet. Gynaecol. 89:694–700, September 1982.

of follicle rupture on the day after hCG administration. All women were between ages 20 and 40 years, had regular cycles, and received no treatment during follicular growth. Patients were placed into one of three groups: group 1, ultrasonography was not performed earlier than 3 days before ovulatory stimulus; group 2, follicular ultrasonography was performed during the 3 days preceding ovulatory stimulus; and group 3, ultrasonography was performed between ovulatory stimulus and the expected time of ovulation.

Ovulation was never observed between 30 and 37 hours after ovulatory stimulus in the 26 cycles studied in group 1; ovulation occurred at 25–36 hours after ovulatory stimulus in 5 of 23 (21.7%) and 8 of 19 (42.1%) cycles studied in groups 2 and 3, respectively ($P < .01$). When ultrasonography is used, ovulation can occur at 25 hours after ovulatory stimulus; ovulation can occur irrespective of the time of the last scan after ovulatory stimulus, the total number of scans, or the follicular size. Among 5 patients in whom several cycles were studied, either ovulation did not occur during the protocols or premature ovulation was observed.

The data show ovarian ultrasonography to be associated with premature follicle rupture when performed immediately before the time of expected ovulation. The mechanism of the phenomena has not been identified, although short variations of either blood volume or ionic balance may be involved in premature ovulation by decreasing resistance of the follicular wall during rapid osmotic alteration. Clinicians are warned against using ovarian ultrasonography during the final days before ovulation if conception is desired. This warning relates to mature oocyte collection as well as control of follicular growth to predict the time for insemination.

▶ [The suggestion here is that ultrasound examinations may be associated with premature (i.e., <36 hours from the ovulatory stimulus) ovulations. Given the current interest regarding in vitro fertilization, this is an issue of considerable practical importance. Other investigators are certain to report their experience. If this phenomenon is real and if it is not explained by anxiety, or by the means used to achieve a full bladder, concerns about the safety of ultrasound will be rekindled.] ◀

15–6 **Pregnancy Following Use of the Cervical Cup for Home Artificial Insemination Utilizing Homologous Semen.** Infertility affects an estimated 10% to 20% of all couples. Michael P. Diamond, Cathy Christianson, James F. Daniell, and Anne Colston Wentz (Vanderbilt Univ. Med. Center, Nashville, Tenn.) report the results in 61 couples with primary or secondary infertility of varying causes of from 1 to 11 years' duration who were instructed in the use of the cervical cup for artificial insemination using homologous semen at home.

Thirty-six pregnancies in 32 women were reported. Overall, 53% of the couples had at least 1 pregnancy, with a pregnancy rate of 43% in women with primary infertility and of 67% in women with secondary infertility. There were 3 spontaneous miscarriages, 2 in 1 couple, but no ectopic pregnancies. All but 6 of the women with continued infertility attempted artificial insemination using homologous semen

---

(15–6) Fertil. Steril. 39:480–484, April 1983.

for at least 6 cycles. Sperm counts and percent motility showed considerable variation, regardless of whether infertility was primary or secondary and regardless of whether pregnancy occurred or not. Postcoital tests improved in 30 of 38 couples, but only 16 of these couples achieved a pregnancy; in 2 couples who showed no improvement on the postcoital test the women became pregnant. No woman developed vaginismus from cup insertion or removal, and there were no reported complications.

In this series, more than 50% of the couples achieved at least 1 pregnancy. This technique of artificial insemination using homologous semen is simple, inexpensive, does not pose significant risks or discomfort, and can be performed by a couple at their convenience and in privacy.

▶ [If artificial insemination with the husband's semen (AIH) is planned, there is no reason that, after appropriate instruction of the couple, it cannot be done at home. The high success rate reported here probably reflects patient selection. As the authors point out in their discussion, many of the men had normal semen analyses. We are not particularly enthusiastic about AIH, but can see the cost and comfort advantages of doing it at home.] ◀

15–7 **Initial Evaluation of a Convection Counter Streaming Galvanization Technique of Sex Separation of Human Spermatozoa.** Many attempts have been made to separate X and Y chromatin-bearing spermatozoa so as to influence the sex of offspring. Using Y-body fluorescence microscopy, James F. Daniell, Carl M. Herbert, John Repp, Charles A. Torbit, and Anne Colston Wentz (Vanderbilt Univ., Nashville, Tenn.) evaluated a new method for separating X and Y human spermatozoa. The process involves the use of a universal semen extender medium, developed by Bhattacharya, and a convection streaming, galvanic cell apparatus. Semen specimens were obtained from 33 men.

Prior to separation, the semen specimens showed normal volume, sperm concentration, and motility and viability percentages. After separation, sperm motility and viability percentages were unchanged, volume collected at each pole was constant at 1 ml, but sperm concentrations were approximately 15% of the original concentration. The distribution of X and Y sperm showed a normal pattern prior to separation (table). After separation, the fractions collected at the anode contained an average of 77% Y-fluorescing spermatozoa (range, 68% to 92%), but the fraction collected from the cathode contained an average of 76% non-Y-fluorescing spermatozoa (range, 67% to 88%). In vitro tests of cervical mucus penetration of sperm showed no significant change in penetrating capacity of the sperm samples after separation.

Fractions of highly motile spermatozoa with good capacity for penetrating cervical mucus can be separated by the Bhattacharya technique. However, the mean recovery concentration in the X- and Y-enriched fractions was only 15% to 16% of the original concentration, and the separation of X and Y spermatozoa was not as high as previously suggested. Nonetheless, this technique may offer hope of an

---

(15–7) Fertil. Steril. 38:233–237, August 1982.

RESULTS OF SEX SEPARATION PROCEDURE ON Y-BODY FLUORESCENCE OF SPERMATOZOA (33 SEPARATIONS)

	Prior to separation		Male-enriched fraction (anode)		Female-enriched fraction (cathode)	
	% Y-BS*	% X-BS†	% Y-BS*	% X-BS†	% Y-BS*	% X-BS†
Mean	48.45	51.55	77.36	22.64	23.39	76.61
SD‡	4.79	4.79	5.29	5.29	5.42	5.42
Range	35–56	44–64	68–92	8–32	12–33	67–88

*Y-bearing spermatozoa.
†X-bearing spermatozoa.
‡Standard deviation.
(Courtesy of Daniell, J., et al.: Fertil. Steril. 38:233–237, August 1982.)

altered sex ratio for couples who specifically desire a male or female child. Further independent evaluations are necessary to determine whether significantly altered birth ratios can be achieved without reduced pregnancy rates or occurrence of abnormal births.

▶ [Sex separation of human spermatozoa with subsequent artificial insemination is apparently feasible. This should improve the 50:50 chance of achieving the "desired" sex of the next offspring. It's proably progress, but it doesn't seem quite right.
A related article follows. Read on . . . .] ◀

15–8 **Male Sex Preselection Through Sperm Isolation.** Ferdinand J. Beernink (Berkeley, Calif.) and Ronald J. Ericsson (Sausalito, Calif.) present the current results of clinical trials using Y sperm-rich fractions of human sperm and discuss the effects of combining this technique with the use of clomiphene citrate. In 1976, couples were gradually enrolled in a clinical study to evaluate the results of insemination with albumin-separated sperm. The study included fertile women of childbearing age who had previously delivered only female infants (26 patients had 59 previous children, 57 girls and 2 boys). The patients were informed of the following uncertainties: whether the 85% Y sperm fraction would translate into the same proportion of male infants, and whether insemination high in the cervix of only a few million spermatozoa would result in pregnancy in a reasonable length of time.

The separation technique used was begun with dilution of ejaculate by Tyrode's solution. Washed sperm was layered over salt-poor human serum albumin (hSA) for 1 hour. After layering, the initial sperm layer was centrifuged for 10 minutes and the resulting sperm disk was resuspended and layered over hSA (12.5% hSA at top; 20.0% hSA at bottom). The 20% hSA sperm sample was centrifuged for 10 minutes, resuspended, and inseminated high in the cervix.

Results showed that, as of October 1981, 66 patients have been inseminated. Twenty-two have discontinued therapy after an average of 3 inseminations. Of the other 44 patients, 30 have conceived (68%). Twenty-four conceived in 3 cycles or less (80%). There were 3 abortions (10%). Five patients are still pregnant. Of the 20 who delivered, 13 had boys and 7 had girls (there were two sets of female twins, one after Clomid treatment). Of the 15 non-Clomid-treated women who delivered, 12 had boys and 3 had girls. This number was statistically

(15–8) Fertil. Steril. 38:493–495, October 1982.

significant only when compared with the number of deliveries after Clomid treatment. Total results from all centers using three-step, three-layer separation were as follows: 53 patients delivered 39 boys and 16 girls, a male birth ratio of 73.5%, excluding Clomid deliveries, 46 patients delivered 38 boys and 9 girls, a male birth ratio of 82.6%. Two-step, two-layer separation, which yields about 70% Y sperm, has produced a male birth ratio of 73%, 19 boys among 26 infants born.

The authors' experience and that of other centers participating in this study show that couples coming for male sex preselection have had only girls. It is not known that this would change the "risk" in either direction for their next offspring. As of April 1982, all centers reported a total of 91 deliveries, 68 boys and 25 girls, a 75% male birth ratio. Non-Clomid deliveries numbered 84, 66 boys and 19 girls, a 79% male birth ratio. Current use of Clomid in patients desiring male sex preselection appears to be contraindicated.

▶ [Isolation of Y-bearing sperm followed by cervical insemination resulted in a higher than expected percentage of births of boys (75%). We don't understand the mechanism (if indeed it's more than chance) of the preponderance of births of girls after clomiphene-induced ovulation.] ◀

15–9 **Relation Between the Luteinizing Hormone Peak, the Nadir of Basal Body Temperature, and the Cervical Mucus Score.** A. A. Templeton, G. C. Penney, and M. M. Lees (Edinburgh) compared assessment of basal body temperature (BBT) and scoring of cervical mucus with the results of a short-incubation radioimmunoassay for LH during 287 nonconceptual menstrual cycles in 87 patients receiving artificial insemination (AID). Of 198 evaluable ovulatory cycles, 17 were induced by clomiphene. An identifiable LH peak occurred in 97% of the ovulatory cycles. An identifiable BBT nadir was found in 65% of 81 evaluable cycles. The BBT nadir and LH peak coincided in a minority of cycles. A mucus score peak was identified in 87% of ovulatory cycles. The mucus score peak and LH peak coincided in less than half of evaluable cycles, but the timing of the maximal cervical mucus score was similar to that of the LH peak in all but 7% of cycles.

Cervical mucus scoring may be useful in identifying the time of ovulation where LH assay is unavailable or speed and economy are important considerations. If a close relation between the timing of the LH and mucus score peaks is confirmed in a prospective series, this simple technique might have advantages over the short LH assay, which is relatively expensive and involves a delay of about 4 hours.

▶ [The cervical mucus score served as a more accurate clinical technique for identifying the day of the LH surge than did the BBT nadir. The latter preceded the LH peak by more than 1 day, and therefore preceded presumed ovulation by more than 2 days, in 35% of cycles.] ◀

15–10 **Correlation Between Serum Antichlamydial Antibodies and Tubal Factor as a Cause of Infertility.** Although salpingitis frequently produces tubal damage and infertility, many women with

(15–9) Br. J. Obstet. Gynaecol. 89:985–988, December 1982.
(15–10) Fertil. Steril. 38:553–558, November 1982.

Relationship Between Serum Antichlamydial Antibodies and Potential Causes of Infertility

Contributing factors	Chlamydial serology S+ No.	S+ %†	S− No.	S− %	Total No.	Total %	Significance*
Tubal disease							
Sole or contributing	46	75	31	28	77	44	< 0.001
Sole	28	46	18	16	46	27	< 0.001
Absent	13	21	64	56	77	45	< 0.001
Unknown	2	3	16	14	18	10	0.03
Male factor	3	5	18	16	21	12	0.05
Ovulatory factor	11	18	35	32	46	27	0.08
Endometriosis	12	20	18	16	30	17	0.72
Recurrent abortions	1	2	0	7	9	5	0.16
Other	1	2	13	12	14	8	0.61
No abnormality	5	8	13	12	18	10	0.21
Total patients	61	100	111	100	172	100	

*P value.
†Percentage refers to columns down, not rows across.
(Courtesy of Jones, R. B., et al.: Fertil. Steril. 38:553–558, November 1982.)

tubal factor as a cause of their infertility do not have a clinical history of salpingitis. In order to investigate whether or not some such cases may be due to subclinical chlamydial infections, Robert B. Jones, Barbara R. Ardery, Siu L. Hui, and Robert E. Cleary (Indiana Univ., Indianapolis) measured antichlamydial antibodies in the serum of 172 women consecutively undergoing evaluation for infertility. Only 16 (9.3%) had a prior history of salpingitis.

Patients were classified according to whether or not they had serum antibodies to *Chlamydia trachomatis;* 61 (35%) of 172 patients were seropositive (S+) and 111 (65%) were seronegative (S−). Among the seropositive patients, 11 (18%) showed both IgG and IgM, and the remainder showed IgG only. The mean ages of both groups was the same. Most patients (97%) were white. Women employed at skilled or semiskilled jobs were more often seropositive than women employed as professionals, administrators, or homemakers. Ten of the 16 women with a history of salpingitis (62%) were seropositive. Among the 172 women, 77 (44%) had tubal factor. A highly significant correlation (table) was observed between a positive chlamydial serologic test and evidence of tubal disease, whether tubal disease was the only factor found or was one of several potential contributing factors. Significant negative correlations were found between seropositivity and other common causes of infertility such as male factor, ovulatory dysfunction, and other miscellaneous causes.

The data from this study in conjunction with the literature, suggest subclinical chlamydial infections are a major cause of tubal infertility in the United States, as well as in Europe. Attempts should be made to diagnose and treat endocervical chlamydial infections in sexually active women before tubal damage can occur.

▶ [This study clearly indicates an association between previous chlamydial infection and infertility secondary to tubal damage. It doesn't establish cause, however. The antichlamydial antibodies may only be an index of sexual activity, i.e. some other sexually transmitted agent(s) may be the responsible pathogen(s). *Chlamydia trachomatis* certainly can cause acute salpingitis (1982 Year Book, pp. 348–349), but we don't think enough is known yet about the natural history of genital infection with this organism to recommend routine screening for it (1980 YEAR BOOK, pp. 344–345). More follows . . . .] ◀

15–11 **Increased Frequency of Serum Antibodies to *Chlamydia trachomatis* in Infertility due to Distal Tubal Disease.** *Chlamydia trachomatis* has been isolated from the cervix of normal nonpregnant and pregnant women and at a greater frequency from women with acute pelvic inflammatory disease (PID). Serologic findings support a role for *Chlamydia* in acute PID. Donald E. Moore, Leon R. Spadoni, Hjordis M. Foy, San-Pin Wang, Janet R. Daling, Cho-Chou Kuo, J. Thomas Grayston, and David A. Eschenbach (Univ. of Washington) investigated whether *Chlamydia* is an important cause of infertility in women with a history of PID. Data on 186 women seen consecutively with infertility for a year or longer were reviewed. Hysterosalpingography (HSG) usually was carried out, and 87 women underwent laparoscopy.

Infertility due to tubal disease was significantly associated with secondary infertility, a history of PID, and a history of intrauterine device (IUD) use (table). *Chlamydia trachomatis* antibody was most prevalent in women with abnormal HSG findings and in those with distal occlusion. Prevalences were similar in women with and those without secondary infertility, but it was greater in patients with a history of PID or of IUD use than in others. Discriminant analysis indicated that antibody to *C. trachomatis* was as predictive of tubal disease in these women as were the HSG findings. Infertility factors other than tubal disease were not associated with an increased prevalence of antibodies to *C. trachomatis*. The organism was not isolated by cervical culture in 11 women or by fallopian tube culture in 18.

The findings suggest that the presence of chlamydial antibody has high predictive value for the presence of hydrosalpinx, peritubal disease, or both in infertile women. It appears to be as accurate as the HSG in predicting tubal disease in this population. The serologic test for chlamydial antibody is rapid and inexpensive, and it should become a routine part of the infertility workup.

▶ [These results from Seattle are consistent with those from Indiana reported previously. The relationship between tubal disease and chlamydial antibody is striking. The authors point out that acute chlamydial salpingitis produces fewer overt clinical signs than does gonococcal salpingitis. The diagnosis may be in doubt, the patient may not be admitted to the hospital or treated with antibiotics, and yet severe tubal damage may result. Rightly or wrongly, these studies are likely to lead to the increased use of tetracycline in outpatient gynecology. Cervical colonization with *Chlamydia trachomatis* is quite common. We don't think enough is known of the natural history of this phenomenon in either pregnant or nonpregnant women to permit firm guidelines as to who should have cultures, treatment, etc.] ◀

15–12 **Microbiologic Study of Infertile Women at Time of Diagnostic Laparoscopy: Association of *Ureaplasma urealyticum* With a Defined Subpopulation.** There is considerable controversy regarding the role of *U. urealyticum* in human infertility. Gail H. Cassell, J. Benjamin Younger, Mary B. Brown, Richard E. Blackwell, Jerry

(15–11) Lancet 2:574–577, Sept. 11, 1982.
(15–12) N. Engl. J. Med. 308:502–505, Mar. 3, 1983.

DEMOGRAPHIC, HISTORICAL, AND SEROLOGIC FINDINGS IN RELATION TO CONDITION OF FALLOPIAN TUBES AS SEEN ON HSG OR AT OPERATION

	Findings on HSG				Findings at surgery			
	Normal (N=84)	Suspicious (N=29)	Abnormal (N=28)	Total (N=141)	No tubal disease (N=35)	Feritubal adhesions (N=19)	Distal occlusion (N=33)	Total (N=87)
Mean± SEM age (yr)	29·5±0·44	28·9±0·69	29·0±0·64	29·3±0·32	29·1±0·62	30·0±0·67	28·7±0·58	29·2±0·52
No. of Caucasion race (%)	77 *(92%)*	27 *(93%)*	23 *(82%)*	127 *(90%)*	31 *(89%)*	17 *(89%)*	30 *(91%)*	78 *(90%)*
No. with secondary infertility (%)	29 *(35%)*	9 *(31%)*	16 *(57%)**	54 *(38%)*	11 *(31%)*	6 *(32%)*	21 *(64%)*†	38 *(44%)*
Duration of infertility:								
Mean± SEM (yr)	45·6±2·3	38·0±4·8	48·6±5·7	44·6±2·3	47·5±4·8	56·2±5·3	47·4±5·4	49·4±3·0
No. and % >2 yr	72 *(86%)*	18 *(62%)*	21 *(75%)**	111 *(79%)*	30 *(86%)*	18 *(95%)*	25 *(76%)*	73 *(84%)*
No. with history of PID (%)	13 *(15%)*	5 *(17%)*	14 *(50%)*§	32 *(23%)*	5 *(14%)*	8 *(42%)**	18 *(55%)*§	31 *(36%)*
No. with history of IUD use (%)	12 *(14%)*	2 *(7%)*	9 *(32%)**	23 *(16%)*	2 *(6%)*	5 *(26%)**	11 *(33%)*‡	18 *(21%)*
No. with positive serology¶ *(%)*	9 *(11%)*	7 *(24%)*	22 *(79%)*§	38 *(27%)*	0 *(0%)*	4 *(21%)*‡	24 *(73%)*§	28 *(32%)*

*$P < .05$ compared with normal group.
†$P < .01$ compared with normal group.
‡$P < .005$ compared with normal group.
§$P < .001$ compared with normal group.
¶Antibody titer ≥ 1/32.
(Courtesy of Moore, D. E., et al.: Lancet 2:574–577, Sept. 11, 1982.)

K. Davis, Pam Marriott, and Sergio Stagno (Univ. of Alabama) examined the role of *Ureaplasma* in a series of 194 women, mean age 30 years, who had histories of involuntary infertility for a year or longer. Sixty-one were primiparous or multiparous women. Laparoscopy was performed in the late luteal phase. Cultures from 56 fertile women undergoing laparoscopy for tubal ligation also were studied.

CERVICOVAGINAL ISOLATION RATE OF *UREAPLASMA UREALYTICUM* IN 194 INFERTILE WOMEN, ACCORDING TO POSTLAPAROSCOPIC DIAGNOSIS

POST-LAPAROSCOPIC DIAGNOSIS *	NO. OF PATIENTS WITH DIAGNOSIS	PER CENT INFECTED
Male factor	23	74 †
Ovulatory disorder	72	40
Endometritis	18	56
Endometriosis	53	30 ‡
Tubal obstruction or adhesions	86	46
Uterine anomaly or tumor	9	22
Cervical factor	17	47
Unexplained causes	18	44

*All diagnostic tests and pathologic evaluations were performed routinely by clinical personnel. The final diagnosis was made without knowledge of culture results. Some patients had multiple factors contributing to their infertility and were included in more than one category.

Diagnosis of a male factor was based on subnormal results of 2 or more semen analyses or the presence of chronic prostatitis with consistently poor results of postcoital tests.

Diagnosis of ovulatory disorders was based on analysis of at least 2 and usually 3 endometrial biopsy specimens combined with evaluation of basal body temperature and pregnanetriol excretion when necessary.

Diagnosis of a cervical factor was based on poor results of mucus or postcoital tests with normal findings on semen analysis.

†Significantly higher ($P < .05$) than any other infertile subpopulation.

‡Less likely to be infected ($P < .05$).

(Courtesy of Cassell, G. H., et al.: N. Engl. J. Med. 308:502–505, Mar. 3, 1983.)

Blacks in all groups and less educated patients were more likely to have cervicovaginal colonization by *U. urealyticum*. No difference in isolation rates was found between fertile and infertile patients, even taking into account the major factors influencing mycoplasmal colonization, e.g., age, race, socioeconomic status, and sexual experience. In women with infertility associated with a male factor, ureaplasmal infection was more prevalent than in any other infertile subgroup (table). *Mycoplasma hominis* was isolated from the endometrium in 2 of 34 infertile women who were cervicovaginally infected by this organism. *Ureaplasma urealyticum* was isolated from 1 of 82 infertile women who were cervicovaginally infected with *Ureaplasma*. Neither organism was isolated from the endometrium of fertile patients. No chlamydiae or toxoplasmas were isolated. Cytomegalovirus was isolated from 2 infertile and 2 fertile women.

These findings suggest that *U. urealyticum* is associated with infertility due to a male factor, but further study is necessary to prove that the relationship is a causal one. In addition to altering sperm motility, adsorption of ureaplasmas to sperm could impair spermatozoal function through interfering with normal metabolism; masking the sperm membrane sites involved in sperm-egg recognition; impairing the ability of the sperm to penetrate the ovum; or producing immunologic damage. The last possibility is intriguing in view of the immunopathologic nature of most mycoplasmal diseases and the propensity of mycoplasmas to induce autoantibody formation.

▶ [This report helps define a possible role for mycoplasmas in infertility. Overall, there was no difference in the isolation rates between fertile and infertile women. The one subset with increased cervicovaginal colonization was the "male factor" group. Presumably, infection with *Ureaplasma urealyticum* adversely affects sperm function. This possibility is not consistent with the reported failure of antibiotic treatment in couples with colonization with mycoplasmas and *unexplained* infertility (1979 YEAR BOOK, pp. 262–263).] ◀

15–13 **Clomiphene Citrate Therapy For Luteal Phase Defect.** Both the diagnosis and treatment of luteal phase defect remain controversial. Kevin A. Downs and Mark Gibson (Univ. of Vermont, Burlington) identified luteal phase defects in 12.7% of a series of 366 infertile patients. Luteal phase defect was diagnosed when a luteal lag of 3 or more days was confirmed by repeated endometrial biopsy and by a midluteal progesterone level of less than 10 ng/ml. Clomiphene citrate was given in a dose of 50 mg orally on days 5 through 9 of the menstrual cycle. Seven patients received a dose of 100 mg, and 1 patient received 150 mg because of continued short luteal phases. Two patients received human chorionic gonadotropin in an intramuscular dose of 5,000 units on day 16 of the menstrual cycle.

Forty-one of the 47 patients with a diagnosis of luteal phase defect received clomiphene, and 16 of them (39%) conceived. Eighteen pregnancies occurred in a total of 44 courses of treatment. Two spontaneous first-trimester abortions and one tubal ectopic pregnancy also occurred. Treatment was more often successful with a lag of 5 days or longer. This finding was confirmed when patients with other possible causes of infertility were excluded. Nine of 12 patients with "pure" luteal phase defect and a deficit of 5 or more days conceived, 2 of them twice, whereas only 1 of 13 patients with a histologic delay of less than 5 days conceived.

Findings from this and previous studies suggest that luteal phase defect is a distinct cause of infertility and that a severe, well-documented luteal phase defect can be expected to respond to clomiphene therapy. Failure to respond may indicate either a milder deficit or the presence of confounding antifertility factors. Reevaluation of infertility and consideration of progesterone supplementation would seem appropriate in such cases.

▶ [Treatment options for luteal phase defect are progesterone vaginal suppositories and clomiphene. This report describes the latter and the results look pretty good—a 40% conception rate—although it's difficult to be certain in the absence of a control group. Paradoxically, the conception rate was better with more marked forms of luteal phase defect (i.e., greater delay in endometrial dating).] ◀

15–14 **Prostaglandin $F_{2}\alpha$ in Peritoneal Fluid of Patients With Endometriosis.** Large amounts of prostaglandins are released by endometrial tissue and may be responsible for altered ovarian function in

(15–13) Fertil. Steril. 39:34–38, January 1983.
(15–14) Int. J. Fertil. 27:73–75, 1982.

patients with endometriosis. Prostaglandins have been implicated in both ovulation and luteolysis. Steven J. Sondheimer and George Flickinger (Univ. of Pennsylvania) determined levels of prostaglandin $F_2\alpha$ in peritoneal fluid in women with and without endometriosis in the follicular phase of the cycle. Dependent peritoneal fluid was obtained from the cul-de-sac at diagnostic laparoscopy or laparotomy for infertility, and the $PGF_2\alpha$ concentration was determined by radioimmunoassay. Ten patients with endometriosis, 7 with pelvic adhesions, and 4 normal women were studied. Four patients had moderate and 3 had severe endometriosis.

Three of 4 patients with moderate endometriosis and 2 of 3 with severe disease had measurable $PGF_2\alpha$ in the peritoneal fluids, as did 1 of the patients with adhesions. Prostaglandin was not found in any clear peritoneal fluids. No evidence of luteal phase defect was found in the patients with endometriosis. One patient with pelvic adhesions but no $PGF_2\alpha$ in peritoneal fluid had an endometrial biopsy 3 days out of phase.

The presence of $PGF_2\alpha$ in peritoneal fluid in patients with endometriosis may be associated with hemorrhage into the abdominal cavity. It seems unlikely that peritoneal fluid $PGF_2\alpha$ mediates infertility in patients with mild endometriosis. Increased $PGF_2\alpha$ in more-advanced endometriosis does not clearly influence corpus luteum function. Prostaglandins might alter tubal or uterine function in the latter cases, thereby contributing to infertility, or they may be unrelated to infertility in this setting.

▶ [An article abstracted in the 1983 YEAR BOOK (p. 370) described high prostaglandin F production rates by endometriotic tissue, suggesting a possible mechanism for pain and infertility (by either luteolysis or altered tubal motility) with endometriosis. This study by Sondheimer and Flickinger found prostaglandin $F_2\alpha$ in peritoneal fluid of patients with endometriosis only if the fluids were grossly discolored, implying that in the absence of old hemorrhage, prostaglandins probably are not involved in the pathogenesis of the disease.] ◀

15–15 **Prolactin Hyperstimulation in Response to Thyrotropin-Releasing Hormone in Patients With Endometriosis.** Ken Muse, Emery A. Wilson, and M. J. Jawad (Univ. of Kentucky) measured baseline serum prolactin (PRL) levels and PRL response to stimulation by thyrotropin-releasing hormone (TRH) to clarify the possible role of hyperprolactinemia in causing infertility in patients with endometriosis. Fourteen infertile women with endometriosis and 13 normal, fertile women were studied. Age range was 21 to 42 years. All patients had a history of normal menses. Preoperative patients were studied on the day of admission and all patients were studied between 4 P.M. and 8 P.M.

Baseline PRL values in the 14 infertile women with endometriosis were twofold greater than levels observed in 10 control patients undergoing tubal fulguration and in 3 normal fertile women, but the mean differences were not significant. Three patients with endometriosis had elevated resting PRL levels, whereas only 1 of 13 fertile women had an elevated baseline value. After stimulation with TRH,

(15–15) Fertil. Steril. 38:419–422, October 1982.

a significant increase in the PRL value was observed at 15 minutes and at 30 minutes in patients with endometriosis, compared with the group having tubal sterilization. A nonsignificant increase in PRL concentration also was observed after 60 minutes in patients with endometriosis. Peak PRL response in patients with moderate endometriosis was significantly greater than that observed in patients with mild endometriosis. The mean baseline level of thyroid-stimulating hormone TSH and peak concentration after administration of TRH in patients with endometriosis did not differ significantly from corresponding TSH values in fertile control patients. Total serum thyroxine concentrations for patients with endometriosis were all normal and did not differ from concentrations in control subjects.

Some infertile patients with endometriosis exhibit a greater capacity for PRL secretion than normal, fertile women. Provocative pituitary studies may be helpful in distinguishing those patients with PRL hypersecretion and, possibly, those patients in whom dopamine agonists would be effective therapy.

▶ [The reason for the association between infertility and endometriosis in some patients with mild disease is unknown. One postulated mechanism is that of the unruptured luteinized follicle (1981 YEAR BOOK, pp. 369–370). Another is suggested in this report. Although patients with endometriosis did not have significantly higher mean basal prolactin levels than those of control patients, they had an exaggerated response to thyrotropin-releasing hormone. The implication here is that certain infertile patients with endometriosis might be helped by bromocriptine. More study of prolactin dynamics in patients with endometriosis is required before such therapy can be recommended.] ◀

15–16 **Sperm Phagocytosis by Human Peritoneal Macrophages: Possible Cause of Infertility in Endometriosis.** The mechanism of infertility in women with endometriosis is unknown, but it is independent of mechanical factors that affect the function of the fallopian tubes. Increased numbers of peritoneal macrophages are present in women with endometriosis, and these macrophages have access to the reproductive tract via the oviducts. Joseph J. Muscato, A. F. Haney, and J. Brice Weinberg (Durham, N.C.) hypothesized that peritoneal macrophages might phagocytize sperm and thereby contribute to infertility in women with endometriosis. In vitro studies were conducted with normal sperm samples and with peritoneal fluid obtained from 10 multiparous women, 10 infertile women with endometriosis, and 12 infertile women without endometriosis.

Fertile women had fewer total peritoneal macrophages (mean, 2.6×10^6) than did infertile women without endometriosis (8.1×10^6) or infertile women with endometriosis (18.2×10^6). Macrophages from infertile women with endometriosis phagocytized more sperm (84%) than did those from fertile women (43%) or infertile women without endometriosis (46%). Sperm phagocytosis occurred rapidly and reached a peak in about 6 hours. Incubating the macrophages at 0 C, lysing them by freezing and thawing, or fixing them with glutaraldehyde inhibited their uptake of sperm. The process occurred in the presence or absence of serum, indicating that sperm phagocytosis did

---

(15–16) Am. J. Obstet. Gynecol. 144:503–510, Nov. 1, 1982.

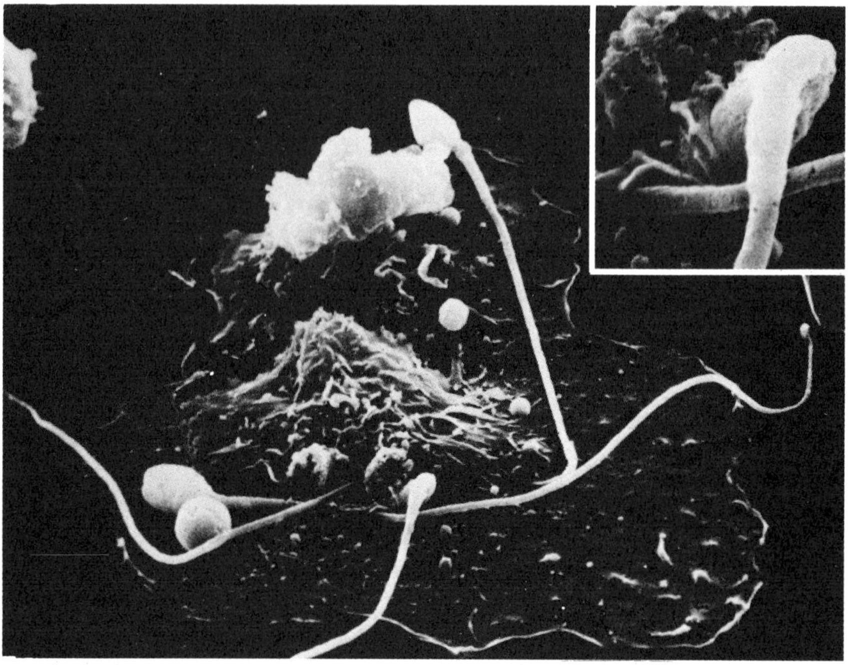

Fig 15–1.—Scanning electron micrograph of human peritoneal macrophage-sperm interaction. Sperm are being phagocytized by macrophage. Inset shows higher magnification of phagocytosis of sperm head. (Courtesy of Muscato, J. J., et al.: Am. J. Obstet Gynecol. 144:503–510, Nov. 1, 1982.)

not depend on sperm opsonization with a serum factor. Electron microscopy (Fig 15–1) showed internalization of the spermatozoa into phagosomes with subsequent intravacuolar degradation.

These observations suggest that, if peritoneal macrophages from women with endometriosis enter the reproductive tract via the oviducts, they might affect fertilization adversely by phagocytosis of sperm. It is also possible that macrophages could inhibit fertilization by mediating injury to oocytes or zygotes. Pathologic conditions other than endometriosis also may reduce fertility via macrophage-mediated injury to gametes. The fact that macrophages from fertile women had some antisperm activity suggests a possible role for macrophages in regulating conception in physiologic circumstances.

▶ [Another possibility that might explain an association between endometriosis and infertility is that of increased intraperitoneal prostaglandin levels causing luteolysis or enhanced tubal contractions or both (see 1983 YEAR BOOK, p. 370). The findings of this study by Muscato et al. point to sperm phagocytosis as yet another potential mechanism. Peritoneal fluid from endometriosis patients was found to contain higher concentrations of macrophages than that from women without the disease, and the macrophages phagocytosed a larger proportion of sperm in vitro.] ◀

15–17 **Postsalpingectomy Endometriosis: A Reassessment.** In 1928, Sampson introduced the term "endosalpingiosis" to describe the local proliferative and invasive properties of tubal mucosa after surgical

(15–17) Obstet. Gynecol. 60:560–570, November 1982.

interruption. R. J. Stock (Naval Regional Med. Center, Portsmouth, Va.) reexamined Sampson's concept of endosalpingiosis in the light of histologic findings in the fallopian tubes of 54 women who underwent elective sterilization and subsequent hysterectomy and bilateral salpingo-oophorectomy. If Sampson's assessment of the aggressiveness of tubal epithelium was correct, then evidence should be found not only in the proximal line of surgical tubal interruption to which Sampson confined his study, but also in the distal line.

Of 75 consecutive patients studied in 1979 to 1981, 54 had tubal ligation procedures that interrupted the tube at one site, leaving a proximal and distal portion available for examination. Thirty-six patients had Pomeroy procedures, 13 had cautery, and 5 had mechanical procedures. Twenty-five procedures had been carried out post partum and 29 were interval sterilizations. Two patients became pregnant after sterilization, 1 of them 2.5 years after a Pomeroy procedure post partum and the other 5 months after an interval laparoscopic bipolar coagulation procedure.

In patients with the Pomeroy procedures, the usual histologic find-

Fig 15–2.—Focus of endometriosis *(arrows)* in terminal portion of proximal tubal lumen. Hematoxylin-eosin; ×42. (Courtesy of Stock, R. J.: Obstet Gynecol. 60:560–570, November 1982. Reprinted with permission from The American College of Obstetricians and Gynecologists.)

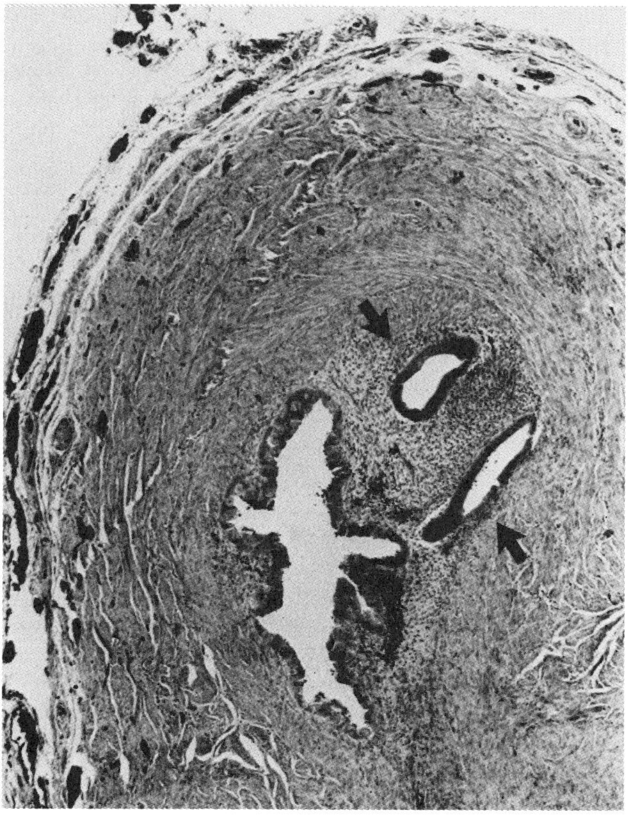

ings showed a remnant of tubal epithelium and smooth muscle adjacent to the blunted ends. Noteworthy was the obvious alteration in tubal epithelium as well as the diminshed smooth muscle in the adjacent remnant. Endometriosis was found only in direct continuity with tubal lumen on the proximal or uterine side. The lesions usually consisted of small foci (Fig 15–2), but well-developed areas occasionally were encountered. No correlation was apparent between the occurrence of localized endometriosis and the timing of sterilization.

The extent of tissue destruction after cauterization procedures was usually much greater than that with other methods. Endometriosis was identified in 8 of the 13 patients who had cautery and was located in the proximal or uterine tubal line of destruction. In patients who were sterilized by the Hulka clip, there was an abrupt termination of epithelium on either side. No endometriosis was encountered.

The occurrence of focal endometriosis appeared to be related to time in the Pomeroy-type procedure, and this might be caused by recurrent bathing of healed and abnormal areas with menstrual products. The occurrence of localized endometriosis was more frequent in patients who also had adenomyosis uteri. Of importance in the present study is the absence of endometriosis within or in continuity with the lumen at the surgical site in the distal tubal remnant. This implies that the endometriosis is not a consequence of a seeded or invading metaplastic tubal epithelium, but is, more plausibly, the result of retrograde menstruation.

▶ [Endometriosis in the proximal portion of the tube, but not in the distal portion, suggests retrograde menstruation as the cause, rather than metaplasia of the tubal epithelium. The increased frequency of association with sterilization by cautery was noted also by Rock and co-workers (1982 YEAR BOOK, pp. 268–269). In constrast to this previous report, the length of the proximal tubal segment was not a factor affecting subsequent focal endometriosis in the present study. The relationship between the localized endometriosis and the risk of subsequent pregnancy in patients who have had tubal sterilization procedures has not been defined. In the current study, pelvic pain was not associated with the presence of endometriosis.] ◀

15–18 **Appendectomy in Surgical Treatment of Endometriosis.** The appendix may be an extragenital site of endometriosis, but guidelines for appendectomy in patients operated on for pelvic endometriosis remain to be established. Donald E. Pittaway (Johns Hopkins Hosp., Baltimore) attempted to determine the prevalence of appendiceal involvement in a series of 500 consecutive patients undergoing appendectomy in a 7-year period at an obstetrics-gynecology department. Pelvic endometriosis was present in 104 patients, 65 of whom were evaluable. Sixty others had surgery for endometriosis without appendectomy.

Thirteen appendices (2.6%) had histologic evidence of endometriosis. In 5 of these cases the appendix had a normal gross appearance. Of patients with pelvic disease, 13% had appendiceal involvement. Five of 13 patients with symptomatic disease who were not interested in future fertility had appendiceal involvement, which in 4 was unrecognized at operation. In 7 of 91 patients undergoing fertility sur-

---

(15–18) Obstet. Gynecol. 61:421–424, April 1983.

gery in whom the appendix was involved, this was recognized at operation. Appendiceal involvement could not be related to the severity of endometriosis or to patient age.

An appendix with clinically evident involvement by endometriosis should be removed as part of the current approach of excising or fulgurating as much of the disease as possible. Routine removal of the appendix from infertile patients because of possible occult endometriosis does not seem to be warranted. No increase in postoperative morbidity was noted in the present series when appendectomy was performed, but many more patients would be needed to detect small differences in morbidity rates. Close attention to meticulous technique in performing appendectomy during infertility surgery should minimize adverse results.

▶ [The high frequency of appendiceal involvement in patients undergoing operations for endometriosis—13%—reported here seems adequate reason for incidental appendectomy in conjunction with endometriosis surgery. The authors feel that routine removal of the normal-appearing appendix when infertility is the indication for operation is not warranted, but it is difficult to see why.] ◀

15–19 **The Effectiveness of Danazol on Subsequent Fertility in Minimal Endometriosis.** Machelle M. Seibel, Merle J. Berger, Frederick G. Weinstein, and Melvin L. Taymor (Harvard Med. School) studied the data on 65 patients with minimal endometriosis in a prospective comparison of conservative medical management with danazol and no therapy in treatment of this disease. After a basic infertility evaluation and the correction of additional factors affecting fertility, diagnostic laparoscopy, dilation and curettage (D & C), and tubal lavage were performed. A randomly selected card determined whether the patient received no treatment for 6 months or danazol for 6 months followed by no treatment for 6 months. The dosage of danazol was 800 mg daily for the first 2 months, 600 mg daily for the next 2 months, and 400 mg daily for the final 2 months. The mean age of patients in both groups was 31 years.

A total of 65 patients entered the study: 32 in the danazol group and 33 in the control group. A number of patients had additional fertility problems, which were correctable. Eleven danazol patients had no other fertility factors, whereas 14 controls had no other such factors. Four (36%) of 11 patients with minimal endometriosis and no other factor conceived after treatment with danazol. Among patients with minimal endometriosis alone not treated with danazol, 8 (57%) of 14 conceived. These differences did not reach statistical significance. Incidence of conception among patients with additional fertility factors was 2 (22%) of 9 in the danazol group and 6 (43%) of 14 in the control group. This difference was not statistically significant.

The results of this study suggest that infertile patients with minimal endometriosis should be given an opportunity to conceive after laparoscopy, D & C, and tubal lavage. This is particularly true in older patients, in whom a 6 months' delay in permitting attempts at conception represents a significant interval of time. That danazol is

---

(15–19) Fertil. Steril 38:534–537, November 1982.

expensive and is associated with side effects further argues against its use initially when infertility is the only symptom.

▶ [Most reports of therapeutic efforts in infertility have the disadvantage of the lack of random assignment of the treatment to the study subjects. The present report is a welcome exception. Danazol offered no advantages over no treatment in patients with mild endometriosis. Indeed, the conception rate was actually lower in the danazol group, most probably reflecting anovulation during the 6 months of drug therapy. A study presented in the 1983 YEAR BOOK (p. 375) indicated that conservative operation likewise was no better than expectant management in this situation.] ◀

15–20 **Effects of Danazol on Plasma Lipid and Lipoprotein Levels in Healthy Women and in Women With Endometriosis.** Danazol is an androgenic substance used to treat fibrocystic disease of the breast, congenital angioneurotic edema, and precocious puberty. Anthony A. Luciano, Katherine S. Hauser, Frederick K. Chapler, William A. Davis, and Robert B. Wallace (Univ. of Iowa, Iowa City) examined the effects of danazol on plasma lipid and lipoprotein levels in 25 infertile women with endometriosis, in 7 normal women, and in a patient with benign fibrocystic disease of the breast. The women with endometriosis received 400 to 800 mg of danazol daily for 6 months. The normal women received 400 mg twice daily for 2 months, and the patient with fibrocystic disease of the breast received 200 mg daily for 2 months.

Most subjects had normal lipid and lipoprotein levels before treatment. The high-density lipoprotein cholesterol (HDL-C) levels declined substantially during danazol therapy, regardless of the dose, and remained suppressed throughout treatment. Pretreatment levels returned within a month of discontinuance of danazol. No consistent changes in total cholesterol, low-density lipoprotein cholesterol (LDL-C), or very low-density lipoprotein cholesterol (VDL-C) levels were observed. Five patients had a substantial reduction in the ratio of HDL-C to LDL-C. Changes in triglyceride levels were insignificant except for a decrease in high-density lipoprotein (HDL) triglycerides.

Danazol has profound effects on lipid metabolism. A distinct reduction in HDL-C and in HDL triglycerides was observed in the present study. Patients with hyperlipoproteinemia before treatment had substantial decreases in plasma lipid and lipoprotein levels and in normal lipoprotein profiles during treatment. The relation between danazol-induced changes in lipoprotein and atherogenic potential is uncertain. Epidemiologic studies and possibly long-term clinical trials will be needed to ascertain the extent of cardiovascular risk associated with danazol therapy.

▶ [This study of lipid and lipoprotein levels with danazol treatment conveys good news and bad news. The good news is that this drug may have some therapeutic effect in certain hyperlipidemias. The bad news is that it seems to lower high-density lipoprotein cholesterol levels selectively, which may increase atherogenic risk.] ◀

15–21 **Peripheral Androgen Levels in Danazol-Treated Premenopausal Women.** In addition to the inhibition of follicular steroidogenesis, danazol has mild anabolic and androgenic effects. Although the effect of danazol on ovarian steroidogenesis is relatively well es-

---

(15–20) Am. J. Obstet. Gynecol. 145:422–426, Feb. 15, 1983.
(15–21) Fertil. Steril. 39:499–504, April 1983.

tablished, data on its effect on adrenocortical steroid biosynthesis are fewer and conflicting. To further elucidate the effects of danazol on adrenal androgen production, Kjell Carlström (Huddinge Univ. Hosp., Huddinge, Sweden) Anton Döberl (Stockholm) and Gunnar Rannevik (Malmö) measured plasma levels of dehydroepiandrosterone (DHEA), dehydroepiandrosterone sulfate (DHEA-S), and testosterone in 18 consecutive, normally menstruating women with endometriosis treated with danazol (600 mg/day) for about 6 months. Blood samples were obtained before and after 2, 4, 8, 12, and 16 weeks of treatment. Serum levels of alanine aminotransferase (ALAT), albumin, creatinine, potassium, and sodium also were determined to assess possible hepatic and renal effects of danazol that may influence steroid homeostasis.

All baseline values were well within normal reference limits. Plasma DHEA-S levels were significantly elevated at 2, 4, and 8 weeks of treatment and DHEA levels were significantly decreased at 8 and 16 weeks. A significant decrease in the DHEA/DHEA-S ratio was observed at 4, 8, 12, and 16 weeks. Testosterone levels were significantly reduced throughout the entire study period. Serum ALAT levels showed a significant increase at 4 weeks and remained significantly elevated for the remainder of the study period. Serum albumin levels did not change significantly. Slight, but significant, increases were observed in the serum creatinine level during the entire study, except for week 4, and in the serum potassium level at weeks 4, 8, and 12. Serum sodium levels were not affected.

It is concluded that, of the two major sources of androgen, the adrenal cortex appears to be relatively unaffected by danazol and the ovary may be affected to a minor degree. Therefore, it is likely that the observed changes are attributable to a combination of mild renal effects and a mild interaction with certain liver enzymes, rather than to an effect on adrenal steroidogenesis.

15–22 **Free Testosterone Levels During Danazol Therapy.** Danazol, an ethinyl testosterone (T) derivative, often is used in the clinical treatment of endometriosis. Its mechanism of action is not known, though its side effects are primarily androgenic. A recent study demonstrated that danazol binds to sex hormone-binding globulin (SHBG) and competes with T for binding sites, thereby displacing T. Using labeled danazol in an aqueous two-phase equilibrium partition system, Bo Nilsson, Ragnar Södergård, Mats-Göran Damber, Jan-Erik Damber, and Bo von Schoultz (Univ. of Umeå) investigated the binding properties of danazol to SHBG and albumin by measuring serum levels of total T, SHBG, and albumin in 16 women with endometriosis undergoing treatment with danazol (600 mg/day for 2 to 3 months). Free and protein-bound T levels were then calculated.

During treatment, all women showed a sharp reduction in SHBG binding capacity, with mean values about 80% lower than pretreatment values ($P < .001$). Albumin and total T levels were unchanged throughout therapy. Prior to treatment, an average of 60.15% of total

---

(15–22) Fertil. Steril. 39:505–509, April 1983.

T was bound to SHBG, 38.57% was bound to albumin, and the fraction of free T was 1.28%. During treatment, however, an average of 17.91% of total T was bound to SHBG, 79.44% was bound to albumin, and the fraction of free T had increased to 2.64%. This reflects an 80% increase in levels of free T during treatment ($P < .001$).

The results suggest that the endocrine effects of danazol can be explained by its ability to displace testosterone and the resulting increase in free testosterone levels during treatment.

▶ [Conflicting results have appeared in the literature concerning the effects of danazol on serum androgen levels. This, in part, relates to cross reactivity between danazol and its metabolites and testosterone (T) in certain assays. The preceding article, by Carlström et al., indicates a fall in T levels with treatment and a dissociation between dehydroepiandrosterone and dehyroepiandrosterone sulfate levels. The authors interpret the latter as indicating hepatic or renal alterations in metabolism or clearance, rather than an effect on adrenal steroidogenesis.

Total T levels were unchanged in the second study, but free T levels were increased, presumably due to displacement of T from sex hormone-binding globulin by danazol. The androgenic side effects of danazol therapy partly may be due to this elevated level of free T. Androstenedione, the "other" ovarian androgen, was not measured in these two studies. Levels reportedly are increased by danazol therapy (*Am. J. Obstet. Gynecol.* 141:723, 1981).] ◀

15–23 **Comparison of Definable Traits in Women Requesting Reversal of Sterilization and Women Satisfied With Sterilization.** Arthur Leader, Neville Galan, Ronald George, and Patrick J. Taylor (Calgary, Alta.) used a questionnaire to devise a profile of readily defined traits of women who request reversal of sterilization and those who appear to be satisfied with the procedure. A total of 159 consecutive women who requested reversal of a previous tubal sterilization were compared with 160 women who were satisfied with sterilization. The respective mean ages were 29.4 and 36.2 years, and the respective ages at sterilization were 25.0 and 31.2 years. The satisfied women had significantly more live children and significantly fewer therapeutic abortions. The largest number of women in both groups had interval sterilization.

Women who requested reversal were likelier than those who were satisfied to have decided on sterilization themselves rather than jointly with their husbands. The most common reasons for sterilization in both groups were completion of the family and the unacceptability of other methods of family planning. Large majorities of both groups reported understanding at the time that the procedure was irreversible. Most women who requested reversal regretted the decision for sterilization within a year after the procedure. The most common reason given for requesting reversal was a combination of remarriage and a desire for more children in the new relation. Fifty-seven women were found at endoscopy to have a repairable condition, and 34 ultimately underwent reversal.

How many patients regret sterilization to the point of requesting a reversal is uncertain. Women who are found when requesting sterilization to share the attributes of those in this study who requested reversal should undergo in-depth assessment of their reasons for

---

(15–23) Am. J. Obstet. Gynecol. 145:198–202, Jan. 15, 1983.

wishing to be sterilized, and the likelihood of a future request for reversal should be assessed. If sterilization is done, the potentially most reversible method should be used.

▶ [With increasingly liberal attitudes regarding sterilization over the past decade or so, it is predictable that we will see increasing numbers of patients who regret having the procedure enough to ask about reversal. This survey compares the characteristics of women requesting reversal with those satisfied with the operation. The results contain no particular surprises; earlier marriage and childbearing and sterilization at a younger age were more likely in dissatisfied patients. These relationships should be kept in mind in counseling patients who request sterilization, but, to take a common example, what (if anything) should the physician do with a 20-year-old woman who married at age 17 and is adamant about being sterilized after her second child?] ◀

15–24 **Circannual Rhythm in Human Sperm Count Revealed by Serially Independent Sampling.** Wilie S. Tjoa, Michael H. Smolensky, Bartholomew P. Hsi, Emil Steinberger, and Keith D. Smith (Univ. of Texas, Houston) reanalyzed previously published data for circannual rhythms in human sperm output as experimentally evaluated by independent serial sampling of more than 4,000 men during a 4-year span. Sperm concentration and total sperm counts from single semen samples from each of 4,435 patients requesting vasectomy between September 1972 and December 1977 were analyzed for circannual (about 1 year) rhythmicity. The sample consisted of men primarily between the ages of 25 and 44. Most were white, married, and fecund.

Results showed a rather large temporal variation, not only from one year to the next, but also within each year. In general, a trend could be seen for higher sperm concentrations during each of the winters, when compared with concentrations during the summers. Similar patterns were discernible for total sperm count. When the data were summarized by average sperm concentration per month, a strong circannual pattern became apparent. Sperm concentration was highest between February and March and lowest during September. A t-test comparison of the values for the months of highest sperm concentration (February and March) versus those of lowest concentration (August and September) showed a statistically significant difference ($P < .05$ to $P < .001$) for each of the years during which the data were collected. An exception was 1974, during which an atypical temporal pattern was observed.

In an interpretation of the data in this report, certain uncontrollable causes of variability must be considered, because it was impossible to insure that sampling instructions were followed rigorously in all cases. However, the large population number should tend to minimize the variation that resulted from random events. The findings of the study indicate that in presumably fertile men the circannual rhythm in sperm count accounts for about 34% (peak-to-trough difference expressed relative to the mensor) of the variance during the year. Accumulating evidence suggests that a type of "breeding season" for human beings may exist. However, the findings presented in this report must be regarded as preliminary.

▶ [This is a new and interesting observation. If it is confirmed, the 34% peak-to-

(15–24) Fertil. Steril. 38:454–459, October 1982.

trough decrease in sperm concentration from January to September must be taken into account when one evaluates therapeutic measures in patients with oligospermia.] ◀

15-25 **Fertilizing Capacity and Sperm Antibodies in Vasovasostomized men.** Pregnancy rates after vasovasostomy in vasectomized men remain substantially below patency rates, for unclear reasons. Elisabeth Requeda, Jules Charron, Kenneth D. Roberts, Alcide Chapdelaine, and Gilles Bleau (Univ. of Montreal) evaluated the fertility of 47 men aged 30–54 years with proved fertility before vasectomy who underwent vasovasostomy. A single-layer macroscopic technique was used in 7 cases and a two-layer microsurgical method in 40 cases. The mean duration of vas obstruction was 5.6 years. Sperm fertilizing capacity was determined and sperm antibody titers were measured in 32 men for longer than 1 year postoperatively.

Sperm reappeared in the ejaculate in 38 of the 47 patients, for a duct patency rate of 80%. Four failures were associated with anatomical difficulties encountered at operation. Two other patients had postoperative complications. Eighteen spouses conceived after vasovasostomy, for a pregnancy rate of 46%. The mean duration of vas obstruction in fertile cases was 4.6 years. Six of 8 fertile patients had low titers of serum agglutinins and normal sperm fertilizing capacity. None had immobilizing antibodies. Six of 7 patients in the group without pregnancy had elevated serum agglutinin titers, and 4 had agglutinating antibody in seminal plasma as well as serum immobilizing antibody. The sperm of all 7 patients failed to fertilize zona-free hamster ova.

Loss of sperm fertilizing ability due to sperm antibodies appears to be an important cause of infertility in vasovasostomized men. The reappearance of spermatozoa in the ejaculate and even normal findings after semen analysis have not been reliable indices of restored fertility, but the zona-free hamster ova assay provides a reliable determination of the likelihood of conception. Sperm antibodies should be measured before as well as after vasovasostomy.

▶ [The normospermic patients whose wives become pregnant after vasovasostomy had lower sperm antibody titers and better performance in the zona-free hamster ova assay than did those normospermic patients whose wives did not conceive. This is consistent with the assumption that the much lower rate of pregnancy than of patency that follows vasovasostomy is due to autoimmunity directed against spermatozoa.] ◀

15-26 **Human Chorionic Gonadotropin in Treatment of the Infertile Man.** Donald J. Mehan and Michael J. Chehval (St. Mary's Health Center, St. Louis) used human chorionic gonadotropin (hCG) to treat 128 men with proved infertility, some of whom had failed to respond to internal spermatic vein ligation of varicocele. Patients received 10 injections of 50,000 units of hCG intramuscularly over 6 weeks, starting with 3 injections on successive days in the first week, 2 in the second and third weeks, and 1 each in the last 3 weeks.

Seventeen of the 40 patients who had failed to respond to operation for varicocele impregnated their partners, including 1 of 5 azoosper-

---

(15-25) Fertil. Steril. 39:197–203, February 1983.
(15-26) J. Urol. 128:60–63, July 1982.

mic patients. Improvements in sperm viability and density were greater in the clinically successful cases. No pregnancies were achieved among 6 patients given hCG in the presence of a varicocele that was not operated on. None of 12 patients with either an increase in FSH concentration or testicular biopsy findings that might preclude successful spermatogenesis responded to hCG therapy. Seven of 23 patients with idiopathic oligospermia impregnated their partners. Significant improvements in spermograms occurred with hCG therapy in patients with initial sperm densities of 20 to 50 million per cc, but only 14% of 21 patients impregnated their partners. Five of 26 patients with initial counts exceeding 50 million per cc did so. No significant increase in either sperm density or viability occurred in this group.

Treatment with hCG is of established value in patients who fail to respond to operation for varicocele and those with idiopathic oligospermia. Normospermia and untreated varicocele are contraindications to the use of hCG for infertility, as are elevated FSH values and significant adverse testicular biopsy findings.

▶ [According to this article, hCG is quite effective in treating male infertility when the condition involves a previously repaired varicocele or idiopathic oligospermia but not an untreated varicocele, high FSH levels, or testicular hyalinization or atrophy. The mechanism presumably reflects the LH-like properties of hCG (due to their common α-subunit).] ◀

15–27 **Incidence of Sperm-Associated Immunoglobulin and C3, the Third Component of Complement, in Infertile Men.** The relative isolation of the male reproductive tract from the circulation may account for the lack of correlation of circulating antisperm antibodies with genital tract antibodies and make it important to examine sperm directly for increased surface immunoglobulin. Gilbert G. Haas, Jr., Alan D. Schreiber, and Luis Blasco (Univ. of Pennsylvania) assayed sperm-associated immunoglobulin and C3 in 104 consecutive men who had semen studies for evaluation of infertility. Ten fertile men also were evaluated. The indirect radioactively labeled antiglobulin test for antisperm antibody was used.

Four of the 87 subjects studied for plasma IgG antisperm antibody had positive tests, but a total of 16 men had increased amounts of IgG detected on their sperm. Two of them also had positive tests for plasma IgG antisperm antibody. Ten of 86 men had increased amounts of sperm-associated IgA, and 1 of them had a rise in sperm-associated IgG values as well. One infertile man gave a weakly positive test for sperm-associated IgM. Only 3 men with increased sperm-associated IgG values had increased amounts of antisperm IgA in the circulating plasma. Increased amounts of sperm-associated C3 were found on the sperm of 5 of 50 infertile men. All men tested who had increased sperm-associated IgG values had decreased sperm penetration on postcoital testing, despite the presence of normal-appearing mucus. Three of the 5 men with increased amounts of sperm-associated IgA had similar findings.

Direct measurements of sperm surface immunoglobulin may be

(15–27) Fertil. Steril. 39:542–547, April 1983.

critically important in evaluation of infertile men. The presence of sperm-associated IgG or IgA in the subjects in this study was not associated with semen abnormalities. The presence of sperm-associated IgG, however, was associated with decreased mucus penetration on postcoital testing despite normal-appearing mucus. This correlation suggests that one of the reproductive steps that may be impaired in these patients is mucus penetration.

▶ [An article abstracted in the 1983 YEAR BOOK (pp. 388–390) indicated that antisperm antibodies in seminal fluid were more important than those in serum. The focus of the present report is on antibody attached to sperm. This sperm-associated nonagglutinating antibody was more common than and unrelated to antibody detected in seminal fluid or serum, but was associated with poor postcoital test results. As more is learned about immunologic factors in male infertility, we become more confused.] ◀

15–28 **The Relationship Between the Postcoital Test and the Sperm Penetration Assay.** Michael R. Soules, Donald E. Moore, Leon R. Spadoni, and Morton A. Stenchever (Univ. of Washington, Seattle) note that although the postcoital test (PCT), which evaluates the sperm-cervical mucus interaction, is one of the basic tests of a standard infertility evaluation, it remains questionable whether the PCT can substitute for a semen analysis. A modified hamster egg sperm penetration assay (SPA) was investigated in relationship to the PCT in infertile couples.

Patients were selected retrospectively from couples attending an infertility clinic. According to the criteria for selection, each male partner had had one or more SPAs and semen analyses performed on a semen sample obtained by masturbation after a 2-day abstinence from ejaculation and each female partner had had one or more PCTs performed within 1 year of her partner's SPA. The PCTs were performed 2–18 hours after coitus after a 2-day abstinence from sexual intercourse. In the SPA, ova were harvested from superovulated female hamsters, the cumulus oophorus was removed with hyaluronidase, and the zona pellucida was removed with trypsin. The human sperm were washed and centrifuged, the concentration was adjusted to 10 million motile sperm per milliliter, and the sperm were mixed with the eggs and incubated for 2 hours. A penetration score of 15% or greater was considered an indication of fertility.

It is generally accepted that fewer than 5 motile sperm per high-power field (HPF) is an abnormal PCT value and that more than 20 motile sperm per HPF is an excellent value. There was a significant correlation between the number of motile sperm per HPF on the PCT in a given patient and the total sperm count and the percentage of sperm motility. Correlation was insignificant between PCT and SPA findings. There was a subgroup of 16 men who had a normal semen analysis value and an SPA score that indicated infertility. In the PCT categories with more motile sperm per HPF, there were higher percentages of men with SPA scores in the fertile range; conversely, when SPA scores were in the fertile range, there was a statistically

---

(15–28) Fertil. Steril. 38:384–387, September 1982.

significant increase in the number of PCTs with 5 or more motile sperm per HPF.

The correlation between SPA and PCT findings was not overwhelming. Of the women with normal cervical mucus but low PCT scores, 54% had male partners with SPA scores in the fertile range. Of the women with excellent PCT scores, 25% had partners with SPA scores that indicated infertility. The relationship between the two tests is not strong enough to recommend exclusion of either test in a complete infertility evaluation.

▶ [This study found some degree of correlation between results of the postcoital and sperm penetration tests, but it wasn't especially close, implying that the two probably measure different things.] ◀

15–29 **Human Sperm Penetration of Zona-free Hamster Eggs After Storage of Semen for 48 Hours at 2 C to 5 C.** Jose R. Bolanos, James W. Overstreet, and David F. Katz (Univ. of California at Davis) attempted to develop a method of short-term storage of human semen permitting its transport to a distant laboratory for testing with the zona-free hamster egg assay. The motility of human spermatozoa and their ability to penetrate hamster eggs were assessed after dilution of semen with N-Tris(hydroxymethyl) methyl-2-aminoethane sulfonic acid (TES) and hydroxymethyl aminomethane (Tris) (TEST) yolk buffer and storage at 2 C to 5 C for 48 hours. Semen samples from 10 fertile donors and 19 infertility patients were studied. More than 65% of spermatozoa that were initially motile in TEST yolk buffer remained active after storage. The mean swimming speed of sperm fell to about 60% of baseline. The proportion of hamster eggs penetrated by spermatozoa from patients and donors increased significantly after storage. Normal and abnormal specimens were equally well preserved.

This method can be used to ship semen samples by commercial transport to specialized laboratories for testing. Low-temperature storage of semen in TEST yolk buffer appears to enhance the fertilizing capacity of human spermatozoa in vitro. Further study may make it possible to define optimal conditions for the zona-free hamster egg assay and to increase the in vitro fertilizing capacity of spermatozoa from subfertile men, permitting treatment by in vitro fertilization and embryo transfer.

▶ [Dr. Roger Williamson, of the University of Iowa, reviewed this paper at our request and commented as follows:

"Semen from fertile men and the male partners of infertile couples, whose semen analyses were either normal or abnormal, was stored in an egg yolk buffer for 48 hours at 2 C to 5 C. Sperm so treated showed a higher percentage of penetration of zona-free hamster ova without a significant reduction of motility or swimming speed relative to fresh semen from the same men in each group. After this low-temperature storage, normal rates of penetration occurred with the sperm of 4 men from infertile couples whose fresh sperm showed low rates or absence of sperm penetration. The significance of these findings lies in the ability to alter in vitro conditions to enhance sperm penetration, suggesting the potential for other methods of treating some infertile couples.

"Properly performed, this bioassay with fresh semen is an accurate indicator of in vivo fertility potential, though more experience and longer follow-up are needed to

(15–29) Fertil. Steril. 39:536–541, April 1983.

assess this question fully. Manipulations of this system will allow a greater understanding of the biology of reproduction and means to enhance in vitro fertilization, but such new wrinkles probably make the assay less useful as a predictor of in vivo fertility."] ◀

15–30 **Who Asks For Vasectomy Reversal and Why?** Geraldine Howard (London) described 76 men who requested reversal of vasectomy between June 1978 and September 1981. Among these 76 men, 31 were still married, and, of 45 who had divorced or separated, 25 had remarried. Eighty percent of the new partners were childless. These men had decided to have a vasectomy during a crisis; a recent pregnancy or financial stress were the most common reasons.

Findings showed that at the time of their request for reversal the men's ages ranged from 21 to 54 years, whereas at the time of the vasectomy, ages had ranged from 20–50 years. These men were significantly younger when compared with a control group, who at the time of vasectomy were aged 22–57 years. Among the group requesting reversal, more men were in social classes I and II and the same number in social classes III (manual) and IV when compared with controls. No men in the study were in social class V, which confirms the lack of interest in vasectomy among the least skilled class. Family size was the same in both groups. The interval between vasectomy and request for reversal varied between 6 months and 12 years. Most men (68%) requested reversal within 5 years of vasectomy.

All men in the study group initially said that they wanted another child, although it later became clear that not all did. Some only wanted to be "put back to normal," and others hoped that reversal would help to relieve marital strains. Among the 76 men seeking reversal, only 4 strongly wished to father more children. Fifteen thought they had been unduly pushed into vasectomy by doctors, and all emphasized it seemed unreasonable to sterilize a healthy partner because of the health problems of a wife. The 31 who were still married often gave more than one reason for requesting a reversal. The divorced men were largely concerned with male infertility in the new marriage or relationship. Many reasons coexisted for the initial vasectomy, including anxiety over pregnancy, postnatal depression, difficulty in birth control, financial and housing problems, and strains developing between the couple.

In vasectomy counseling, reversal should be described realistically—vasectomy reversal is a major operation requiring a stay in the hospital and is not always possible or successful. Pregnancy after reversal occurs in only 25% to 50% of cases. Consequently, for most men, vasectomy is likely to mean permanent infertility.

▶ [Most gynecologists are all too familiar with the woman who regrets having had a tubal sterilization. This report indicates that the same phenomenon can occur in her husband (or former husband) after a vasectomy, and for basically the same reasons.] ◀

(15–30) Br. Med. J. 285:490–492, Aug. 14, 1982.

16. Contraception

16–1 **Factors Associated With Compliance to Oral Contraceptive Use in an Adolescent Population.** The number of adolescent girls engaging in premarital intercourse is increasing and this, with early age at menarche and the societal tendency to delay marriage, increases the risk of premarital pregnancy. P. W. Scher, S. J. Emans, and E. M. Grace (Harvard Med. School) examined factors contributing to contraceptive compliance in a group of adolescents who had made an initial decision to use oral contraception. Age range at the start of oral contraception was 13 to 19 years. A total of 101 adolescents participated in the study; 68% were blacks. The mean time from initial prescription of oral contraception to interview was 26 months.

Patients tended to recall their initial contraceptive visits in great detail. Sixty-two percent of the subjects were classed as being compliant. Differences in compliance could not be correlated with race, city or suburban residence, or method of payment. Active parental involvement at the initial visit, however, was an important factor, and there was striking improvement in compliance when a parent accompanied the adolescent to the clinic for the first visit. Patient satisfaction with the health care visit significantly influenced contraceptive compliance. Concern about medical effects of pill use did not significantly influence compliance, but compliance followed satisfaction with use of the pill as a contraceptive method and was better if side effects did not occur. Noncompliant patients reported side effects and inconvenience to be primary concerns. Adolescents who wished to attend college did better than the others. Forty-two percent of noncompliant patients had an unplanned pregnancy after discontinuing use of the pill.

Nearly 40% of adolescents in this study were erratic in their use of the contraceptive pill and at risk of pregnancy. Concerns about weight gain should be considered. Patients should receive written instructions about proper pill use. Where indicated, patients should be seen frequently to encourage compliance. Adequate information on nonprescription methods of birth control also should be given.

▶ [Given the findings reported here, education and reassurance provided to adolescents concerning the side effects of the pill should improve patient compliance.] ◀

16–2 **Effects of Ampicillin on Oral Contraceptive Steroids in Women.** Different drugs can interfere with the efficacy of oral contraception by a variety of mechanisms. Ampicillin causes a fall in the plasma ethinyl estradiol (EE) concentration in animals by interfering with its enterohepatic recirculation. D. J. Back, A. M. Breckenridge,

---

(16–1) J. Adolesc. Health Care 3:120–123, September 1982.
(16–2) Br. J. Clin. Pharmacol. 14:43–48, July 1982.

M. MacIver, M. Orme, P. H. Rowe, Ch. Staiger, E. Thomas, and J. Tjia (Univ. of Liverpool) examined the effects of co-administration of ampicillin in 7 women aged 19–27 years who were using long-term oral contraception. Five were taking Eugynon 30 (30 μg of EE and 250 μg of levonorgestrel); 1 was taking Ovranette (30 μg of EE and 150 μg of levonorgestrel); and 1 was taking Minovlar (50 μg of EE and 1 mg of norethisterone acetate). Ampicillin was given in a dose of 500 mg 3 times daily for 8 days. Volunteer studies were done in 6 women aged 21–24 years who had used oral contraception for at least 3 months, usually Eugynon 30. The same dose of ampicillin was administered.

No patient experienced side effects or menstrual disturbance during the study. Changes in plasma EE and levonorgestrel levels in the patient group are shown in the table. No significant changes in plasma EE, levonorgestrel, follicle-stimulating hormone, or progesterone concentrations occurred during ampicillin administration. Plasma ampicillin levels up to 1.5 μg/ml were observed 6–8 hours after dosing in 3 of the 7 patients. Comparable findings were obtained in the volunteer group, in whom the mean plasma ampicillin levels was 0.6 μg/ml.

Ampicillin did not significantly alter plasma EE or levonorgestrel levels in women using long-term oral contraception in this study. Apparently women using oral contraceptive steroids need not take alternative contraceptive precautions when ampicillin is prescribed.

▶ [A report presented in the 1981 YEAR BOOK (p. 384) described a patient who conceived while taking oral contraceptives, due perhaps to an interaction with tetracy-

PLASMA CONCENTRATIONS OF ETHINYLESTRADIOL AND LEVONORGESTREL (NORETHISTERONE IN 1 PATIENT) ON 4 DAYS DURING AND AFTER AMPICILLIN THERAPY (MEAN ± SE MEAN)

	Plasma ethinyloestradiol concentration (pg/ml)		*Plasma levonorgestrel concentration (ng/ml)*	
Patient	*During ampicillin*	*After ampicillin*	*During ampicillin*	*After ampicillin*
1	60.3 ± 0.3	88.7 ± 6.1*	2.4 ± 0.08	3.0 ± 1.0
2	32.6 ± 2.6	31.7 ± 0.9	1.4 ± 0.07	1.3 ± 0.05
3	9.3 ± 2.6	92.3 ± 33.7*	2.3 ± 0.13	1.7 ± 0.06
4	35.7 ± 2.9	23.7 ± 0.7	2.8 +	2.8 +
5	130.0 ± 20.1	119.5 ± 10.3	0.7 ± 0.06	0.7 ± 0.07
6	38.7 ± 7.7	45.0 ± 5.6	2.4+	3.0 +
		Mean ± s.e mean	2.0 ± 0.3	2.05 ± 0.4
			Plasma norethisterone concentration (ng/ml)	
7	18.5 ± 5.4	20.5 ± 6.0	7.4 ± 0.9	9.3 ± 0.6
Mean ethinyloestradiol (pg/ml)	46.4 ± 15.2	60.2 ± 14.8		

+ = mean of 2 samples.
*$P < .05$ paired t test for individual patients.
(Courtesy of Back, D. J., et al.: Br. J. Clin. Pharmacol. 14:43–48, July 1982.)

cline. We noted that estriol-lowering effect of ampicillin during pregnancy, due perhaps to interference with the enterohepatic metabolism of estrogen, and wondered if concomitant antibiotic treatment might be a common cause of failure of oral contraceptives. This study by Back et al. found no apparent effect of ampicillin on blood hormone levels, so the problem seems to be more theoretical than real. However, although none of the mean levels was affected to a statistically significant degree, 2 of the 7 subjects (numbers 1 and 3) had quite remarkably lower plasma ethinyl estradiol levels during ampicillin than after. Maybe this isn't the last word.] ◀

16–3 **Effects of Oral Contraceptives on Respiration.** The effect that the synthetic progestins currently used in oral contraceptives (OC) may exert on respiratory function has not been investigated thoroughly. Ana Montes, David Lally, and Ralph W. Hale (Univ. of Hawaii, Honolulu) assessed the potential changes in pulmonary function in 12 nulliparous women before and after OC administration (10 patients taking 1 mg of norethindrone with 0.035 mg of mestranol and 2 patients taking 1 mg of ethynodiol diacetate with 0.05 mg of ethinyl estradiol). Changes in respiratory values were monitored at rest and during programmed exercise at 3 and 6 months after starting drug administration.

During treatment, significant increases were observed only in tidal volume during static and timed spirometric maneuvers ($P = .01$). Four values were assessed during monitoring of the ventilatory response to treadmill exercise at each of four workloads: oxygen uptake, carbon dioxide elimination ($\dot{V}_{CO_2}$), minute ventilation ($\dot{V}_E$), and respiratory exchange ratio. Analysis of the covariance (ANCOVA) for the slopes of each of the values showed no significant variation between test periods. The ANCOVA of the means of these values during exercise revealed increases in $\dot{V}_{CO_2}$ and $\dot{V}_E$.

The results indicate that norethindrone in the dose used is a moderate stimulator of ventilation in normal subjects. It is suggested that progestins increase $\dot{V}_E$ during exercise by a pathway that affects tidal volume without significantly changing breathing frequency.

▶ [Minute ventilation is increased in pregnancy; progestins have been used in the treatment of patients with hypoventilation disorders. This report indicates that patients taking oral contraceptives have increased tidal volumes at rest and increased minute ventilation with exercise. The effect is presumably a central one. No adverse effects on lung or airway mechanics were noted.] ◀

16–4 **Renin-Angiotensin System and Total Body Sodium and Potassium in Hypertensive Women Taking Estrogen-Progestagen Oral Contraceptives.** Nearly all women who take such oral contraceptives have an increase in blood pressure, and occasionally this increase is marked. It appears that the estrogenic component is chiefly responsible. D. McAreavey, A. M. M. Cumming, K. Boddy, J. J. Brown, R. Fraser, B. J. Leckie, A. F. Lever, J. J. Morton, J. I. S. Robertson, and E. D. Williams assessed the renin-angiotensin-aldosterone system and levels of whole body electrolytes in 6 women presenting with hypertension while taking a combination oral contraceptive containing 30 to 50 μg of estrogen. Age-matched women with essential hypertension also were evaluated.

(16–3) Fertil. Steril. 39:515–519, April 1983.
(16–4) Clin. Endocrinol. (Oxf.) 18:111–118, February 1983.

Arterial pressure fell spontaneously within 2 years of withdrawal of the oral contraceptive in 5 of 6 study patients. The remaining patient also had a fall in pressure to normal, but a β-blocker was given for angina. Levels of plasma renin substrate were significantly higher in the study group than in women with essential hypertension. Concentrations of plasma active renin were similar in the two groups. Levels of plasma angiotensin II were significantly elevated in the study group, but plasma aldosterone levels were similar in the two groups. Mean total body potassium and sodium levels also were similar in the two groups, as were mean plasma electrolyte levels.

These findings are consistent with the view that elevated arterial pressure in women on combination-type oral contraceptives may be due at least in part to an elevation in levels of plasma angiotensin II in relation to total body sodium. There is no evidence that the increased blood pressure is dependent on elevated mineralocorticoid activity. The findings are consistent with reports of an acute reduction in blood pressure when an infusion of saralasin is given to hypertensive women who are taking oral contraceptives.

▶ [In this study, women who developed hypertension while taking oral contraceptives were compared with women with essential hypertension. Plasma angiotensin II levels were increased in the hypertensive pill users, but total body sodium levels were normal. The authors think this angiotensin II elevation may be responsible for hypertension associated with oral contraceptives. What are angiotensin II levels in normotensive women on the pill?] ◀

16–5 **Results of a Study to Determine the Effects of Three Oral Contraceptives on Serum Lipoprotein Levels.** Samuel A. Pasquale, Robert J. Murphy, Paula K. Norwood, and Leon C. McBride conducted a multicenter, double-blind investigation with random allocations of subjects to Ortho-Novum 1/50 tablets, Ortho-Novum 1/35 tablets, or Modicon tablets. Each subject received the same oral contraceptive (OC) for at least 4 cycles. Serum high-density lipoprotein cholesterol (HDL), low-density lipoprotein cholesterol (LDL), triglyceride, and total cholesterol concentrations were measured prior to initiation of OC use and were repeated after treatment cycles 2 and 4. The 74 subjects were normal, healthy women of reproductive age (18–38 years) who had regular menstrual cycles, either had never used OCs or had discontinued use of OCs at least 3 months prior to enrollment, and were using no other method of contraception.

There were no significant changes in serum levels of HDL, LDL, or cholesterol for any of the three regimens. There was a significant increase in triglyceride levels at cycle 2 for all three regimens. At cycle 4, all subjects in all three regimens continued to demonstrate a mean increase. These increases, however, were not significant for Ortho-Novum 1/35 or Ortho-Novum 1/50. The mean increase for Modicon was statistically significant.

The medical significance of changes in serum lipoprotein levels in OC users is not clear. Whether women whose HDL levels decrease while taking OCs are at greater risk for arterial disease cannot be

---

(16–5) Fertil. Steril. 38:559–563, November 1982.

determined at this time. However, in these patients, there was no significant effect of the drugs on HDL or LDL levels.

▶ [None of these three combined oral contraceptive preparations affected high-density or low-density lipoprotein cholesterol levels after 4 months use. The pill with the highest estrogen-progestin ratio (Modicon) did increase triglyceride levels.] ◀

16–6 **Fibrinolytic Activity in the Walls of Foot Veins in Women Using Combined Contraceptive Pills.** Fibrinolytic activity in the vessels of superficial vein walls plays an important role in the fibrinolytic defense system against thrombosis. A. Kjaeldgaard and B. Larsson (Huddinge Univ. Hosp., Stockholm) histochemically determined the fibrinolytic activity of dorsal foot veins (FAV) in 46 healthy young (aged 17–35) and middle-aged (aged 36–55) women, 26 of whom were using combined oral contraceptive (OC) agents.

Low FAV scores (less than 6.5 arbitrary units) were recorded in 37% of the women using OCs—including all ages, without predisposing factors. However, most of the pathologic values were found in the middle-aged group, with 54% of these women having subnormal FAV scores, compared with 25% of the younger OC users. Compared with normal young women, FAV values were significantly lower in middle-aged OC users ($P < .025$) and in women with predisposing factors (history of previous thrombophlebitis or family manifestation of deep venous thrombosis) ($P < .01$), but not in younger OC users, whether smokers or not. Younger OC users who smoked had insignificantly higher FAV scores than nonsmokers, however, middle-aged OC users who smoked had significantly lower FAV values than younger OC users who smoked ($P < .05$). The lowest mean FAV value (5.6 arbitrary units) was found in middle-aged OC users who smoked and in women with predisposing factors, regardless of age.

The results confirm a previous finding of low FAV in patients with a history of deep venous thrombosis or recurrent superficial thrombophlebitis and suggest that combined OC agents are unsuitable for middle-aged female smokers.

▶ [The results reported here fit nicely with the epidemiologic studies that suggest that the cardiovascular mortality risk is increased in the "older" user of oral contraceptives who smokes.] ◀

16–7 **Oral Contraceptives and Gallbladder Disease: Royal College of General Practitioners' Oral Contraception Study.** Sally J. Wingrave and Clifford R. Kay report that prior studies of gallbladder disease provided strong evidence of an increased incidence associated with use of oral contraceptives. The rate of reporting of gallstones rose steadily after 2 years of oral contraceptive use, with the suggestion of a plateau after 4–5 years, when the rate in users was just over twice that of controls.

This study suggests that there is no overall long-term increased risk and that the previously demonstrated short-term increase in risk may be due to an acceleration of gallbladder disease only in women susceptible to it. The acceleration may be associated with the dose of estrogen in the combined oral contraceptives. In controls, the rate of

---

(16–6) Gynecol. Obstet. Invest. 15:223–229, April 1983.
(16–7) Lancet 2:957–959, Oct. 30, 1982.

reporting of gallbladder disease increased significantly with parity, smoking, and social class, but not with age.

If, as the studies suggest, an increase in reporting of symptomatic gallbladder disease can occur within the first year of oral contraceptive use, it is likely that the women concerned were already in the presymptomatic stage of the disease before the use of oral contraceptives began, because a considerable lag normally exists between the formation of lithogenic bile and the appearance of symptoms of the disease.

▶ [A common, although not uniform, view is that oral contraceptive use predisposes women to gallbladder disease. The variation in incidence by duration of use reported here is consistent with the authors' opinion that there is no overall increase in the risk of gallbladder disease in patients on the pill, but, rather, that the disease is accelerated in those women who are inherently susceptible to it.] ◀

16–8 **Oral Contraceptives and Pelvic Inflammatory Disease.** George L. Rubin, Howard W. Ory, and Peter M. Layde (Centers for Disease Control, Atlanta) analyzed data from a large multicenter case-control study of contraceptive use and serious gynecologic disorders to study the association of use of oral contraceptives and pelvic inflammatory disease (PID). The analysis included data from interviews of 648 women hospitalized with an initial episode of PID and 2,516 hospitalized control subjects. Women who used a contraceptive method for at least 1 month were considered users of that method. The current method was defined as that used any time during the 3 months prior to interview.

Compared to the control subjects, women in the case group were more likely to be younger, to be black, to have lower educational status, to have a higher number of sexual partners, and to have a greater frequency of sexual activity. The estimated risk of PID for women who had ever used oral contraceptives relative to that for women who had never used them was 0.8 (95% confidence interval). Estimated risk for past oral contraceptive users compared to that for those who had never used oral contraceptives was 0.9. Current oral contraceptive users had a risk of 0.5 relative to current nonusers of contraceptives. The relative risk remained constant when those women who had used oral contraceptives in the past were excluded from the group of current nonusers. Among current users, long-term (13–24 months) oral contraceptive users had 0.3 times the risk of PID and short-term (1–12 months) users had 1.1 times the risk of PID compared with current nonusers of contraceptives. This apparent protective effect of oral contraceptives was present in women both younger and older than age 24 years.

These results indicate that among women currently using oral contraceptives, those who have used them for more than 1 year have only one third the risk of having an initial episode of PID compared with women who use no contraceptive method. These findings are consistent with previous data and are probably not due to selection bias. The mechanism of a protective effect of oral contraceptives against PID is speculative. From these data, it can be calculated that users of

(16–8) Am. J. Obstet. Gynecol. 144:630–635, Nov. 15, 1982.

oral contraceptives in the United States experience about 50,000 fewer cases of PID per year and 12,500 fewer hospitalizations for PID per year than they would if they used no contraception.

▶ [As faithful YEAR BOOK readers know, case-control studies can never "prove" anything. An advantage of this study is that apparent potentially confounding variables are controlled for. The pill may be protective against the development of pelvic inflammatory disease. The authors suggest altered cervical mucus and decreased menstrual flow as possible mechanisms.] ◀

16–9 **Pituitary Adenomas and Oral Contraceptives: Multicenter Case-Control Study.** There is evidence of a causal relation between endogenous estrogens and development of pituitary adenomas, and the incidence of these tumors appears to have increased in recent years in young women in parallel with the increasing use of oral contraceptives.

The Pituitary Adenoma Study Group undertook a case-control study of this relationship in 212 women aged 18–39 years, who were seen at four centers with symptoms of secondary amenorrhea or galactorrhea, or both, due to prolactin-secreting pituitary adenomas. A total of 140 adenomas were confirmed surgically. Control subjects were matched with patients for age, race, and place of residence. In addition, 119 patients with hyperprolactinemia who had amenorrhea or galactorrhea, or both, but normal or equivocal findings on tomograms were interviewed along with 205 normoprolactinemic women with amenorrhea or galactorrhea, or both. All were matched with neighborhood control subjects.

There was no increase in relative odds for any group for use of oral contraceptives (pituitary adenoma cases versus controls). The risk of pituitary adenoma was significantly associated with a history of infertility, menstrual problems such as amenorrhea or galactorrhea, or both, and nulliparity. There was no evidence that use of oral contraceptives by women with a history of menstrual disorder or infertility was associated with an increased risk of pituitary adenoma.

These findings and those of previous studies indicate that use of oral contraceptives is not associated with increased risk of developing pituitary adenoma. Further studies are needed to determine whether the use of oral contraceptives can aggravate an existing adenoma.

▶ [The issue of whether oral contraceptive usage predisposes to hyperprolactinemia–pituitary adenoma is one of continuing controversy (see 1983 YEAR BOOK, p. 417–419). This report from the Pituitary Adenoma Study Group describes a large collaborative investigation using a case-control design. No association was found.] ◀

16–10 **Long-term Oral Contraceptive Use and Risk of Breast Cancer: The Centers for Disease Control Cancer and Steroid Hormone Study.** It has been proposed that the long-term use of oral contraceptives or their use in the presence of other risk factors increases the risk of breast cancer, although most reported studies indicate a minimal overall effect of oral contraceptive use on the risk of cancer. Data are available from the Centers for Disease Control Cancer and Steroid Hormone Study, a multicenter case-control study of women aged 20–54 years with a first diagnosis of breast cancer, ascertained

---

(16–9) Fertil. Steril. 39:753–760, June 1983.
(16–10) JAMA 249:1591–1595, Mar. 25, 1983.

at eight population-based cancer registries. Women representing the first 689 cases were matched with 1,077 control women selected randomly from the general populations of the study areas. The two groups had similar age and race distributions. Women in the case group were more likely to be nulliparous, to have a family history of breast cancer and a history of benign breast disease, and to be premenopausal.

The relative risk of breast cancer in oral contraceptive users was 0.9, and the duration of use did not influence the risk even when it exceeded 10 years. Analysis of time elapsed from the first oral contraceptive use indicated no association with breast cancer. The lack of association was evident for all age groups. No association was evident in women with different family histories of breast cancer or in those of differing menopausal status. Oral contraceptive use had little effect on the breast cancer risk in women who had had operations for benign breast disease.

These preliminary results are reassuring to women who have used oral contraceptives. Neither short-term nor long-term use of oral contraceptives appears to increase the risk of breast cancer. Future analyses will focus on oral contraceptive use before the first pregnancy and on the effects of various types and doses of oral contraceptives.

▶ [This case-control study found no association between oral contraceptive use and the risk of development of breast cancer. The risk of development of two other cancers is apparently decreased in pill users. Read on.] ◀

16–11 **Oral Contraceptive Use and Risk of Endometrial Cancer: The Centers for Disease Control Cancer and Steroid Hormone Study.** The results of previous case-control studies suggest that the risk of endometrial cancer in ever-users of combination-type oral contraceptives is half that in never-users. Results are now available from the first 10-month phase of the Cancer and Steroid Hormone Study, an ongoing multicenter case-control study of the effects of oral contraceptive use on various gynecologic cancers. Cases were women aged 20–54 years with a first diagnosis of endometrial cancer ascertained at one of eight population-based cancer registries. Findings in 187 cases were compared with those in 1,320 randomly selected population controls.

The relative risk of endometrial cancer in women who had used combination-type oral contraceptives at some time was 0.5, with 95% confidence limits of 0.4–0.8, compared with never-users. A protective effect was evident in women using contraceptives for at least a year, and it persisted for at least 10 years after cessation of oral contraceptive use. Protection was most evident in nulliparous women, who had a relative risk of 0.4 associated with oral contraceptive use. The results could not be attributed to differences in health status, parity, infertility, or other potentially confounding variables.

These preliminary findings are important to women who have used oral contraceptives of the combination type, especially nulliparous

---

(16–11) JAMA 249:1600–1604, Mar. 25, 1983.

women, who are at an increased risk for the development of endometrial cancer. Endometrial cancer may be averted in an estimated 2,000 women each year in the United States by the past and current use of oral contraceptives. Further study is needed of the influence of various brands and doses of oral contraceptives and of the administration of exogenous estrogens for perimenopausal symptoms.

▶ [Given the well-known effects of postgestational agents on normal endometrium, oral contraceptive usage should protect against endometrial cancer. Such are the findings of this case-control study from the Centers for Disease Control.] ◀

16–12 **Oral Contraceptive Use and Risk of Ovarian Cancer: The Centers for Disease Control Cancer and Steroid Hormone Study.** Several epidemiologic studies report a reduced risk of ovarian cancer in women who have used oral contraceptives. This risk was estimated in an ongoing multicenter population-based case-control study of the effects of oral contraceptive use on gynecologic cancers. In a 10-month period, 179 women aged 20–54 years with newly diagnosed ovarian cancer, ascertained at eight population-based cancer registries, were entered into the study; findings in these women were compared with those in 1,642 control women having intact ovaries.

Oral contraceptive users had an age-adjusted risk of ovarian cancer of 0.6 compared with never-users, with 95% confidence limits of 0.4–0.9. The risk of cancer decreased with increasing duration of oral contraceptive use and remained low for some time after cessation of use. The results could not be attributed to parity, infertility, or other possibly confounding factors.

Women in this survey who used oral contraception at any time had a significantly reduced risk of ovarian cancer compared with never-users, and the risk declined with duration of oral contraceptive use. Oral contraceptives may exert a protective effect against the development of ovarian cancer. The relative risk is lowest for nulliparous oral contraceptive users. Ovarian cancer may be averted in an estimated 1,700 or more women yearly in the United States through the past and current use of oral contraceptives. Further study of the epidemiology of ovarian cancer and its relationship with oral contraceptive use clearly is warranted.

16–13 **Factors Affecting Association of Oral Contraceptives and Ovarian Cancers.** It has been suggested that a decreased risk for ovarian cancer is associated with the use of oral contraceptives, but some such studies have not provided details on how the risk may be modified by such factors as age at first use, length of use, recentness of use, and type of formulation. Daniel W. Cramer, George B. Hutchison, William R. Welch, Robert E. Scully, and Robert C. Knapp (Boston) attempted to overcome these defects in a case-control study of histologically verified ovarian cancer. Oral contraceptive usage was compared in 144 white women younger than age 60 years who had primary epithelial ovarian cancer and 139 randomly selected women matched for age and race.

Oral contraceptives had been used at some time by 34 study pa-

---

(16–12) JAMA 249:1596–1599, Mar. 25, 1983.
(16–13) N. Engl. J. Med. 307:1047–1051, Oct. 21, 1982.

tients (24%) and 48 controls (34%). The relative risk for ovarian cancer associated with oral contraceptive use, adjusted for age and parity, was 0.38, with 95% confidence limits of 0.15 to 0.96. Oral contraceptives had been used by 30 (71%) of the 42 study patients younger than age 40 years and by 25 (60%) of the 42 controls younger than age 40. In this younger group, the relative risk for ovarian cancer associated with oral contraceptive use, adjusted for parity, was 1.98, with 95% confidence limits of 0.74 to 5.27. In contrast, oral contraceptives had been used by only 4 (4%) of 102 study patients aged 40 to 59 years, compared with 23 (24%) of 97 controls aged 40 to 59. In this older group, the relative risk was 0.11, with 95% confidence limits of 0.04 to 0.33. Thus, age at the time of the study was an important modifier of the association between ovarian cancer and oral contraceptive use.

No significant heterogeneity in the association of oral contraceptives and ovarian cancer was observed between parous and nonparous women. The risk for malignant ovarian cancers associated with oral contraceptives in women younger than age 40 was close to unity, 1.28, whereas the risk for ovarian tumors of borderline malignancy associated with oral contraceptives in women in that age group was 2.95. The risk for ovarian cancer appeared to decrease with increasing age at first use, but the trend was not significant after adjustment for age, duration of use, and interval since last use. There appeared to be a decreased risk after more than 3 years of use, but there was no consistent linear trend. A decreased risk for ovarian cancer appears to occur primarily after oral contraceptive usage was discontinued, but after adjustment for age, age at first use, and duration of use, the trend was of borderline significance.

Too few women could recall the exact type of pill they had taken to permit a breakdown by dosage of the estrogen or progestogen. No significant differences in formulations used by study patients and controls were observed. The predominent type of estrogen used by both groups was mestranol, and the predominant progestogen was norethindrone. Formulations containing ethynodiol diacetate were used by 4 of 8 study patients younger than age 40 who were current or recent users at the time of their diagnosis, but by none of 4 similar controls. Although intriguing, this finding remains within the realm of chance ($P = .14$).

The lowest risk for ovarian cancer associated with the use of oral contraceptives was found in older parous women and in those who had discontinued use more than 10 years previously.

▶ [Because oral contraceptives suppress pituitary gonadotropins, and therefore ovarian activity, it would seem theoretically that any association with ovarian cancer would be negative. In other words, if prior oral contraceptive usage has any effect on the development of ovarian cancer, it should be protective. This hypothesis is confirmed by this article and the preceding one. This study of Cramer and colleagues suggests that the "protection" is limited to women aged 40–59 at the time of cancer diagnosis; for women younger than age 40, there was actually an increased risk.

In related studies, Rosenberg and associates (*JAMA* 247:3210, 1982) also found an apparent "protective" effect of prior oral contraceptive use against epithelial cancers of the ovary, and Risch and colleagues (*Am. J. Epidemiol.* 117:128, 1983) found a similar association for pregnancy and lactation as well as for oral contraceptives. Thus, the evidence seems to be unanimous.] ◀

16–14 **Risk of Breast, Uterine Corpus, and Ovarian Cancer in Women Receiving Medroxyprogesterone Injections.** Animal studies have failed to give clear results regarding the carcinogenicity of long-acting progestins. Over 1½ million women worldwide are receiving injections of depot medroxyprogesterone acetate (MPA). Arthur P. Liang, Aliza Greenspan Levenson, Peter M. Layde, James D. Shelton, Robert A. Hatcher, Malcolm Potts, and Marcia J. Michelson reviewed data on gynecologic cancers in 5,003 black women attending a family planning clinic at a metropolitan hospital who received injections of MPA for contraception between 1967 and 1976. Median age at initial injection was 26 years. Injections generally were given every 3 months. Most women were treated for less than a year. Median follow-up was 9 years.

The numbers of breast, uterine, and ovarian cancers observed in over 43,000 woman-years of follow-up were compared with the expected numbers based on annual age-, race-, and sex-specific rates from National Cancer Institute data. No evidence of an increased risk of any of the cancers was obtained. After adjustment for incomplete follow-up, the relative risks for MPA users were 0.7 for breast cancer, 1.2 for uterine corpus cancer, and 0.8 for ovarian cancer.

No evidence of increased risk of gynecologic cancers was found in this survey of women receiving MPA injections. A weak carcinogenic effect or one appearing only after a long latent period would not have been detected, but a strong association between medroxyprogesterone injections and cancers of the breast, uterine corpus, or ovary is unlikely.

▶ [There has been much concern about the oncogenic potential of medroxyprogesterone because of the findings in dogs, and this is probably the major reason that release of the drug as an injectable contraceptive has been held up. This study should do something to allay these concerns. The follow-up rate of 72% is pretty good and gives some confidence regarding the negative findings. On the other hand, nearly 60% of the subjects received the drug for less than 12 months and only 4.3% received it for longer than 5 years, so there must be some lingering doubt about the effects of long-term exposure.] ◀

16–15 **Risk of Uterine Perforation Among Users of Intrauterine Devices.** To determine which attributes of the intrauterine contraceptive device (IUD) and which user characteristics contribute to the risk of uterine perforation and incarceration, Stephen F. Heartwell and Sarah Schlesselman (Women's Health Study) analyzed data on 32 women with uterine perforation requiring transperitoneal IUD removal, 106 women with uterine incarceration of an IUD removed transcervically, and 497 controls who used an IUD in a collaborative multicenter study.

Among women with at least one live birth, those lactating at the time of IUD insertion were found to have an estimated tenfold increased risk of perforation when compared with women not lactating at the time of insertion. Women with at least one live birth were

---

(16–14) JAMA 249:2909–2912, June 3, 1983.
(16–15) Obstet. Gynecol. 61:31–36, January 1983.

found to be at increased risk of perforation even in the absence of lactation. An incarcerated IUD resulting in difficult removal was 2.3 times as likely among women lactating at the time of insertion as among women not lactating at the time of insertion. The likelihood of uterine perforation and uterine incarceration were unchanged regardless of the type of IUD used.

▶ [This analysis indicates that the IUD in the lactating woman carries a relatively high risk of uterine perforation and incarceration of the device. The absolute risk cannot be determined from these data, so it does not seem to us, at least at this point, that the IUD is contraindicated in the breast-feeding mother. However, there clearly is a need for special thought in selecting this form of contraception, and special care in inserting the device, in a nursing woman.] ◀

16–16 **Comparison Between Antifibrinolytic and Antiprostaglandin Treatment in Reduction of Increased Menstrual Blood Loss in Women With Intrauterine Contraceptive Devices.** Antifibrinolytic drugs are effective in reducing menstrual blood loss; prostaglandin synthesis inhibitors also reduce bleeding in women with essential menorrhagia and menorrhagia associated with use of an intrauterine device (IUD). Olavi Ylikorkala and Lasse Viinikka (Univ. of Oulu, Finland) compared the efficacy of the antifibrinolytic agent tranexamic acid (TA) and the prostaglandin synthesis inhibitor diclofenac sodium (DS) in reducing heavy menstrual bleeding in 31 women using an IUD. Of the 19 women who remained in the trial, 15 lost more than 80 ml of blood, and 4 lost from 70 to 80 ml. All patients but 1 had used a copper-containing IUD for a year or longer; 1 had used an inert device for 10 years. The mean age was 35 years, and physical findings were normal in all. The patients received TA orally in a dose of 1.5 gm 3 times daily for 5 days in 2 cycles; DS in a dose of 50 mg 3 times on the first day, followed by 25 mg 3 times daily for 4 days in 2 cycles; and a placebo for 5 days in 1 cycle.

Treatment with TA significantly reduced mean blood loss by about 50%, and DS reduced it by 20%. The effect of TA was significantly superior to that of DS. Neither drug altered the duration of menstrual bleeding or abolished pelvic discomfort. Most patients reported side effects with both drugs. Tranexamic acid caused mostly gastrointestinal tract disturbances. The women discontinued iron supplements during the trial, but there were no significant changes in hemoglobin, packed cell volume, or serum ferritin level.

Tranexamic acid appears generally to be more effective than DS in reducing menorrhagia in women wearing IUDs. Diclofenac, however, markedly reduces bleeding in some patients and causes side effects less frequently. The authors suggest that an antiprostaglandin be tried for 2 cycles and that an antifibrinolytic agent be tried if this fails. Blood loss should be quantitated before any treatment is instituted.

▶ [This report isn't really very encouraging. The fibrinolytic inhibitor did a better job in reducing blood loss than did the antiprostaglandin, but the former was associated with more side effects (12 of 19 women). Why not pull the IUD?] ◀

(16–16) Br. J. Obstet. Gynaecol. 90:78–83, January 1983.

16–17 **Two Years' Experience With Two Levonorgestrel-Releasing Intrauterine Devices and One Copper-Releasing Intrauterine Device: A Randomized Comparative Performance Study.** Carl Gustaf Nilsson, Hannu Allonen, Juan Diaz, and Tapani Luukkainen report data from a study comparing two levonorgestrel intrauterine devices (IUD) and a copper device, the Nova-T, at two clinics in Finland and one in Brazil during 24 months. The 100 women in the study provided 6,000 woman-months of use of the levonorgestrel devices and 3,000 woman-months of use of the Nova-T. The two levonorgestrel devices released 20 and 30 μg daily, respectively. All subjects were aged 18–38 years when entering the study and had not used any long-acting hormonal preparation or had not received hormonal therapy in the past 6 months.

Pregnancy rates after 2 years of use were 0.6 and zero with the levonorgestrel IUDs and 3.3 with the Nova-T. Rates of removal because of bleeding or pain, or both, were low with all three devices, ranging from 7.1 to 7.6 after 2 years. Significantly fewer days of bleeding occurred with use of the levonorgestrel devices from the second month of use and afterward. Use of a Nova-T IUD was terminated in 1 case because of infection. Continuation rates of use after 2 years were 66.6 and 60.7 for the levonorgestrel IUDs and 71.9 for the Nova-T; the differences were not significant.

Bleeding and pain were the most common causes for removing a copper-medicated IUD. The use of levonorgestrel-releasing IUDs in the present study was associated with low rates of removal because of bleeding or pain, or both, in the first 2 years and with a decline in the rate of removal for these reasons in the second year of use.

The IUDs used in this study have an estimated lifetime of 7 years. Their use does not seem to be associated with an increased risk of pelvic infection. These devices may provide protection against infection similar to that obtained with oral contraceptives. Only one pregnancy occurred in association with a levonorgestrel device in the first year of use, and none occurred in the second year of use.

▶ [This study population was evaluated at 1 year (1982 YEAR BOOK, pp. 449–451). The present report provides information through the second year of IUD use. It's a good news, bad news situation concerning the progestin device. High efficacy and less blood loss are on the plus side, but on the minus side are more removals because of amenorrhea, especially in the second year of use. One can argue that less bleeding is more important, particularly in nutritionally deprived women in developing countries, but the fact remains that many women are reassured by the regular occurrence of menses. More experience is needed, but the potential importance of this side effect on continuation rates shouldn't be minimized.] ◀

16–18 **Treatment of Menorrhagia With Intrauterine Release of Progesterone.** Iron deficiency is prevalent in both developed and developing countries. The Progestasert is a T-shaped intrauterine contraceptive device that has reduced blood loss substantially in women with losses within the normal range. A. Bergqvist and G. Rybo investigated whether intrauterine release of progesterone can reduce blood loss in women with menorrhagia. Twelve healthy parous women who

---

(16–17) Fertil. Steril. 39:187–192, February 1983.
(16–18) Br. J. Obstet. Gynaecol. 90:255–258, March 1983.

reported the loss of over 80 ml of blood in at least one of two menstrual periods were included in the study. Parity ranged from 1 to 4, and mean age was 34 years. Three women had their intrauterine devices removed during the 12-month study. Another had a hysterectomy mainly because of excessive intermenstrual bleeding.

Menstrual blood loss declined after insertion of the Progestasert from a median of 83 ml to 49 ml during the last study cycle, a significant effect. Intermenstrual bleeding usually was most frequent in the first postinsertion cycles and gradually decreased. In most cases the amount of blood lost through spotting was reported to be small. The serum iron concentration was higher after 1 year, whereas the hemoglobin concentration and total iron-binding capacity were not changed significantly. Several women who initially had avoided going out on some days because of heavy blood loss were able to be less restricted when using the Progestasert.

The Progestasert is a useful treatment for menorrhagia. The chief disadvantages of intrauterine progesterone application are intermenstrual spotting and prolongation of the menstrual period, but these effects were mostly tolerated by the patients in this study. Women who are more tolerant of menstrual irregularities may prefer the reduction in blood loss. It has been suggested that use of the Progestasert may be associated with an increased risk of ectopic pregnancy. The women in this study were instructed to use barrier contraception.

▶ [Why not? The hypomenorrhea or amenorrhea that detracts from the general appeal of the progesterone-releasing intrauterine device, as noted in the preceding editorial comment, might make it just the ticket for selected women with menorrhagia for whom the pill is not a good choice.] ◀

16–19 **Interval IUD Insertion in Parous Women: Randomized Multicenter Comparative Trial of the Lippes Loop D, TCu220C, and Copper 7.** Outside the People's Republic of China, the most commonly used intrauterine device (IUD) is the Lippes Loop D. Recently, increasing numbers of family-planning programs have begun to use "second-generation" IUDs such as the TCu200. The results of a multicenter randomized clinical trial of the TCu220C, Lippes Loop D, and Copper 7 IUDs undertaken in nine World Health Organization (WHO) Collaborating Centers for Clinical Research in Human Reproduction by the WHO's Special Program of Research, Development and Research Training in Human Reproduction are now reported. A total of 2,970 subjects were recruited into the study. There were 984 insertions of the TCu220C, 992 of the Lippes Loop D, and 994 of the Copper 7. The study was terminated at 2 years, at which time 18,743, 17,013, and 17,927 woman-months' experience had been accumulated with each device, respectively.

In the first 48 hours after insertion, there were 12 insertion failures, 9 of which involved the Lippes Loop D. During this time, there were 3 expulsions (2 Lippes Loop and 1 Copper 7) and 4 removals (3 Lippes Loop and 1 Copper 7) for pain or bleeding, or both, but no perforations. At both 1- and 2-year follow-ups, the pregnancy and ex-

(16–19) Contraception 26:1–22, July 1982.

	Cumulative Net Probabilities of Discontinuation					
	TCu220C vs	Lippes Loop	Lippes Loop	vs Copper 7	TCu220C	vs Copper 7
At 390 days						
Intrauterine pregnancy	0.5	1.9*			0.5	1.9†
Expulsions	3.7	7.8‡			3.7	6.3*
Removals for bleeding	2.2	4.5*				
Use-related discontinuations	10.4	17.3‡			10.4	15.8‡
Total non-medical removals			4.3	6.8*		
Wish to become pregnant			1.5	3.3*		
Continuation rate	76.3	68.8‡			76.3	70.6†
At 750 days						
Intrauterine pregnancy	1.7	3.7*			1.7	3.6*
Expulsions	6.1	10.0†				
Total medical removals					11.4	15.3*
Removals for bleeding	3.9	7.9†			3.9	6.5*
Other medical removals			1.4	3.7†		
Use-related discontinuations	18.4	25.8‡			18.4	25.3‡
Total non-medical removals	14.3*	10.8	10.8	15.2*		
Wish to become pregnant	8.8*	5.9				
Continuation rate	60.3	54.8*			60.3	55.5*

Significant differences between devices (standard pairwise chi-square test).
$*P < .05$.
$\dagger P < .01$.
$\ddagger p < .001$.
(Courtesy of The World Health Organization's Special Program of Research, Development and Research Training in Human Reproduction: Contraception 26:1–22, July 1982.)

pulsion rates, as well as the rate of removals for bleeding irregularities, were significantly lower for the TCu220C, compared with the Lippes Loop. The TCu220C also performed significantly better than the Copper 7 with respect to pregnancy and expulsion rates (table). Use-related discontinuations were fewer for the TCu220C than for either the Lippes Loop or Copper 7. The pregnancy and expulsion rates for the Lippes Loop and Copper 7 did not differ significantly. Removal rates for nonmedical reasons were higher for the TCu220C and Copper 7, primarily because the subjects wished to have another pregnancy.

With the Lippes Loop and Copper 7, there was a significantly higher expulsion rate and use-related discontinuation rate and a considerably lower continuation rate in subjects aged 16 to 24 years than in the older age groups. In women of parity 1 and 2, the Lippes Loop had a significantly higher rate of expulsion and use-related discontinuation than the TCu220C. In women of parity 3 or more, the TCu220C had significantly lower rates for total medical removals, removals for bleeding, and use-related discontinuation than the Copper 7.

It is concluded that of the three IUDs studied, the TCu220C is the IUD of choice.

▶ [This study was controlled, randomized, and huge! The TCu220C performed better than did either the Copper 7 or the Lippes Loop D.] ◀

16–20 **Effect of Different Types of Intrauterine Devices on the Risk of Pelvic Inflammatory Disease.** Many studies have shown that use of an intrauterine contraceptive device (IUD) increases the risk of pelvic inflammatory disease (PID), but it remains unclear whether the risk differs with the particular IUD used. David W. Kaufman, Jane Watson, Lynn Rosenberg, Susan P. Helmrich, Donald R. Miller, Olli S. Miettinen, Paul D. Stolley, and Samuel Shapiro examined the effects of various types of IUDs on the risk of PID in a case-control study of 155 women with PID and 305 control women at several metropolitan areas in the United States and Canada in 1976 to 1981.

The age-adjusted relative risk estimate for use of any IUD within a month of admission to the study was 8.6, with 95% confidence limits of 5.3 and 13.8. For past use of an IUD, the estimate of relative risk was 1.6. Estimated risk was highest for users of the Dalkon Shield, lowest for users of copper-containing IUDs, and intermediate for users of other devices, principally the Lippes Loop (table.) The relative risk estimate for the Dalkon Shield, compared with the copper-containing IUDs, was 6.5. Nine of 11 women using the Dalkon Shield had severe PID, compared with 12 of 40 women using copper-containing IUDs and 9 of 32 using the Lippes Loop. The risk of PID did not appear to be related to the duration of use of any of the devices.

These findings confirm an increased risk of PID associated with the use of IUDs. The Dalkon Shield appears to be more harmful than other devices. Direct information on sexual activity was not obtained in this study. Another possible source of bias is that although patients were not eligible for the study if they had a past history of PID, this information was not available for controls.

Age-Adjusted Relative Risk for PID Among Users of IUDs Within Month of Admission to Study

Type of IUD	PID	Control	Age-Adjusted Relative Risk Estimate (95% Confidence Limits)
Never used IUDs	44	192	1.0*
Copper-containing	40	34	6.8 (3.7-12.3)
Dalkon Shield	11	2	78.7 (22.7-272)
Lippes Loop	32	23	13.3 (6.7-26.5)
Saf-T-Coil	8	6	24.1 (7.5-77.9)
Other	3	4	11.4 (1.5-85.3)
Unknown	10	23	

*Reference category.

(Courtesy of Kaufman, D. W., et al.: JAMA 250:759–762, Aug. 12, 1983; copyright 1983, American Medical Association.)

(16–20) JAMA 250:759–762, Aug. 12, 1983.

▶ [The results of this case-control study seem to confirm an association between IUD usage and risk of PID. However, the finding of an eightfold to 11-fold increased risk may be an overestimate because of two features of the study: (1) women with PID, but not controls, were asked about previous pelvic infections and (2) the level of sexual activity was not controlled for. With respect to the comparison among different IUD types, the data are more solid and indicate that the risk is highest with the Dalkon Shield, lowest with copper-containing devices, and intermediate with others. From the clinical perspective, it seems clear that any woman still harboring a Dalkon Shield should have it removed.

Almost exactly the same findings were reported by Lee and associates (*Obstet. Gynecol.* 62:1, 1983) in a survey from the Women's Health Study.] ◀

16–21 **Factors Associated With *Actinomyces*-Like Organisms on Papanicolaou Smear in Users of Intrauterine Contraceptive Devices.** Diana B. Petitti, David Yamamoto, and Nathan Morgenstern (Kaiser-Permanente Med. Center, Oakland Calif.) examined the relation between *Actinomyces*-like organisms on the cervicovaginal Papanicolaou smear in users of intrauterine devices (IUDs) with the type of device used, the duration of use, and symptoms. A case-control study was carried out including about 80,000 smears examined in a 1-year period in a large cytology laboratory. *Actinomyces*-like organisms were seen on 107 smears, all but 3 of which were from IUD users. Two of the latter patients had foreign bodies in the cervix or vagina.

Neither age nor race was significantly associated with the presence of *Actinomyces*-like organisms on the smear. The duration of continuous IUD use after 7 years was a significant factor. More women with organisms used the Dalkon Shield, and fewer used the Cu-7, but the relation with type of device was not significant when allowance was made for duration of IUD use. Gynecologic symptoms were not significantly correlated with the presence of organisms.

The presence of *Actinomyces*-like organisms on the Papanicolaou smear in IUD users is correlated with the duration of IUD use, but not with the presence of symptoms or disease. It is possible that a finding of *Actinomyces*-like organisms on a smear is a marker for heavy bacterial colonization of the genital tract, since some apparently positive smear findings actually may represent only bacterial debris.

▶ [This report differs from one presented in the 1982 YEAR BOOK (pp. 451–452), as in the current study there was no clear association between the type of intrauterine device and *Actinomyces*-like organisms identified on the Papanicolaou smear. The vast majority of patients with this finding were asymptomatic (see also 1983 YEAR BOOK, pp. 425–426).] ◀

(16–21) Am. J. Obstet. Gynecol. 145:338–341, Feb. 1, 1983.

17. Abortion

17–1 **Chromosome Polymorphism in 110 Couples With Reproductive Failure and Subsequent Pregnancy Outcome.** Whether chromosomal variants can increase the risks of repeated pregnancy wastage, abnormal progeny, and reduced fertility capacity is uncertain. Sandra P. T. Tho, J. Rogers Byrd, and Paul G. McDonough (Med. College of Georgia, Augusta) compared the roles of heterochromatic polymorphism and balanced translocation in a series of 110 couples seen for reproductive failure in a 3-year period. They had had 2 or more spontaneous abortions, 1 or more abortions plus a malformed child, or 1 or more abortions with interval infertility of 2 or more years' duration. The trypsin-Giemsa banding method of chromosomal analysis was used, with supplemental studies by the Q, C, and silver staining methods where indicated.

Chromosomal anomalies were found in 17% of couples. Thirteen had a chromosomal variant and 6, a gross structural rearrangement. Seven of the former couples had chromosome variants with telomeric addition of fluorescent heterochromatin or duplication of centromeric nonfluorescent heterochromatin, and 6 had chromosome variants with inversion of the pericentromeric heterochromatin. None of these 13 couples had had defective viable children. Six of the 7 former couples subsequently had normal children, but only 1 of the 6 couples with inversion of the pericentromeric heterochromatin was successful. Three couples with balanced major chromosomal rearrangements attempted further conception, and all were successful.

Pericentric inversion may have an adverse effect on reproductive performance. Karyotypes of abortus material are critical in determining the causal relation of chromosome polymorphism to reproductive failure. This study was limited by the scarcity of abortus karyotypes and by a lack of cytogenetic data on relatives of propositi and their reproductive performance.

▶ [In this study, 17% of couples with a history of reproductive difficulties (spontaneous abortion ± fetal malformations ± infertility) had some type of chromosomal abnormality in one or the other partner. Two thirds of the cases were relatively minor "chromosome variants" and one third of them were more severe problems such as balanced translocation or large pericentric inversion. Most of the couples with anomalies in the former group subsequently achieved a normal pregnancy, whereas most of the latter did not. The incidence of abnormalities reported here is greater than that noted previously and suggests that the diagnostic yield of parental karyotyping may be large enough to justify the considerable expense involved. Of course, there is no therapy to be administered if an abnormality is found, except to advise amniocentesis if a pregnancy reaches 16 weeks.] ◀

(17–1) Fertil. Steril. 38:688–694, December 1982.

17-2 **Mixed Lymphocyte Reactivity Nonresponsiveness in Couples With Multiple Spontaneous Abortions.** Some studies but not others have suggested that, in cases of habitual abortion, the partners more frequently share common human leukocyte antigen (HLA) antigens. Jorge R. Oksenberg, Emanuel Persitz, Albert Amar, Joseph Schenker, Shraga Segal, David Nelken, and Chaim Brautbar undertook HLA analysis and mixed lymphocyte reactivity studies in 33 couples seen at Hadassah University Hospital, Jerusalem, with histories of at least 3 consecutive spontaneous abortions and 30 control couples matched for age and country of origin.

No significant differences were found between patient and control groups in the distribution of HLA A, B, and C antigens. No significant deviation from control mating frequencies was found in the habitual abortion group in the degree of HLA A and B sharing. Seventy percent of husbands in the infertile group had a low mixed lymphocyte culture (MLC) response when challenged with cells from their wives, but the MLC responses of aborting wives to their husbands' stimulations did not deviate from that of the control group. Male lymphocytes from the abortion group responded normally to cells from randomly selected women, including other women from the habitual abortion group. Cells from habitually aborting women stimulated lymphocytes from randomly selected men normally.

The combination of a husband's responder lymphocytes with his wife's irradiated stimulating lymphocytes in the one-way MLC gave a lower mitotic reaction in the habitual aborter group than in the control group in this study. This may be significant in the etiology of some cases of habitual abortion. The finding may be explained by the presence of a suppressor lymphocyte subpopulation in women who have multiple spontaneous abortions. The suppressor cells or their products may inhibit in vivo the enhancing protective factors of fetal and maternal origin involved in successful pregnancies. Alternatively, specific suppressor mechanisms might develop as a result of repeated abortions.

▶ [Immunologic mechanisms have been sought as explanations for habitual abortion in certain couples (1983 YEAR BOOK, pp. 432–433). In contrast to earlier reports, the authors of this study did not find more frequent sharing of HLA antigens by husband and wife in cases of habitual abortion than in control couples. The significance of the observation that husbands' lymphocytes showed a depressed response to stimulation by their wives' lymphocytes in the habitual abortion group is hard to understand. Does this mean that the fetus normally does "something" to prevent rejection and that in these couples the mother is suppressing that "something"?] ◀

17-3 **Outcome of Delivery Subsequent to Induced Vacuum-Aspiration Abortion in Parous Women.** Olav Meirik, Karl-Gösta Nygren, Reinhold Bergström, and Anna Gunsjö (Univ. Hosp., Uppsala, Sweden) evaluated the outcome of delivery to 429 parous women subsquent to a legally induced first-trimester vacuum-aspiration abortion during 1970–1975 in Uppsala County, Sweden, in a historical prospective study for 1970–1978. The outcome of delivery in women in this study was compared with the outcome of delivery in

---

(17–2) Fertil. Steril. 39:525–529, April 1983.
(17–3) Am. J. Epidemiol. 116:415–429, September 1982.

391 randomly chosen, matched parous women and with that of all parous women in Sweden in 1975. Confounding variables were controlled for in multiple regression analysis using infant birth weight and gestational duration as dependent variables.

Results show no association between induced first-trimester vacuum-aspiration abortion in parous women and an unfavorable outcome of subsequent delivery. On the contrary, results of multiple regression analysis showed that infants born to women who had had a previous induced abortion had significantly higher birth weights than infants born to women who had had no previous induced abortion. Perinatal death rate was 0.5% for both the abortion group and controls. Cesarean section was performed in 7.2% of the abortion group and in 8.2% of controls. Infants born to women who had had a previous vacuum-aspiration abortion were on the average about 100 gm heavier than those born to women who had had no induced abortion. With regard to gestational age, only cigarette smoking had statistical significance; each extra cigarette smoked per day during pregnancy shortened the pregnancy on the average of another 0.05 weeks.

Induced first-trimester vacuum-aspiration abortion in parous women, performed under proper medical conditions, was not found to exert any harmful effect on the outcome of subsequent delivery.

▶ [The study subjects described here were parous and had had first-trimester suction curettage procedures. No adverse effects of induced abortion on subsequent length of gestation or birth weight were demonstrable.] ◀

17–4 **Relationship Between Induced Abortion and Outcome of Subsequent Pregnancies.** Previous study has suggested an increased risk of spontaneous abortion in women having 2 or more previous induced abortions, and also a possible increased risk of ectopic pregnancy in this group. Shai Linn, Stephen C. Schoenbaum, Richard R. Monson, Bernard Rosner, Phillip G. Stubblefield, and Kenneth J. Ryan (Harvard Univ.) examined the relationship between previous induced abortion and subsequent late pregnancy outcome in a series of 9,823 deliveries in women with no past history of spontaneous abortion, stillbirth, or ectopic pregnancy. The women with no, 1, or 2 previous induced abortions were comparable in age. Past abortions were related to being single, black, and Protestant; to receiving welfare; and to smoking tobacco and marihuana. Women with past induced abortions were more likely to be having an unplanned pregnancy currently.

First-trimester bleeding was significantly more frequent in women with previous induced abortions. Cervical incompetence, third-trimester bleeding, and abruptio placentae also were more frequent, but not significantly so. Premature rupture of the membranes and abnormal presentations were more frequent in women with 2 or more past induced abortions. Major malformations, stillbirths, and neonatal deaths were not significantly related to past induced abortions. The only factor associated with 1 past induced abortion was first-trimester bleeding (table). Two or more past induced abortions were signifi-

---

(17–4) Am. J. Obstet. Gynecol. 146:136–140, May 15, 1983.

ODDS RATIO (OR) AND 95% CONFIDENCE INTERVAL (CI) ESTIMATION BY LOGISTIC REGRESSION ANALYSIS*

	1 Abortion		*2+ Abortions*	
Characteristic	*OR*	*CI*	*OR*	*CI*
Abnormal presentation	0.83	0.38, 1.83	3.02	1.34, 6.79
Premature rupture of membranes	0.95	0.71, 1.27	1.90	1.26, 2.87
Bleeding in first trimester	1.45	1.20, 1.76	1.80	1.29, 2.51
Gestational age <37 wk	1.07	0.86, 1.34	1.31	0.91, 1.89
Birth weight <2,500 gm	0.93	0.74, 1.17	1.25	0.88, 1.79
Major malformation	0.76	0.51, 1.13	1.28	0.71, 2.32

*Listed are the ORs and CIs for a woman with 1 or with 2 or more induced abortions having a particular characteristic. For each characteristic, a separate logistic regression analysis was performed with simultaneous controlling for age ≥35, being black, smoking 3+ cigarettes per day at delivery, being on welfare, and being multiparous.

(Courtesy of Linn, S., et al.: Am. J. Obstet. Gynecol. 146:136–140, May 15, 1983.)

cantly associated with abnormal presentations and premature rupture of the membranes, as well as first-trimester bleeding. Similar findings were obtained in an analysis of 1,361 women who had a proximate induced abortion.

Although more research is needed, these findings are generally reassuring. One or more past induced abortions appear not to increase substantially the risk of adverse late outcomes in subsequent pregnancies. Most induced abortions in the present series of patients were done in the first trimester by the suction technique.

▶ [Although details concerning length of gestation at induced abortion, degree and method of cervical dilatation, and various other characteristics were not collected in this study, the reported results suggest that induced abortion is not an important risk factor for late pregnancy adverse outcome. When correction is made for demographic and other variables, a history of two or more induced abortions was associated with an increased likelihood of abnormal presentation and premature rupture of the membranes, but not with low birth weight or premature delivery. First-trimester bleeding was more common in women with a history of one or more induced abortions.] ◀

17–5 **Clinical Test For Placenta in 300 Consecutive Menstrual Aspirations.** Robert A. Munsick (Indiana Univ., Indianapolis) analyzed the results of menstrual aspirations in 300 consecutive patients. The study method included the removal of placenta when it appeared and its immersion in water. The gross appearances of placenta and decidua are compared in Figure 17–1. Figure 17–2 shows a typical wet-mount photomicrograph of placenta.

When pregnancy tests were not required, 21 of the first 200 patients were not pregnant. When a positive pregnancy test was required, 2 of the last 100 patients were not pregnant. Infection was never severe; it followed aspiration in 4 (1.4%) of the pregnant pa-

(17–5) Obstet. Gynecol. 60:738–741, December 1982.

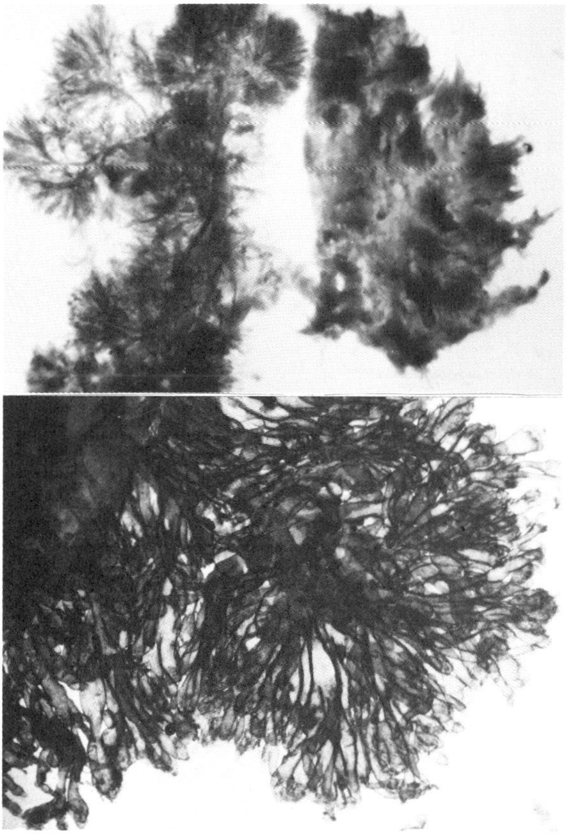

Fig 17–1 (top).—Typical fluffy villi of placenta *(left)* and shaggy decidua *(right)* are seen immersed in water.

Fig 17–2 (bottom).—Wet-mount microscopic appearance of placental villi.

(Courtesy of Munsick, R. A.: Obstet. Gynecol. 60:738–741, December 1982. Reprinted with permission from The American College of Obstetricians and Gynecologists.)

tients. Aspiration was incomplete in 4 (1.4%) patients. In each case, the gross test for placenta was questionable, but the microscopic test was positive and was confirmed by histopathologic examination. It is noteworthy that each of these patients was 7–10 weeks' pregnant.

In 7 of the initial 200 women (4% of those pregnant), curettage was performed because of hemorrhage 3–5 days after aspiration. All had positive gross tests for placenta. No villi were identified from the curettaged material, but necrotic tissue was found in each patient. Because of this early decidual shedding with hemorrhage, all of the last 100 patients were counselled to stay in bed for 12–24 hours if worrisome bleeding occurred in the first 6 days, when results of their gross test was positive. Four patients had negative results of gross and microscopic tests for placenta, a subsequent positive sensitive blood test for human chorionic gonadotropin, and either decidua or Arias-Stella reaction observed histologically. Among the 21 nonpregnant patients, endometrial histology was proliferative in 3, secretory in 7, decidual in 2, and inactive or noncyclic in 9. Except for a patient with an incomplete abortion, the combined results of gross and microscopic tests proved reliable.

The placental tests were nearly 100% reliable and their use improves not only the practice of early abortion but also the diagnosis and management of suspected ectopic pregnancy and problematic situations in which tissue is passed vaginally.

▶ [The technique described here seems to be a useful one for identifying placenta in menstrual extractions or other forms of early abortion. If no products of conception are evident, the patient is either still pregnant (in the uterus or elsewhere) or was not pregnant in the first place.] ◀

17–6 **Hypertonic Saline as an Abortifacient in a Select Group of Patients.** J. A. Garbaciak, Jr., and R. J. Benzie reviewed the clinical course of 40 patients with a uterine scar who were undergoing second-trimester abortion induced with either hypertonic saline or prostaglandin $F_{2\alpha}$ ($PGF_{2\alpha}$). Abortions were carried out at between 16 and 20 weeks' gestation. A 20% hyperosmolar saline solution was the principal abortifacient used; $PGF_{2\alpha}$ was also available for intra-amniotic instillation. No special attempt was made to withdraw fluid before infusion of saline.

About 1,000 second-trimester abortions are performed at the Toronto General Hospital annually. During 1972–1979, intra-amniotic saline injection was used in more than 90% of these procedures. Of the 40 patients with a uterine scar, 38 had intra-amniotic infusion of 2 dl of 20% hypertonic saline. There was no evidence of suspicion of uterine rupture in these patients. Twelve (31.6%) required curettage for complete removal of placental tissue. In 2 (5.3%), antibiotic therapy was started after the uterine cavity was completely emptied. One patient complained of abdominal pain after passage of the uterine contents; the pain resolved after 4 days of antibiotic therapy.

Uterine rupture in the second trimester is a catastrophe and in some cases is fatal. The safest technique for termination of a second-trimester pregnancy in patients who have had a previous cesarean delivery or a prior uterine operation has not been proved conclusively. However, in this experience with 38 successive patients with a scarred uterus who underwent hypertonic saline instillation at between 16 and 20 weeks' gestation, no evidence of uterine rupture was seen when the stated guidelines for oxytocin use were followed. Oxytocin was used in the absence of strong, regular contractions and softening of the cervix 24 hours after infusion time; in the absence of contractions 4 hours after rupture of the membranes; and in the management of incomplete abortion.

▶ [The patient with a scarred uterus in whom a second trimester abortion is to be done presents a special problem. There were no uterine ruptures in this series of 38 patients in whom amnioinfusion of hypertonic saline was used for abortion. It is not clear from the data given whether any received oxytocin as well, but the protocol called for oxytocin to be given only if contractions had not begun 24 hours after instillation or 4 hours after membrane rupture. The literature reviewed contains cases

(17–6) Obstet. Gynecol. 61:37–41, January 1983.

of uterine rupture after the use of saline only when oxytocin was given *before* membrane rupture, as well as cases after the use of prostaglandin regardless of whether or not oxytocin was used. Thus, it seems that the safest approach is saline and no oxytocin until the membranes have ruptured.] ◀

17–7 **Dilatation and Evacuation Procedures and Second-Trimester Abortions: The Role of Physician Skill and Hospital Setting.** Willard Cates, Jr., Kenneth F. Schulz, David A. Grimes, Arthur J. Horowitz, Fred A. Lyon, Fred H. Kravitz, and Melvin J. Frisch note that some clinicians have hesitated to perform dilatation and evacuation (D&E) procedures at 13 weeks' gestation or later because such procedures are more difficult to carry out safely than are suction-curettage procedures. Many clinicians also still believe all second-trimester abortion procedures should be performed in a hospital. To evaluate these concerns, the authors analyzed 24,664 abortions performed between 1973 and 1978 by 4 physicians associated with a large outpatient abortion facility; 3,711 (15%) of the abortions were second-trimester procedures.

The overall serious complication rate for procedures at the abortion facility was low. About 1 in 400 D&E procedures, 1 in 80 dinoprost instillation procedures, and 1 in 40 saline instillation procedures led to a temperature greater than 38 C for more than 3 days. Fewer than 1 in 1,000 women undergoing suction-curettage procedure suffered serious complications. Of those procedures available at 13 weeks' gestation or later, D&E was the safest. Instillation of saline was related to a higher serious complication rate, but this was not statistically significant. Gestational age, the physician, and the type of facility had no great effect on the relatively low risks of D&E.

The authors conclude that their data, collected over 6 years, document a 90% decrease in serious complication rate accompanying the gradual shift of second-trimester abortion procedures from instillation methods to D&E. The abortion facility physicians, who already were skilled in first-trimester suction-curettage, could safely perform D&E by cautiously advancing their gestational age threshold. Dilatation and evacuation procedures can be safely performed in nonhospital facilities, thus decreasing the cost and increasing the convenience to the patient.

▶ [This large series indicates that in experienced hands the D&E procedure is a safe means of pregnancy termination early in the second trimester.] ◀

(17–7) JAMA 248:559–563, Aug. 6, 1982.

18. Sexuality, Breast Diseases, Primary Care

18–1 **Relationship Between Sexual Arousal Experience and Genital Response.** Previous studies of the relation between subjective and genital measures of sexual arousal have given conflicting results. Janice Korff and James H. Geer (SUNY at Stony Brook) used psychophysical scale methods to obtain ratings of subjective arousal in 36 undergraduate women and assessed the effects of attending to body cues on the subjective-genital relationship. Experimental subjects received instructions suggesting that they attend to either genital or nongenital body signals of sexual arousal while viewing erotic slides. Control subjects received no attentional instructions. Subjects set sound and light intensities to match the intensity of arousal and used a rating scale. A vaginal photometer was used to measure physiologic responses to the stimuli.

Group computed correlations were extremely high, and individually computed subjective-genital correlations were highest in the attention-instructed groups. Paying attention to body cues had significant positive effects on the subjective-genital relationship.

The findings cast doubt on previous assumptions of low subjective-genital correlations in women. Attention to body cues appears to influence the relationship between subjective and genital measures of sexual arousal in women. The low correlations reported in earlier studies might have resulted in part from reduced attention to physiologic cues. Improved self-report methods appear to be needed, because self-reports of subjective experience are a critical component of sexual arousal. Those investigating subjective-physiologic relationships must be aware that the correlations obtained should be viewed as a function of the factors affecting the particular experiment.

▶ [These results indicate that a close correlation exists between subjective perceptions and an objective index of sexual arousal in female undergraduate students. It would be interesting to know how these indices related to previous sexual experience and attitudes about sex.] ◀

18–2 **Sexual Responsiveness in Diabetic Women.** An association between diabetes and impotence in men is recognized, but little attention has been given to sexual responsiveness in diabetic women. G. Tyrer, J. M. Steel, D. J. Ewing, J. Bancroft, P. Warner, and B. F. Clarke (Edinburgh) evaluated sexual and autonomic nerve function in 82 insulin-dependent diabetic women aged 18–45 years, all married or cohabiting for at least a year and living with their partners; 47 healthy women attending a family-planning clinic served as con-

(18–1) Psychophysiology 20:121–127, March 1983.
(18–2) Diabetologia 24:166–171, March 1983.

trols. The mean duration of diabetes was 13.5 years. Thirteen diabetic patients were pregnant and in the third trimester at the time of study.

The diabetic patients and healthy women reported similar frequencies of sexual intercourse in the previous 3 months. The diabetic women less often reported negative feelings concerning intercourse. The frequencies of orgasm were similar. More than 80% of diabetic women were satisfied with their sexual relationships. The 14 women with symptomatic autonomic neuropathy resembled the other diabetic women with respect to sexual function, although they reported slightly less sexual arousal during sexual activity. Sexual function also was similar in patients with and those without retinopathy.

Very little difference is apparent in the sexual responsiveness of women with diabetes and symptomatic autonomic neuropathy and other diabetic women. Diabetic patients in the present study did not exhibit sexual dysfunction in comparison with healthy women. Any modest physiologic deficit in diabetic women may be countered by a tendency for their marriages to be more caring, or for the women to feel less resentment toward their spouses. More attention should be given to the quality of sexual relationships in future studies of sexuality in diabetic individuals.

▶ [A relatively high incidence of impotency is found in diabetic men, presumably reflecting either vascular disease or autonomic neuropathy. This study explored the effect of diabetes on sexual functioning in women and found relatively little difference between diabetics and controls selected from a family-planning clinic. Because the sexual response of women is more "psychologic" and less "physiologic" than is that of the men, these results are probably what would be predicted.] ◀

18–3 **Vaginal Atrophy in the Postmenopausal Woman: Importance of Sexual Activity and Hormones.** It is generally thought, but unproved, that ongoing coital activity helps maintain vaginal elasticity and reduces coital discomfort postmenopausally. Sandra Leiblum, Gloria Bachmann, Ekkehard Kemmann, Daniel Colburn, and Leora Swartzman (New Jersey-Rutgers Med. School, Piscataway) examined the effects of sexual activity on vaginal status in 52 postmenopausal women not receiving estrogen replacement therapy. They were aged 50–65 years and had been postmenopausal for at least a year at the time of study. None had major physical or mental disorders, and none had undergone hysterectomy or bilateral oophorectomy. Active women reported a coital frequency of 2.4 times weekly, whereas sexually inactive women had a frequency of 0.2 times weekly.

Current coital activity was not significantly related to hormone levels. Significantly less vaginal atrophy was noted in sexually active women. Mean estrone and estradiol levels were similar in women with high and low vaginal atrophy scores, but those with less vaginal atrophy had higher levels of androgens and gonadotropins. The difference in luteinizing hormone (LH) levels was most pronounced. These levels correlated closely with labia and pubic hair scores and moderately with skin elasticity and vaginal mucosa status. Androstenedi-

(18–3) JAMA 249:2195–2198, Apr. 22/29, 1983.

one and testosterone levels correlated only with vaginal mucosa scores.

Women in this study who had less vaginal atrophy in the postmenopausal period had significantly higher circulating androgen levels and LH levels. Androgens may have a role in retarding senile vaginal changes in postmenopausal women. Androgens appear to be more important than sexual activity per se in preventing vaginal atrophy. Androgens would seem to be more important than estrogens in the maintenance of sexual interest both before and after the menopause.

▶ [In this study, postmenopausal women who were sexually active were found on examination to have less vaginal atrophy that those who were inactive sexually, consistent with the adage "use it or lose it." However, the problem is somewhat of a chicken and egg nature. Does coitus lead to a "healthier" (i.e., less atrophic) vagina or do women with less vaginal atrophy have more coitus because they find it more pleasant? Another interesting point in this study is the apparent inverse correlation between blood androgen concentrations and vaginal atrophy.] ◀

18–4 **Hormonal Treatments of Sexual Unresponsiveness in Postmenopausal Women: Comparative Study.** Although it is not certain that declining sexual interest and responsiveness occur with the menopause, many menopausal clinic patients report symptoms of sexual dysfunction. M. G. T. Dow, D. M. Hart, and C. A. Forrest (Glasgow) examined the effects of a combined testosterone-estradiol implant and of estradiol alone in 40 postmenopausal women, with a mean age of 47, who reported loss of libido, had a regular sexual partner, and had no gross primary marital disturbance or significant psychopathologic change or physical illness. Six patients had had a natural menopause; the other 34 had undergone hysterectomy and bilateral oophorectomy an average of 3½ years previously. Twenty patients had implants providing 50 mg of estradiol, and 20 received implants containing 100 mg of testosterone besides estradiol.

Both treatment groups showed a significant improvement in most measures after 2 months. No evidence of a differential response to the treatments was obtained. Improvement was largely maintained after 6 months. The treatments had comparable effects in patients without significant dyspareunia. Psychologic, somatic, and vasomotor symptoms improved in both treatment groups. Sexual interest and responsiveness increased significantly.

No advantage of supplemental testosterone over treatment with estradiol alone was apparent in this study of sexually unresponsive postmenopausal women. Testosterone was of no substantial added benefit either in patients with or those without significant dyspareunia.

▶ [According to this study, the addition of testosterone to estradiol gave no further improvement in libido in postmenopausal women complaining of sexual unresponsiveness. It's a pity, though certainly understandable, that no placebo controls were included.] ◀

18–5 **Psychologic and Hormonal Factors in Treatment of Female Sexual Dysfunction.** Despite extensive use and evidence for the ef-

(18–4) Br. J. Obstet. Gynaecol. 90:361–366, April 1983.
(18–5) Psychol. Med. 13:83–92, February 1983.

fectiveness of behavioral counseling for psychosexual dysfunction, little is known about the mechanisms underlying such treatment. Using a balanced factorial design, Andrew Mathews, Antonia Whitehead, and John Kellett (St. George's Hosp., London) assessed the therapeutic contribution of treatment variables in a controlled study of 48 couples presenting with complaints of female sexual unresponsiveness. The couples were randomly assigned to treatment conditions consisting of all eight possible combinations of testosterone or placebo, weekly or monthly sex therapy sessions, and one female therapist or a male-female therapist pair. Treatment was for a 3-month period in all cases. All counseling was adapted from the work of Masters and Johnson (1970) and Heiman et al. (1976). The results were evaluated by a "blind" assessor and by the couple before treatment, at the end of treatment, and after 6 months of follow-up.

Assessor's ratings showed significant improvements in 5 ratings of female sexual response (increased enjoyment, interest, orgasm, lubrication, and reduced aversion), 1 male rating (ejaculatory control), and on the 2 general ratings of marital and sexual relationship. Contrary to expectations from earlier work, the best posttreatment outcome was in the subgroup receiving placebo who had attended weekly sex therapy sessions ($P < .05$). The next most improved subgroup had received testosterone, but attended monthly sex therapy sessions. Only 33 couples completed the follow-up assessment at 6 months. Analysis of covariance indicated that follow-up attenders who had received testosterone showed less improvement than those who had received placebo ($P < .02$). Related differences further supporting the placebo group were found in the ratings of general marital relationship ($P < .03$) and male ejaculatory control ($P < .03$), and supporting trends were found in ratings of female enjoyment ($P < .1$) and decreases in aversion ($P < .1$). Male partners seemed to indicate negative reactions to some aspects of sex therapy when it involved a male-female therapist team, especially when weekly sessions were involved. Ratings by the female partners reflected a strong preference for the weekly mode of sex therapy.

It is concluded that testosterone, in the dose used, is not likely to be of value in the treatment of sexually unresponsive women, though weekly counseling sessions with one therapist is a reasonably effective and economic form of sex therapy. Further research into the mechanisms underlying improvement could provide a better understanding that will lead to a more complete response to treatment.

▶ [This study assessed several treatments of couples presenting with the complaint of female sexual unresponsiveness. The most important results were negative—testosterone therapy (10 mg daily) did not help and there was some indication that one female therapist was more effective (or at least preferred by the male partner of the couple) than the co-therapy team popularized by Masters and Johnson 15 years ago. Not surprisingly, weekly therapy sessions seemed to work better than monthly sessions.] ◀

18–6 **Immunodeficiency in Female Sexual Partners of Men With Acquired Immunodeficiency Syndrome.** The development of op-

(18–6) N. Engl. J. Med. 308:1181–1184, May 19, 1983.

portunistic infections or Kaposi's sarcoma has been associated with acquired immunodeficiency syndrome (AIDS) in previously healthy persons, chiefly male homosexuals in urban areas. Carol Harris, Catherine Butkus Small, Robert S. Klein, Gerald H. Friedland, Bernice Moll, Eugene E. Emeson, Ilya Spigland, and Neal H. Steigbigel examined the female sexual partners of male patients with AIDS in an attempt to define further the populations affected. Seven female partners of drug-abusing patients were evaluated. Five of the women were Hispanic. Their mean age was 31 years. All were long-term residents of New York City. None had a history of serious, recurrent, venereal, or opportunistic infections. All of the male partners had had opportunistic infections and cellular immunodeficiency diagnosed within the past 18 months, and all had abused intravenous drugs, except for 1 who reported homosexual encounters.

One woman had full-blown AIDS; another had an illness consistent with the prodrome of AIDS, including generalized adenopathy, lymphopenia, and a reduced ratio of helper to suppressor T cells. Four other women had generalized adenopathy or lymphopenia, with or without a reduced helper-suppressor T cell ratio. Only 1 woman was without abnormality. *Pneumocystis carinii* infection was confirmed in the woman having the full syndrome.

Women who are sexual partners of heterosexual men with AIDS are apparently at risk of acquiring the syndrome. The present findings suggest that AIDS may be sexually transmitted between heterosexual men and women. One of 7 women in the present study had the full syndrome, 1 had prodromal features, and 4 had some of the clinical, immunologic, or virologic features associated with AIDS. Recent findings indicate that an agent transmissible by sexual contact may be responsible for the abnormalities in cellular immunity present in AIDS.

▶ [The acquired immunodeficiency syndrome (AIDS) has taken the spotlight from toxic shock syndrome in the mass media in the United States. Perhaps by the time of publication of the 1984 YEAR BOOK the information presented here will be old hat. This report suggests the possibility that AIDS may be caused by a transmissible biologic agent.] ◀

18–7 **Profile of Women Practicing Breast Self-examination.** Retrospective studies indicate that frequent breast self-examination (BSE) can lead to early detection of breast cancers, especially in women not screened by other modalities. Susan E. Bennett, Robert S. Lawrence, Katharine H. Fleischmann, Carolyn S. Gifford, and Warner V. Slack examined factors that influence the practice of BSE in a series of 616 women interviewed by Beth Israel Hospital, Boston, 155 of them nurses, physicians, or paraprofessionals and the rest patients waiting for a routine visit at an ambulatory care department. The interview was conducted by interactive computer dialogue.

Seventy-eight percent of respondents reported practicing BSE, over a third of them at least monthly. Women living with their sexual partners, those who had been shown how to perform BSE, and those confident in their examination technique were likelier than others to

(18–7) JAMA 249:488–491, Jan. 28, 1983.

practice BSE frequently, as were women with a maternal history of breast disease. Monthly BSE could not be correlated with degree of formal education. No relation was apparent between BSE and the practice of other preventive health activities. Fear that breast surgery would decrease attractiveness was associated with infrequent practice of BSE.

It appears that the number of women who practice BSE frequently could be increased by showing women how to perform the examination and by reinforcing their confidence in their BSE technique. Women who have been shown how to perform BSE are more confident in their technique, and reinforcement may involve simply the repeated demonstration of BSE. These measures could be incorporated into the routine breast examination.

▶ [Regular breast self-examination (BSE) is associated with earlier detection of breast cancer and improved survival (1982 YEAR BOOK, pp. 463–465). The present report examines the characteristics of women who do or do not perform BSE. The hypothesis that women who practice other health-promoting activities would be more likely to perform BSE was not supported by the data. The important finding is that women who are instructed in BSE and who are confident in their technique are more likely to do it on a regular basis. The implications for the practicing gynecologist are clear.] ◀

18–8 **Thermography in Breast Diagnosis.** Ernest E. Sterns, Arthur C. Curtis, Sally Miller, and John R. Hancock (Kingston, Ont.) studied the role of two types of thermography in diagnosis of breast disease. Thermography was performed under standard conditions in 502 women seen during a 2-year period. The infrared thermogram (IRT) was performed first, followed by the plate thermogram (PT). Clinical examination followed.

A total of 792 IRTs and 718 PTs were performed. Of the 502 patients, 11 were proved to have breast cancer. Two had bilateral disease. Each type of thermogram correctly detected only 4 cancers. The true positive rate (sensitivity) was 33.3% for the IRT and 36.4% for the PT. The true-positive rate for clinical impression was 69%. Both forms of thermography gave abnormal results in 3 of 11 patients with cancer. Neither thermogram was interpreted as abnormal in 5 patients with cancer. Thermograms were interpreted by 2 observers on two separate occasions. Normal thermograms were reported in a consistent fashion, with the same diagnosis being made in 83%–90% of cases. There was far more variation in interpretation of thermograms that were reported as equivocal; the consistency varied from 30%–63%. Interpretation was least efficient for abnormal thermograms, with reproducibility of interpretation ranging from 21% to 77%.

In this study, the thermogram failed to identify cancers that were diagnosed incorrectly clinically. Also, fewer than half the thermograms that were considered abnormal when the clinical data were known to the reporter were interpreted in the same manner on another occasion when the clinical information was not provided. At this point, thermography cannot be recommended for breast diagnosis or as an indication for mammography.

(18–8) Cancer 50:323–325, July 15, 1982.

▶ [Neither infrared nor plate thermography performed well in this study. Half of the cancers were missed, many patients with benign changes had abnormal thermograms, and the intraobserver consistency of reporting left much to be desired. It doesn't seem that these techniques have a place in breast diagnosis. Thermography is apparently not too hot!] ◀

18–9 **Nipple Discharge: Diagnostic Value of Testing for Occult Blood.** Nipple discharge usually is evidence of abnormality within the breast. Murid A. Chaudary, Rosemary R. Millis, Gerald C. Davies, and John L. Hayward (Guy's Hosp., London) examined the significance of detecting hemoglobin in spontaneous nipple discharge from a single identifiable duct in 270 patients without an associated lump who underwent microdochectomy. In this series, 292 microdochectomies were carried out. Hemoglobin was detected using Bililabstix reagent strips. The patients represented 4.5% of all those with breast symptoms who were operated on during a 10-year period. The mean age was 45.5 years.

The pathologic findings are related to the hemoglobin status of the nipple discharge in the table. The incidence of cancer was 5.9%. All of the occult cancers were accompanied by a hemoglobin-positive discharge. The most common lesion was intraductal papilloma. Cancer developed subsequently in the same breast in 3 patients in this group. In 2 patients with no histologic abnormality, cancer later developed in the same breast. Six of the 16 patients with cancer had a frankly bloodstained discharge. All cancers were of the ductal type. The overall rate of development of cancer in the same breast after microdochectomy in 177 patients followed up who initially had benign disease was 3.3%.

Close follow-up is necessary of all patients with a hemoglobin-positive nipple discharge in whom no cause is found at the microdochectomy.

▶ [This study indicates that more than 90% of patients presenting with nipple dis-

PATHOLOGY OF 292 MICRODOCHECTOMIES IN 270 PATIENTS

Type of Lesion	Number of lesions	Haemoglobin Status Positive	Negative	Not Known
Benign intraduct papilloma	132	107	19	6
Duct ectasia	94	67	25	2
Cystic disease	17	9	8	—
Cystic disease with epithelial hyperplasia	11	4	7	—
Carcinoma	16	16	0	—
No abnormality found	22	12	10	—
Total number of operations	292	215	69	8

(Courtesy of Chaudary, M. A., et al.: Ann. Surg. 196: 651–655, December 1982.)

(18–9) Ann. Surg. 196:651–656, December 1982.

charge from a single duct but without a palpable mass will have a histologic abnormality. The most common lesion, found in 45% of all patients, was intraductal papilloma. Cancer was present in 5.5%. Testing the discharge for occult blood yielded positive results in 75% of the series and was invariably positive in the presence of malignancy. Thus, it appears that a negative hemoglobin test result in this situation may rule out cancer, but positive findings are not particularly helpful.] ◀

18–10 **Role of Fine-Needle Aspiration Cytology in Management of Solid Breast Tumors.** The staged management of breast cancer requires data on tissue histology before plans for definitive treatment can be established. Angelos A. Kambouris (Henry Ford Hosp., Detroit) evaluated fine-needle aspiration cytology in 38 patients with breast masses who were seen in 1979 to 1982. In many cases the study was part of the initial office evaluation. Cytologic study indicated cancer in 23 of 29 patients with clinical and mammographic findings of carcinoma. In 4 cases the reports were suspicious or atypical, and all these patients were proved to have cancer on open biopsy. Two patients with unsatisfactory specimens had infiltrating lobular carcinoma on open biopsy. There were no false positive cytologic reports. In 9 patients with clinical and mammographic findings of benign disease, aspiration cytology indicated normal cells in 2 cases, atypical cells in 2, abnormal cells in 2, unsatisfactory cells in 2, and suspicious findings in 1. Six of these patients were proved on biopsy to have benign disease. In no case has there been a delayed diagnosis of cancer.

Fine-needle aspiration cytology is a rapid, easy, and reliable ancillary procedure that aids in the diagnosis and treatment planning for patients with breast masses. When cytology is positive for cancer and is accompanied by consistent clinical and mammographic findings, open biopsy may not be necessary before mastectomy. Otherwise, the decision regarding mastectomy is based on the open biopsy findings. If the cytology report indicates "suspicious," "atypical," or "abnormal" cells, tissue biopsy is necessary. Patients with a report indicating "normal," "ductal," or "apocrine" cytology should remain under observation.

▶ [Advocates of needle-aspiration cytology of breast masses believe it to be the most important step in diagnosis. In the small series of solid breast tumors presented here, the correlation between cytologic and subsequent histologic diagnosis was quite good. In a much larger series of 865 cases of both solid and cystic tumors (Dua et al.: *N.Y. State J. Med.* 83:867, 1983), the incidence of cancer was 86% with positive cytology, 56% with suspicious cytology, and 2% with negative smears; however, in the last group, not all patients later had biopsy, so the figure given must be regarded as a minimum.

How can one inexperienced in performance and interpretation of fine-needle aspiration of the breast acquire the skills needed without compromising patient care? For a description of a staged program of implementation, see the description by Abele and associates (*Arch. Surg.* 118:859, 1983).] ◀

18–11 **Aspiration Cytology Is Superior to Tru-Cut Needle Biopsy in Establishing the Diagnosis of Clinically Suspicious Breast Masses.** M. Michael Shabot, Irwin M. Goldberg, Peter Schick, Roberta Nieberg, and Yosef H. Pilch compared the diagnostic accuracy of

---

(18–10) Am. Surg. 49:310–313, June 1983.
(18–11) Ann. Surg. 196:122–126, August 1982.

physical diagnosis, mammography, Tru-Cut (Travenol Labs., Inc.) needle biopsy, and thin-needle aspiration cytology in evaluation of clinically suspicious breast masses.

Breast masses clinically suspected of malignancy were evaluated prospectively in 81 consecutive patients. There were 31 benign lesions and 50 malignancies. Clinical diagnosis was correct in 85% (2.5% false negative, 12.5% false positive). Mammography was diagnostic in 52.8% (31.5% false negative, 15.7% false positive). Needle biopsy was accurate in 78.9% (21.1% false negative, 0% false positive). Aspiration cytology was diagnostic in 96.2% (3.8% false negative, 0% false positive). Statistical comparison of all four tests showed that aspiration cytology was slightly more accurate than physical examination for all lesions and significantly more accurate for benign lesions. Overall, aspiration cytology was significantly more accurate than mammography and needle biopsy. Only one minor complication, a superficial infection, occurred with the use of aspiration cytology and needle biopsy.

In this study, the diagnosis of malignancy was established in 45 of 50 cases (90%) by combining the use of aspiration cytology and needle biopsy. Thin-needle aspiration cytology was found to be a rapid, simple procedure that was 96.2% accurate and was superior to physical examination, mammography, and Tru-Cut needle biopsy in establishing a diagnosis in clinically suspicious breast masses. This technique deserves further evaluation as a method for screening clinically benign lesions for unsuspected malignancy.

▶ [These findings that aspiration cytology was more accurate than needle biopsy, mammography, and clinical findings in diagnosing breast lesions are somewhat surprising to us. We have aspirated a number of breast cysts and have found few, if any, positive cytologic results, suggesting that obtaining fluid from a breast "mass" is reassuring. Perhaps the discrepancy might be one in perspective. The authors of this article are surgeons and pathologists affiliated with various branches of the University of California, and maybe their patients came to them by referral; thus, 50 of their 81 consecutive patients had breast cancer, a much higher percentage than would be found in a primary-care setting.] ◀

18–12 **Postmenopausal Breast Abscess.** Breast abscess is considered to be rare in premenopausal, nonlactating women and even rarer in postmenopausal women. Jeanne Petrek (Emory Univ.) reviewed the records of 18 postmenopausal women treated for breast abscess between 1975 and 1978. Median age was 56 years. No patient was using estrogenic preparations. All patients had had a natural menopause. No patient had had a previous breast abscess. One had had a biopsy at the abscess site, and 15% of patients had a long-standing inverted nipple on the breast with the abscess. Only 3 of 6 mammographic studies suggested the possibility of an abscess. Abscess was not suspected even at operation in many patients; edema and induration were lacking in these cases. Most patients had subareolar abscesses. Half the patients had adult-onset diabetes. The most common organism was *Staphylococcus aureus*. Associated conditions included 1 case each of simple duct ectasia, cystic duct dilatation with apocrine metaplasia, and dilated ducts lined with squamous epithelium.

(18–12) South. Med. J. 75:1198–1200, October 1982.

Breast abscess in a postmenopausal woman can be confused with cancer because of its indolent characteristics. The physical and mammographic findings and white blood cell count are not diagnostically helpful. Although abscesses generally are incised and drained, in this age group the excision of the total mass may help make the diagnosis and prevent recurrence. If left in place, the thick, fibrotic wall of the abscess will not readily collapse and resolve.

▶ [Abscess formation in the nonlactating breast is unusual, and in the postmenopausal woman it must be rare indeed. In fact, we don't recall ever seeing such a case. This review of 18 cases encountered on a large surgical service during a 3-year period indicates that the clinical features are certainly far from typical.] ◀

18–13 **The Physician-Patient Accommodation: A Central Event in Clinical Medicine.** Mark Siegler (Univ. of Chicago) believes that there is no single adequate theoretical description of the nature of clinical medicine. The determination of what will be recognized as a problem for clinical medicine depends on three separate but interdependent events. The first is the patient's decision to consult a physician about a problem thought to be medical in nature. The distinction between health and nonhealth matters often is obscure at this stage. Social, cultural, and psychologic factors strongly influence judgments of whether a "problem" is present. The second clinical moment is the physician's analysis of the patient's complaint, leading to a determination of whether or not a clinical medical problem is actually present. Finally, a negotiated accommodation is reached, involving acquiescence by the patient in care by the physician and an agreement by the physician to care for the particular patient. This is the central event in contemporary American clinical medicine. The accommodative process depends on all of the particulars of the medical encounter. The model of medicine inherent in the emphasis on the need to reach an accommodation is one of mutuality, voluntariness, noncoercion, and respect for autonomy.

The freedom of both the patient and the physician to enter an accommodation is at the heart of morally acceptable medical practice. The physician-patient accommodation is a dynamic relationship that is constantly in flux. Some accommodations are stronger than others. What is considered a relationship may be viewed more accurately as repeatedly negotiated physician-patient accommodations. Medicine today is becoming increasingly bureaucratic and political, and these changes may transform the physician-patient encounter from a negotiated accommodation to an impersonal contract between client and provider. Clinical medicine will never be the same if this occurs.

▶ [This article was reviewed by Dr. Susan R. Johnson of the University of Iowa, who commented:

"In this article, Siegler has attempted to put the notion of the physician-patient relationship in terms of the realities of modern medicine. The first key concept is that a situation only becomes a problem for the clinician when the patient believes that she has a problem and the doctor agrees. As we know, the perceptions of these two parties often differ. The second key concept is the dynamic nature of the physician-patient accommodation. These days, it will be rare for a patient to see a single physician throughout her entire life or to accept the advice of a particular physician

---

(18–13) Arch. Intern. Med. 142:1899–1902, October 1982.

without question. The theoretical analysis of medical practice that this kind of article offers can be helpful in understanding some of the social and medicolegal dilemmas we find ourselves in these days."] ◀

18–14 **Rubella Vaccination: Persistence of Antibodies for up to 16 Years.** Siobhan O'Shea, Jennifer M. Best, J. E. Banatvala (St. Thomas' Hosp. and Med. School, London), W. C. Marshall, and J. A. Dudgeon (Inst. of Child Health, London) tested serum from 123 volunteers vaccinated from 6 to 16 years previously with one of four rubella vaccines (Cendehill, RA27/3, HPV77-DE5, and To-336) for rubella antibodies by using single radial hemolysis and radioimmunoassay.

Low concentrations of antibody (≤15,000 IU/L) were detected in 19 vaccinees (15.4%) by single radial hemolysis and in 13 (10.6%) by radioimmunoassay. Low concentrations of antibody occurred more frequently among subjects given Cendehill vaccine. None of those with naturally acquired immunity had low concentrations of antibody. Low concentrations occurred more commonly among those vaccinated 11–16 years previously than among those vaccinated 6–8 years previously.

Titers of rubella-specific IgG, measured by radioimmunoassay, were significantly higher after naturally acquired infection than vaccination. Among volunteers vaccinated 6–8 years previously, RA27/3 and HPV77-DE5 induced the highest geometric mean titers and Cendehill the lowest. In contrast, volunteers vaccinated 11–16 years previously with RA27/3 vaccine had a lower geometric mean titer than those given Cendehill, but this difference was not significant. Those receiving RA27/3 vaccine 11–16 years previously had a significantly lower geometric mean titer than those vaccinated 6–8 years previously. Those given Cendehill 11–16 years previously had a higher geometric mean titer than those vaccinated 6–8 years before, but this difference was not significant.

The authors stress the importance of further long-term surveillance (for 30–40 years) for women receiving these vaccines so that vaccination policies may be reviewed and revaccination considered if an appreciable number of vaccinees lose detectable antibody within this time.

▶ [In the United States, RA27/3 is the rubella vaccine available. This report indicates that only 1 of 46 persons vaccinated with the strain 11–16 years previously was seronegative by radioimmunoassay, and she had a low concentration of antibody when tested by single radial hemolysis. Although antibody persistence is good, several vaccinees had low titers. The authors point out that it remains to be determined whether infection with viremia can occur in this circumstance. Congenital rubella has been reported after successful vaccination with the Cendehill strain (Bott, L., and Eizenberg, D.: *Med. J. Aust.* 1982; 1:514). Obviously, more long-term surveillance is in order. The individual patient should be managed on the basis of her antibody titer and not her vaccination history.] ◀

18–15 **Body Weight and Subsequent Diabetes Mellitus.** John B. O'Sullivan (Boston Univ.) prospectively evaluated the 10- to 16-year predictive value of body weight for diabetes mellitus in two groups of

---

(18–14) Br. Med. J. 285:253–255, July 24, 1982.
(18–15) JAMA 248:949–952, Aug. 27, 1982.

women with initially normal results of glucose tolerance tests. Initial selection for the high-risk group required two or more of the following oral glucose tolerance test values: fasting, 110 mg/dl; 1 hour, 170 mg/dl; 2 hours, 120 mg/dl; and 3 hours, 110 mg/dl.

The mean age for the high-risk group of 602 patients was 30.8 years and that for the control subjects not at high risk, 25.1 years. The number of subjects in whom diabetes developed among the overweight and normal-weight control subjects not at high risk did not differ significantly. The incidence of diabetes in the 602 high-risk (previous transient gestational glucose intolerance) participants was significantly higher for overweight subjects (46.7%) than for those of normal weight (25.6%). In 328 concurrently selected control subjects not at high risk (without previous intolerance), the difference was not significant (4.5% vs. 1.9%). Use of another definition of diabetes, which indicated further deterioration, gave similar results, although high-risk overweight women had disproportionately higher incidence rates. Being overweight had no substantial predictive value for diabetes mellitus during this period unless the additional evidence for a high-risk classification was present. Among such persons at high risk, excess weight also predicted the severity of subsequent diabetic conditions. Figure 18–1 shows the cumulative incidence of diabetes for each of the four subgroups.

The data in this study indicate the predictive capacity of transient gestational blood glucose elevations for subsequent diabetes. The predictive ability of initial gestational classification greatly exceeds that contributed by obesity. The parallels between the roles of obesity and that of pregnancy are, however, striking. The tolerance for glucose

Fig 18–1.—Cumulative incidence of diabetes in high-risk and control subjects (*open squares,* overweight control subjects; *open triangles,* normal-weight control subjects; *solid squares,* overweight high-risk subjects; *solid triangles,* normal-weight high-risk subjects). (Courtesy of O'Sullivan, J. B.: JAMA 248:949–952, Aug. 27, 1982; copyright 1982, American Medical Association.)

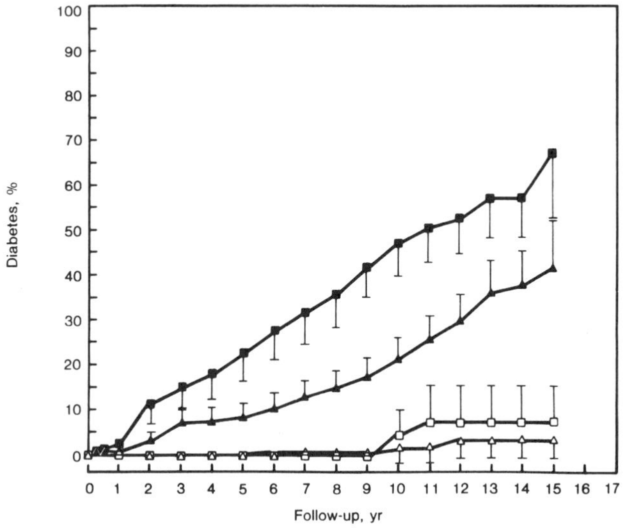

improves or returns to normal with the removal of the conceptus, and with the elimination of obesity in overweight subjects. The resultant return to normal, however, does not eliminate the risks of subsequent diabetes, at least as shown by the continued observation of persons in whom the transient condition of gestational diabetes is demonstrated. Results of this study also suggest that the great majority of overweight persons may not be at significant risk for diabetes.

▶ [This follow-up study of women who had glucose tolerance tests performed during pregnancy sheds some light on the obesity-diabetes relationship. The subsequent development of diabetes was independent of obesity in those subjects with normal glucose tolerance tests during pregnancy. In those women with abnormal tests, however, obesity was an important predictor of the later development of diabetes. Whether weight loss after pregnancy in obese women with gestational diabetes would decrease the risk of diabetes subsequently developing was not addressed in this study.] ◀

18–16 **Guidelines for Providing Medical Care to Southeast Asian Refugees** are presented by Giao N. Hoang (Univ. of Connecticut) and Roy V. Erickson (UConn-Burgdorf Clinic, Hartford, Conn). Almost 500,000 refugees from Vietnam, Kampuchea, and Laos have arrived in the United States since 1975. Although they have not presented substantial public health problems, they have important personal health problems that often require medical attention. Physicians should be aware of disease patterns and prevalence among these refugees and also should be aware of their cultural and religious background and previous medical practices that may influence their ability to obtain and maintain medical services provided in the United States.

Most recent refugees suffered hardships during their escape and are likely to be uneducated, of low socioeconomic class, and often illiterate even in their native language. Religious beliefs have great influence in their lives. Some religions such as Buddhism and Confucianism attribute physical suffering to inability to be righteous rather than to physical illness, and this may make patients appear impassive. The family unit is very important and separation from it may cause depression. The Indochinese lack a sense of time urgency and punctuality and may be very early or very late for appointments. Women are shy and modest, and unmarried women may refuse a pelvic examination, at least initially.

Many of these people believe that disease is caused by imbalance (deficiency or excess of bodily fluids or airs), malevolent spirits, or bad winds. Western medicine is mostly practiced in large cities. Modern Indochinese medicine is rooted in 19th century French medicine and often relies on "shotgun therapy" and "placebo effect." Traditional medicine includes Chinese and folk medicines. One study of Vietnamese refugees found that 80% wait at least 5 days after the onset of illness before seeking a physician, and 75% fail to return for follow-up care. They distrust hospitals and often believe that surgery and hospitalization are preludes to imminent death.

To care for this population properly, appropriate interpreters, well

(18–16) JAMA 248:710–714, Aug. 13, 1982.

versed in Indochinese cultures, are an absolute necessity. Clerks should be trained in Indochinese names and name order. Practices to be avoided during the health assessment include complete disrobing of female patients, mandatory pelvic examination of every female patient on a first visit, visible presence of an interpreter of opposite sex during breast or genital examination, forceful indoctrination in family planning during the first visit, negative judgmental attitudes toward traditional healing practices, and withdrawal of numerous tubes of blood without careful explanation. The medical history should be brief because refugees tend to minimize or deny previous illness or symptoms. A history of diet and self-medication with remedies brought from Southeast Asia should be elicited. The physical examination should be as complete as possible, with a tactful approach to the anogenital area. Aspects to be emphasized include the skin, teeth, eyes, ears, and endocrine and cardiovascular systems. Screening should include complete blood cell count, urinalysis, and stool examination for parasites, as well as tests for venereal disease, hepatitis B surface antigen, and tuberculosis.

▶ [This essay points out the marked cultural and attitudinal differences that exist between the citizens of the United States and the nearly 500,000 recent refugees from Southeast Asia. Apparently, stoicism, passivity, modesty concerning the physical examination, and a distrust of Western medicine are common in the Indochinese. Medical conditions that often are encountered include parasitic infestations, tuberculosis, syphilis, and the hepatitis B carrier state.] ◀

Subject Index

H

T

U

Index to Authors

D

E

Y

Z